Practical Sports Nutrition

Louise Burke, PhD

Department of Sports Nutrition
Australian Institute of Sport

Belconnen
Australia

HUMAN KINETICS

Library of Congress Cataloging-in-Publication Data

Burke, Louise.
    Practical sports nutrition / Louise Burke.
        p. cm.
    Includes bibliographical references.
    ISBN-13: 978-0-7360-4695-4 (hard cover)
    ISBN-10: 0-7360-4695-X (hard cover)
    1. Athletes--Nutrition. 2.   Sports--Physiological aspects.   I. Title.

    TX361.A8B89 2007
    613.2'024796--dc22

                                                    2006037750

ISBN-10: 0-7360-4695-X (hard cover)
ISBN-13: 978-0-7360-4695-4 (hard cover)

The Web addresses cited in this text were current as of February 5, 2007, unless otherwise noted.

Acquisitions Editor: Michael S. Bahrke, PhD; **Developmental Editor:** Judy Park; **Assistant Editor:** Lee Alexander; **Copyeditor:** Julie Anderson; **Proofreader:** Anne Rogers; **Indexer:** Bobbi Swanson; **Permission Manager:** Dalene Reeder; **Graphic Designer:** Nancy Rasmus; **Graphic Artist:** Dawn Sills; **Photo Manager:** Laura Fitch; **Cover Designer:** Keith Blomberg; **Photographer (cover):** Monitz Winde/Bongarts/Getty Images; **Art Manager:** Kelly Hendren; **Illustrator:** Accurate Art; **Printer:** Sheridan Books

Printed in the United States of America   10   9   8   7   6   5   4   3   2

Human Kinetics
Web site: www.HumanKinetics.com

United States: Human Kinetics
P.O. Box 5076
Champaign, IL 61825-5076
800-747-4457
e-mail: humank@hkusa.com

Canada: Human Kinetics
475 Devonshire Road Unit 100
Windsor, ON N8Y 2L5
800-465-7301 (in Canada only)
e-mail: orders@hkcanada.com

Europe: Human Kinetics
107 Bradford Road
Stanningley
Leeds LS28 6AT, United Kingdom
+44 (0) 113 255 5665
e-mail: hk@hkeurope.com

Australia: Human Kinetics
57A Price Avenue
Lower Mitcham, South Australia 5062
08 8372 0999
e-mail: info@hkaustralia.com

New Zealand: Human Kinetics
Division of Sports Distributors NZ Ltd.
P.O. Box 300 226 Albany
North Shore City
Auckland
0064 9 448 1207
e-mail: info@humankinetics.co.nz

For Jack and for John, the loves of my life.

This book is also dedicated to the memory of two important mentors in my career in sports nutrition: Richard SD Read, who introduced me to this developing science and to his love of academic pursuits, and "Coach" (Terry Gathercole), who opened many doors to my work at the coal face of sport. I am eternally grateful for the generosity of your knowledge and the opportunities you provided me.

contents

preface

In March 1990, I commenced work at the Australian Institute of Sport, with the brief of setting up a program and later, department, of sports nutrition. Within the first week, I consulted runners, gymnasts, and rowers; met with residential swimming and basketball programs to devise a year-long nutrition education program; and provided sports nutrition lectures to a visiting soccer team and the coaches undertaking a national accreditation scheme for ten pin bowling. Despite a background that included a doctorate in sports nutrition and 10 years of experience as a dietitian specializing in sport, I was overwhelmed by the breadth and complexity of the situations to which my knowledge of sports nutrition needed to be applied. The final task of my first week was to provide an education session to the national futsal team—a sport I'd never heard of! What were the nutritional demands of this sport? What kinds of nutritional strategies were likely to enhance competition performances? What did these athletes normally eat, and how important did they think their nutrition was? How could I engage their interest? I was terrified as I walked in to face the room of futsal players. This book is a result of my experiences and of the general explosion of interest in the real-life practice of sports nutrition that has occurred over the past 15 years.

Our knowledge and practice of sports nutrition have become increasingly sophisticated over the last 15 years. Today, we expect specialized nutrition information for various sports or exercise activities. It is no longer sufficient to consider the generic athlete or general issues in sports nutrition, such as the preevent meal or eating for recovery. Instead, we now appreciate that basketball players, swimmers, distance runners, gymnasts, and bodybuilders all have different nutritional needs. These differences are a consequence of the diversity in everyday requirements for nutrients (training needs) as well as specific nutrition strategies used to optimize performance in a single exercise session (especially in competition situations). To work with an athlete or team, we must understand fully the unique demands of their training and competition schedules. The preparation of these athletes, the way they train, and their physique needs reflect the requirements of competition. As such, competition is discussed first within each chapter. Particular consideration is given to the physical and physiological determinants of successful performance in each sport. In some cases, these details need to be fine-tuned even further to recognize the specific challenges of

a particular event, playing position, or playing style. These factors underpin the nutritional requirements and nutrition goals for each athlete.

The next step is to consider how the athlete can turn his or her unique nutritional goals into the practical use of foods, fluids, and special supplements. The food choices and eating habits of athletes are influenced by their life-styles and the practical considerations of their sports. These issues are, of course, individual to the athlete concerned. However, some nutritional challenges occur in a predictable way because of the characteristics of a sport—for example, coping with early-morning training sessions that interfere with the goals of preexercise nutrition, managing nutrition goals while undertaking a demanding travel schedule, finding a way to meet hydration and refueling goals within the rules and practical constraints of a sporting competition, or balancing the need to refuel with the need to remain lean. In some sports, certain issues occur so frequently that they become synonymous with the specific nutrition considerations for that activity. In other sports, the practical challenges of achieving a nutritional goal are so demanding that creative solutions deserve to be highlighted rather than hidden behind the banner of general sports nutrition—for example, how do you fuel the extreme demands of the Tour de France, where competitors cycle about 4,000 km in 3 weeks, over some of the most mountainous sections of Europe?

Finally, we need to consider the strong cultural influence attached to participation in some sports. Many sports provide a "closed environment" for their participants, promoting certain messages and values via the close interaction between athletes and the handing down of knowledge from coaches and trainers. Most sports have their own "literature" in the form of specialized magazines, club newsletters, and Web sites. The culture of a sport may influence nutrition beliefs and attitudes to food. The content and delivery of sports nutrition education need to be tailored to the culture of the individual athlete or specific group. This might include targeting the nutrition myths or poor eating practices that have become embedded in the folklore of the sport, using the language that is familiar to the athletes, or using case histories or situations that have occurred in that sport. Such practices will help to make sports nutrition information more interesting and effective.

Practical Sports Nutrition extends other textbooks on sports nutrition by examining sports nutrition information and practice in the context of actual sports. This book examines specific nutrition issues arising in various categories of sports that share common physiological and lifestyle characteristics. Each section takes the following format:

1. A comprehensive review of the physiological, nutritional, and cultural characteristics of the sports, and a summary of the sport-specific nutrition research that has been undertaken

2. Discussion of special issues in sports nutrition research, including topics related to the existing research and directions for research in these sports

3. Discussion of practical issues, providing a summary of practical strategies and information that is useful for achieving sports nutrition goals in these sports

All chapters are fully referenced by state-of-the-art research as well as the cutting-edge practice of the world's best athletes and teams.

Practical Sports Nutrition provides the next step in sports nutrition research and education. This unique book translates information that is generic and theoretical into advice that is specific and practical. It will help you to take sports nutrition from the page or classroom onto the court, field, or track—and, ultimately, the victory dais!

acknowledgments

Many people have contributed directly and indirectly to the publication of this book; it would take a separate chapter to fully acknowledge all these contributions. My attempt to simplify this process should not imply any underestimation of the role that all have played or my gratitude for their assistance. I thank those at Human Kinetics who guided this book to the shelves, and the countless number of colleagues who contributed information, feedback, proof-reading and general support for the process. Special thanks are extended to Nanna Meyer and Susie Parker-Simmons for contributing the chapter on winter sports; there are not enough mountains or snow in Australia to provide me with their level of experience in such sports.

Much of the information contained in *Practical Sports Nutrition* is the result of the time I have spent with people in sport—from scientists, to coaches and athletes themselves. A general goal in sport is to create an environment in which excellence is possible. I am grateful to all the people who have provided me with such an environment for the 25 years of my professional life, as well as fun and friendship. In particular, I thank the amazing team at the Australian Institute of Sport, and highlight the energy, creativity and loyalty of the past and present members of my Department of Sports Nutrition, particularly my long serving second-in-command, Greg Cox. Ron Maughan and Mark Hargreaves have been instrumental in opening doors to research and international collaboration. Melinda Manore and Linda Houtkooper have been special friends along the road. My husband, John Hawley, continues to be my primary collaborator, co-author and supporter, and wields the red pen in our family.

credits

chapter 1

Training and Competition Nutrition

The aim of this book is to examine sports nutrition in the context of real-life practice. In the following chapters we examine principles of sports nutrition as they apply to the training and competition performances of specific athletes and sporting teams. Before we tackle such variations and specialized applications, we need to discuss the background that underpins them. This chapter provides an overview of current nutrition guidelines for athletes and physically active people, separated into goals for the training diet and strategies for competition nutrition.

Goals of Training Nutrition

The benefits of a sound diet are most obvious in the area of competition performance, where nutrition strategies help athletes perform their best by reducing or delaying the onset of factors that would otherwise cause fatigue. However, daily eating patterns are probably even more important, because they help athletes achieve the platform from which they are ready to compete. The major role of the daily diet is to supply athletes with fuel and nutrients needed to optimize the adaptations achieved during training and to recover quickly between workouts. Athletes must also eat to stay in good health and to achieve and maintain an optimal physique. A summary of the goals of the training diet is provided in the highlight box on page 2.

Goal 1

Meet the energy and fuel requirements needed to support a training program.

The energy requirements of individual athletes are influenced by their body size, growth, pursuit of weight loss or gain, and, most important, the energy cost of their training load (frequency, duration, and intensity of training sessions). The training programs of athletes vary according to their event, their caliber, and the time of the athletic season. An athlete's energy intake is of interest for several reasons (Burke 2001b) :

- Energy intake determines the potential for achieving the athlete's requirements for energy-containing macronutrients (especially protein and carbohydrate) and the food needed to provide vitamins, minerals, and other non-energy-containing dietary compounds required for optimal function and health.

- Energy intake assists the manipulation of muscle mass and body fat levels to achieve the specific physique that is ideal for athletic performance

- Energy intake affects the function of hormonal and immune systems.

- Energy intake challenges the practical limits to food intake set by issues such as food availability and gastrointestinal comfort.

Results from dietary surveys reveal that male athletes typically report daily energy intakes varying from 12 to 20 MJ (~4,000-5,000 kcal) over prolonged periods, with endurance-training athletes reporting higher energy intakes when these values are expressed relative to body mass than those in nonendurance sports (Burke, Cox, et al. 2001). The expected (absolute) energy requirements of a female athlete should be ~20% to 30% less than her male counterpart, principally to take into account her smaller size. However, most dietary surveys report that even when energy intake is expressed per kilogram of body mass, the reported energy intakes of female athletes are still substantially lower than those reported by an equivalent male group (Burke, Cox, et al. 2001). Of course, the results of dietary surveys do not necessarily represent the actual and habitual energy intakes of athletes. Rather, these surveys provide an estimation of what athletes report eating during a particular period of time. Dietary surveys are limited by athletes' abilities to accurately report what they consumed as well as degree to which the study period provides a true representation of usual eating patterns. In general, dietary surveys

Goals of Sports Nutrition

For training, athletes should do the following:

1. Meet the energy and fuel requirements needed to support a training program
2. Achieve and maintain an ideal physique for their event; manipulate training and nutrition to achieve a level of body mass, body fat, and muscle mass that is consistent with good health and good performance
3. Enhance adaptation and recovery between training sessions by providing all the nutrients associated with these processes
4. Refuel and rehydrate well during each training session to perform optimally at each session
5. Practice any intended competition nutrition strategies so that beneficial practices can be identified and fine-tuned
6. Maintain optimal health and function, especially by meeting the increased needs for some nutrients resulting from heavy training
7. Reduce the risk of sickness and injury during heavy training periods by maintaining healthy physique and energy balance and by supplying nutrients believed to assist immune function (e.g., consume carbohydrate during prolonged exercise sessions)
8. Make well-considered decisions about the use of supplements and specialized sport foods that have been shown to enhance training performance or meet training nutrition needs
9. Eat for long-term health by following healthy eating guidelines
10. Enjoy food and the pleasure of sharing meals

For competition, athletes should do the following:

1. In weight-division sports, achieve the competition weight division with minimal harm to health or performance
2. Fuel up adequately before an event by consuming carbohydrate and tapering exercise during the days before the event according to the importance and duration of the event; use carbohydrate-loading strategies when appropriate before events of greater than 90 min duration
3. Top up carbohydrate stores with a preevent meal or snack during the 1 to 4 hr before competition
4. Keep hydration at an acceptable level during the event by drinking appropriate amounts of fluids before, during, and after the event
5. Consume carbohydrate during events of greater than 1 hr duration or where body carbohydrate stores become depleted
6. Achieve fluid and food intake before and during the event without causing gastrointestinal discomfort or upsets
7. Promote recovery after the event, particularly during multiday competitions such as tournaments and stage races
8. During a prolonged competition program, ensure that competition eating does not compromise overall energy and nutrient intake goals
9. Make well-considered decisions about the use of supplements and specialized sport foods that have been shown to enhance competition performance or meet competition needs

underestimate the true intakes of most people, because many participants undereat or underreport their usual intake while being investigated (Schoeller 1995).

Although most individuals are able to achieve remarkable energy balance over long periods, the athlete is often faced with the challenge of managing energy intakes that are either extremely high or extremely low. High energy intakes are expected where athletes have a large body mass to support, extremely high training or exercise loads, or the additional energy requirement for growth or purposeful increase in lean body mass. Such athletes are often recommended to consume extra energy, particularly in the form of carbohydrate or protein, at special times or in greater quantities than would be provided in an everyday diet or dictated by their appetite and hunger. These athletes may also need to consume energy during and after exercise when the availability of foods and fluids, or opportunities to consume them, are limited. Practical issues interfering with the achievement of energy intake goals during postexercise recovery include loss of appetite and fatigue, poor access to suitable foods, and distraction from other activities.

Conversely, other athletes need to restrict energy intake to reduce or maintain low levels of body mass and fat. This can be difficult to achieve in the face of hunger, customary eating patterns, or the eating habits of peers. These athletes may also need to address their requirements for other nutrients within a reduced energy allowance. Specialized advice from a sports dietitian often helps athletes achieve their optimal energy intake. Principles that may assist in achieving such goals include being organized to have suitable foods on hand in a busy day, choosing foods that are either compact and easy to eat or high in satiety value, and considering the micronutrient and macronutrient content of food within the framework of total energy allowances.

Dietary surveys reveal that some athletes report large energy intakes, commensurate with energy requirements of prolonged daily training or competition sessions or efforts to gain muscle size and strength. However, many endurance athletes, particularly females, appear to consume lower energy intakes than would be expected; in fact, their reported intake often appears to be insufficient to support their training loads let alone basal energy requirements (for review of studies, see Barr 1987; Manore and Thompson 2006).

Apparently low energy intakes can be explained as an artifact of dietary survey methodology or because the athlete was observed during a period of loss of body weight or fat—negative energy balance (Burke 2001b). However, an alternative and more worrying explanation is that some athletes are energy efficient—that is, they can balance their basal metabolic needs and the energy cost of eating and exercise at a substantially lower than predicted energy intake (Manore and Thompson 2006). Most sports dietitians are familiar with the frustration voiced by athletes who claim that they can't reduce their weight or body fat levels despite "hardly eating anything." The situation may be worse for female athletes, who already face strong societal pressure to be lean yet naturally carry higher levels of body fat despite undertaking substantial training loads.

There is research evidence both to support (Thompson et al. 1995) and to contradict (Edwards et al. 1993) the presence of energy efficiency in groups of athletes. Some athletes may truly have low energy requirements attributable to a reduction in resting metabolic rate accompanying energy restriction, low activity levels outside the training program, or an efficient exercise technique. In some cases, however, the energy discrepancy exists or is exacerbated by underrecording or undereating during the period of investigation (Edwards et al. 1993; Schulz et al. 1992). It is suspected that athletes who are conscious of weight and physique or dissatisfied with their body image are at highest risk of significant underestimation errors when completing dietary surveys (Edwards et al. 1993; Fogelholm

et al. 1995; Schulz et al. 1992). Reporting errors can be minimized when athletes are motivated to receive a true dietary assessment and when they have been trained to enhance record-keeping skills. Nevertheless, researchers and practitioners should be cautious in interpreting self-reported assessments of dietary intake.

Adequate energy intake is important to maintain health and achieve sound eating practices; there is evidence that restricted energy intake, or energy drain, is a direct cause of metabolic and reproductive disorders in female and possibly male athletes (Loucks 2004). Adequate energy intake is also important in providing adequate quantities of macronutrients and micronutrients needed to achieve most of the other goals of training and competition.

Goal 2

Achieve and maintain an ideal physique for their event; manipulate training and nutrition to achieve a level of body mass, body fat, and muscle mass that is consistent with good health and good performance.

Physical characteristics, including height, limb lengths, body mass, muscle mass, and body fat, can all play a role in sports performance. An athlete's physique is determined both by inherited characteristics and by the conditioning effects of his or her training program and diet. A number of techniques are available to assess body fat levels or other aspects of physique. These range from techniques that are best suited to the laboratory (e.g., hydrodensitometry and dual-energy X-ray absorptiometry scans) to protocols that can be taken into the field. Useful information about body composition can be collected from anthropometric data such as measurements of skinfold (subcutaneous) fat, body girths, and circumferences (Kerr 2006). Coaches or sports scientists who make these assessments on athletes should be trained appropriately to minimize their measurement error and to understand the limitations of their assessments.

Often, coaches or athletes set rigid criteria for an ideal physique, based on the characteristics of other successful competitors. Although such information is useful, it fails to take into account the considerable variability in the physical characteristics of athletes, even between individuals in the same sport. It also fails to acknowledge that some athletes need many years of training and maturation to achieve their ideal shape and body composition. Therefore, it is dangerous to establish rigid physique prescriptions for individuals. A preferable strategy is to determine a range of acceptable values for body fat and body mass within each sport and then monitor the health and performance of individual athletes within this range. Sequential profiling of an athlete can be used to monitor the development of physical characteristics that are associated with good performance for that individual as well as identify the changes in physique that can be expected over a season or period of specialized training.

Some athletes easily achieve the body composition that is best suited to their sport. Others may need to manipulate characteristics such as muscle mass or body fat levels through changes in diet and training. An increase in muscle mass is desired by many athletes whose performance is linked to size, strength, or power. In addition to the increase in muscle mass and strength that occurs during adolescence, particularly in males, specific muscle hypertrophy is sometimes pursued through a program of progressive muscle overload. An important nutritional requirement to support such a program is adequate energy. Energy is required for the manufacture of new muscle tissue as well as to provide fuel for the training program that supplied the stimulus for this muscle growth. Many athletes do not achieve a sufficiently positive energy balance to optimize muscle gains during a strength-training program. Specialized nutrition advice can help the athlete improve this situation by making energy-dense foods and drinks accessible and easy to consume (Burke 2001b). Despite the interest in gaining muscle size and strength, there is little rigorous scientific study of the amount of energy required, the optimal ratio of macronutrients supplying this energy, and the requirements for micronutrients to enhance this process.

Because protein forms the most significant structural component of muscle, it is tempting to hypothesize that an increase in dietary protein will stimulate muscle gain. Many strength-trained athletes consume very large amounts of protein, in excess of 2 to 3 g per kilogram of body mass per day (two to three times the recommended intakes for protein in most countries), in the belief that this will enhance the gains from resistance training programs. However, the value of very high protein intakes in optimizing muscle gains remains unsupported by the scientific literature (Lemon 1991b). Instead, there is recent evidence that timing the intake of protein after or even before a resistance training session is a useful strategy to increase net protein balance (Rasmussen et al. 2000; Tipton et al. 2001). Issues related to the protein needs of athletes are discussed separately, within goals 3 and 6.

A reduction in body mass, particularly through loss of body fat, is a common nutritional goal of athletes. There are situations when an athlete is clearly carrying excess body fat and will improve his or her health and performance by reducing these levels. Loss of body fat should be achieved through a program based on a sustained and moderate energy deficit. Counseling from a sports nutrition expert can help the athlete to decrease dietary energy intake and, perhaps, increase energy expenditure through aerobic exercise or daily physical activity. Athletes are not immune to fad diets and other quick weight loss gimmicks promoted to the general community, often preferring the scales to reflect an immediate reduction rather than undertaking the steps to achieve a slower but consistent reduction of body fat. The disadvantages of many quick weight loss strategies range from failure to achieve any loss of fat to the impairment of performance attributable to inadequate fuel intake or dehydration. Recently, attention has been drawn to the deaths of several high-profile athletes in association

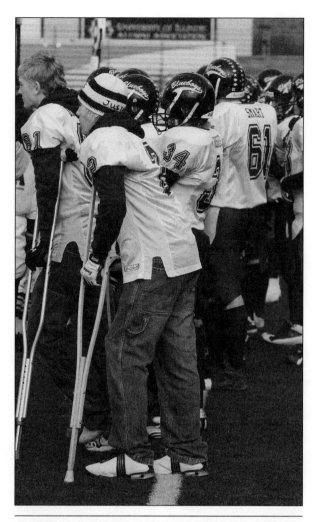

Excess body fat may occur because of heredity or lifestyle factors or because the athlete has suddenly altered energy expenditure without making a compensatory change in energy intake—for example, failing to reduce energy intake while injured or taking a break from training.

with their attempts to lose weight. Although these athletes were believed to have preexisting medical conditions, other practices in common included severe restriction of fluid and food intake while in heavy training.

In some sports, a low body mass or body fat level offers distinct advantages to performance. Such benefits can be seen in terms of the energy cost of movement (e.g., distance running, cycling), the physics of movement in a tight space or against gravity (e.g., gymnastics, diving, cycling uphill), or aesthetics (e.g., gymnastics, bodybuilding). In many such weight-conscious or body fat–conscious sports, athletes strive to achieve minimum body fat levels or at least try to reduce their body fat below the level that seems natural or healthy for them. In the short term, this may improve performance. However, the long-term disadvantages include outcomes related to having very low body fat stores as well as the problems associated with unsound weight loss methods. Excessive training, chronically low intakes of energy and nutrients, and psychological distress are often involved in fat loss strategies and may cause long-term damage to health, happiness, or performance. The special issues related to making weight in weight-category sports will be discussed separately (goal 11).

Ideal weight and body fat targets for a sporting group should be set in terms of ranges, and weight control for an individual athlete should consider measures of long-term health and performance as well as the athlete's ability to eat a diet that is adequate in energy and nutrients and free of unreasonable food-related stress. Some racial groups or individuals are naturally light and have low levels of body fat or can achieve these without paying a substantial penalty. Furthermore, some athletes vary their body fat levels over a season so that very low levels are achieved only for a specific and short time. In general, however, athletes should not undertake strategies to minimize body fat levels unless they can be sure there are no side effects or disadvantages. Although it is difficult to get reliable figures on the prevalence of eating disorders or disordered eating behavior and body image among athletes, there appears to be a higher risk of problems among female athletes and among athletes in sports that require specific weight targets or low body fat levels (Beals and Manore 1994; Sundgot-Borgen 2000; Wilmore 1991). Even where clinical eating disorders do not exist, many athletes appear to be restrained eaters, reporting not only energy intakes that are considerably less than expected energy requirements but also considerable stress related to food intake (Beals and Manore 1994). The female athlete triad, the coexistence of disordered eating or energy restriction, menstrual dysfunction, and osteopenia (Loucks and Nattiv 2005), has received considerable publicity as a potential outcome of the excessive pursuit of thinness by female athletes; this is discussed in greater detail in goal 7. Expert advice from sports medicine professionals, including dietitians, psychologists, and physicians, is important in the early detection and management of problems related to body composition and nutrition.

Goal 3

Enhance adaptation and recovery between training sessions by providing all the nutrients associated with these processes.

There is some evidence, or at least sound theories, that the requirements for many nutrients are increased as a result of prolonged exercise. Acute requirements for carbohydrate and fluid in relation to exercise are relatively easy to identify and are discussed in greater detail in goals 4 and 6. However, to maintain optimal health and function, the athlete will also need to meet any increases in protein and micronutrient requirements arising from their commitment to regular prolonged exercise. In general, two dietary factors underpin the athlete's success in achieving increases in nutrient intakes: adequate intake of total energy, and focus on a wide variety of nutrient-rich foods. When these factors are in place, most athletes will be able to achieve their increased needs for protein and micronutrients.

Prolonged daily training may increase protein requirements, not only to support muscle gain and repair of damaged body tissues but also to meet the small contribution that protein oxidation makes to the fuel requirements of prolonged exercise (for reviews, see Lemon 2000; Tarnopolsky 2006). Although athletes undertaking recreational or light training activities will normally meet their protein needs within the daily recommendations prepared for the general population, sports nutrition guidelines often recommend higher protein intakes for athletes in heavy training. Table 1.1 summarizes some of the recommendations for both strength and endurance athletes in heavy training or competition, with the acknowledgement that athletes experiencing growth spurts (e.g., adolescent athletes) will also have an increased protein need. These recommendations are somewhat equivocal (Tipton and Wolfe 2004), because they have been derived from short-term studies of athletic populations, using methods with recognized

Table 1.1   Guidelines for Protein Intakes for Athletes and Physically Active People

Population	Estimates of maximum protein need for males ($g \cdot kg^{-1} \cdot day^{-1}$)
Sedentary people	0.8-1.0
Recreational exercisers	0.8-1.0
Serious resistance athletes: early phase of training	1.5-1.7
Serious resistance trained athletes: established training program	1.0-1.2
Serious endurance athlete	1.2-1.6
Adolescent athletes	1.5-2.0
Female athletes	15% lower than males

Data from Lemon 2000; Tarnopolsky 2006.

shortcomings. Furthermore, they may not take into account such issues as long-term adaptation to a training stimulus or dietary intake. However, it is likely that these recommendations reflect the range of maximal protein needs for athletes who are not undertaking pharmacological stimulation of muscular development. Negative energy balance (Butterfield 1987) and inadequate carbohydrate intake during heavy training (Brouns et al. 1989) can both increase the protein intake required to maintain nitrogen balance.

Although the higher protein needs of athletes continue to be debated, current sports nutrition guidelines do not promote the need for special high-protein diets or protein supplements (Tipton and Wolfe 2004). Dietary surveys of free-living athletes find that most sports people already report protein intakes within or above the raised protein intake targets summarized in table 1.1, largely as a result of the increased energy allowances that accompany training. Athletes at risk of inadequate protein intakes are those with restricted energy intakes and unusual dietary practices (e.g., excessively high carbohydrate diets with poorly chosen vegetarian practices). Although large amounts of protein-rich foods or expensive protein supplements are considered unnecessary, sport foods such as liquid meal supplements and sport bars may allow the athlete to achieve high intake of energy or protein at strategic times. Nutritional strategies that promote the protein response to exercise are discussed under goal 6.

Vitamins and minerals play important roles as co-factors for key reactions in energy metabolism or the synthesis of new tissues. Athletes need to know whether a heavy program of exercise increases their requirement for micronutrients and whether the intake of additional amounts of vitamins and minerals will enhance performance by supercharging these key reactions. Dietary surveys of athletes show that when moderate to high energy intakes are consumed from a wide variety of nutrient-rich foods, reported intakes of vitamins and minerals are well in excess of population recommendations and are likely to meet any increases in micronutrient demand caused by training. In addition, research has failed to show clear evidence of an increase in performance following vitamin supplementation, except in the case where a preexisting deficiency was corrected (see Fogelholm 2006).

This information indicates no justification for routine vitamin and mineral supplementation by athletes. However, not all athletes achieve variety or adequate energy intake in their eating plans. Suboptimal intake of micronutrients may occur in athletes who are restrained or disordered eaters and those following fad diets. Other risk factors for a restricted food range include poor practical nutrition skills, inadequate finances, and an overcommitted lifestyle that limits access to food and causes erratic meal schedules. The best long-term management plan is to educate athletes to improve the quality and quantity of their food intake. However, a vitamin and mineral supplement, providing a broad range of micronutrients in doses similar to daily recommendations, may be useful when the athlete is unwilling or unable to make dietary changes or is traveling to places with an uncertain food supply.

An inadequate iron status is the most likely micronutrient deficiency among athletic populations, just as it is within the general community. Inadequate iron status can reduce exercise performance via suboptimal levels of hemoglobin and perhaps also via changes in the muscle including reduced myoglobin and iron-related enzymes (Hood et al. 1992). Because exercise itself alters many of the measures of iron status, because of changes in plasma volume or the acute phase response to stress, it is sometimes hard to distinguish between true iron deficiency and the normal effect of strenuous training or competition. Reduction of blood hemoglobin concentrations that results from the expansion of plasma volume in response to endurance training, often termed *sports anemia*, does not impair exercise performance (for review, see Deakin 2006). It can be useful to collect a long-term history of iron status results from the individual athlete to establish what is normal for him or her and how parameters may vary across the training season or with different interventions. Athletes often believe that more is better regarding hemoglobin levels. However, in the absence of hemoconcentration secondary to dehydration, very high hemoglobin levels are usually explained by genetic individuality or banned practices such as blood-doping or the use of the drug erythropoietin. As such they are not possible for most athletes to achieve.

Despite initial conflict in the literature, there is now evidence that iron depletion in the absence of anemia (i.e., reduced serum ferritin concentrations) may impair exercise performance (for review, see Deakin 2006). In addition, athletes with reduced iron stores complain of feeling fatigued and failing to recover between a series of competition or training sessions. Because low ferritin levels may become progressively lower and eventually lead to iron-deficiency anemia, there is merit in monitoring athletes deemed to be at high risk of iron depletion and implementing an intervention as soon as iron status appears to decline substantially or to symptomatic levels. Many experts and practitioners use the cutoff point of a ferritin concentration of less than 20 to 30 ng/ml.

The evaluation and management of iron status in athletes should be undertaken by a sports physician and considered on an individual basis. The publicity during the 1990s surrounding iron deficiency in athletes probably led to an overestimate of the true prevalence of the problem. It is tempting for the fatigued athlete and his or her coach to self-diagnose iron deficiency and to self-medicate with iron supplements that are available over the counter. However, there are dangers in self-prescription or long-term supplementation in the absence of medical follow-up. Iron supplementation is not a replacement for medical and dietary assessment and therapy, because it typically fails to correct underlying problems that have caused iron drain—iron requirements and losses exceeding iron intake. Chronic supplementation with high doses of iron carries a risk of iron overload, especially in males for whom the genetic traits for hemochromatosis are more prevalent. Iron supplements can also interfere with the absorption of other minerals such as zinc and copper.

Of course, prevention and treatment of iron deficiency may include iron supplementation. However, the manage-

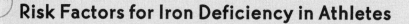

Risk Factors for Iron Deficiency in Athletes

Predictors of Increased Iron Requirements

- Recent growth spurt in adolescents
- Pregnancy (current or within the past year)

Predictors of Increased Iron Losses or Iron Malabsorption

- Sudden increase in heavy training load, particularly running on hard surfaces, causing an increase in intravascular hemolysis
- Gastrointestinal bleeding (e.g., some anti-inflammatory drugs, ulcers)
- Gastrointestinal diseases involving malabsorption (e.g., Crohn's disease, ulcerative colitis, parasitic infestation, coeliac disease)
- Heavy menstrual blood losses
- Excessive blood losses such as frequent nosebleeds, recent surgery, substantial contact injuries
- Frequent blood donation

Predictors of Inadequate Intake of Bioavailable Iron

- Chronic low energy intake (<2,000 kcal or 8 MJ per day)
- Vegetarian eating—especially poorly constructed diets in which alternative food sources of iron are ignored (e.g., legumes, nuts, and seeds)
- Fad diets or erratic eating patterns
- Restricted variety of foods in diet; failure to match iron-containing foods with dietary factors that promote iron absorption
- Overconsumption of micronutrient-poor convenience foods and sport foods (e.g., high-carbohydrate powders, gels)
- Very high carbohydrate diet with high fiber content and infrequent intake of meats, fish, and chicken
- Natural food diets: failure to consume iron-fortified cereal foods such as commercial breakfast cereals and bread

ment plan should be based on long-term interventions to reverse iron drain—reducing excessive iron losses and increasing dietary iron. Risk factors for iron depletion in athletes are summarized in the highlight box on this page. Dietary interventions to improve iron status need not only to increase total iron intake but also to increase the bioavailability of dietary iron. The heme form of iron found in meat, fish, and poultry is better absorbed than organic or nonheme iron found in plant foods such as fortified and whole-grain cereal foods, legumes, and green leafy vegetables (Hallberg 1981, Monsen 1988). However, iron bioavailability can be manipulated by matching iron-rich foods with dietary elements that promote iron absorption (e.g., vitamin C and other food acids, "meat factor" found in animal flesh) and by reducing the interaction with iron inhibitory factors (e.g., phytates in fiber-rich cereals, tannins in tea) (Hallberg 1981, Monsen 1988). Changes to iron intake should be achieved with eating patterns that are compatible with the athlete's other nutrition goals (e.g., achieving fuel requirements for sport, achieving desired physique). Such education is often a specialized task, requiring the expertise of a sports dietitian.

Some athletes are at risk of problems with calcium status and bone health. Low bone density in athletes seems contradictory, because exercise is considered to be one of the best protectors of bone health. However, a serious outcome of the menstrual disturbances frequently reported by female athletes is the high risk of either direct loss of bone density or failure to optimize the gain in peak bone mass that should occur during the 10 to 15 years after the onset of puberty (for review, see Kerr et al. 2006). Because this problem is primarily related to an abnormal hormonal environment rather than inadequate calcium intake, it is discussed in more detail under goal 7.

Goals 4 and 5

Refuel and rehydrate well during each training session to perform optimally at each session. Practice any intended competition nutrition strategies so that beneficial practices can be identified and fine-tuned.

The maintenance of fuel status and fluid balance plays an important role in the performance of exercise and forms the basis of most of the special nutrition strategies undertaken for competition. Of course, many of the same physiological challenges that cause fatigue also occur during exercise sessions undertaken in the training phase. Therefore, the nutritional strategies for competition (goals 14 and 15) should also be built into the training program. This will allow the athlete to achieve optimal performance and adaptations to training. In addition, he or she can practice any intended competition strategies to identify and fine-tune a successful plan.

There is considerable variability between athletes and events, even in the same sport, in relation to nutritional challenges, opportunity for nutritional support, and response to nutritional intake. Therefore, the training situation offers each athlete a chance to find the intake of fluid and food that will be practical and valuable for future competitive events. For example, by monitoring changes in body mass over training sessions undertaken in simulation of an event, athletes can gauge their predicted competition sweat losses. They can then experiment with the types of drinks that are made available in an event under the same conditions or regulations and assess the outcomes in terms of fluid balance, gastrointestinal comfort, and performance. A number of practical issues prevent the theoretical ideal of achieving a fluid intake that matches most of the athlete's sweat losses (e.g., 80% of the body weight that is lost during the session). Sometimes, these issues can be addressed—for example, to train with a gradually increasing fluid intake

or new drinking plan, so that the skills of drinking on the run are improved or gastrointestinal tolerance is increased. On other occasions, the barriers to fluid replacement are insurmountable, and the athlete must then be prepared for such consequences. Issues related to refueling during exercise can be tackled with a similar logic.

Goal 6

Maintain optimal health and function, especially by meeting the increased needs for some nutrients resulting from heavy training.

Recovery is a major challenge for the elite athlete, who undertakes two or even three workouts each day during certain phases of the training cycle, with 4 to 24 hr between each session. But it can also be a concern for recreational athletes who train once or twice a day in preparation for a special endurance event such as a marathon or triathlon. Recovery involves a complex range of processes of restoration and adaptation to physiological stress of exercise, including these:

- Restoration of muscle and liver glycogen stores
- Replacement of fluid and electrolytes lost in sweat
- Synthesis of new protein following the catabolic state and damage induced by the exercise
- Responses of the immune system

Issues of Postexercise Recovery

Recovery nutrition goals are specific to each athlete and each workout and may be determined by some of the following factors:
The physiological or homeostatic challenges caused by the workout, including
- the extent of fuel depletion (principally glycogen),
- the extent of dehydration, and
- the extent of muscle damage or protein catabolism
The goals associated with enhanced performance or adaptation to the exercise session, including
- increases in muscle size or strength,
- reductions in body fat levels,
- increases in content of functional proteins (e.g., enzymes) or manufacture of functional cells or tissues (e.g., red blood cells, capillaries), and
- the importance of fuel or hydration status in the subsequent exercise bout
The duration of the period between workouts, including
- total recovery time and
- other commitments or needs during the recovery period (e.g., sleep, drug testing, travel)
The availability of nutrients for intake during the recovery period, including
- the athlete's total energy budget,
- food availability, and
- the athlete's appetite and opportunity to consume foods and drinks during recovery period

In the training situation, with correct planning of the workload and the recovery time, such adaptation allows the body to become fitter, stronger, faster, or otherwise better suited to the chosen exercise task.

Recovery has become a buzzword used ubiquitously throughout the sporting world, and recovery eating strategies are often promoted to athletes with an almost "one size fits all" approach. In fact, recovery can encompass a variety of different priorities or goals according to the individual athlete and his or her specific training or competition session (see the highlight box on this page for a summary). Athletes and coaches should be educated to better recognize the specificity of postexercise nutrition goals and to plan a strategy for postworkout eating practices. Detailed information regarding postexercise refueling (Burke, Kiens, et al. 2004) and rehydration (Shirreffs et al. 2004) strategies is available and is summarized next, along with the accumulating information on practices that enhance net protein balance following exercise.

Despite improved fluid intake practices during exercise (see goal 14), most athletes can expect to be at least mildly dehydrated at the end of their session. Ideally, the athlete should aim to fully restore fluid losses after workouts so that the next workout can be commenced in fluid balance. This is difficult in situations where moderate to high levels of hypohydration have been incurred (e.g., a fluid deficit equivalent to 2-5% body mass or greater) and the interval between sessions is less than 6 to 8 hr. In normal circumstances, the daily replacement of fluid losses and maintenance of fluid balance are well regulated by thirst and urine losses. However, under conditions of stress such as exercise, environmental heat, and cold or altitude, thirst may not be a sufficient stimulus for maintaining euhydration (Greenleaf 1992) There may be a lag of 4 to 24 hr before body fluid levels are restored in an acute situation of hypohydration, and success of postexercise rehydration depends on how much the athlete drinks and then how much of this fluid is retained and re-equilibrated within body fluid compartments.

After exercise, many people fail to drink sufficient volumes of fluid to restore fluid balance. This is known as involuntary dehydration in recognition of the fact that the dehydrated individual has no desire to rehydrate even when fluids and opportunity are available (Nadel et al. 1990). Numerous factors have been involved in determining the voluntary fluid intake of individuals, including behavioral patterns and social customs, as well as a genetic predisposition to be a "reluctant" or "good" drinker (Greenleaf 1992). Flavoring of drinks is known to contribute to voluntary fluid intake, with studies reporting greater fluid intake during postexercise recovery with sweetened drinks than with plain water (Carter and Gisolfi 1989) (see figure 1.1). The intake of sodium in or with a fluid helps to maintain plasma osmolality while plasma volume is being restored, thus preserving thirst (Nose et al. 1988). The temperature of drinks is also important, and although very cold fluids (0 °C) may be regarded as the most pleasurable, cool drinks (15 °C) are more likely to be consumed quickly and in larger quantities (Hubbard et al. 1990).

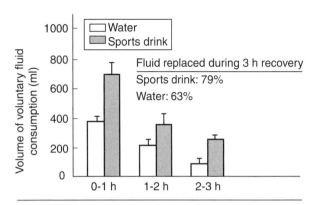

Figure 1.1 Participants who were observed over the 3 hr following dehydrating exercise consumed larger volumes of fluid when a flavored carbohydrate–electrolyte beverage (sport drink) was provided than in another trial providing only water. Regardless of drink choice, voluntary fluid intake decreased with time and failed to replace total fluid losses by the end of the 3 hr period.

* = P<0.05

Reprinted from Carter and Gisolfi 1989.

Because sweating and obligatory urine losses continue during the recovery phase, athletes must replace more than their postexercise fluid deficit to achieve fluid restoration. Typically, a volume of fluid equivalent to ~150% of the postexercise fluid deficit must be consumed to compensate for these ongoing losses and ensure that fluid balance is achieved over the first 4 to 6 hr of recovery (Shirreffs et al. 1996). Whether the pattern of fluid intake influences rehydration has been investigated, where intakes of larger amounts of fluid in the immediate postexercise period were compared with the same total volume of fluid being spread equally over 5 to 6 hr of recovery (Kovacs et al. 2002). Early replacement of large volumes of fluid was associated with better restoration of fluid balance during the first hours of recovery despite an increase in urinary output; however, differences in fluid restoration between hydration patterns disappeared by 5 to 6 hr of recovery. In another study, spacing fluid intake over several hours of recovery after exercise was more effective in restoring fluid balance because of lower urine losses than was consuming fluid as a large bolus immediately after the exercise (Archer and Shirreffs 2001). Of course, factors such as gastric comfort need to be considered in postexercise rehydration practices, especially if the athlete needs to perform another exercise session within the next hours.

Fluid replacement alone will not guarantee that rehydration goals are achieved. Unless there is simultaneous replacement of the electrolytes lost in sweat, particularly sodium, consumption of large amounts of fluid will simply result in large urine losses (Shirreffs et al. 1996). The addition of sodium to rehydration fluids has been shown to better maintain equilibrium between plasma volume and plasma osmolality, reduce urine losses, and enhance net fluid balance at the end of 6 hr of recovery (Maughan and Leiper 1995; Shirreffs et al. 1996). In contrast, with no or little sodium replacement, participants were still substantially dehydrated at the end of the 6 hr recovery period, despite drinking 150% of the volume of their postexercise fluid deficit (see figure 1.2). On a practical note, fluid replacement without sodium intake may return a false positive for good hydration status, at least in the acute phase of recovery. The production of copious amounts of clear urine, or urine with a low osmolality and specific gravity, may be useful as an overall sign of euhydration, particularly when early morning urine is used to monitor day-to-day variations in hydration (Shirreffs and Maughan 1998). However, during the hours immediately after a substantial fluid deficit is replaced without attention to sodium losses, athletes are likely to produce large amounts of urine with characteristics suggesting the return of fluid balance, when in reality they are still in substantial fluid deficit (Kovacs et al. 1999). An additional disadvantage of

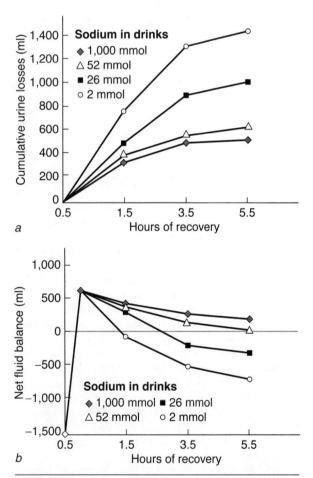

Figure 1.2 *(a)* Effect of sodium replacement on hydration. The presence of sodium in fluids consumed after exercise (replacing 150% of the fluid deficit) reduced urine losses and *(b)* enhanced net fluid balance at the end of 6 hr of recovery. The optimal level of sodium appears to be about 50 mmol/L, because a greater sodium concentration did not further enhance the effect. With little or no sodium replacement, participants were still dehydrated at the end of the 6 hr recovery period.

Reprinted from Maughan and Leiper 1995.

failing to replace sodium losses when rehydration occurs in the late part of the day is that large urine losses may occur overnight, causing frequent trips to the restroom and interrupted sleep.

The optimal sodium level in a rehydration drink appears to be ~50 to 80 mmol/L (Maughan and Leiper 1995), as is provided in oral rehydration solutions manufactured for the treatment of diarrhea. This is considerably higher than the concentrations found in commercial carbohydrate–electrolyte drinks, or sport drinks (typically 10-25 mmol/L), and may be unpalatable to many athletes. Sport drinks may confer some rehydration advantages over plain water, in terms of palatability as well as fluid retention (Gonzalez-Alonso et al. 1992). Nevertheless, where maximum fluid retention is desired, there may be benefits in increasing the sodium levels of rehydration fluids to levels above those provided in typical sport drinks (Maughan and Leiper 1995). Alternatively, sodium may be ingested during postexercise recovery via everyday foods containing sodium or by adding salt to meals. These methods are all effective in enhancing rehydration (Maughan et al. 1996; Ray et al. 1998). In addition, food consumption may provide a social or psychological stimulus to increase voluntary fluid intake and further enhance rehydration goals (Hubbard et al. 1990).

Because caffeine and alcohol increase diuresis, consumption of alcoholic and caffeine-containing drinks during postexercise recovery may result in greater fluid losses compared with other fluids (Gonzalez-Alonso et al. 1992; Shirreffs and Maughan 1997). Athletes are often told that caffeine-containing beverages such as tea, coffee, and cola or guarana drinks are not suitable rehydration fluids and should be avoided in situations where there is a risk of developing dehydration, such as during and after exercise or during air travel. However, a recent review of caffeine and hydration status found that there is a lack of rigorously collected data to show that caffeine intake impairs fluid status (Armstrong 2002). This report concluded that the effect of caffeine on diuresis is overstated and may be minimal in people who are habitual caffeine users. In addition, increased fluid losses from caffeine-containing or low-alcohol drinks may be more than offset by the increased voluntary intake of fluids that are well liked by the athlete or part of social rituals and eating behaviors. If athletes are suddenly asked to remove such beverages from their diets, or postexercise meals, they may not compensate by drinking an equal volume of other less familiar or well-liked fluids. Of course, the intake of large amounts of alcoholic beverages after exercise will interfere with recovery, particularly by distracting the athlete from following recommended dietary practices and by promoting high-risk behavior (Burke and Maughan 2000).

The depletion of muscle glycogen provides a strong drive for its own resynthesis (Zachwieja et al. 1991). Muscle glycogen synthesis follows a biphasic response consisting of a rapid early phase for 30 to 60 min (non–insulin dependent) followed by a slow phase (insulin dependent) lasting up to several days (Ivy and Kuo 1998; Piehl 1974). The restoration of muscle glycogen takes priority over that of liver glycogen, and even in the absence of carbohydrate intake after exercise it occurs at a low rate (hourly rate of 1-2 mmol/kg wet weight [ww] muscle), with some of the substrate being provided through gluconeogenesis (Maehlum and Hermansen 1978). High-intensity exercise, resulting in high postexercise levels of lactate, is associated with rapid recovery of glycogen stores in the absence of additional carbohydrate feeding (Hermansen and Vaage 1977). After moderate-intensity exercise, however, high rates of muscle glycogen synthesis are dependent on provision of a dietary source of carbohydrate.

Maximal rates of muscle glycogen storage reported during the first 12 hr of recovery are within the range of 5 to 10 mmol/kg ww/hr (for review, see Jentjens and Jeukendrup 2003a). Given a mean storage rate of 5 to 6 mmol/kg ww/hr, 20 to 24 hr of recovery is required following exercise depletion for normalization of muscle glycogen levels (100-120 mmol/kg ww) (Coyle 1991). However, because the training and competition schedules of many athletes often provide considerably less time than this, these athletes may compromise subsequent performance by beginning with inadequate muscle fuel stores. Several factors that are within the control of the athlete can enhance or impair the rate of muscle glycogen storage (see highlight box on this page).

The major dietary factor involved in postexercise refueling is the amount of carbohydrate consumed. As long as total energy intake as adequate (Tarnopolsky et al. 2001), increased carbohydrate intake promotes increased muscle glycogen storage until the threshold for glycogen synthesis is reached (figure 1.3). Until recently, guidelines for athletes stated that optimal glycogen storage is achieved when ~1 to 1.5 g of carbohydrate is consumed every hour in the early stages of recovery, leading to a total carbohydrate of 6 to 10 g/kg of body mass (BM) over 24 hr (American College of Sports Medicine et al. 2000). However, these guidelines were developed on the basis of maximum glycogen storage during a passive recovery period and may both overestimate the carbohydrate needs of athletes who do not substantially deplete glycogen stores in their daily training and underestimate the daily refueling needs of athletes with extremely high training or competition workloads. For example, cyclists undertaking 2 hr of training each day were found to have higher muscle glycogen stores after 7 days of a daily carbohydrate intake of 12 g/kg BM compared with an intake of 10 $g \cdot kg^{-1} \cdot day^{-1}$ (Coyle et al. 2001). In addition, cyclists in the Tour de France, who compete in daily stages lasting at least 6 hr, have been reported to consume 12 to 13 g of carbohydrate per kilogram of BM each day (Saris et al. 1989). These situations have been incorporated into revised guidelines for the carbohydrate needs of athletes that recognize different carbohydrate needs based on exercise load (see table 1.2).

Factors That Influence the Rate of Muscle Glycogen Restoration

Factors that enhance the rate of restoration

- Depletion of glycogen stores—the lower the stores, the faster the rate of recovery
- Immediate intake of carbohydrate after exercise—starts effective recovery immediately
- Adequate amounts of carbohydrate and total energy intake
  - About 1 g per kilogram of the athlete's body mass within first hour of recovery
  - 7 to 12 g/kg over 24 hr
- Focus on carbohydrate-rich foods with a high glycemic index
- Perhaps, frequent intake of carbohydrate (every 15-60 min) during first hours of recovery
- In the situation where carbohydrate intake is below threshold for glycogen storage, addition of protein to carbohydrate meals and snacks

Factors that have minimal effect on rate of restoration

- Gentle exercise during recovery
- Over long-term recovery, frequency of meals and snacks (provided total amount of carbohydrate is adequate)
- When total carbohydrate intake meets threshold for glycogen storage, intake of other macronutrients (e.g., protein or fat)

Factors that reduce the rate of restoration

- Damage to the muscle (contact injury or delayed-onset muscle soreness caused by eccentric exercise)
- Delay in intake of carbohydrate after exercise (postpones the start of effective recovery)
- Inadequate intake of carbohydrate
- Inadequate total energy intake
- Reliance on carbohydrate-rich foods with a low glycemic index
- Prolonged, strenuous exercise during the recovery period

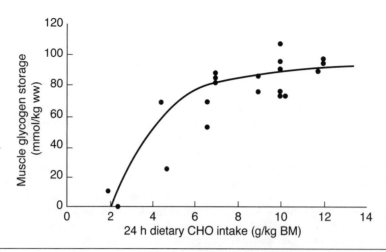

Figure 1.3 Amount of carbohydrate intake and muscle glycogen storage. The relationship between daily carbohydrate intake and muscle glycogen storage during 24 hr of passive recovery from glycogen-depleting exercise is plotted from data taken from Burke et al. (1993, 1995); Burke, Collier, et al. (1996, 2003); Costill et al. (1981); Kiens and Richter (1998); Parkin et al. (1997); and Starling et al. (1997). These data suggest an increase in glycogen storage with increasing dietary carbohydrate intake until the muscle storage threshold is reached.

Reprinted from Burke, Kiens, and Ivy 2004.

Table 1.2 Guidelines for Carbohydrate Intake by Athletes

Situation	Recommended carbohydrate intake
ACUTE SITUATION	
Optimal daily muscle glycogen storage (e.g., for postexercise recovery or to fuel up or carbohydrate load before an event)	7-12 g·kg^{-1} body mass·day^{-1}
Rapid postexercise recovery of muscle glycogen, where recovery between sessions is <8 hr	1-1.2 g/kg immediately after exercise; repeated each hour until meal schedule is resumed. There may be some advantages to consuming carbohydrate as a series of small snacks every 15-60 min in the early recovery phase.
Preevent meal to increase carbohydrate availability before prolonged exercise session	1-4 g/kg eaten 1-4 hr before exercise
Carbohydrate intake during moderate-intensity or intermittent exercise of >1 hr	0.5-1.0 g·kg^{-1}·hr^{-1} (30-60 g/hr)
CHRONIC OR EVERYDAY SITUATION	
Daily recovery or fuel needs for athletes with very light training program (low-intensity exercise or skill-based exercise). These targets may be particularly suited to athletes with large body mass or a need to reduce energy intake to lose weight.	3-5 g·kg^{-1}·day^{-1}
Daily recovery or fuel needs for athlete with moderate exercise program (i.e., <1 hr)	5-7 g·kg^{-1}·day^{-1}
Daily recovery or fuel needs for endurance athlete (i.e., 1-3 hr of moderate- to high-intensity exercise)	7-12 g·kg^{-1}·day^{-1}
Daily recovery or fuel needs for athlete undertaking extreme exercise program (i.e., >4-5 hr of moderate- to high-intensity exercise such as Tour de France)	≥10-12 g·kg^{-1}·day^{-1}

Adapted from Burke, Kiens, and Ivy 2004.

The type and timing of carbohydrate intake may affect the rate of glycogen restoration, and it is hypothesized that strategies that enhance blood glucose availability or insulin levels might enhance glycogen synthesis. For example, moderate and high glycemic index carbohydrate-rich foods and drinks appear to promote greater glycogen storage than meals based on low glycemic index carbohydrate foods (Burke et al. 1993). However, the mechanisms may include additional factors such as the malabsorption of low glycemic index carbohydrate rather than differences in the glycemic and insulinemic response to such foods alone (Burke, Collier, et al. 1996). The form of the carbohydrate—fluids or solids—does not appear to affect glycogen synthesis (Keizer et al. 1986; Reed et al. 1989) .

Early research indicated that glycogen synthesis was enhanced by the addition of protein to carbohydrate snacks consumed after exercise, an observation that was explained by the protein-stimulated enhancement of the insulin response (Zawadzki et al. 1992). However, these findings have been refuted in other studies (Jentjens et al. 2001; Van Hall, Shirreffs, et al. 2000), especially when the energy contents of protein or amino acids included in recovery feedings were matched (Burke et al. 1995; Carrithers et al. 2000; Roy and Tarnopolsky 1998; Tarnopolsky et al. 1997; Van Loon et al. 2000). The current consensus is that co-ingestion of protein or amino acids with carbohydrate does not clearly enhance glycogen synthesis. Any benefits to muscle glycogen storage are limited to the first hour of recovery (Ivy et al. 2002) or to situations where protein is added to an amount of carbohydrate or pattern of intake that is below the threshold for maximal glycogen synthesis. Of course, the intake of protein within carbohydrate-rich recovery meals may allow the athlete to meet other nutritional goals including the enhancement of net protein balance after exercise. Nevertheless, excessively large amounts of protein and fat in an athlete's diet may displace carbohydrate foods within the athlete's energy requirements and gastric comfort, thereby indirectly interfering with glycogen storage by preventing adequate carbohydrate intake.

Athletes have been advised to enhance recovery by consuming carbohydrate as soon as possible after the completion of a workout. The highest rates of muscle glycogen storage occur during the first hour after exercise (Ivy et al. 1988), attributable to activation of glycogen synthase by glycogen depletion (Wojtaszewski et al. 2001) and exercise-induced increases in muscle membrane permeability and insulin sensitivity (Richter et al. 1989). Carbohydrate feeding immediately after exercise takes advantage of these effects, with higher rates of glycogen storage during the first 2 hr of recovery, slowing thereafter to the more typical rates of storage (Ivy et al. 1988). The most important consideration, however, is that failure to consume carbohydrate in the immediate phase of postexercise recovery leads to very low rates of glycogen restoration until feeding occurs. Therefore, early intake of carbohydrate following strenuous exercise is valuable because it provides an immediate source of substrate to the muscle cell to start effective recovery, and it takes advantage of a period of moderately

enhanced glycogen synthesis. Although early feeding may be important when there is only 4 to 8 hr between exercise sessions (Ivy et al. 1988), it may have less impact over a longer recovery period. For example, there was no difference in glycogen storage after 8 and 24 hr of recovery whether carbohydrate consumption was begun immediately after exercise or delayed for 2 hr (Parkin et al. 1997) (see figure 1.4, a and b). It appears that when the interval between exercise sessions is short, athletes should begin to consume carbohydrate as soon as possible to maximize the effective recovery time. However, when longer recovery periods are available, athletes can choose their preferred meal schedule as long as total carbohydrate intake goals are achieved. It is not always practical to consume substantial meals or snacks immediately after the finish of a strenuous workout.

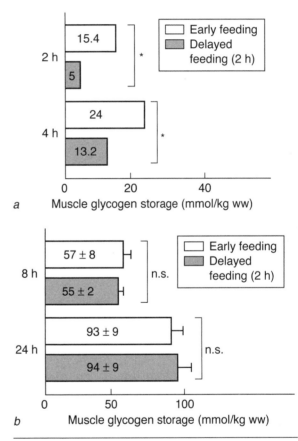

Figure 1.4 (a) Delaying intake of carbohydrate until 2 hr after the finish of a prolonged exercise session has a significant effect on short recovery periods (e.g., up to 6-8 hr). Because effective refueling does not occur until substantial amounts of carbohydrate are consumed, recovery after 4 hr is impaired with delayed feeding compared with intake of the same amount of carbohydrate immediately after and during recovery. (b) When recovery periods are long enough (8-24 hr), immediate intake provides no further enhancement of glycogen storage as long as total carbohydrate intake is adequate.

* = $P < 0.05$

Reprinted from Burke, Kiens, and Ivy 2004.

The frequency of food intake has also been studied. Restoration of muscle glycogen over 24 hr was the same whether a given amount of carbohydrate was fed as two or seven meals (Costill et al. 1981) or as four large meals or 16 hourly snacks (Burke, Collier, et al. 1996) despite differences in insulin and glucose responses. In contrast, very high rates of glycogen synthesis during the first 4 to 6 hr of recovery have been reported when large amounts of carbohydrate were fed at 15 to 30 min intervals (Doyle et al. 1993; Jentjens et al. 2001; Van Hall, Shirreffs, et al. 2000; Van Loon et al. 2000) and have been attributed to the higher sustained insulin and glucose profiles achieved by such a feeding protocol. The effects of enhanced insulin and glucose concentrations on glycogen storage may be important during the first hours of recovery or when total carbohydrate intake is below the threshold of maximum glycogen storage. However, during longer periods of recovery or when total carbohydrate intake is above this threshold, manipulations of plasma substrates and hormones within physiological ranges do not add further benefit. In summary, meeting total carbohydrate requirements is more important than the pattern of intake, at least for long-term recovery, and the athlete is advised to choose a food schedule that is practical and comfortable. Small frequent meals may be useful in overcoming the gastric discomfort often associated with eating large amounts of bulky, high-carbohydrate foods, but additional benefits to glycogen storage may also occur directly during the early recovery phase.

Many of the adaptations stimulated by exercise are underpinned by changes in various proteins in the muscle cell, including regulatory proteins, found in the mitochondria and sarcoplasma, and the structural or myofibrillar proteins. The body protein pool is highly dynamic, undergoing constant synthesis from, and breakdown to, free amino acids that are exchanged between intracellular and plasma pools. During exercise there is a change in the balance, with rates of breakdown exceeding those of synthesis; a goal of postexercise recovery is to reverse this situation so that over time, the magnitude of positive protein balance outweighs that of negative protein balance. This reversal can occur through an increase in protein synthesis, a decrease in protein breakdown, or a combination of both. Although the exact processes are not well explained, experience suggests that endurance exercise increases muscle oxidative capacity by preferentially stimulating the net synthesis of the mitochondrial and sarcoplasmic proteins, whereas a net increase in myofibrillar proteins explains the hypertrophy following resistance training.

The specific study of muscle protein balance is complex and relatively new (Tipton and Wolfe 2001). Our knowledge is based on studies of the acute response to exercise and dietary interventions, although fortunately, recent research shows that the first few hours following an exercise or dietary intervention provide a representative picture of 24 hr muscle protein balance (Tipton et al. 2003). The majority of studies have been undertaken using resistance training as the mode of exercise, using untrained participants. Although the postexercise period is characterized by an improvement in net protein balance, in the absence of nutritional support, net protein balance in the muscle remains negative (Phillips et al. 1997; Phillips et al. 1999). In contrast, the delivery of a source of amino acids following resistance exercise causes a net gain in muscle protein balance, principally attributable to an increase in rates of muscle protein synthesis rather than changes in muscle protein breakdown (Tipton et al. 1999). This effect can be produced by the intake of essential amino acids alone (Borsheim et al. 2002) and is further enhanced when the amino acids are provided immediately before the resistance training session, rather than after exercise (Tipton et al. 2001). The minimum amount of amino acids needed to produce an effect and the amount required for an optimal effect are currently unknown; however, there are dramatic responses to the intake of as little as 3 to 6 g of essential amino acids—10 to 20 g of high-quality protein (Borsheim et al. 2002; Tipton et al. 2001)—and there is evidence of both a dose response (Borsheim et al. 2002) and continued responses to repeated intake of recovery snacks (Miller et al. 2003).

Intake of carbohydrate after resistance exercise stimulates insulin secretion and decreases the normal stimulation of muscle protein breakdown (Biolo et al. 1999). The combination of carbohydrate and amino acids after exercise might optimize muscle protein synthesis by increasing synthesis and reducing breakdown; however, the available research suggests that the enhancement of protein synthesis is small (Miller et al. 2003). The major effect of carbohydrate intake on protein synthesis appears to be delayed for several hours (Borsheim, Cree, et al. 2004), and there may be value in delaying the intake of amino acids to coincide with the peak of the insulin action. Such protocols need to be studied. Nevertheless, the combined intake of carbohydrate and protein is a sensible strategy for recovery from resistance training because it addresses needs for refueling as well as the protein response. There is less information regarding nutritional interventions for postexercise protein balance following endurance exercise. However, there is some evidence that protein and carbohydrate intake enhances net protein balance following prolonged cycling and that early intake of recovery meals (1 hr) has greater benefits than delayed intake (3 hr) (Levenhagen et al. 2001).

More research is needed to elucidate optimal feeding practices for postexercise protein recovery. Issues that should be addressed include the amounts of amino acids needed to achieve desired outcomes, the effects of different types of whole proteins (i.e., foods), the interaction of protein and carbohydrate, the optimal timing of intake of nutrients, differential effects in well-trained athletes versus untrained subjects, and the response to different exercise stimuli. Also needed are the complex end-point studies that can prove that various interventions enhance training adaptations and competition performance. Until such research is completed, it makes sense for the athlete to address recovery goals with an integrated nutritional approach, which includes choosing foods and drinks that provide valuable sources of both protein and carbohydrate in post- and preevent meals (see table 1.3).

Table 1.3   Carbohydrate-Rich Choices Suitable for Special Issues in Sport

Carbohydrate-rich choices for preevent meals	Carbohydrate-rich foods suitable for intake during exercise (50 g of carbohydrate portions)

• Breakfast cereal + low-fat milk + fresh or canned fruit
• Muffins or crumpets + jam or honey
• Pancakes + syrup
• Toast + baked beans (this is a high-fiber choice)
• Creamed rice (made with low-fat milk)
• Rolls or sandwiches
• Fruit salad + low-fat fruit yogurt
• Spaghetti with tomato or low-fat sauce
• Baked potatoes with low-fat filling
• Fruit smoothie (low-fat milk + fruit + yogurt or ice cream)
• Liquid meal supplement
	• 600-800 ml of sport drink
	• 2 sachets of sport gel
	• 1-1.5 sport bars
	• 2 cereal bars or granola bars
	• Large bread roll filled with
	  -jam, honey, or cheese
	  -2 bananas or 3 medium pieces of other fruit
	  -60 g of jelly confectionery
	• 450 ml of cola drinks
	• 80 g chocolate bar
	• 100 g of fruit bread or cake
	• 80 dried fruit or 120 g of trail mix

Recovery snacks, to be eaten postexercise, or preexercise in the case of resistance training to promote refueling and protein responses (Each serving provides 50 g of carbohydrate and at least 10 g of protein.)	Portable carbohydrate-rich foods suitable for the traveling athlete
• 250-350 ml of liquid meal supplement, milk shake, or fruit smoothie • 500 ml of flavored low-fat milk • Sport bar + 200 ml of sport drink • 60 g (1.5-2 cups) of breakfast cereal with 1/2 cup of milk • 1 round of sandwiches with cheese, meat, or chicken filling, and 1 large piece of fruit or 300 ml of sport drink • 1 cup of fruit salad with 200 g of fruit-flavored yogurt or custard • 200 g of fruit-flavored yogurt or 300 ml of flavored milk and 30 to 35 g cereal bar • 2 crumpets or English muffins with thick spread of peanut butter • 250 g of baked beans on 2 slices of toast • 250 g (large) baked potato with cottage cheese or grated cheese filling • 150 g thick-crust pizza	• Breakfast cereal (and skim milk powder) • Cereal bars, granola bars • Dried fruit, trail mixes • Rice crackers, dry biscuits • Spreads: jam, honey • Sport bars • Liquid meal supplements: powder and ready-to-drink forms • Sport drink

Goal 7

Reduce the risk of sickness and injury during heavy training periods by maintaining healthy physique and energy balance and by supplying nutrients believed to assist immune function.

An athlete's ability to train consistently rests on remaining healthy and injury-free. Meeting known nutrient needs is important for general health and well-being. However, several issues related to sport and exercise merit special comment. The first involves the immunosuppression that is known to accompany prolonged and strenuous training, whereas the other concerns disturbances of the athlete's

hormonal system with potential implications for illness and bone integrity.

Prolonged exhaustive exercise is known to cause a transient impairment of various immune system parameters and the potential for an increased risk of illness (for review, see Pedersen et al. 1999). Various nutritional interventions such as supplementation with glutamine, echinacea, and antioxidants have failed to provide a clear and consistent improvement to the athlete's immune status or health (Gleeson and Bishop 2000). Recent studies have found that carbohydrate status may play an important role in maintaining effective immune function in athletes. Disturbed immune function may occur through two principal mechanisms related to low carbohydrate intake: direct immunosuppression attributable to the depletion of glucose, which is a key substrate for the high metabolic needs of immune cells, and indirect impairment via increased concentration of stress hormones (Gleeson et al. 2001). Studies in which carbohydrate is consumed during prolonged continuous exercise (Henson et al. 1999; Nehlsen-Cannarella et al. 1997) or in high amounts in the preexercise diet (Gleeson et al. 1998) have shown that there is less disturbance to immune system parameters during the postexercise period than when the athlete is deprived of carbohydrate. However, not all studies have found an enhancement of the distribution and function of immune parameters, especially when the exercise involves a intermittent high-intensity protocol (Bishop et al. 1999) or is carried out to the point of fatigue (Henson et al. 2000). The ideal study to find that long-term dietary practices correlate with reduced frequency or severity of illness in athletes is yet to be undertaken. Notwithstanding these limitations, the current literature supports the importance of adequate carbohydrate intake for the health of the athlete. Although the primary benefit is the availability of fuel supply, leading to better training or competition performance, protection of the immune system may be a secondary but substantial benefit of carbohydrate intake strategies.

Lengthy periods of restricted energy intake by female athletes are associated with menstrual dysfunction, hormonal disturbances, and energy conservation (Loucks 2001), with the hormone leptin providing a potential link between energy availability and the hormones responsible for reproductive and metabolic function (Thong and Graham 1999). Male athletes who undertake periods of severe energy restriction are also likely to suffer some of these effects. A variety of causes of menstrual dysfunction in female athletes have been suggested, and there is a large degree of individuality in response to risk factors (for review, see Manore 2002). Nevertheless, energy drain, or low energy availability—chronic periods of restricted energy intake in conjunction with high energy expenditure—appears to be an underlying factor in many cases of menstrual dysfunction (Loucks et al. 1998). Disordered eating and food-related stress are frequently related to menstrual dysfunction. Recent research has shown that low energy availability directly impairs bone formation and resorption (Ihle and Loucks 2004) as well as having an indirect effect on bones arising from menstrual dysfunction and altered hormonal environment. The cluster of disordered eating, amenorrhea, and osteopenia became known during the 1990s as the female athlete triad (Yeager et al. 1993), in recognition that female athletes are at increased risk of developing one or more of these problems and that the causes and outcomes are often closely linked. Individually, or in combination, these problems can directly impair athletic health. Significantly, they will reduce the athlete's career span by increasing her risk of illness and injury, including stress fractures. Long-term problems such as an increased risk of osteoporosis in later life and chronic suboptimal nutritional status might also be expected.

Although awareness of the female athlete triad has focused attention on menstrual dysfunction and has highlighted the seriousness of the triad, criticism of the initial "packaging" of the syndrome (Khan et al. 2002; Nattiv 2002) has helped broader definitions and recommendations to evolve. A diagnosis of the first definition of the female athlete triad required extreme cutoff points for the following:

- Eating disorders: described as a wide range of harmful eating behaviors used to achieve a reduction of weight or body fat, with the spectrum ranging from restricted food intake to frank cases of eating disorders
- Amenorrhea: described as primary or secondary amenorrhea according to standard definitions
- Osteoporosis: described as a bone mineral density more than 2.5 standard deviations below the mean value for young adults

The more recent concept of the female athlete triad (Loucks and Nattiv 2005) targets energy availability, menstrual health, and bone density. It considers that each of these issues involves a continuum between optimal health and frank disorder and that the athlete should be alert to any change in her status of any issue. In other words, athletes must be educated about the benefits of early diagnosis and treatment of problems and the likelihood that negative outcomes occur at a much earlier stage than previously considered. The detection, prevention, and management of the female athlete triad, or individual elements within it (Beals and Manore 2002), require expertise and, ideally, the teamwork of sports physicians, dietitians, psychologists, coaches, and fitness advisors. Dietary intervention is important to correct factors that underpin menstrual dysfunction as well as those that contribute to suboptimal bone density. Dietary goals include adequate energy intake and the reversal of disordered eating or suboptimal intake. Adequate calcium intake is important for bone health, and requirements may be increased to 1,200 to 1,500 mg/day in athletes with impaired menstrual function. Where adequate calcium intake cannot be met through dietary means, usually through use of low-fat dairy foods or calcium-enriched soy alternatives, a calcium supplement may be considered. There is some doubt about the degree of reversibility of bone loss and in particular the restoration of a strong bone formation, particularly in cases of long-term loss (Drinkwater et al. 1986). Prevention or early intervention is clearly the preferred option.

Goal 8

Make well-considered decisions about the use of supplements and specialized sport foods that have been shown to enhance training performance or meet training nutrition needs.

Sport foods and supplements represent a multibillion dollar industry, supported by aggressive marketing from manufacturers and word of mouth between athletes and coaches. Exercise scientists and sports nutrition practitioners believe that well-controlled research should underpin the promotion of any sports nutrition practice and are understandably frustrated that producers of supplements often make impressive claims about their products without adequate, or in some cases any, proof. However, in most countries, legislation regarding supplements or sport foods is either minimal or not enforced, allowing unsupported claims to flourish or products to be manufactured with poor compliance to labeling and composition standards. Athletes are usually unaware of these lapses.

Before making a decision to use a supplement or sport food, athletes and coaches should consider the likely benefits, balanced against the cost of the product and the risk of negative outcomes. Problems include the risk of side-effects or inadvertent intake of a substance that is banned in sport, leading to a positive doping outcome. Athletes and coaches should be empowered to make a decision by having unbiased information about any scientifically documented benefits of the use of the supplement or sport food, as well as the potential risk of short- and long-term harmful effects. Athletes and coaches should also be well educated about the specific ways in which the supplement or sport food can be used to achieve nutritional goals or enhance performance. The advice of sport scientists or sports nutrition authorities should be sought to provide such information.

The ever-growing range of sports nutrition products can be divided into two separate groups. Some supplements and sport foods address the special nutritional needs of athletes and offer a simple or practical way to meet known nutritional goals. This group includes sport drinks, sport bars, liquid meal supplements, and micronutrient supplements that are part of a prescribed dietary plan. Many of these products are specially designed to help an athlete meet specific needs for energy and nutrient, including fluid and carbohydrate, in situations where everyday foods are not practical to eat. This is particularly relevant for intake immediately before, during, or after exercise. These supplements can be shown to improve performance when they allow the athlete to achieve well-defined sports nutrition goals (for review, see Burke, Cort, et al. 2006). However, these supplements are more expensive than normal food, a consideration that must be balanced against the convenience they provide. In some cases, the athlete may decide to limit the use of these products to competition or to key training sessions that are used to simulate competition practices.

In contrast, some produce claim a direct ergogenic benefit to sport performance. These products, which continually change in popularity, include megadoses of vitamins and some minerals, free-form amino acids, ginseng and other herbal compounds, bee pollen, coenzyme Q10, inosine, and carnitine. In general, these supplements have been poorly tested or have failed to live up to their claims when rigorous testing has been undertaken (for review, see Burke, Cort, et al. 2006). Exceptions to this are bicarbonate and citrate (McNaughton 2000), creatine (Hespel et al. 2001), caffeine (Graham 2001a and b), and glycerol (Robergs and Griffin 1998), each of which may enhance the performance

of certain athletes under specific conditions. Other products that have some, but at present inconclusive, evidence in support of benefits include β-hydroxy β-methylbutyrate (HMB) (Slater and Jenkins 2000) and bovine colostrum. Athletes should seek expert advice about such supplements to see if their sport or exercise warrants experimentation with these products in the training phase and to ensure that a correct protocol is tried. Athletes should realize, however, that supplements and sport foods are neither a shortcut to optimal performance nor a replacement for the sound principles that underpin good training.

Goals 9 and 10

Eat for long-term health by paying attention to healthy eating guidelines. Enjoy food and the pleasure of sharing meals.

Although athletes tend to focus on their immediate competition pursuits, they should remembered that there is life after a sporting career! Therefore, athletes are included in the healthy nutrition guidelines prepared for the general population. Dietary guidelines recommend a reduced intake of fats and oils, increased intake of nutrient-rich carbohydrate foods, and moderation with alcohol intake. These principles are compatible with the strategies for optimal training nutrition that have already been discussed. Although this provides further incentive to the athlete to follow a healthy training diet, his or her opportunity to provide a role model for the community should also be considered: High-profile athletes can provide a good example of the potential benefits of a well-chosen diet.

Although some athletes may need to modify their eating patterns, they are encouraged to avoid extreme dietary changes and the exclusion of all their favorite foods. Moderation and variety are key elements in preserving nutritional adequacy, but the pleasure derived from food and eating should also be valued and preserved. Unfortunately, some athletes experience dietary extremism rather than flexibility and enjoyment of food. This problem arises most often in relation to issues of body fat and weight but can simply reflect the rigid and perfectionist personalities of many athletes. The athlete should always seek a balance between meeting his or her nutritional goals and enjoying the social and hedonistic aspects of eating.

Goals of Competition Eating

The nutritional challenges of competition vary according to the length and intensity of the event, the environment, and factors that influence opportunities to eat and drink during the event or in recovery afterward. To achieve optimal performance, the coach and athlete should identify factors that are likely to cause fatigue during the event and undertake nutritional strategies before, during, and after the event that minimize or delay the onset of this fatigue. Of course, competition nutrition strategies need to be undertaken with consideration of practical issues such as avoiding gastrointestinal problems during the event or finding access to suitable food supplies when competition takes place away from home.

Goal 11

In weight-division sports, achieve the competition weight division with minimal harm to health or performance

In some sports, competition regulations exist to match competitors of equal size and strength via the setting of weight divisions or weight limits. Weight-regulated sports include combative sports (boxing, judo, and wrestling), lightweight rowing, handicapped horse races, and weightlifting. In such sports, the culture and common practice are to try to compete in a weight division that is considerably lighter than the athlete's usual training weight (Brownell et al. 1987; Steen and Brownell 1990). Athletes achieve their weight loss over a number of days before competition by dehydrating (by using saunas, exercising in sweat clothes, or ingesting diuretics) and restricting food and fluid intake (Steen and Brownell 1990). A number of disadvantages arise from these weight-making practices. The acute penalties include the negative effects of dehydration and inadequate fuel status on performance, whereas the long-term penalties include psychological stress, chronic periods of inadequate nutrition, and effects on hormone status (Walberg-Rankin 2006). The potential problems associated with extreme weight-making practices should not be underestimated and have led some sports to develop programs combining education and testing to deter acute weight loss practices (Oppliger et al. 1995). The worst-case scenario is the death of the athlete, as occurred in 1997 in three separate situations involving college wrestlers in the United States (Centers for Disease Control and Prevention 1998). Athletes in these sports should be guided to choose the appropriate competition weight division and to achieve necessary weight loss by safe and long-term strategies to reduce body fat levels (Walberg-Rankin 2006).

Where a small reduction in body mass (e.g., 1-2% BM) is needed to allow the athlete to achieve the weight target at the official competition weigh-in, this may be achieved by acute strategies such as the short-term use of a low-residue diet to reduce the mass of gastrointestinal contents and, perhaps, mild dehydration. The period between the weigh-in and the start of the event varies between sports and may range from an hour to a day (Walberg-Rankin 2006). Therefore, the rules of each sport offer their athletes different opportunities to rehydrate or refuel after the weigh-in. Strategies for such rapid recovery were covered in goal 6. The penalties of failing to completely restore fluid balance or to optimally fuel up for an event will vary according to the conditions of performance in a sport; for example, the duration and intensity of the event, the environmental conditions, and the number of times the athlete is required

to perform. However, the best approach will always be to minimize the physiological and psychological stress that the athlete must face before the event.

Goal 12

Fuel up adequately before an event by consuming carbohydrate and tapering exercise during the days before the event according to the importance and duration of the event; use carbohydrate-loading strategies when appropriate before events of greater than 90 to 120 min duration.

The usual resting glycogen concentrations of the trained athlete (100-120 mmol/kg ww) appear adequate to meet the fuel needs of events lasting up to 60 to 90 min (Hawley, Schabort, et al. 1997). In the absence of severe muscle damage, such stores can be achieved by 24 hr of rest and an adequate carbohydrate intake (7-10 g · kg BM^{-1} · day^{-1}) (Costill et al. 1981). For many athletes, this might be as simple as scheduling a day of rest or light training the event while continuing to follow high-carbohydrate eating patterns. However, not all athletes eat sufficient carbohydrate in their usual diets to maximize glycogen storage, particularly females who restrict their total energy intake to control body fat levels (Burke, Cox, et al. 2001b). These athletes may need education or encouragement to relax temporarily their dietary restraint and prioritize refueling as the major dietary goal on the day before competition. Similarly, some athletes may need to reorganize their training programs to allow a lighter training day or rest on the day before their event.

The term *carbohydrate loading* describes practices that aim to maximize or supercompensate muscle glycogen stores before a competitive event that would otherwise deplete these fuel reserves. Carbohydrate-loading protocols, which can elevate muscle glycogen stores to 150 to 250 mmol/kg ww, evolved in the late 1960s from studies in which muscle biopsy techniques were first used to investigate muscle fuel stores. Researchers found that muscle glycogen content could be manipulated by various dietary and exercise strategies and that preexercise stores of this substrate were an important determinant of endurance or capacity to sustain prolonged moderate-intensity exercise (Ahlborg et al. 1967; Bergstrom et al. 1967). Specifically, several days of a low-carbohydrate diet depleted muscle glycogen stores and reduced cycling endurance compared with a normal carbohydrate intake. However, the subsequent intake of a high-carbohydrate diet over several days caused a supercompensation of glycogen stores and prolonged cycling time to exhaustion. Glycogen supercompensation was shown to be localized to the muscle that had been previously depleted, and the activity of an enzyme, glycogen synthase, was found to be important in glycogen synthesis (Bergstrom and Hultman 1966). These pioneering studies produced the classic 7-day model of carbohydrate loading: a 3- to 4-day depletion phase of hard training and low carbohydrate intake followed by a 3- to 4-day loading phase of high-carbohydrate eating and exercise taper. Early field studies of prolonged running events showed that carbohydrate loading could enhance sport performance, not by allowing the athlete to run faster but by prolonging the time that race pace could be maintained (Karlsson and Saltin 1971).

Carbohydrate loading strategies were modified when trained muscle was later shown to be able to supercompensate glycogen stores without a severe depletion, or glycogen-stripping, phase. Well-trained runners elevated their muscle glycogen stores with 3 days of taper and high carbohydrate intake, regardless of whether this was preceded by a depletion phase or a more typical diet and training preparation (Sherman et al. 1981). Carbohydrate loading was repositioned as an extension of fueling strategies (rest and high carbohydrate intake) over ~3 days. This modified protocol was offered as a more practical strategy for competition preparation, avoiding the fatigue and complexity of extreme diet and training requirements associated with the previous depletion phase. More recent studies showed that maximal glycogen storage can be achieved by well-trained athletes in as little as 36 to 48 hr following the last exercise session, at least when the athlete rests and consumes adequate carbohydrate intake (Bussau et al. 2002). Of course, it isn't always desirable for athletes to achieve total inactivity in the days before competition, because even in a taper, some stimulus is required to maintain previously acquired training adaptations (Mujika and Padilla 2000a and b).

Theoretically, carbohydrate loading could enhance performance in exercise or sporting events that would otherwise be limited by glycogen depletion, typically activities of greater than 90 min duration (Hawley, Schabort, et al. 1997). An increase in preevent glycogen stores prolongs the duration for which moderate-intensity exercise can be undertaken before fatiguing and may enhance the performance of a set amount of work by preventing the decline in pace or work output that would otherwise occur. Typically, carbohydrate loading postpones fatigue and extends the duration of steady-state exercise by ~20%, and it improves performance over a set distance or workload by 2% to 3% (Hawley, Schabort, et al. 1997).

Many athletes undertake prolonged events of a less predictable nature—for example, tennis matches or football games that extend for at least 80 to 90 min of playing time, featuring intermittent passages of high-intensity exercise with high rates of glycogen utilization. Although it is intuitive that games that cause glycogen depletion would benefit from supercompensation of muscle glycogen stores, it is extremely difficult to undertake studies that measure the performance of such complex and variable sports. A preevent increase in glycogen stores has been shown to enhance the performance of the movement patterns in a soccer-simulated trial (Bangsbo et al. 1992), an indoor soccer game (Balsom, Wood, et al. 1999), and a real-life

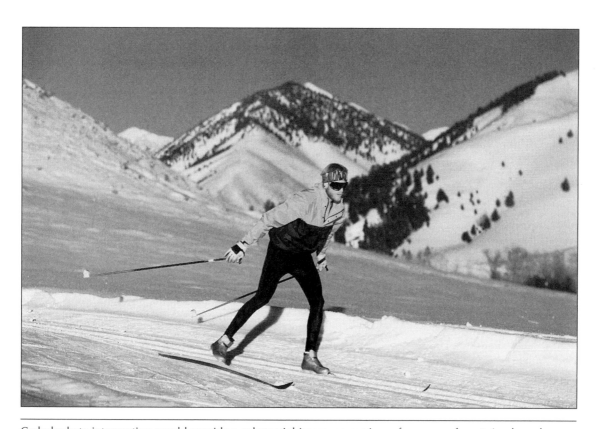

Carbohydrate intervention would provide a substantial improvement in performance of most simple endurance events such as marathons, prolonged cycling and triathlon races, and cross-country skiing events.

ice hockey match (Akermark et al. 1996). In contrast, such a glycogen increase failed to significantly improve the performance of skill-based tasks in a simulated soccer match (Abt et al. 1998). Decisions about the benefits of carbohydrate loading may be specific not only to the sport but also to the individual athlete, depending on the requirements of his or her position or style of play. Of course, the logistics of competition in many of these sports, where games may be played every day or every second day, might prevent preevent optimization of glycogen stores. Indeed, a recent study showed that it is not possible to glycogen-load several times within a short time period, although continuing a high carbohydrate diet maintained the performance advantages (McInerney et al. 2005). Athletes in these sports should fuel up before each competition as well as possible and perhaps experiment with an extended preparation before the most important games, such as the final of the tournament. Finally, the ~2 kg gain in body mass that accompanies carbohydrate loading (Brotherhood and Swanson 1979) may not be desirable in some weight-sensitive sports, although it should be seen as a temporary outcome of the increase in the muscle content of carbohydrate and water. Presumably, there is a weight decrease throughout the event as these nutrients are liberated from the muscle.

Goal 13

Top up carbohydrate stores with a preevent meal or snack during the 1 to 4 hr before competition.

Foods and drinks consumed in the 4 hr before an event have a role in fine-tuning competition preparation and should achieve the following goals:

- Further enhance muscle glycogen stores if they have not been fully restored or loaded since the last exercise session.

- Restore liver glycogen content, especially for events undertaken in the morning when liver stores are low after an overnight fast.

- Contribute to fluid balance to ensure that the athlete is well hydrated.

- Prevent hunger and avoid of gastrointestinal discomfort and upset often experienced during exercise.

- Include foods and eating practices that are important to the athlete's psychology or superstition.

The preevent meal menu should include carbohydrate-rich foods and drinks (see table 1.3 for suggestions), especially in the case where body carbohydrate stores are suboptimal because of inadequate recovery from the previous workout, or where the event is of sufficient duration and intensity to challenge these stores. Carbohydrate consumed during the hours before the event enhances carbohydrate availability by increasing muscle and liver glycogen stores (Coyle et al.

1985) as well as by storing glucose in the gastrointestinal space for later release. Because liver glycogen stores are labile and may be substantially depleted by an overnight fast, carbohydrate intake on the morning of an event may ensure that hepatic glucose output is able to maintain blood glucose levels during the latter stages of prolonged exercise. Compared with trials undertaken after an overnight fast, the intake of a substantial amount of carbohydrate (~200-300 g) in the 2 to 4 hr before exercise has been shown to prolong cycling endurance (Wright et al. 1991) and enhance performance of an exercise test undertaken at the end of a standardized cycling task (Neufer et al. 1987; Sherman et al. 1989).

In the field it is not always practical to consume a substantial carbohydrate-rich meal or snack in the 4 hr before a sporting event. For example, it is unlikely that an athlete will want to sacrifice sleep to eat a large meal before an early-morning race start. In this situation, many athletes will settle for a lighter meal or snack before the event and consume carbohydrate throughout the event to balance missed fueling opportunities (goal 15). The size and composition of the preevent meal may need to be modified for athletes who are at risk of gastrointestinal discomfort or upset during exercise (see goal 16). Athletes should also be conscious of fluid needs and consume adequate fluid to ensure that they are well hydrated at the start of the event (see goal 14). Because competition often occurs away from home, the preevent eating plan should be able to be adapted to the available food supply and catering options. Many special or important foods can be taken by the athlete to the competition location (see table 1.3). Above all, each athlete should choose a strategy that suits his or her situation and past experiences and that can be fine-tuned with further experimentation.

Despite the benefits previously discussed, the issue of carbohydrate intake before exercise is not straightforward. Carbohydrate eaten in the hours before exercise causes a series of metabolic perturbations. The stimulation of insulin following carbohydrate intake suppresses lipolysis and subsequent fat utilization during exercise while increasing carbohydrate oxidation compared with that seen during exercise undertaken in a fasted state. These effects can be seen when carbohydrate is consumed up to 4 hr before exercise (Coyle et al. 1985) but are most pronounced when carbohydrate is consumed in the final hour before exercise. Typical outcomes of consuming carbohydrate before exercise include a transient decrease in plasma glucose levels at the start of exercise and an increased rate of muscle glycogen utilization. In one well-publicized study, glucose consumed in the hour before submaximal exercise was shown to reduce exercise capacity (Foster et al. 1979). In most athletes, however, these metabolic perturbations are either minor or transient and are not detrimental to performance. Instead, the decline in blood glucose observed during the first 20 min of exercise is self-corrected with no apparent effects on the athlete. In fact, most studies show that carbohydrate intake in the hour before exercise can enhance performance by enhancing body carbohydrate availability (for review of the literature, see Hawley and Burke 1997).

Nevertheless, a small proportion of athletes appear to respond negatively to carbohydrate feedings in the hour before exercise. These athletes experience an exaggerated increase in carbohydrate oxidation and decrease in blood glucose concentrations at the start of exercise, suffering symptoms of hypoglycemia and a rapid onset of fatigue. The exact reasons that some athletes experience such an extreme reaction are unclear. Risk factors identified in one study include the intake of small amounts of carbohydrate (<50 g), increased sensitivity to insulin, a lower sympathetic induced counterregulation, and a low or moderate workload in the subsequent exercise bout (Kuipers et al. 1999). However, Jeukendrup and colleagues more recently conducted a series of studies in which these factors in pre-exercise feeding were systematically manipulated before a 20-min bout of steady-state exercise in a group of trained cyclists. The researchers found that the amount of carbohydrate (range 20-200 g) fed 45 min before exercise (Jentjens et al. 2003) and the intensity of subsequent exercise (55-90% $\dot{V}O_2$max; Achten and Jeukendrup 2003) affected neither the degree of the mild decline in blood glucose during exercise nor the prevalence of blood glucose concentrations defined as hypoglycemic (<3.5 mmol/L). Changing the timing of intake of 75 g of carbohydrate before exercise (15-75 min) caused differences in blood glucose concentrations at the beginning of exercise. Later feeding times (45 and 75 min) were associated with a greater prevalence of hypoglycemic levels of blood glucose, but differences self-corrected within 10 minutes of cycling (Moseley et al. 2003). Intake of trehalose or galactose, sugars with a lower glycemic index, was associated with a reduced prevalence of hypoglycemic levels of blood glucose compared with glucose feedings (Jentjens and Jeukendrup 2003b). Finally, cyclists who developed hypoglycemic blood glucose levels did not differ in insulin sensitivity, measured from an oral glucose tolerance test, compared with participants whose lowest blood glucose level remained above 3.5 mmol/L (Jentjens and Jeukendrup 2002).

Not all athletes who experience a major decline in blood glucose concentrations experience classical symptoms of hypoglycemia and fatigue; sensitization to low glucose levels may adapt the athlete to an increased threshold before symptoms are reported (Kuipers et al. 1999). Neither does a decline in blood glucose at the onset of exercise necessarily impair performance. In the study series described previously, performance of a time trial following the steady-state exercise did not differ between trials in which mild hypoglycemia was noted compared with control trials, for either the whole group or the subgroup who developed hypoglycemic blood glucose levels with various treatments (Jentjens et al. 2003; Jentjens and Jeukendrup 2002, 2003b; Moseley et al. 2003). Nevertheless, the effects of severe fatigue in some symptomatically hypoglycemic athletes are so clear-cut that at-risk athletes will be easily identified. Following are some potential strategies for athletes who experience an extreme reaction to carbohydrate consumed in the hour before exercise:

- Experiment to find the critical time before exercise that carbohydrate intake should be avoided.

- Consume a substantial amount of carbohydrate in the preevent snack or meal (>1 g/kg BM) to compensate for the increase in carbohydrate oxidation during exercise.

- Choose low glycemic index, carbohydrate-rich choices in the preevent menu, which have an attenuated and sustained blood glucose and insulin response.

- Include some high-intensity sprints during the warm-up to the event to stimulate hepatic glucose output.

- Consume carbohydrate during the event.

It has been proposed that preevent meals based on low glycemic index carbohydrate sources will improve the performance of prolonged exercise (Thomas et al. 1991), by attenuating the postmeal insulin response and maintaining carbohydrate availability throughout the exercise bout. Overall, such preevent meal choices achieve a lower postprandial blood glucose response and a smaller decline in blood glucose concentrations at the onset of exercise compared with high glycemic index carbohydrate foods (see Burke 2006a). There is also some, but not complete, evidence that carbohydrate availability and oxidation are better maintained throughout the exercise. However, most studies fail to show performance differences arising from the differences in glycemic index of carbohydrates in the preevent meal, even when metabolism has been altered throughout the exercise bout (Burke 2006a). One study has shown that when carbohydrate is consumed during exercise according to sports nutrition guidelines, any effects of differences in preexercise meals on both metabolism and cycling performance are abolished (Burke et al. 1998).

Each athlete must judge the benefits and the practical issues associated with preexercise meals and snacks in his or her own sporting situation. In cases where athletes are unable to consume carbohydrate during a prolonged event or workout, they may find it useful to choose a preevent menu based on low glycemic index carbohydrate foods to promote a more sustained release of carbohydrate throughout exercise. However, there is no evidence of universal benefits from such menu choices, particularly where athletes are able to refuel during the session, or where favored and familiar food choices happen to be high in glycemic index. In the overall scheme, preevent eating needs to balance a number of factors including the athlete's food likes, availability of choices, and gastrointestinal comfort.

Goal 14

Keep hydration at an acceptable level during the event by drinking appropriate amounts of fluids before, during, and after the event.

Some degree of dehydration is inevitable in most sports because of the mismatch between the athlete's sweat losses and his or her capacity to replace fluids during the event. Sometimes, the athlete may even start competition with a fluid deficit, because of the deliberate use of dehydration to reduce body mass (make weight) or the failure to replace sweat losses arising from an unaccustomed environment or previous exercise. The disadvantages of dehydration are most apparent when prolonged or high-intensity exercise is undertaken in the heat (Sawka and Pandolf 1990). A fluid deficit of less than 2% of the athlete's body mass has been shown to reduce exercise capacity and performance by a detectable amount (Walsh et al. 1994). In addition, the degree of thermoregulatory and cardiovascular impairment, and the increased perception of effort associated with the exercise, both appear to be directly related to the size of fluid deficit (Montain and Coyle 1992). Dehydration has been shown to reduce the rate of gastric emptying (Rehrer et al. 1990), which may further compromise exercise performance by decreasing the opportunity for fluid replacement or increasing the risk of gastrointestinal upset. Dehydration may also reduce skill and decision-making abilities (Gopinathan et al. 1988).

Although it may not be possible to avoid some level of dehydration, the athlete should aim to keep the fluid deficit associated with his or her event to an acceptable level by developing a hydration strategy for before, during, and after the event. Before competition, the athlete should be aware of deliberate or involuntary dehydration and ensure that hydration practices during the hours or days leading up to the event address any residual fluid deficit. General drinking practices may need to be targeted to meet increased fluid requirements in a hot climate or at altitude. Aggressive rehydration strategies may be needed to reverse the fluid deficit deliberately incurred while making weight in weight-division sports (see goal 11) or from a previous exercise bout. Tactics of hyperhydration in preparation for an event in which an unavoidably large fluid deficit is expected should be undertaken under supervision and after appropriate experimentation.

During events lasting longer than 30-60 min, there is usually both a need and an opportunity for intake of fluid during the exercise to offset sweat losses. Evaporation of sweat provides a key mechanism for dissipating the heat generated as a by-product of exercise, and sweat rates vary across and between sports according to factors such as the intensity of exercise, the environmental conditions, the athlete's individual characteristics, and his or her level of acclimatization (Sawka and Pandolf 1990). A range of factors influence fluid intake during events, but across a range of sports and exercise activities, athletes typically drink at a rate that offsets only 30% to 70% of their sweat losses (Broad et al. 1996; Noakes et al. 1988). The following factors influence fluid intake during exercise:

- Individual variability—genetic predisposition to be an avid or reluctant drinker
- Awareness of sweat losses and fluid needs
- Awareness of benefits of good hydration
- Availability of fluids
- Palatability of fluids (flavor, temperature, sodium content)
- Opportunity to drink
- External cues or encouragement to drink
- Gastrointestinal comfort
- Fear of urination
- Weight loss issues (fear of energy content of sport drinks, belief that change in body mass after exercise reflects weight loss)

It is not always possible, and perhaps not even always desirable, to replace all sweat losses during exercise. Once sweat rates exceed 800 to 1,000 ml/hr it becomes difficult to drink to keep pace with such losses; in some events, sweat rates exceeding 2 L/hr are commonly reported. However, many athletes can improve their fluid intake practices and reduce the fluid deficit that accumulates during exercise.

The guidelines for athletes regarding hydration during exercise have evolved over the past 30 years. The initial focus on fluid needs evolved to the realization that strategies to supply both fluid and fuel needs during exercise can be successfully integrated. Many investigations have demonstrated that the intake of carbohydrate drinks of 4% to 8% concentration promotes effective rehydration during exercise and provides a useful source of fuel for the muscle and central nervous system. In fact, voluntary intake of fluid, which is an important determinant of rehydration in real-life activities, is enhanced by adding sodium and a palatable flavor to water. As a result, recent guidelines on rehydration during exercise support the use of commercially available sport drinks (4-8% carbohydrate, 10-25 mmol/L sodium) during a range of prolonged sports and exercise activities (American College of Sports Medicine 1996; 2007), although water is still positioned as a suitable choice of beverage for exercise of less than 60 min duration.

Guidelines for fluid intake during prolonged exercise have also evolved in terms of how athletes are educated to achieve optimal practice. Early guidelines focused on distance running and provided prescriptive advice about drinking practices in terms of recommended volumes to be consumed at aid stations or time points. Although these guidelines might have been intended as an example of good practice, they were often interpreted as a definite rule. In fact, a literal application of such figures has been shown to be impractical—leading to severe dehydration in some athletes and excessive fluid intake in others (Coyle and Montain 1992). Furthermore, the guidelines did not take into account the wide variety of sports and exercise activities in which fluid intake will benefit the safety, enjoyment, or performance of the session.

Accordingly, recent guidelines recognize the variable nature of sport and exercise activities and individual differences that occur between athletes (American College of Sports Medicine 1996; 2007)). Issues that must be taken into account include individual sweat rates and fluid needs, sport-specific opportunities for fluid intake, and practical challenges such as making fluid available, preventing gastrointestinal discomfort, and being aware of fluid needs. Because we now recognize that dehydration has a progressive effect on exercise performance and that an improvement in fluid balance is generally worthwhile, the emphasis is no longer on absolute fluid intakes but rather on individual opportunities to improve fluid intake practices. Newer guidelines emphasize attitudes and behaviors that can be changed to improve fluid intake practices and enhance fluid balance during sport and exercise. There is also consideration that the individual can experiment with his or her own fluid intake and learn to make this a comfortable habit.

The most recent addition to fluid guidelines during exercise involves the recognition that some athletes overhydrate during exercise (Noakes 2003b). This is not a common occurrence in most sports lasting less than 2 to 3 hr, but observational studies of sporting events show that it can occur in certain individuals who are overzealous with their interpretation of hydration guidelines and drink at a rate that exceeds their rates of sweat loss (Almond et al. 2005; Noakes et al. 2005; Noakes and Speedy 2006). Risk factors for this syndrome, which can lead to the potentially fatal condition of symptomatic hyponatremia (low plasma sodium concentrations), include being female and undertaking endurance and ultraendurance events at a slow pace, the latter of which both reduces the rate of sweat loss and provides opportunity to drink multiple servings of fluid provided at aid stations throughout the event (Almond et al. 2005; Noakes et al 2005; Noakes and Speedy 2006). Mathematical modeling shows that this syndrome may also occur as a result of large salt losses in individuals who excrete salty sweat (Montain et al. 2006), although probably to a less extreme level. Several deaths have occurred among athletes and military personnel as a result of encephalopathies and other events associated with severe hyponatremia. Some sport scientists have taken the controversial stance of criticizing guidelines to athletes that promote fluid intake during exercise, claiming that such advice is not necessary and is potentially dangerous (Noakes 2003b; Noakes and Speedy 2006). Although this stance will draw attention to this rare but serious condition, most sport scientists prefer the view that balances the risk of overhydration (low risk, serious outcomes) and underhydration (high risk, mild to serious outcomes) in most sports and exercise activities. In other words, athletes should be warned against the behaviors that lead to problems at both ends of the spectrum. It is useful to add clear statements in guidelines for hydration practices during exercise, particularly those targeted at endurance and ultraendurance sports, that fluid intake during an event should not exceed rates of sweat loss.

Goal 15

Consume carbohydrate during events of >1 hr in duration or where body carbohydrate stores become depleted.

Many sports and exercise activities challenge the availability of body carbohydrate stores. Carbohydrate depletion can manifest as central fatigue (hypoglycemia), peripheral fatigue (glycogen depletion in the working muscles), or a combination of these. When carbohydrate is consumed during exercise to enhance or maintain body carbohydrate availability, there is clear evidence of an enhancement in endurance or exercise capacity (for review, see Hargreaves 1999). It is more difficult to undertake studies that measure the effect on exercise performance, especially in the field or when the activity involves complex decision making and motor skill. Nevertheless, studies have shown that carbohydrate intake during exercise enhances the performance of prolonged events involving cycling (Edwards et al. 1986; Febbraio, Chiu, et al. 2000) and running (Tsintzas, Liu, et al. 1993; Tsintzas et al. 1995) as well as the intermittent high-intensity running as found in team sports (Welsh et al. 2002) and the movement patterns during actual team games (Muckle 1973). Studies in field situations, or in laboratory settings simulating competition, have shown that carbohydrate ingestion during team and racket games sometimes (Ostojic and Mazic 2002; Vergauwen et al. 1998), but not always (Zeederberg et al. 1996), enhances mental and physical skills by reducing the impairment usually associated with fatigue. Even when benefits are not found, carbohydrate intake during exercise does not impair exercise performance.

Evidence of the beneficial effects of carbohydrate intake during exercise is not new. In fact, descriptions of performance enhancements associated with carbohydrate intake during sport date back to the 1920s and the Boston marathon (Gordon et al. 1925; Levine et al. 1924). Scientists reported that when runners were fed candy, they felt and performed better than in the previous year's event, where they suffered from a marked decline in postrace plasma glucose concentrations (2.8 mmol/l) which was manifested as "astenia, nervous irritability, extreme pallor and prostration" (Levine et al. 1924, p. 1779). However, it has taken time for sport scientists to fully understand the effects of carbohydrate intake during exercise and to integrate the dual needs for rehydration and fuel intake during exercise.

Today, during exercise of greater than 60 to 90 min duration, athletes are encouraged to consume a source of carbohydrate to provide an available glucose supply of at least 30 to 60 g/hr (Coyle 2004). A range of carbohydrate of moderate and high glycemic index appears to provide a suitable fuel supply, reaching a maximal rate of oxidation of ~1 g/min after ~60 min of exercise, at least in the case of single carbohydrate sources (for review, see Jeukendrup and Jentjens 2000). Recent studies feeding multiple sources of carbohydrate in the same drink have reported maximal oxidation rates of 1 to 1.3 g/min with the consumption of very large carbohydrate amounts (Jentjens, Achten, et al. 2004; Jentjens, Moseley, et al. 2004). The optimal rate of carbohydrate intake during exercise has not yet been determined and is likely to vary according to the event and the individual athlete. Although only small amounts of exogenous carbohydrate (~20 g) are used during the first hour of exercise (Hawley et al. 1992), athletes are advised to begin intake of carbohydrate from the start of exercise (McConell et al. 1996) or at least well before the onset of feelings of fatigue (Coyle et al. 1983). Sport drinks provide a convenient form of carbohydrate intake during exercise for most athletes. However, the culture and conditions of many sports allow a range of carbohydrate-containing foods and drinks to be consumed to meet fuel needs during the event (see table 1.3)

A variety of mechanisms explain the benefits of the ingestion of carbohydrate during exercise, including the prevention or correction of hypoglycemia (Coggan and Coyle 1987; Gordon et al. 1925). Although the oxidation of exogenous carbohydrate was first thought to spare the utilization of muscle glycogen (Coyle et al. 1983; Hargreaves et al. 1984), at least in cycling, the role of carbohydrate feedings during prolonged exercise is to maintain high plasma glucose concentrations and provide substrate to sustain high rates of carbohydrate oxidation once muscle glycogen stores become depleted (Coyle et al. 1986). Carbohydrate intake during exercise, however, spares the utilization of liver glycogen (Bosch et al. 1994). There is some controversy regarding the effect of carbohydrate intake on glycogen utilization during constant pace running, with some (Tsintzas, Williams, et al. 1993) but not all (Arkinstall et al. 2001) studies reporting glycogen sparing, perhaps confined to certain muscle fibers (Tsintzas, Williams, Boobis, et al. 1996). Glycogen sparing, or net resynthesis of muscle glycogen, may occur when carbohydrate is consumed during intermittent high-intensity bouts of running (Nicholas et al. 1999) and cycling (Yaspelkis et al. 1993) or during low-intensity cycling within nonactive muscle fibers that have been previously depleted (Kuipers et al. 1987).

Of considerable interest is the growing number of studies to report benefits of carbohydrate ingestion during performance of high-intensity exercise lasting about 1 hr (Below et al. 1995; Jeukendrup et al. 1997; Millard-Stafford et al. 1997). These findings are puzzling because muscle carbohydrate stores are not considered to be limiting in events of this duration. Further research is needed to con-

firm and explain the effects, but it is possible that benefits to central performance, involving the brain and nervous system, are implicated (Carter, Jeukendrup, and Jones 2004; Carter, Jeukendrup, Mann, et al. 2004). One study found that the benefits of carbohydrate ingestion, at least to the performance of 1 hr of high-intensity cycling, are independent and additive to the effects of fluid ingestion (Below et al. 1995; see fig 1.5). There is also some evidence that the benefits of combining two strategies that enhance carbohydrate availability—for example, eating a high-carbohydrate meal before the event and consuming carbohydrate during the event—are also additive (Chryssanthopoulos and Williams 1997; Wright et al. 1991). However, another study found that ingestion of carbohydrate before exercise is only beneficial to the performance of a time trial late in exercise when there is further intake of carbohydrate during the session (Febbraio, Chui, et al. 2000) Studies of carbohydrate intake during exercise, alone or in combination with other strategies to promote carbohydrate availability, need to be conducted over a greater range of sport events and exercise activities so that scientists can give more detailed advice to athletes.

Goal 16

Achieve fluid and food intake before and during the event without causing gastrointestinal discomfort or upsets.

One reason for consuming solid foods before or during ultra-endurance events is to prevent the discomfort of hunger that would otherwise occur when eating is delayed for prolonged periods. However, foods and drinks consumed before or during an event can exacerbate the gastrointestinal problems and discomfort experienced by some athletes during exercise. Gastrointestinal problems

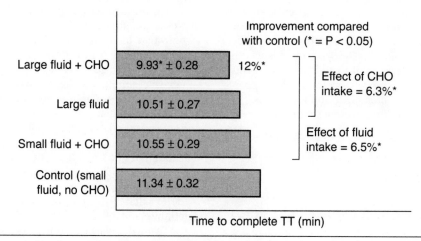

Figure 1.5   Well-trained cyclists undertook four trials in random order of cycling at 80% $\dot{V}O_2$max followed by a time trial. Treatments involved replacement of either fluid, carbohydrate (CHO), or both fluid and carbohydrate, compared with a trial in which placebo capsules were consumed. Results show that fluid and carbohydrate replacement independently enhanced time trial performance and that the effects of these strategies were additive. (Data drawn from Below et al. 1995.)

can reduce the athlete's performance and enjoyment of exercise and in extreme cases can prevent the athlete from completing the event. Some athletes appear to suffer from chronic problems.

Gastrointestinal problems during exercise can occur both in the upper gastrointestinal tract (e.g., belching, vomiting) and in the lower gastrointestinal tract (e.g., diarrhea, gastrointestinal bleeding, flatulence, cramping). The prevalence and severity of problems vary across sports, with reports being greater among female athletes and in sports involving running or other activities that cause "joggling" of the body (for reviews, see Fallon 2006; Peters et al. 2001). Risk factors that appear to increase the occurrence of complaints, particularly in susceptible athletes, include the following:

- Gender (female)
- Running and other activities involving joggling of gastrointestinal system
- High-intensity exercise (i.e., race situation or race-pace training)
- Lack of training
- Dehydration
- Intake of certain foods or fluids before or during exercise (fiber, lactose, fat)
- Preexisting or underlying gastrointestinal problems (e.g., Crohn's disease, parasitic infection, irritable bowel disease)

Nutritional issues include excessive intake of fiber, fat, and protein in the preevent meal (Rehrer et al. 1992) as well as moderate to severe levels of dehydration (Rehrer et al. 1990). Some people experience malabsorption of lactose (found in milk) and fructose (found in fruits, some sport drinks and sweetened beverages) and may need to curtail their intake of these sugars, particularly in relation to exercise. Of course, many food intolerances are specific to the individual. Athletes with gastrointestinal problems should seek expert medical and, where appropriate, dietary intervention. Treatment of underlying medical problems is important, and in some cases, pharmacological intervention is needed to eliminate or alleviate the symptoms and allow the athlete to participate in sports.

Goal 17

Promote recovery after the event, particularly during multiday competitions such as tournaments and stage races.

In some sports, competition is conducted as a series of events or stages. In sports such as swimming or track and field, athletes can be scheduled to compete in a number of brief races or in a series involving heats, semifinals, and finals, often performing more than once each day. In tennis and team sport tournaments, or cycle stage races, competitors may be required to undertake one or more

lengthy events each day, with the competition extending for up to 1 to 3 weeks. Even where athletes compete in a weekly fixture, optimal recovery is desired to allow the athlete to train between matches or races. In training, the coach can plan the macro- and microcycles of workouts so that with appropriate recovery strategies there is a gradual enhancement of specific fitness and performance. In the competition scenario, however, there may be less control over the work-to-recovery ratio. Indeed, it may not be possible to completely recover between events. A simpler but more realistic goal for postevent recovery is to ensure that the athlete is ready to face the next opponent, or the next round or stage in a competition, as well prepared as possible.

Recovery encompasses a complex range of nutrition-related issues including restoration of muscle and liver glycogen stores, replacement of fluid and electrolytes lost in sweat, and regeneration, repair, and adaptation processes following the catabolic stress and damage caused by exercise (see goal 6). In competition, particularly, recovery will only occur with a nutrition plan that addresses the athlete's postexercise intake of fluid and food. This is particularly important for the traveling athlete, who may have limited access to familiar food.

Goal 18

During a prolonged competition program, ensure that competition eating does not compromise overall energy and nutrient intake goals.

During competition phases, eating strategies that promote refueling and rehydration in preparation for, or recovery from, each exercise bout are likely to be the athlete's top priority. To achieve these goals, the athlete may choose palatable and easy-to-consume foods and drinks and may consume them in amounts that reach the threshold of storage or utilization. Such eating strategies may contrast with the athlete's everyday nutritional requirements. For example, energy intake may exceed energy requirements during competition phases, especially in sports where the energy costs of the taper and competitive event are considerably less than everyday training (e.g., swimming). In addition, available food choices may be low in protein and micronutrients, meaning that the athlete will fail to meet his or her nutrient intake goals when reliant on these foods. The travel associated with competition, or postevent celebrations, may also cause athletes to alter their usual dietary practices. Finally, an athlete in a weight division sport may severely restrict his or her energy or nutrient intake in order to rapidly shed weight before a competition weigh-in.

When competition is infrequent or lasts only for several days, such dietary aberrations are unlikely to compromise overall nutritional status and energy balance. However, this is not the case for athletes who have a frequent competition cycle, such as those who compete in a weekly schedule (e.g., the wrestling season) or on a continuous tour (e.g., the professional tennis or road cycling circuit). In other cases, a single competitive event may last for 2 to 3 weeks (e.g., tennis tournaments and cycling stage races) and carry the potential for undermining overall nutritional status. Athletes who fall into such categories will need to find a balance between their competition nutrition goals and long-term nutrition goals. Expert nutrition advice will be valuable to find this balance between goals: for example, to select practical carbohydrate sources that are also nutrient-dense or to eat enough carbohydrate to adequately but not excessively refuel.

Goal 19

Make well-considered decisions about the use of supplements and specialized sport foods that have been shown to enhance competition performance or meet competition needs.

The milliseconds and millimeters that separate the winners of sporting competitions from their colleagues provide a powerful incentive to search for any product or intervention that might improve performance. However, even recreational athletes devote large amounts of their resources in the pursuit of a personal best. Although supplements and sport foods carry many claims that they can enhance an athlete's performance, in reality only a small proportion of the available products are supported by credible scientific support (for review, see Burke 2006a).

Some supplements and sport foods offer real advantages to the athlete. Of course, the appropriate use of the product as much as the product itself leads to the beneficial outcome. Therefore, education about specific situations and strategies for the use of supplements and sports foods is just as important as the formulation of the product. Any decision to use sport supplements or foods should consider the evidence for real or even placebo-driven benefits versus the risk of side effects or a positive doping outcome. Supplement use, even when it provides a true performance advantage, is an expense that athletes must acknowledge and prioritize within their budget.

chapter 2

Practical and Cultural Factors

Each sport and each athlete have a unique set of nutritional requirements and goals. Although sports nutrition research has allowed us to make generic guidelines for sports nutrition practice, as summarized in chapter 1, the application of these guidelines varies between and even within sports. It is easy to recognize that cyclists have different nutritional needs than bodybuilders or that basketball players eat differently than gymnasts. An in-depth review of carbohydrate-loading strategies will reveal that these strategies assist a marathon runner but are of little use to an archer and perhaps are even detrimental for a lightweight rower preparing for a regatta. But why is this so?

It is useful to examine a sport from three separate angles, because the common nutrition issues in a sport usually arise from these factors:

- The physiological requirements of training and competition
- The athlete's lifestyle
- The culture of the sport

Physiological requirements of daily training underpin the athlete's baseline needs for energy and various nutrients. The physiological costs of performance require special nutrition strategies that enhance the outcome of an exercise session, particularly in competition. The athlete's lifestyle and other special characteristics of the sport determine food choices, eating patterns, and the use of special sport foods and supplements. Finally, the culture of the sport also influences eating habits, attitudes to nutrition, and nutrition beliefs. In this chapter we develop a systematic approach to understanding these features, which in turn will help to identify and manage the specific nutritional challenges faced by various athletes and teams.

Physiological Basis of Training and Competition

The starting point, when working with an athlete or sporting team, is to understand fully the demands of their training and competition schedules. Daily requirements for energy and nutrients are determined by both the athlete's training program and the specific challenges of a particular event, playing position, or playing style. For example, athletes may need to alter their nutritional intake to change their physiques (to gain lean body mass or lose body fat) or to provide the fluid and fuel needs of specific training sessions. Specific nutrition strategies used to optimize performance in a single exercise session are most relevant to competition but may also be undertaken daily to enhance training outcomes and to fine-tune the practices intended for the competition arena. These factors, which underpin the nutritional requirements and goals of the athlete, will vary over the sporting season but also between athletes even in the same sport because of genetic, physiological, medical, or other differences between individuals.

Examining the preceding issues will help to determine the athlete's everyday and competition requirements for energy, protein, micronutrients, and fluid and the optimal fuel for exercise. Fluid and carbohydrate requirements may be assessed over a day or in terms of specific needs for replacement before, during, and after an exercise session. An assessment of the physiological factors that limit performance will identify these and other nutritional strategies that reduce or delay fatigue and thus enhance performance. This may include the use of sport foods to achieve nutritional goals or strategic application of certain ergogenic aids.

Although we have tried to cover the basic training and competition features of a wide range of sports, numerous sports are not specifically discussed. However, most sports will fit into at least one of the categories that we have included, and the information from related sports should be used to construct a detailed overview of any sport in which you have an interest. Information about the training and competition characteristics of a sport can be found in the scientific and general sports literature, but your sources should also include official sporting organizations, coaches, and athletes themselves. With regard to the sport science literature, we will find over the course of this book that surprisingly few studies have investigated the effect of various sports nutrition strategies in an appropriate *sport-specific* context. Even fewer studies have been conducted with elite athletes. Therefore, we must rely on the results of laboratory studies conducted

Nutrition for Optimal Training Adaptation and Performance in Training: Physiological, Practical, and Cultural Issues

The following questions may help you to identify an athlete's nutritional requirements and challenges during training.

- *What are the typical exercise requirements of the athlete's training schedule?* Type of training sessions? Frequency? Duration? Intensity? How are training sessions periodized over the week, month, season, and year? What total energy and fuel requirements do such exercise patterns set?
- *What is the environment in which training sessions are undertaken?* What are the typical sweat losses and fuel requirements of training sessions? What opportunities are available to consume fluid or foods during the session? How are such foods or fluids made available?
- *What are the opportunities to practice competition intake strategies in a training session?*
- *What are the typical exercise patterns during the off-season or during an injury break?*
- *How important are body mass and composition to performance in this sport?* What are the typical characteristics of elite athletes in this sport—body mass, lean body mass, body fat levels? What is the current physique of the athlete, and what is his or her history of physique changes? What physique characteristics should allow the athlete to achieve optimal training and competition performances? Will these physique goals be achieved as a result of genetics and training, or must a special dietary program be followed to gain muscle mass or lose body fat?
- *What is the typical domestic situation in which the athlete lives?* Where does the athlete eat most of his or her meals? Who does the cooking?
- *What are the typical dietary intakes and practices of athletes (or a particular athlete) in this sport?*
- *What is the risk of the athlete developing any of the following problems?*
  - Iron deficiency (low iron intake, increased iron requirements, increased iron losses)
  - Menstrual dysfunction or compromised bone status
  - Disordered eating
  - Other nutrient deficiencies?
- Does the athlete undertake special training programs? Altitude training? Heat acclimatization?
- Is there direct or indirect evidence that supplementation with ergogenic aids will enhance training adaptation and performance? For example, creatine? Caffeine? Antioxidant vitamins?
- What are the practical considerations or difficulties in arranging food intake during a typical training day?
  - At what times does the athlete train?
  - What other activities need to be scheduled into the day?
  - What factors limit access to food during the day?
  - Do gastrointestinal considerations or appetite limit food intake, particularly at strategic times?
  - How often or how far does the athlete need to travel to fulfill training commitments?
  - Is the athlete's nutrition influenced by other factors such as financial constraints or religious or social customs?
- What are the current beliefs of athletes from this sport?
- Where do athletes in this sport commonly seek dietary advice or information?
- What is the typical level of nutrition awareness of athletes in this sport?

under a variety of conditions and apply them to the world of competitive sport. At various times we will discuss the limitations of this approach.

Whether your interest lies in a sport that is covered in this book or a totally unfamiliar sport, it pays to systemati-

cally assess the potential nutritional influences affecting that sport. Strategic questions that help to determine an athlete's nutritional needs are provided in the highlight box for training issues and the box for competition issues on this page.

Nutrition for Competition Performance: Physiological, Practical, and Cultural Issues

The questions that may help you to identify the nutritional strategies that will optimize the athlete's competition performance.

- *What are the exercise requirements of competition?* What are the frequency, duration, and intensity of the specific activity? Is this specialized into individual events or different playing positions or styles?
- *Is competition undertaken as a single event or a series of activities?* For example, is it a tournament, schedule of heats and finals, multiday stages, or weekly fixture?
- *What are the typical environmental conditions in which competition is undertaken?* What is the heat? Humidity? Airflow?
- *How often is major competition undertaken by the athlete?*
- *Are there competition weight limits that dictate the class of competition or overall eligibility to compete?* How often does the athlete need to weigh in? What is the time interval between weigh-in and competition?
- *What is the indirect or direct evidence that any of the following factors might limit competition performance?*
  - Dehydration
  - Carbohydrate availability
  - Gastrointestinal problems
- What is the indirect or direct evidence that sports nutrition strategies such as the following may affect competition performance?
  - Carbohydrate loading
  - Carbohydrate refueling before or between events
  - Carbohydrate intake in the 1 to 4 hr before the event
  - Fluid intake during the event
  - Carbohydrate intake during the event
  - Hydration strategies before the event
  - Hydration strategies between events
  - Acute use of supplements such as caffeine, bicarbonate, or creatine
  - Strategies to promote fat availability and utilization
- What time of day does competition occur?
- Are the athletes in familiar surroundings or have they traveled to undertake competition? What food is available in these surroundings?
- What other practical considerations affect competition nutrition strategies? Is the athlete's nutrition affected by financial constraints or religious or social practices?
- Do gastrointestinal problems commonly occur? Are these affected by preexercise intake? Is hydration status markedly affected during exercise? What amount and type of fluid or food might be required during exercise?
- What opportunities does the athlete have to consume fluid and foods during the event? How is such food or fluid made available? What strategies can improve availability of food and fluid?
- What factors interfere with postexercise eating? How can foods and fluids be made available to the athlete?
- What are the beliefs of athletes in this sport?
- What are the competition practices of the athletes, or a particular athlete, in this sport?
- Where do athletes in this sport commonly seek their nutrition information and advice?

Lifestyle Challenges and Cultural Factors

Athletes' food choices and eating habits are influenced by lifestyle and practical considerations. These issues are, of course, individual to each athlete. However, some factors that prejudice good eating habits or call for special nutrition strategies arise in a predictable way in response to the characteristics of a sport. For example, two almost universal features of competitive swimming are that swimmers undertake heavy training programs at an early age and that training sessions are undertaken early in the morning. As a result, nutritional considerations for a swimmer can include nutritional needs for adolescence, support for a heavy training program, and the lifestyle issues of adolescence. Typical problems for this sport and age group range from fitting food into a busy school or university timetable to following good sports nutrition practice while participating in peer-group patterns of skipping meals or eating fast foods. Early-morning training sessions impose constraints on ideal eating strategies; for example, it is impractical to consume substantial amounts of carbohydrate before the training session, despite research evidence pointing to

probable performance and endurance benefits. It is also difficult to devise a posttraining recovery meal that can be consumed by the swimmer while traveling from training to school.

Finally, we should also consider the strong cultural influence attached to participation in some sports. Many sports provide a closed environment for their participants, with tradition being handed down from coaches and trainers and information and values being spread via interaction between athletes. Most sports have their own literature in the form of specialized magazines, club newsletters, and Web sites. The culture of a sport can strongly influence nutrition beliefs and attitudes to food. In such a situation, sports nutrition activities should be tailored, both in content and style, to this culture. This might include targeting the nutrition myths or poor eating practices that have become embedded in the folklore of the sport, using language that is familiar to the athletes, or using case histories or situations that have occurred in that sport. Such practices will help to make sports nutrition information more interesting and effective.

In summary, a systematic approach to developing a sports nutrition program for an athlete or team should encompass the practical and cultural factors that ultimately determine eating behaviors and food choices. Questions

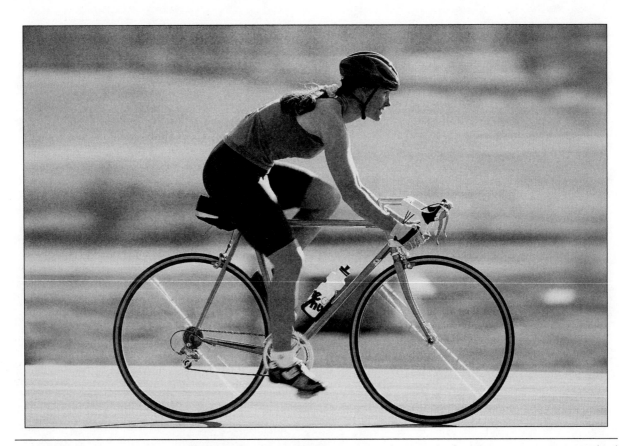

When issues such as managing nutrition goals while undertaking a demanding travel schedule, arranging access to food and fluid intake when undertaking prolonged training sessions in a wilderness area, or finding a preevent meal routine that overcomes the risk of exercise-related gastrointestinal disturbance occur frequently within a sport, they can be integrated into the specific nutrition considerations for that sport.

that help to elicit these factors are included in the lists previously provided.

Sports Nutrition Practice

A range of people, including nutrition professionals such as dietitians, are involved in sports nutrition. Many colleges, universities, and professional groups are experiencing the popularity of sports nutrition as an area of study and intended career choice. The training options or requirements to become a sports dietitian or sports nutritionist vary around the world. However, sports nutrition can be seen as an intersection of the sciences of food, human nutrition, exercise physiology, metabolism, and sport and should be underpinned by a sound background in all areas. To assist in the practice of sports nutrition, it is ideal to have additional training in clinical nutrition practice, counseling and education techniques, and dietary assessment methodology. For the remainder of this book, we refer to a person

who undertakes sports nutrition activities with athletes or sporting teams as a sports nutritionist or dietitian. This term acknowledges that the background training or the professional allegiances of this person may vary.

Working in a Multidisciplinary Sports Nutrition Team

The ideal approach to the nutrition of an athlete or sporting team is a holistic and team-based approach, involving the input of a range of sports medicine and science professionals. This is because a range of issues often intersect with the athlete's nutritional status or achievement of his or her nutrition goals, and in the field, a range of professionals work with the athlete. The sports nutritionist or dietitian may need to collect information and opinions from this range of professionals and, at times, may need to engage them in the delivery or organization of the athlete's nutrition plan. Table 2.1 summarizes the role that various

Table 2.1 Professional Nutrition Roles in a Sports Nutrition Team

Professional	Expertise or Opportunities in Sports Nutrition	Roles in the Delivery of Sports Nutrition Program
Sports dietitian/sports nutritionist (abbreviated in this table to sports dietitian)	Specialist qualifications or expertise in <ul><li>assessment of nutrient needs and nutrient status</li><li>dietary survey methodology,</li><li>diet therapy in disease</li><li>counseling</li><li>food composition</li><li>food and supplement standards</li><li>food preparation and handling</li></ul>	<ul><li>Nutrition screening or dietary survey of team</li><li>Nutritional assessment and counseling of individual athletes</li><li>Organization of appropriate catering and food provision for training, competition, and travel</li><li>If not directly involved in team travel or competition, delegation of implementation of plan to other sports science/medicine network members who have "hands-on" role</li><li>Setting nutrition policies for team or sporting group (e.g., supplement use, fluid intake practices)</li><li>Development of nutrition education resources and activities</li><li>Education of other members of sports medicine/science network regarding best practice in sports nutrition</li><li>Cooperation with sport scientist to plan and implement projects/studies monitoring the effect of various nutrition interventions on training and competition performance</li></ul>
Sports physician	<ul><li>Often the primary appointment of a sporting team, or first point contact of an athlete seeking help for problem.</li><li>Often appointed as head of multidisciplinary sports medicine/science support team for athletic group or team, or case management of individual athlete</li><li>Often travels with team or is sited at field of play during team training or competition, thus seeing nutrition practice firsthand</li></ul>	<ul><li>Identification of need for specialized nutrition activities leading to referral to sports dietitian</li><li>Organization of appropriate diagnostic tests to allow or confirm diagnosis of nutrition-related medical problems (e.g., iron deficiency, poor bone status, menstrual dysfunction)</li><li>Case management of individuals with complex medical problems (e.g., female athlete triad), as head of multidisciplinary team providing holistic approach to treatment</li></ul>

(continued)

Table 2.1 *(continued)*

Professional	Expertise or Opportunities in Sports Nutrition	Roles in the Delivery of Sports Nutrition Program
Sports physician *(cont'd)*	• Able to approve a variety of relevant diagnostic tests (e.g., hematology, biochemistry, bone density tests) • May not have studied nutrition or sports nutrition in depth	• Where in close access to athletes during travel or competition, implementation or monitoring of team nutrition plan—often acting as the "eyes" or "hands" of the team sports dietitian who has organized plan
Sports physiotherapist or physical therapist	• Lengthy individual treatments often provide rapport between athlete and therapist, and an environment where athlete's lifestyle, behaviors, and beliefs are discussed • Often travels with team or attends team training or competition, thus seeing nutrition practice firsthand	• Referral of athlete to sports dietitian for assessment and counseling • Where in close access to athletes during travel or competition, implementation or monitoring of team nutrition plan—often acting as the "eyes" or "hands" of the team sports dietitian who has organized plan
Sport psychologist	• Clinical expertise in diagnosis and management of athletes with eating disorders/disordered eating • Work often identifies athletes with food-related stress or poor nutrition practices	• Work within sports medicine/science team to provide treatment to athletes with eating disorders/disordered eating • Referral of athlete to sports dietitian for assessment and counseling • Work with multidisciplinary team to develop resources and implement activities related to prevention and early intervention of disordered body image and eating
Sport scientist/exercise physiologist	• Often has expertise in monitoring of body physique • Undertakes routine monitoring of physiological, metabolic, and performance status of athletes	• Monitoring of nutrition-related factors underpinning training and competition performance • Cooperation with sports dietitian to plan and implement activities to monitor the effect of various nutrition interventions on training and competition performance • Referral of athlete to sports dietitian for assessment and counseling
Coach	• Has day-to-day contact with athlete or team, and may observe poor nutritional practice • Surveys indicate strong influence on many nutritional beliefs and practices of athletes (e.g., supplement use, weight management) • Optimal weight and weight management is a sensitive area between athlete and coach • In some situations has final say in nutritional practices of team/athlete during training and competition • Ultimate observer of performance changes in athletes, identifying situations caused by poor nutrition practice, or enhancements potentially caused by positive nutrition interventions	• Support for best nutrition practice by athletes • Encouragement of use of experts to develop and implement sports nutrition programs, policies, and activities within team or sporting group • Recognition of poor nutrition practice or need for nutrition education, leading to referral to sports dietitian • Work as part of sports medicine/science team in management of athletes with complex problems (e.g., eating disorders)
Trainer	• Has contact with athlete or team during training and competition and may observe poor nutritional practice • Is responsible for many nutritional practices or implementation of nutritional plan during training and competition	• Support for best nutrition practice by athletes • Recognition of poor nutrition practice or need for nutrition education, leading to referral to sports dietitian • During training or competition, implementation or monitoring of team nutrition plan—often acting as the "eyes" or "hands" of the team sports dietitian who has organized plan

professionals may play. Clearly, best practice will occur when there is regular contact between all the professionals who work with an athlete or sporting team and when there is understanding and respect with regard to the roles that each person plays. Most well-organized teams, athletes, or sporting organizations implement a service team structure that promotes such interaction and regard. However, this might also be achieved by regular meetings and case history discussions within a multidisciplinary sports medicine center, gym, or human performance laboratory.

Even where a sports nutritionist or dietitian is working in isolation, for example, in his or her own private practice, it is useful to participate in sports medicine or sport science networks or to contact significant professionals working with the athletes with whom he or she consults. Such a collaboration will provide shared experience and knowledge and will also enhance the overall perspective of the sports nutrition practitioner. In a business sense, it is valuable to have a source of referrals, particularly from people who value and support the ways in which you practice sports nutrition.

Keeping Up to Date in Sports Nutrition

Knowledge and practice are evolving concepts. It is not sufficient, in any profession, to rely on the information that was provided in primary or even specialized training courses. For young sports nutritionists or dietitians, there is great value in having an official mentor, an experienced practitioner who is prepared to provide guidance, feedback, and even structured learning opportunities. In some countries, professional organizations for sports nutritionists or dietitians run continuing education programs and mentoring schemes to ensure that their members develop their knowledge and practical skills throughout the entire duration of their careers. But even with this foundation, each sports nutritionist or dietitian needs to have his or her own plan for staying abreast with new developments in sports nutrition research, education, or practice. This should include regular monitoring of key journals and new textbooks, attendance at conferences or seminars, and access to valuable Web sites.

RESEARCH TOPIC

Measuring Energy Expenditure: How Much Do Athletes Need to Eat?

The central role of energy intake in sport performance is understood by most athletes. Indeed, a frequently asked question by athletes is "How many kilojoules (or Calories) should I eat each day?" The athlete expects the response be precise and correct to the second decimal place. Of course, such information cannot be determined to such a degree of accuracy. Nevertheless, achieving an adequate of supply of energy or knowing how to manipulate energy intake to achieve alterations in body mass and composition is important for most athletes and warrants some method to determine general needs. The energy requirement, or total energy expenditure (TEE), of each athlete is unique and arises from the contribution of the following four components (see figure 2.1):

- Basal metabolic rate (BMR), which is determined by body size, body composition, sex, age, and inherited characteristics and typically accounts for 60% to 70% of total energy expenditure
- Thermogenesis (including thermic effect of food and nonshivering thermogenesis), which typically accounts for 10% of total energy expenditure
- Physical activity (typically 15-30% of total energy expenditure)
- Energy cost of growth (including muscular development), pregnancy, and lactation

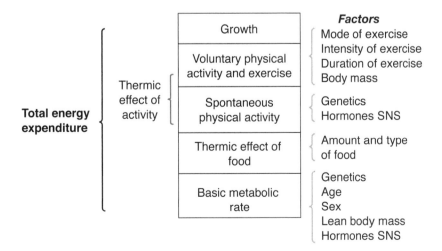

Figure 2.1   The energy requirements, or total energy expenditure (TEE), of each athlete is unique and arises from the contribution of the following four components.

The variability in these components leads to a considerable range in the energy needs in different types of sports and between individuals within sporting groups. Of course, there are some predictable patterns. In some sports with a commitment to prolonged high-intensity training sessions (e.g., road cycling, triathlon, swimming, distance running), the energy cost of exercise may double total daily energy requirements. Other athletes (e.g., gymnasts) may undertake lengthy training sessions yet have low total energy requirements. This is because training sessions focus on low-intensity skill and flexibility work, with only short bursts of high-intensity exercise. The low energy cost of training for athletes may be exacerbated by a low level of general activity in their everyday lives. Some athletes, such as swimmers and rowers, must meet the energy cost of a large muscle mass and body size, in addition to their training load. High energy requirements are also experienced by adolescent athletes who are undergoing a rapid growth spurt (e.g., the basketball player who is on his way to his 210 cm height potential) or by athletes undertaking programs designed to stimulate rapid gain of muscle mass.

Several methods are available to estimate an athlete's energy expenditure. The most common laboratory-based method is indirect calorimetry, in which energy expenditure is indirectly calculated from the measurement of the rates of oxygen consumption ($\dot{V}O_2$) and production of carbon dioxide ($\dot{V}CO_2$) in breath samples. This relationship of $\dot{V}CO_2$ to $\dot{V}O_2$ is termed the respiratory exchange ratio (RER) and is considered an accurate reflection of what is happening in the cells under steady-state conditions. Respiratory gases can be collected in a variety of ways—for example, in a metabolic chamber over a day or more, or using a ventilation hood, mask, or mouthpiece for shorter time periods. Various published formulas are available for estimating energy expenditure from the data measured on these gases: RER and the amount of oxygen consumed and carbon dioxide produced. Disadvantages of indirect calorimetry techniques include the expense and the need for trained personnel and specialized equipment to collect and analyze respiratory gases. Most important, the technique usually interferes with the normal daily living and exercise activities, creating an artificial situation in which daily energy expenditure is measured. On the other hand, in addition to measuring TEE over longer periods, this method can be used to measure the individual components of energy expenditure, such as resting metabolic rate, the thermic response to a meal, and the energy cost of various exercise activities. This might be useful to explore the case of an individual athlete who appears to have unusual issues in achieving energy balance.

More recently, the doubly labeled water (DLW) technique has been developed and validated to estimate TEE (Schoeller et al. 1986). In this technique, the participant ingests a sample of water ($^2H_2^{18}O$) that has been labeled with stable (nonradioactive) isotopes of both hydrogen and oxygen. Energy expenditure can be calculated by periodically monitoring the concentration of these isotopes in body fluids such as urine, to compare the differential rates of disappearance of these isotopes. Because deuterium ($^2H_2$) is eliminated as water, whereas the ^{18}O is eliminated as both water and carbon dioxide, the difference between the two elimination rates is a measure of carbon dioxide production. This technique has no effect on the daily activities of the participant, so it is particularly useful for monitoring energy expenditure in the field over a period of days or weeks. Nevertheless, the cost and availability of the DLW sample and analyses restrict the use of this method to the realms of research. Indirect calorimetry and DLW estimates are rarely used in the management of individual athletes, unless perhaps they are used to investigate the case of an athlete who has an apparent disturbance of energy balance. However, a number of studies have used these techniques to monitor energy expenditure compared with reported energy intake in groups of athletes. The findings of these studies are summarized in the appendix table 2.a and show several examples where energy balance is well achieved, as well as situations of apparent energy imbalance where there is a mismatch of >5% of total energy expenditure. In most cases, the mismatch is toward an energy deficit—reported energy intakes that are substantially less than estimated expenditure. Changes in body mass and composition measured over the period of investigation need to be factored into energy balance considerations. Such changes allow estimation of how much an apparent energy deficit reflects undereating (participant consumes less than usual during the period and loses body mass) and underrecording (participant fails to record all food intake during the period and underestimates actual energy intake). There is a tendency to overestimate energy expenditure by these DLW techniques as well as to underestimate energy intake by dietary survey methods (see the second research topic).

An accessible and practical way to assess the TEE of an athlete is the factorial method, using prediction equations based on assessments of resting metabolic rate (RMR) and the energy cost of daily activities (Manore and Thompson 2006). Several equations are available to predict RMR (which provides an approximation of BMR) from factors such as age, height, weight, or lean body mass. However, these equations have been derived from populations of essentially sedentary adults and may differ in their validity when applied to specialized groups such as athletes. One study has attempted to determine which of the commonly available equations works best for active individuals and athletes (Thompson and Manore 1996). In this study, the resting metabolic rate of a group of 37 endurance-trained male and female athletes was measured in the laboratory and compared with the results achieved by the common prediction equations. The Cunningham equation was shown to provide the best prediction of RMR for both male and female endurance athletes, although the utility of this equation is limited by the need to have a measurement of lean body mass (Cunningham 1980). The Harris–Benedict equation, using commonly available factors of age, height, and weight, was the next best predictor (Harris and Benedict 1919). These equations are presented next and can be converted to kilojoules by multiplying by 4.2.

Harris–Benedict (1919):

> Males: RMR (kcal) = 66.47 + 13.75 (body mass in kg) + 5 (height in cm) − 6.76 (age in years)

> Females: RMR (kcal) = 655.1 + 9.56 (body mass) + 1.85 (height) − 4.68 (age)

Cunningham (1980):

> RMR = 500 + 22 (lean body mass in kg)

Other commonly used equations such as the WHO equation (World Health Organization 1985) and the Schofield equation (Schofield et al. 1985) were not involved in this study and should also be considered. However, it is also recommended that studies be undertaken on groups of highly trained athletes to derive population-specific equations using a range of commonly available factors. Only one such study is currently available, deriving a prediction equation from 51 male athletes involved at high levels of training in water polo, judo, and karate (De Lorenzo et al. 1999). The equation derived from this study is presented next and requires further validation:

De Lorenzo and colleagues (1999):

> Males: RMR (kcal) = −857 + 9.0 (body mass in kg) + 11.7 (−height in cm)

Once RMR is estimated from one of the available prediction equations, it must then be multiplied by various activity factors (see table 2.3) to determine the daily TEE (Manore and Thompson 2006). At the simplest level, an overall activity factor is applied to the whole day to represent the athlete's typical exercise level. At the most complex level, an athlete might complete an intricate activity diary, with the predicted cost of each activity undertaken over the day being estimated (time spent × energy cost of activity) and then summed to predict overall TEE for the day. In some cases, the athlete may have accurate measurements of the energy cost of training-related activities to improve the

validity of energy costs for at least part of the day's activities, especially where these make a major contribution to TEE. Although this protocol can provide a general estimation of an athlete's energy requirements, the considerable possibility for error should be taken into account.

Finally, in the clinical setting, a sports nutrition practitioner may want to assess an athlete's energy availability. This is a relatively new concept that can be used to assess whether an athlete's energy intake is likely able to support a healthy and well-performing body or whether restricted energy intake is likely to impair health and performance. Energy availability is defined as the dietary energy that is available to the body once the energy cost of daily exercise is taken into account (Loucks 2004). Typically, this should be around 45 kcal (189 kJ) per kilogram of the athlete's lean body mass per day. Elegant studies in females have shown that when energy availability drops below a threshold of 30 kcal (126 kJ) per kilogram of lean body mass per day, there are negative consequences to metabolism and menstrual function (Loucks and Thuma 2003) and to the resorption and formation of bone (Ihle and Loucks 2004). These outcomes are particularly found in young females, but appear to disappear in older females, at least when menstrual function has been established for greater than 14 years (Loucks 2006). Studies on males also show negative consequences of low energy availability on metabolic and reproductive hormones (Friedl et al. 2000), although dose–response relationships have not been explored.

The calculation of energy availability may be useful when you work with athletes who restrict their energy intake to achieve a certain body mass or body fat. In such athletes, severe energy deprivation may reduce resting metabolic rate; therefore, calculations of energy expenditure and requirement from factorial methods may substantially overestimate the athlete's true energy expenditure and provide an impractical benchmark for energy balance. Although the human body's ability to adapt to some degree of accidental or intentional energy restriction is robust, all athletes should aim to consume sufficient energy to achieve an energy

Table 2.3   Approximate Energy Cost of Different Activities

Activity Grade	Examples	Activity Factor (per unit of time)
Resting	Sleeping, reclining	RMR × 1
Very light	Seated and standing activities, driving, cooking	RMR × 1.5
Light	Slow walking on level surface (2.5-3 miles per hour), house cleaning, table tennis, recreational golf and tennis	RMR × 2.5
Moderate	Walking 3.5-4 miles per hour, carrying a load, tennis, slow cycling	RMR × 4 (3-5)
Strenuous	Jogging/running, fast tennis, moderate swimming, weight training, walking up hill with a load, soccer	RMR × 7 (5-9)
Very strenuous	Race pace swimming, race pace rowing, race pace cycling, running (10-15 km/h)	RMR × 10 (7-13)

Data from Manore and Thompson 2006

Energy availability = energy intake - training energy expenditure

Athlete One: Male Lightweight Rower

Body mass = 73 kg
Body fat = 5%
Lean body mass = 95% of 73 kg = 69.3 kg
Mean daily energy intake = 2750 kcal (11.55 MJ)
Energy cost of daily training: 800 kcal (3.36 MJ)
Energy availability = 1950 kcal/d (8.19 MJ) = 28 kcal/kg LBM/d (118 kJ/kg LBM/d)

> *Interpretation: This athlete has low energy availability that is likely to impair health performance.*

Athlete Two: Female Distance Runner

Body mass = 55 kg
Body fat = 15%
Lean body mass = 85% of 55 kg = 46.75 kg
Mean daily energy intake = 2750 kcal (11.55 MJ)
Energy cost of daily training: 800 kcal (3.36 MJ)
Energy availability = 1950 kcal/d (8.19 MJ) = 42 kcal/kg LBM/d (175 kJ/kg LBM/d)

> *Interpretation: This athlete has suitable energy availability.*

Figure 2.2   Calculations of energy availability.

availability above 30 kcal (126 kJ) per kilogram of lean body mass per day. Figure 2.2 provides examples of calculations of energy availability for some fictional athletes, including a case where an athlete should be encouraged to increase energy intake.

RESEARCH TOPIC

Measuring Dietary Intake: What Do Athletes Actually Eat?

In each of the sport-specific chapters of this book, information from dietary surveys of serious athletes is presented to illustrate the apparent energy and nutrient intakes and typical eating patterns of these groups. This information has been sourced from the published literature. However, it often appears to have been collected in quick and "low-tech" studies, undertaken primarily to take advantage of the authors' access to a group of interesting athletes. Many authors do not appear to have had specific training in dietary survey methodology, and, in most cases, the article provides few details of special characteristics built into the survey methodology to optimize the reliability and validity of results. Most of the results are discussed without any reference to the inherent limitations or inaccuracies of self-reported data on dietary intake. Despite the apparent simplicity of most dietary surveys, assessment of the typical eating patterns of an individual athlete or group is a time-consuming process that requires special expertise. A number of methods are available to monitor dietary intake; each has specific advantages and disadvantages and each adds a particular bias to the information collected. The dietary survey method chosen to monitor the intake of an individual athlete or group of athletes should reflect on

the type of information that is sought and the resources and opportunities available to collect it (Burke, Cox, et al. 2001).

The dietary history is the most popular retrospective technique used in individual counseling situations. In this technique, the athlete is asked by a skilled interviewer to describe his or her food intake during a typical day over recent times. The interviewer, using prompts and probing questions, ascertains the athlete's whereabouts and activities over each section of the day and the food and drink that is usually consumed at these times. Aids such as food models may help the athlete to accurately describe his or her usual portion sizes. In most situations, the athlete will be assisted to build a composite of *usual* eating patterns, which includes a summary of how different options might be chosen weekly, monthly, or seasonally. This technique is valuable because it captures information about usual intake and does not affect ongoing eating patterns. The interviewer also has the opportunity to probe the athlete regarding factors that influence his or her present nutrition and underpin the ability to make changes, for example, motivation, finances, food availability, nutrition beliefs, domestic skills, and daily schedule. A thorough interview can collect information from athletes such as where they live, who cooks their meals, how often they travel, how and why they have chosen their present eating patterns, what supplements they take, and how much of their time is committed to various activities in a typical day. The interview is relatively quick and places fewer burdens on the athlete than prospective techniques. On the other hand, the dietary history technique is reliant on the skills of the interviewer and assumes that athletes can provide an accurate (and truthful) recall of their intake.

The dietary recall technique involves questioning about actual intake of foods and fluids on a previous occasion, usually the last 24 hr. Again, a skilled interviewer is needed and should use prompts and aids to stimulate the athlete to provide accurate information about the type and amounts of foods and drinks consumed. Although most people will find it easier to remember what they ate yesterday rather than create an overview of what is typically eaten, a major disadvantage of this technique is that it doesn't provide a picture of usual intake. After all, we eat differently from day to day, and the athlete may have followed a totally unrepresentative eating plan the day before an interview. The 24 hr recall is often used in dietary surveys of large groups where a number of separate accounts of a day's eating can build a picture of the typical eating habits of a population. Alternatively, this method may be undertaken on a number of separate occasions with the same individual to build a picture of daily or weekly changes in intake.

A food frequency questionnaire (FFQ) is a checklist of commonly eaten foods and drinks, with each item requiring one response denoting the size of the serving that the athlete typically consumes and another response listing the frequency of consumption of this item. This list is often supplemented with questions on other foods eaten by the respondent but not found in the list as well as questions about food preparation, supplement use, and other food-related behaviors. FFQs can be undertaken by interview or as a self-administered questionnaire. In its early form, the FFQ was designed as a *qualitative* method, seeking information on the frequency of consumption of specific food items. More recent versions of FFQs focus on portion sizes so that a quantitative determination of food and nutrient intake can be achieved. The accuracy of FFQs is dependent on how well the checklist has been prepared to include the foods and drinks consumed by the athlete and how well and accurately the athlete can summarize his or her usual intake. Many FFQs are developed to focus on the intake of a specific nutrient (e.g., carbohydrate or calcium) and are validated against the results achieved by other dietary survey techniques. A particular advantage of the FFQ is that it is relatively quick and easy for both the athlete and the interviewer.

All recall or retrospective techniques are limited by the athlete's memory, insight, and cooperation. Furthermore, people deliberately or unconsciously rewrite their usual food intake to downplay the foods they see as undesirable (e.g., snacks, sweets, and second helpings) and increase their stated intake of foods seen as desirable (e.g., fruit and salads). Many athletes give biased responses in fear of revealing inappropriate dietary behavior to a coach or investigator or to impress the investigator. Studies have shown that most people have poor skills in recalling portion sizes of foods and fluids. Retrospective methods of assessing food and nutrient intake tend to overestimate true intake, although they may underestimate the true intake of large eaters. Research shows that young people and adolescents have limited insight into their food intake and that a typical day is difficult to picture in an erratic and chaotic lifestyle.

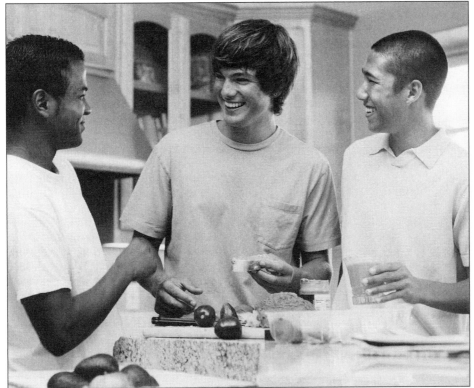

© BananaStock/Robertstock.com

A 3 to 7 day food diary is a common choice to balance reporting reliability with compliance in an athlete's busy lifestyle.

The food record, a prospective method of assessment, involves a complete account of all food and fluid intake over a specified period of time; this record is usually kept by the participant, but in special cases (such as the monitoring of children or athletes in extreme competition such as a cycling tour) a designated food handler records intake. The period of recording is considered to reflect usual intake or a specialized eating practice (e.g., carbohydrate loading before an event). As in all dietary survey methods, accuracy in describing the type and amount of food and fluid intake is critical. In some food record protocols, the athlete is required to use scales to weigh all food and drinks, whereas other techniques ask the athlete to estimate portion sizes using a combination of household measures and measuring grids. The weighed food record is sometimes considered the gold standard of dietary survey techniques, and although the use of scales improves the accuracy of the record, the extra burden of having to weigh all food items may reduce compliance or alter usual eating patterns.

All dietary surveys are hampered by errors of accuracy (how well they measure the participant's actual intake) and validity (how closely the period of monitoring reflects the athlete's usual intake). Prospective techniques carry a disadvantage in that athletes may deliberately or subconsciously alter their eating habits during the period of recording so that it no longer reflects their usual intake. This may happen, as in the case of recall techniques, because an athlete is embarrassed about his or her true intake and wants to appear to eat better than usual. On the other hand, the requirement to record all food and fluid intake is intrusive and time-consuming, and the athlete may subconsciously try to simplify the demands by choosing to eat foods that are easier to record or by simply omitting to record or eat any meals or snacks that are inconvenient.

Extensive study of the accuracy of food diaries in the general population shows a bias toward widespread and significant underreporting of true intake; comparisons of energy intakes estimated from food diaries and other techniques such as doubly-labeled water show that food records typically underestimate true intake by about 20% (Black et al. 1993; Mertz et al. 1991). Although it is tempting to try to apply a correction factor to every dietary record, not all participants underreport and some individuals underreport to an even greater extent. People who are most prone to underreporting include those who are overfat and dissatisfied with their body mass and body image and those who have a strong sense of what they should be eating (Heitmann and Lissner 1995; Johansson et al. 1998; Muhlheim et al. 1998). Underreporting errors can be divided into undereating (reducing food intake during the period of recording) and underrecording (failing to record all food consumed during the observation period), but few studies have tried to measure the relative contribution of each aspect to the total error. Theoretically, each of these errors could be estimated by using independent measures of energy expenditure of the participants during the period of recording, changes in body composition to estimate energy surplus or deficit, and, ideally, a marker of the accuracy of recording. For example, a dietary study was conducted on

female dietitians who were characterized as lean individuals with a high degree of motivation and knowledge about food (Goris and Westerterp 1999). Using labeled water to measure water loss, the authors of this study found a high correlation between recorded and predicted water intake, suggesting a high precision in dietary recording. However, weight loss measured during the recording period indicated that the dietitians under-ate their energy needs by a mean of 16%, with this discrepancy almost entirely explaining the underreporting error.

Several sophisticated energy balance studies have also been carried out on athletes, and most, but not all, have found discrepancies between reported energy intakes and energy requirements, particularly among female athletes and those in weight-conscious sports (see appendix table 2.a). It is likely that discrepancies in energy balance in these athletic groups reflect errors both in the estimation of energy expenditure and in energy intake. It is not known whether the underreporting of all nutrients mirrors the underreporting of energy intake—this may not occur if particular foods or eating occasions are more likely to be selectively reported. This means that even if a correction factor for energy could be ascertained from energy balance studies, it may not be valid to use this factor across the board for all nutrients.

Typically, food records are kept for periods of 1 day to 7 days, although there have been rare studies that have monitored food intake over several years. The duration of the food diary is important both for the reliability of the estimate of energy or nutrient intake (a longer period of recording reduces the variability in estimation of daily intakes) and for the compliance of the participant (longer periods reduce the attention and compliance of the participant). In the general population, a 3- to 4-day record is considered a reasonable compromise, although it is limited in being able to accurately estimate typical intakes of only the stable dietary components such as energy and carbohydrate. Other, more variable nutrients such as vitamin A and cholesterol may require up to 4 weeks of recording to accurately estimate the daily intake of an individual to within the 95% confidence interval of true intake (Marr and Heady 1986). In athletic populations, where individuals are highly motivated and familiar with documenting other aspects of their training, many researchers and clinicians like to use a 7-day food diary, because this usually represents a complete microcycle in the athlete's training program. Extending the length of the food diary from 3 to 7 days greatly improves the reliability of the estimate of energy and nutrient intake by athletes (Braakhuis et al. 2003). An alternative method to increase the reliability of monitoring is to have the athlete complete a number of food diaries over shorter periods (e.g., 4-day food diaries completed two to three times over a period of training). If 3- to 4-day food diaries are used, they should be undertaken over a period that is representative of the different influences on food intake (e.g., 1 weekend day and 3 weekdays, or 3 days of heavy training and 1 light day or rest day).

Finally, the information collected in dietary surveys relates to intakes of fluids and foods. Sometimes this is judged against food-related benchmarks, for example, the recommended daily number of servings from various food groups. Most often, however, this information is analyzed quantitatively and converted into intakes of energy and nutrients using computerized dietary analysis programs incorporating food composition tables. This process is a major source of error in dietary surveys and reflects the skills and knowledge of the researcher, the method of data collection, and the available food composition database.

Care should be taken to minimize and standardize the errors involved in processing a food diary and to understand the limitations that they add to the assessment process (Braakhuis et al. 2003). An assessment of the reported dietary intake of an individual athlete or group or athletes provides information that should be regarded as an *estimate of true likely intake* and the *likelihood* of success or failure to meet nutritional goals, rather than an exact measure of true intake.

chapter 3

Sport Foods and Supplements

According to surveys, athletes are major consumers of supplements and an important target group for the multi-billion dollar supplement industry (for review, see Burke et al. 2000). Health food stores, supermarkets, sports stores, network marketing, mail order companies, and the Internet all provide access to an increasing number of products that claim to prolong endurance, enhance recovery, reduce body fat, increase muscle mass, minimize the risk of illness, or achieve other goals that enhance sport performance. It is understandable that the claims of improved performance are attractive to athletes and coaches in elite competition,

where very small differences separate the winners from the rest of the field (Hopkins et al. 1999). Athletes provide each other with testimonials or hearsay about the benefits attributed to supplements and sport foods. Many athletes fear that their opponents might have a secret weapon, and even in the absence of scientific evidence to support the claims for a certain supplement they often feel compelled to use the product to maintain a level playing field.

Although some athletes and coaches believe that sport scientists have a closed mind and dismiss the use of supplements as unnecessary, in fact most sport scientists

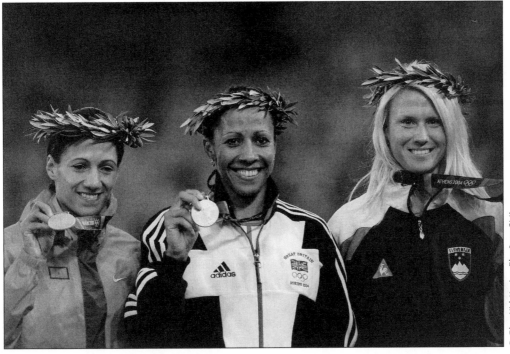

© Glyn Kirk/Action Plus/Icon SMI

The drive to achieve an Olympic gold medal or a world record provides only part of the incentive to search for a magic bullet, because even non-elite and recreational athletes are avid consumers of sport foods and supplements (Burke et al. 2000).

are interested in supplements and sport foods as part of their search for new strategies to enhance training, recovery, and competition performance. Many scientists undertake the applied sports nutrition research that has helped to develop new products and investigate the specific ways in which these products can be used to optimize performance. Unfortunately, the many challenges to undertaking such research mean that it is impossible to keep pace with the number of new products that appear on the market. Thus, the majority of products used by athletes are either untested or have failed to live up to expectations in the preliminary studies that have been conducted. Scientists believe that well-controlled research should underpin the promotion of any sports nutrition practice and are understandably frustrated that producers of supplements often make impressive claims about their products without adequate or, in some cases, any proof. In most countries, legislation regarding supplements or sport foods is either minimal or unenforced, allowing unsupported claims to flourish and products to be manufactured with poor compliance to labeling and composition standards. Athletes and coaches are usually unaware of these lapses.

This chapter provides a brief overview of some of the most popular nutritional products or compounds available to athletes, noting items that have true value as part of an athlete's nutrition program and compounds that have been proven to be ergogenic (work enhancing) by rigorous scientific testing. An overview of the consensus from supplementation studies involving athletes and sport-specific protocols is provided, but details of individual studies are provided in following chapters of the book.

Manufacture and Regulation of Sport Foods

Although we are able to provide athletes with sophisticated guidelines for sports nutrition (see chapter 1), many dietary surveys find that athletes fail to achieve appropriate food choices and eating plans. This is often because of practical challenges associated with the consumption of everyday foods, creating a need for foods and drinks with special properties. Such characteristics could include a serving size or composition that delivers a special amount of a key nutrient and good portability or ease of consuming while exercising. A characteristic that appears alluring to manufacturers is the inclusion of special ingredients claimed to enhance sport performance. In theory, the composition and practical characteristics of sport foods might be fine-tuned to meet a specific need in sport or even a specific type of sport; however, it is often impossible to turn such a niche food into a commercially viable product.

In some countries, the national or state food standards codes make a provision for sport foods. Standards might make provision for a range of acceptable formulations and permitted additives as well as a list of permitted or compulsory education messages for presentation on product packaging. Although such standards might exist, the

responsibility for adopting them into laws or enforcing these laws is often dispersed. In reality, some sport foods do not meet the relevant standards, either by containing ingredients that are in contravention to the code or by carrying claims that are not permitted. This is generally not the case for mainstream products, such as commercial sport drinks and bars. However, some sport foods, usually produced by smaller manufacturers targeting a niche market of athletes, fail to comply. When food standards codes rely on a largely self-regulated industry of food manufacture and marketing, there is a greater likelihood that sport foods will contain nonpermitted substances and incomplete or inaccurate labeling information.

Manufacture and Regulation of Sport Supplements

The availability and marketing of dietary supplements fitting the description of pills, powders, or other nonfood forms vary between countries. Athletes need to have a global understanding of the regulation of dietary supplements, because regular travel and modern conveniences such as mail order and the Internet provide easy access to products that fall outside the scrutiny of their own country's system. In Australia, a country with more comprehensive regulation, these products fall within the jurisdiction of the Therapeutic Goods Administration (TGA) under the Australian Therapeutic Goods Act of 1989. Although dietary supplements may be packaged in a way suggesting medical or scientific rigor, most are considered listable products, meaning that they receive considerably less regulation and attention than prescription pharmaceutical products. Although these products need to comply with relevant statutory standards (e.g., to exclude ingredients banned by Australian Customs laws), they are considered low-risk self-medications and are not subjected to a comprehensive review of quality, safety, and efficacy. They are expected to comply with good manufacturing practice and, according to advertising regulations, to make limited therapeutic claims. In practice, these products receive little investigation of quality and advertising claims unless they are the subject of serious complaints regarding health and safety issues.

In other countries, nonfood forms of supplements fall under the same regulatory bodies as food products. For example, in the United States, supplements fall under the jurisdiction of the Food and Drug Administration (FDA) and the Dietary Supplement Health and Education Act of 1994. This act reduced the regulation of supplements and broadened the category to include new ingredients, such as herbal and botanical products, and constituents or metabolites of other dietary supplements. Most important, the act shifted responsibility from the manufacturer to the FDA to enforce safety and claim guidelines. Since then, products and manufacturers have been free to flourish unless there is specific intervention by the FDA.

In the absence or minimization of rigorous government evaluation, the quality control of supplement manufacture is trusted to supplement companies. Large companies that produce conventional supplements, such as vitamins and minerals, particularly to manufacturing standards used in the preparation of pharmaceutical products, are likely to achieve good quality control. This includes precision with ingredient levels and labeling and avoidance of undeclared ingredients or contaminants. However, this does not appear to be true for all supplement types or manufacturers, with many examples of poor compliance to labeling laws and quality control of ingredients (Gurley et al. 1998; Hahm et al. 1999; Parasrampuria et al. 1998). The presence of contaminants and undeclared ingredients can cause a number of problems including inadvertent doping outcomes (see practical issue).

Although manufacturers are not supposed to make unsupported claims about health or performance benefits elicited by supplements, product advertisements and testimonials show ample evidence that this aspect of supplement marketing is underregulated and exploited. Most consumers are unaware that such advertising is not closely regulated. Therefore, athletes are likely to believe that claims about supplements are medically and scientifically supported, simply because they believe that untrue claims would not be allowed to exist.

Balancing the Pros and Cons Associated With Sport Foods and Supplements

The decision to use a supplement is a personal choice made by athletes, often in consultation with their coach or, in the case of younger athletes, their parents. Before making a decision, athletes and coaches should consider likely benefits balanced against the cost of the supplementation program and the risk of negative outcomes such as side effects or a positive doping outcome. The advice of sport scientists or sports nutrition authorities should be sought to provide such information. By gathering unbiased information about any scientifically documented benefits of the supplement use, as well as the potential risk of short- and long-term harmful effects, the athlete and coach are empowered to make a decision. They should also be well educated about the specific ways in which the supplement or sport food can be used to achieve nutritional goals or enhance performance.

Benefits

Some supplements and sport foods offer real advantages to the athlete. Benefits may arise from some or all of the following outcomes:

- Use of the product to meet known nutritional needs
- Direct ergogenic (performance-enhancing) effect
- Placebo effect

Some ergogenic effects or guidelines of sports nutrition are so well known and easily demonstrated that beneficial uses of sport foods or supplements arising from these first two outcomes are clear-cut. But even when indirect nutritional benefits or true ergogenic outcomes from supplement use are small, these supplements are often worthwhile in the competitive world of sport (see research topic). Of course, athletes need to be aware that it is the correct use of the product as much as the product itself that leads to the beneficial outcome. Therefore, education about specific situations and strategies for the use of supplements and sport foods is just as important as the formulation of the product.

Even when a sport food or supplement does not produce a true physiological or ergogenic benefit, an athlete might attain some performance benefit because of a psychological boost or placebo effect. The placebo effect describes a favorable outcome arising simply from an individual's belief that she has received a beneficial treatment. In a clinical environment, a placebo is often given in the form of a harmless but inactive substance or treatment that satisfies the patient's symbolic need to receive a therapy. In a sport setting, an athlete who receives enthusiastic marketing material about a new supplement or hears glowing testimonials from other athletes who have used it is more likely to report a positive experience. Despite our belief that the placebo effect is real and potentially worthwhile, only a few studies have tried to investigate the application of the placebo effect in sport (Ariel and Saville 1972; Clark et al. 2000). Additional well-controlled studies are needed to better describe the potential size and duration of this effect and whether it applies equally to all athletes and across all types of performance. In the meantime, we can accept that the placebo effect exists and may explain, at least partially, why athletes report performance benefits after trying a new supplement or dietary treatment.

Problems

The use of supplements and sport foods by athletes can be associated with a number of disadvantages and costs. For example, in deciding to set up its Sport Supplement Program, experts at the Australian Institute of Sport assessed the supplement use by athletes in its sporting programs and identified a list of problems (see the highlight box on this page and practical issue). An obvious issue with extensive supplement use is the expense, which in extreme cases can equal or exceed the athlete's weekly food budget. The situation is compounded for teams and sport programs that need to supply the needs of a group of athletes. Supplements and sport foods generally provide nutrients or food constituents at a higher price than everyday foods. This is understandable and often justified as the result of the costs of special ingredients, research and development, marketing, specialist packaging or processing, and higher unit costs for niche products. However, products are sometimes priced to provide an extravagant profit margin, simply to take advantage of the money that many athletes are willing to pay for their dreams of winning performances.

Supplement use, even when it provides a true performance advantage, is an expense that athletes must acknowledge and prioritize appropriately within their total budget. At times, it may be deemed money well spent, particularly when the supplement or sport food provides the most practical and palatable way to achieve a nutrition goal or when ergogenic benefits have been well documented. On other occasions the athlete may choose to limit the use of expensive products to the most important events or training periods. There are often lower-cost alternatives to some supplements and sport foods that the budget-conscious athlete can use on less critical occasions. This strategy is explored in more detail in chapter 11 in regard to protein and energy supplements.

The possibility of side effects and negative reactions to supplements and sport foods should also be considered. These include allergic reactions to some products, toxicity, overexposure as a result of self-medication, and poisoning caused by contaminants. Because most supplements are considered by regulatory bodies to be relatively safe, in many countries there are no official or mandatory accounting processes to document adverse side effects arising from the use of these products. Nevertheless, information from medical registers (Bent et al. 2003; Dennehy et al. 2005; Kozyrskyj 1997; Perharic et al. 1994; Shaw et al. 1997) shows that although the overall risk to public health from the use of supplements and herbal and traditional remedies is low, definite problems do occur. During the 1980s, deaths and medical problems resulted from the use

of tryptophan supplements (Roufs 1992). More recently, products containing ephedrine or ephedra have been linked to medical problems (Bent et al. 2003), including death in susceptible individuals (Charatan 2003).

Inadvertent doping through supplement use has emerged as a major concern for athletes who participate in sporting competitions governed by an antidoping code. Some supplements and sport foods contain ingredients from the list of banned substances provided by the World Anti-Doping Agency (WADA) or the national and international governing bodies of sport, and an athlete may record a positive drug test after unintentionally consuming a banned substance found in such products. Because supplements are regarded as harmless or as alternatives to drugs, some athletes may not carefully check product labels for banned substances. In addition, there is now growing evidence that many supplements or sport foods contain banned substances as undeclared ingredients or contaminants (see practical issue). Because sporting codes apply strict liability to athletes who test positive for banned substances, regardless of the source of their ingestion or intention of use, an inadvertent doping outcome can have major consequences for an athlete.

Finally, a more subtle outcome of reliance on supplements is the displacement of the athlete's real priorities. Successful sport performance is the product of a large number of factors, including superior genetics, long-term training, optimal nutrition, state-of-the-art equipment, and a committed attitude. These factors cannot be replaced by the use of supplements but often appear less exciting or more demanding than the use of supplements and sport foods, which may be marketed with enthusiastic and emotive claims. Athletes can sometimes be sidetracked from the true elements of success in search of shortcuts from bottles and packets.

Problems With Current Supplement Practices by Athletes, As Evaluated by the Australian Institute of Sport's Sport Supplement Program

- Strategies that genuinely enhance performance (e.g., specialized training, sound nutrition practice, good equipment, adequate rest and sleep, mental preparation) are overlooked in favor of supplement use.
- Athletes are drawn to new supplements with marketing hype rather than supplements and sport foods that might have true value in achieving nutrition goals.
- Ad hoc use of supplements often means that valuable products are not used in a manner that achieves optimal outcomes.
- Products with little value are a drain of resources (i.e., money, time, and interest are all limited assets).
- Use of unproven supplements by well-known or successful athletes (and institutions) provides endorsement in the eyes of other athletes and continues false expectations.
- Supplements carry a risk of side effects.
- Supplements carry a risk of inadvertent positive doping outcome.

RESEARCH TOPIC

Characteristics
of Well-Designed Studies

The scientific trial is the gold standard for investigating the benefits of dietary supplements and nutritional ergogenic aids for athletes. Sport scientists who undertake such scientific trials should test the effects of the supplement in a

setting that mimics real-life sport as much as possible. The challenges of measuring changes in sport performance should not be underestimated. Additional studies might be needed to elucidate the mechanisms by which any effects occur. Many factors interfere with the outcomes of research. A researcher must design a protocol that eliminates extraneous or confounding variables and monitors a set of carefully chosen independent and dependent variables. It is beyond the scope of this book to fully explore the characteristics of good research design. Table 3.1 summarizes a number of

Table 3.1   Features of Well-Designed Research on Sport Supplements and Ergogenic Aids

Feature	Strategies
1. Appropriate experimental design and sample size	• Incorporate the use of a placebo treatment or trial to overcome the psychological effect of supplementation. It is also interesting, if practical, to add a control (no treatment) trial so that the magnitude of the placebo effect can be determined. • Where possible, use a repeated-measures or crossover design, in which each participant acts as his own control by undertaking both the treatment and placebo trials. This is a stronger statistical design than an experimental–placebo design (two separate groups of participants who receive either the treatment or the placebo) and requires a smaller sample size. • Randomly assign participants to treatment and placebo groups, balancing for participant features (e.g., sex, age, fitness, or training characteristics) that could interact with the treatment. • In a crossover study, provide each of the treatments to participants in a randomized counterbalanced order to remove the effect of time or training on study outcomes. In other words, have equal numbers of participants receive all treatments in the various possible sequences of order. Allow a suitable washout period in a crossover-designed study so that the effects of a treatment are removed before the next trial begins. • Where possible, use a double-blind allocation of treatments to remove the subjective bias of both researcher and participants. The placebo effect has been most identified in terms of participant expectations. It is not always possible to blind the treatment to participants. When this is the case, use a single-blind presentation in which key researchers who measure performance outcomes are not aware of the treatment received by participants. Blinding of the researchers will help to control the occurrence of the "halo effect," where an observer who believes an effect is likely "marks up" or encourages the performance of participants. • Choose the sample size after considering the likely range of changes in the measurements of interest. Power analysis of changes in outcome measures will determine the minimum number of participants needed to detect changes that are worthwhile.
2. Appropriate treatment protocol	• Choose a supplementation protocol—timing, amount, and duration of supplement use—that maximizes the likelihood of a positive outcome. This may not always be the dose recommended by the manufacturer. Other information can be found from pilot investigations. • Alternatively, replicate a supplementation protocol that represents the popular use patterns among athletes. • If a positive effect is found, manipulate doses in further trials to refine the optimal supplementation protocol.
3. Appropriate choice of participants	• Recruit participants who represent the population for whom recommendations about supplement use are needed. • Be aware that effects seen with untrained or recreational participants may not apply to well-trained or elite athletes. Training status may affect the outcomes of supplementation. Characteristics that make athletes elite may also cause them to react differently to a treatment. • Be aware that the performances of highly-trained athletes are typically more reliable than those of recreational participants, especially when athletes are familiar with an exercise protocol. A reduction in intra- and interparticipant variability in performance will increase the statistical power of the study and increase the chance of detecting small but worthwhile changes in performance.

(continued)

Table 3.1   *(continued)*

Feature	Strategies
4. Appropriate exercise stimulus and performance protocol	• Develop laboratory or field protocols that mimic the demands and environments in which a real-life sport is played. • Ensure that the exercise protocol provides the physiological stimulus that the supplement is suggested to address. • Ensure that athletes are familiar with the exercise or performance protocol. If this is not a field or laboratory test that is already incorporated into the athlete's training or competition program, allow participants to undertake familiarization training until they are able to undertake reliable performances. Participants may need time to experiment with new equipment and with appropriate pace judgment. • Consider all strategies to standardize or supervise the test protocol so that reliability is optimized. A reliable test will increase the change of detecting small changes in performance that are worthwhile in real life.
5. Consideration of variables to explain performance changes	• Where possible and practical, collect data that can explain or support observations of performance changes. Although the athlete may only be interested in performance outcomes, the sport scientist will be interested in physiological and psychological factors that underpin performance changes. This understanding is more than an academic interest; proof of an underlying mechanism can corroborate the observed performance benefits and offer insight to fine-tune protocols for using the supplement. • Choose parameters that are directly relevant to the hypothesis that is being tested and sufficiently reliable to detect important changes. These parameters should only be measured if this does not interfere with the athlete's ability to perform in the exercise protocol. Otherwise, studies should be separated into those that measure performance and those that monitor mechanisms explaining performance changes. It is not always possible to monitor both simultaneously.
6. Standardization of conditions	• Standardize extraneous variables that can affect metabolism and performance during exercise, to reduce inter- and intratrial variability and enhance the likelihood of detecting the effects of the supplement. Such variables include overall training status of participants, acute diet and training on the day(s) before each trial, pretrial hydration, participant fatigue, and environmental conditions. • Choose standardized conditions that mimic the real-life practices in sport.
7. Appropriate analysis and interpretation of results	• Undertake a valid statistical analysis of the data. • Interpret results in light of the changes that are worthwhile to an athlete and a specific sport.

ideas that are useful in designing trials to test the effects of supplements on sport performance. This summary includes encouragement to present results in light of changes that would be meaningful to sport. This issue is worthy of further discussion because the views of athletes and coaches are extremely different than the hypotheses tested in most current studies.

In the world of sport, the differences between winning and losing and the margins between the winners on a podium and the rest of the field are often tantalizingly small. To the athlete or coach, that hundredth of a second or millimeter seems a meaningful improvement in performance. This helps to explain the enthusiasm with which supplements and ergogenic aids that promise a performance boost are greeted. Many athletes believe they can't afford to miss out on an edge, however tiny, that might be found in a pill or potion. The chance of the tiniest improvement seems worth their investment. Unfortunately, scientists who undertake controlled trials on supplements and ergogenic

aids operate at almost the opposite end of the spectrum of performance changes. The traditional framework of such research is that the scientist aims to detect or declare an effect as statistically significant, with acceptably low rates of detection of nonexistent effects (5%) and failed detection of a real effect (20%). Most scientific investigations of supplements are biased toward rejecting the hypothesis that the product enhances performance, because of small sample sizes and performance testing protocols with low reliability. In practice, most intervention studies are only able to detect large differences in performance outcomes. Changes that are smaller than this large effect are declared to be not statistically significant and are dismissed.

This dilemma was addressed by Hopkins and colleagues in a discussion of ways to detect worthwhile performance enhancements in elite sport (Hopkins et al. 1999). These authors considered the need to find middle ground between what scientists and athletes consider significant. The first point to be addressed was that an athlete's required improvement is *not* the small margin between place-getters in race (also known as *between*-athlete variation). Each athlete has her own day-to-day or event-to-event variability in performance, known as the *within*-athlete variation or coefficient of variation (CV) of performance. This variation would influence the outcome of an event if it were to be rerun without any intervention. By modeling the results of various sporting events in track and field, Hopkins and colleagues suggested that worthwhile changes to the outcome of most events require a performance change equal to ~0.4 to 0.7 times the CV of performance for that event. Simulating the results of a mythical event with typical between- and within-athlete variability produced a range in changes in outcome according to the true place that an athlete would get without any intervention. For example, the athlete who averages 10th place in a field would be expected to win 1% of events, but the chance rises to 11% with an enhancement of 1.3 of the CV. The athlete who averages 4th place needs an enhancement of 0.6 of the CV to increase the frequency of winning from 9% to 19%. The 1st place-getter normally wins 38% of the time, but with an enhancement of 0.3 of the CV the chance rises to 48%. Therefore, a worthwhile change does not guarantee that an athlete would win an event but would make a reasonable change to an athlete's likelihood of winning. Across a range of track-and-field events, Hopkins and colleagues noted that the CV of performance of top athletes was within the range

of 0.5 to 5%, thus making performance changes of up to 3% important to detect (Hopkins et al. 1999).

Even though worthwhile performance differences are larger than the tiny margins considered important by athletes, these changes are still outside the realms of detection for many of the studies commonly published in scientific journals. As discussed by Hopkins and colleagues (1999), a change of 0.7 of the CV in a parameter requires a sample size of about 32 for detection in a crossover study in which every athlete receives an experimental and control treatment. For a experimental–placebo or parallel group–designed study, in which performance is assessed before and after either an experimental treatment or control in two separate groups of participants, the necessary sample size is four times as large—128 participants. To detect changes of ~0.35 CV, the sample sizes must be increased again by four: 128 for a crossover and 520 for a fully controlled study. Such sample sizes are beyond the resources of most sport scientists (Hopkins et al. 1999).

Hopkins and colleagues have proposed a new approach to undertaking and interpreting intervention studies—focusing on the precision of estimation of the magnitude of effect of a treatment. To encourage greater understanding of research on performance enhancement among sport scientists, coaches, and athletes, the following recommendations for presentation of findings have been made (Hopkins et al. 1999; Batterham and Hawkins 2006):

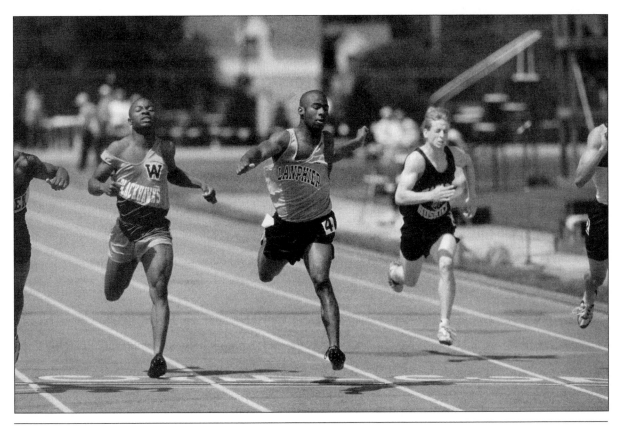

Games are won in the last seconds by the smallest possible score; hundredths of seconds and millimeters separate athletes in many races.

- Report the outcome as a percent change in a measure of athletic performance and in mean power outputs, where possible. For example, a study may find a 2% enhancement in time, caused by a 1.5% improvement in mean power, as a result of the use of a supplement.

- Report the 95% confidence limits for the outcome; these provide the likely range of the true effect of the treatment on the average participant. For example, in this study, the 95% confidence interval (CI) for the change in time might be –1% to +4%.

- Interpret the magnitude of the outcome and confidence limits in terms of the likely effect on athletes in an event. For example, the outcome in this study includes the possibility of a small decrement in performance as well as a substantial improvement in performance. Both possibilities could change the outcome of an event, and the athlete needs to consider the small risk of a negative outcome as well as the more likely chance of a noticeable improvement in finishing order. A refined magnitude-based interpretation of the results would divide the real-world significance of changes in zones of negative, trivial, and positive. Then, the result and the spread of its confidence intervals would be plotted within these zones. Such a plot would show the most likely outcome of a study, and how certain you were of the results. The final interpretation of the change seen in a study might range from "unclear" (if it overlaps all zones), to probably positive (if it was mostly in the positive zone but overlapped into the trivial zone), and to almost certainly positive (if the range was all within the positive zone). Resist making conclusions that a treatment does not cause a change, even when the observed effect is too small to be of interest to well-trained athletes. Unless the study has been performed with an adequate sample size, consider that the 95% CI may not be able to exclude the possibility of important decrements or enhancements in performance. Be prepared to conclude that the study could not detect a substantial change, but neither could it rule it out as a possibility.

- Discuss the possibility of different outcomes for athletes who differ in caliber, training, dietary practices, and other characteristics.

- Consider the possibility that the experiences of individuals within a group differ, and that a treatment might be beneficial for some but harmful or trivial for others.

PRACTICAL ISSUE

Supplements and Doping

During the late 1990s, there was an apparent increase in the number of positive drug tests in sport for the steroid nandrolone, or at least an increased awareness of these outcomes because of the involvement of high-profile athletes across a range of sports. These athletes denied the use of banned substances, claiming that their use of performance aids was limited to supplements. However, these claims helped to force the recognition that supplements can be a source of substances banned by the various antidoping codes of sport. In addition to containing banned prohormones (steroid-related compounds) that can cause a positive test for nandrolone metabolites or other indicators of steroid use (e.g., an increase in testosterone–epitestosterone ratio greater than 6:1), supplements may also provide a source of banned stimulants such as ephedrine or related substances (Green et al. 2001). Some supplements contain caffeine or guarana, which might contribute to high urinary caffeine levels in athletes; however, caffeine was removed from the list of banned substances on the World Anti-Doping Agency code in 2004. Athletes may be unaware that their supplement use could cause them to test positive for banned substances—because they have not read the product labels to note the presence of these substances or because the products they are ingesting contain these substances as undeclared ingredients. The claim of inadvertent doping outcomes via supplementation has steadily increased over time. Within the National Collegiate Athletic Association, supplement use has become the most common cause of positive drug tests and underpins most of the appeals against such findings (Burke 2001a)

Drug education programs now highlight the need for athletes to read the labels of supplements and sport foods carefully to ensure that they do not contain banned substances. This is undoubtedly a responsibility that athletes can master to prevent inadvertent doping outcomes. The antidoping codes under which many sports operate place strict liability with the athlete for ingestion of banned substances, regardless of circumstances and the source of ingestion. As such, full penalties can be expected for a positive doping test arising from the ingestion of a banned substance that is a contaminant or an undeclared ingredient of a supplement. Poor manufacturing practices within the supplement industry have been identified as a cause of mislabeling of ingredients, the presence of undeclared substances, and the absence or altered dosages of stated ingredients. The following studies provide evidence of problems:

- An herbal supplement used by a Dutch cyclist who tested positive for ephedrine contained ephedra as a stated ingredient but also contained significant amounts of another alkaloid stimulant that was not declared as an ingredient (Ros et al. 1999).

- A ginseng supplement was found not to contain any ginsenosides (the active ingredient in ginseng) but instead contained ephedrine. This supplement was used by a Swedish athlete who tested positive for ephedrine (Cui et al. 1994).

- An over-the-counter prohormone product (androstenedione) was contaminated with 19-norandrostenedione, which produces a positive urine test for nandrolone. Furthermore, some brands of androstenedione were grossly mislabeled (Catlin et al. 2001).

- An International Olympic Committee (IOC)–accredited laboratory in Cologne (Geyer, Henze, et al. 2000) reported the detection of testosterone and various forms of androstenedione and 19-norandrostenedion–diol in three different commercial preparations from the United States. The supplements were not named but were listed as a chrysin, *tribulus terrestris*, and a guarana product. All products failed to declare these compounds as ingredients. Furthermore, urinary excretion studies undertaken on volunteers showed that the consumption of even one capsule of these supplements could produce a positive test for the metabolites of nandrolone.

- A larger follow-up study from this Cologne laboratory analyzed 634 supplements from 215 suppliers in 13 countries, with products being sourced from retail outlets (91%), the Internet (8%), and telephone sales (Geyer et al. 2004). None of these supplements declared prohormones as ingredients, and they came both from manufacturers who produced other supplements containing prohormones and from companies who did not sell these products. Ninety-four of the supplements (15% of sample) were found to contain hormones or prohormones that were not stated on the product label, and a further 10% of samples provided technical difficulties in analysis such that the absence of hormones could not be guaranteed. Of the positive supplements, 68% contained prohormones of testosterone, 7% contained prohormones of nandrolone, and 25% contained compounds related to both. Forty-nine of the supplements contained only one steroid, but 45 contained more than one, with eight products containing five or more different steroid products. According to the labels on the products, the countries of *manufacture* of all supplements containing steroids were the United States, the Netherlands, the United Kingdom, Italy, and Germany; however these products were *purchased* in other countries. In fact, 10% to 20% of products purchased in Spain and Austria were found to be contaminated. Just over 20% of the products made by companies selling prohormones were positive for undeclared prohormones, but 10% of products from companies that don't sell steroid-containing supplements were also positive. Again, the brand names of the positive products were not provided in the study but included amino acid supplements, protein powders, and products containing creatine, carnitine, ribose, guarana, zinc, pyruvate, β-hydroxy β-methylbutyrate, *tribulus terrestris*, herbal extracts, and vitamins and minerals. It was noted that a positive urinary test for nandrolone metabolites occurs in the hours following uptake of as little of 1 μg of nandrolone prohormones. The positive supplements contained steroid concentrations ranging from 0.01 to 190 μg per gram of product.

- An IOC-accredited laboratory in Vienna conducted analyses on 54 supplements purchased in Austria (dopinginfo.de 2000). The lab reported that 22% of products contained prohormones not stated on the label. The names of the individual products manufacturers were identified in this report provided on the Internet.

- The IOC-accredited Cologne laboratory undertook analysis of 110 supplements that did not declare the presence of stimulants on the label (Parr et al. 2003). The analysis revealed that 14 contained caffeine and 2 contained ephedrine, which remains a banned substance in many antidoping codes.

- Three supplements manufactured in the United States but sold by a UK company promoting an ingredient called 1-T Matrix were analyzed (Geyer et al. 2003). Other ingredients declared on the labels of these powders and capsules were ribose, creatine, branched-chain amino acids, and taurine. One of the powders contained caffeine, ephedrine, and pseudoephedrine, which were not declared on the label. All of the products contained metandienone, a prescription-only anabolic steroid commonly known as Dianabol. The concentrations of this steroid varied from capsule to capsule in one of the products, but all products would have provided supratherapeutic levels of the steroid if taken according to the manufacturer's recommendations (10-40 mg/day compared with the recommended therapeutic dose of 5-10 mg/day). In addition to causing a positive doping test, the use of metandienone is associated with adverse medical and health effects.

- One hundred three dietary supplements, categorized as creatine, prohormone, mental enhancers, or branched-chain amino acids, were bought on the Internet and analyzed for stimulants and anabolic steroid compounds (Baume et al. 2006). Three products were found to contain the anabolic steroid metandienone in a very high amount. One creatine product and three mental enhancers contained traces of hormones or prohormones not claimed on the labels, and 14 prohormone products contained substances other than those indicated by the manufacturer.

Although the presence of undeclared ingredients is often suggested to reflect poor manufacturing processes that allow contamination from one product to another, there is also a reasonable theory that at least some manufacturers deliberately add ingredients to their products to enhance the effects and improve sales. For example, the presence of stimulants to a supplement might be associated with a feeling of well-being or energy. The presence of high levels of a controlled steroid also suggests deliberate contamination to produce a measured effect on gains in muscle size and strength.

In summary, athletes who compete in sports under an antidoping code must recognize that supplement use exposes them to a real risk of a positive doping outcome.

Because the problem seems widespread and underpinned by a complicated system involving government regulations and business manufacturing processes, it is difficult to find easy or universal solutions to offer athletes. Various countries and sporting bodies have tried to bring the problem to the attention of athletes in different ways, including advising athletes that they should not take any dietary supplements:

- "We would like to caution the athletes of the world that recent findings show that supplements may contain drugs that will cause the athletes to test positive for substances that are currently on the banned list. Moreover, we as a commission fully endorse that athletes must take complete responsibility for all drugs that are found in their bodies due to the use of nutritional supplements" (Athletes' Commission of the International Olympic Committee, 2000).

- A 2004 publication from the World Anti-Doping Agency offers the following advice: "Athletes who believe that they need supplements should first consult a competent sport science professional such as a sport nutritionist or a sports physician to ensure they are professionally advised as to whether their needs can be met from normal foods. If supplements are used, they should be suitable for their nutrient needs, safe for their health, and should not lead to a positive doping test."

In 2004, a symposium was held in Montreal by the World Anti-Doping Agency, in cooperation with the Canadian Centre for Ethics in Sport, the Canadian Olympic Committee, and Sport Canada, to deal with the consequences of the use and misuse of nutritional supplements by athletes. Participants from within sport, antidoping organizations, medical and scientific fields, industry, and governments, together with elite athletes and coaches, discussed and made specific recommendations for action in the short, medium, and longer term. Those recommendations (www.wada-ama.org) include the following:

- Agreement on a common definition of dietary supplements

- Implementation of a coordinated research program to identify what supplements are being used and misused by athletes and why

- Establishment of a global database on supplements to ensure that access to all current and reliable information on supplements is made available

- Consideration of a product testing and certification program of supplements that could be supported by the industry

- Agreement by industry to implement self-regulation programs that would include stringent standards and third-party, independent auditing and monitoring to improve quality, minimize contamination, and provide accurate labeling

- Enactment by governments of appropriate regulations on the industry because of their responsibilities for public health, consumer protection, and education

- Organization of a follow-up symposium to ensure that recommendations turn into concrete and coordinated actions

The outcomes of these initiatives are eagerly awaited.

PRACTICAL ISSUE

An Approach to Supplements and Sport Foods

Since 2000, the Australian Institute of Sport (AIS) has implemented a supplement program for athletes within its funding program with the following goals:

- Allowing its athletes to focus on the sound use of supplements and special sport foods as part of their nutrition plans

- Ensuring that supplements and sport foods are used correctly and appropriately to deliver maximum benefits to the immune system, recovery, and performance

- Giving its athletes the confidence that they receive cutting-edge advice and achieve state-of-the-art nutrition practices

- Minimizing the risk that supplement use leads to an inadvertent doping offence

A key part of the AIS program is a ranking system for supplements and sport foods, based on a risk–benefit analysis of each product by a panel of experts in sports nutrition, medicine, and science. This ranking system has four tiers or groups, each of which has a prescribed level of use by AIS-funded athletes. Although the hierarchy of categories was developed for long-term use, there is a regular assessment of supplements and sport foods to ensure that they are placed in the category that best fits the available scientific evidence. The Sports Supplement Panel recognizes the limitations in the quantity and quality of the current supplement research. For example, evidence from a small number of studies showing that a product enhances the exercise capacity of healthy or active people may not translate into benefits to the sport-specific performance of elite athletes. Alternatively, a few studies that have reported a lack of benefits from the use of a compound may not adequately address the potential for a small but worthwhile enhancement of performance when the compound is used to its best effect. The main aim of the program is to prioritize the resources of the AIS for supplying supplements and sport foods to its athletes (and delivering research and education programs in this area) so that the main focus is given to the products that are likely to provide the greatest outcomes.

Table 3.2 provides a summary of the AIS supplement program at the time of publication. The program is reissued annually following a review of the updated literature on various supplements and sport foods and of issues that

Table 3.2 Australian Institute Sport (AIS) Supplement Program 2007

Supplement category and explanation of use within the AIS supplement program	Products included in category
GROUP A: APPROVED SUPPLEMENTS	
• Provide a useful and timely source of energy and nutrients in the athlete's diet. • Or have been shown in scientific trials to provide a performance benefit, when used according to a specific protocol in a specific situation in sport.	• Sport drinks • Liquid meal supplements • Sport gels • Sport bars • Caffeine • Creatine • Bicarbonate/citrate • Antioxidants: vitamin C, vitamin E • Sick pack (zinc and vitamin C) • Multivitamin and mineral supplement • Iron supplement • Calcium supplement • Glycerol (for hyperhydration) • Glucosamine

AIS Sports Supplement Panel position:

We know that athletes and coaches are interested in using supplements to achieve optimal performance. Our supplement program aims to focus this interest on products and protocols that have documented benefits, in the following ways:

- Making some of these supplements available and accessible to the AIS athletes who will benefit from their appropriate use. In particular, to provide these supplements at no cost to AIS sport programs, through systems managed by appropriate sport science and sport medicine departments. Strategies to provide products will range from individual "prescription" of supplements requiring careful use (e.g., creatine) to creative programs that make valuable sport foods and everyday foods accessible to athletes in situations of nutritional need (e.g., postexercise recovery); see chapter 6).
- Providing education to athletes and coaches about the beneficial uses of these supplements and sport foods and their appropriate use, with the emphasis on state-of-the-art sports nutrition.
- Ensuring that supplements and sport food used by AIS athletes carry a minimal risk of doping safety problems.

GROUP B: SUPPLEMENTS UNDER CONSIDERATION	
Supplements may be classified category B if they have no substantial proof of health or performance benefits, but • remain of interest to AIS coaches or athletes, • are too new to have received adequate scientific attention, or • have preliminary data that hint at possible benefits.	• Glutamine • β-hydroxy β-methylbutyrate (HMB) • Colostrum • Probiotics • Ribose • Melatonin

AIS Sports Supplement Panel position:

These supplements can be used at the AIS under the auspices of a controlled scientific trial or a supervised therapeutic program.

GROUP C: SUPPLEMENTS THAT HAVE NO CLEAR PROOF OF BENEFICIAL EFFECTS	
• This category contains the majority of supplements and sport products promoted to athletes. Supplements not specifically listed within this system probably belong here. • These supplements, despite enjoying a cyclical pattern of popularity and widespread use, have not been proven to enhance sport performance or recovery. In some cases these supplements have been shown to impair sport performance or health, with a clear mechanism to explain these results.	• Amino acids (these can be provided by everyday foods or sport foods in group A) • Ginseng • Cordyceps • Rhodiola rosea • Inosine • Coenzyme Q10 • Cytochrome C • Carnitine • Bee pollen

(continued)

Table 3.2   *(continued)*

Supplement category and explanation of use within the AIS supplement program	Products included in category
GROUP C: SUPPLEMENTS THAT HAVE NO CLEAR PROOF OF BENEFICIAL EFFECTS	
	• γ-oryzanol and ferulic acid • Chromium picolinate • Pyruvate • ZMA supplements • Vitamin supplements when used in situations other than summarized in Group A • Nitric oxide–stimulating supplements • Oxygenated waters • Most of the other supplements not listed in this system

AIS Sports Supplement Panel position:

In the absence of proof of benefits, these supplements should not be provided to AIS athletes from AIS program budgets.

If individual athletes or coaches wish to use a supplement from this category, they may do so providing
  • they are responsible for payment for this supplement,
  • any sponsorship arrangements are within guidelines of AIS marketing,
  • the supplement brand has been assessed for doping safety and is considered "low risk," and
  • they report their use to their AIS sport physician.

GROUP D: BANNED SUPPLEMENTS	
These supplements are either directly banned by the World Anti-Doping Agency code or provide a high risk of producing a positive doping outcome.	• Androstenedione • DHEA • 19-norandrostenedione and 19-norandrostenediol • *Tribulus terristris* and other herbal testosterone supplements • Ephedra • Strychnine

AIS Sports Supplement Panel position:
These supplements should not be used by AIS athletes.

The AIS does not support the use of supplements sold under network marketing schemes.

Adapted from Australian Institute of Sport. www.ais.org.au/nutrition.

occurred during the previous 12 months. Resources that explain the program and outline how individual sport programs can access supplements and sport foods are provided to athletes and coaches via the AIS Department of Sports Nutrition Web site (www.ais.org.au/nutrition). Many education and research activities within the AIS are organized to support and develop the Sports Supplement Program. These activities include undertaking sport-specific research to investigate the exact conditions under which category A and B supplements and sport foods benefit athletes. These activities also include the production of education resources and the delivery of lectures and discussions for specific athletic groups related to using these products well—such as consuming them at the right time and in the right amounts. The AIS program states that the use of supplements carries a small risk of inadvertent doping and that AIS athletes should not purchase their own supplements

outside the system without discussing this with their team doctor and without considering the level of risk associated with the specific product.

OVERVIEW OF COMMON SPORT FOODS AND SUPPLEMENTS

Sport Drinks (Carbohydrate-Electrolyte Drinks)

Sport drinks are flavored drinks, typically providing carbohydrate (6-8% or 6-8 g/100 m), sodium (10-25 mmol/L), and potassium (3-5 mmol/L), to rapidly deliver fluid and fuel during and after exercise.

- Sport drinks increase voluntary intake of fluid compared with water, even when athletes claim not to like the taste (Minehan et al. 2002). Athletes are likely to match fluid intakes with sweat losses during exercise and recovery when offered sport drinks compared with water.

- Sport drinks are rapidly emptied from the stomach and absorbed through the small intestine. Solutions of 4% to 8% carbohydrate can deliver an effective source of carbohydrate without interfering with rehydration goals.

- Replacement of electrolytes, particularly sodium, is useful for maintaining thirst drive and may help to reduce urine losses during postexercise recovery.

Potential Situations for Use

- During exercise: Athletes should use the opportunities provided by their sport and training activities to drink sufficient sport drink to replace ~80% of sweat losses, or as much of the sweat loss as is practical and comfortable. The concentration of the sport drink can be changed to increase delivery of carbohydrate in sports where the need for fuel replacement takes priority over hydration (e.g., distance events in cold conditions) or to decrease carbohydrate concentration where fluid delivery is of priority (e.g., events in very hot conditions).

- Use after exercise: Typically, athletes will finish a training or competition session with mild to severe fluid deficit. Monitoring changes in body mass can provide an estimate of levels of dehydration. Rehydration requires a fluid intake of ~150% of the volume of the postexercise fluid deficit over the next 1 to 2 hr and may not occur voluntarily. Use of a palatable drink and the replacement of electrolytes are important strategies in this process.

Research Support

- Replacement of fluid and carbohydrate during many types of exercise has a substantial independent and additive effect on performance. Benefits have been seen in the following situations:

- Performance of prolonged continuous sports (endurance sports)—see chapter 4 (cycling and triathlon) and chapter 5 (middle- and long-distance running)

- Performance of movement patterns and skills in prolonged intermittent sports such as team and racket sports (see research topics, chapter 9)

- Performance of high-intensity sports lasting about 1 hr (see chapter 5, research topic)

Concerns Associated With Use

- For athletes who must remain lean or meet weight (body mass) targets, overuse of energy-containing fluids may create problems of energy balance or overall nutrient density in a restricted energy diet.

- Sport drinks should be mixed properly, according to the manufacturer's directions or special strategies

suggested by a sport scientist, to ensure that fluid and carbohydrate intake goals are met. Alterations in concentration should be carefully considered, because dilution may change flavor characteristics and reduce voluntary intake of the drink.

- Drinks should be kept cool to promote palatability and encourage intake.

- Athletes should not consume excessive amounts of sport drinks during exercise, for example, intakes in excess of sweat losses that cause a substantial increase in body mass.

- Individuals who lose very large amounts of sodium in sweat may find it useful to consume sport drinks with a higher sodium concentration during exercise. Similarly, the reversal of moderate to severe levels of dehydration usually requires replacement of sodium losses, and a sport drink with higher sodium concentrations may be useful. While some commercial sport drinks offer a higher sodium concentration (30-35 mmol/L), additional sodium may need to be consumed from dietary sources or from purpose-built electrolyte supplements (see below).

Electrolyte Replacement Supplements

Several types of products can provide a higher and measured dose of sodium and other electrolytes for replacement during and after exercise:

- Sport drink with higher sodium content (>25 mmol/L sodium)

- Oral rehydration solution (50-80 mmol/L sodium, 10-30 mmol/L potassium)

- Electrolyte sachets (30 mmol of sodium, 10 mmol of potassium)

Potential Situations for Use

Situations may occur in sport where focused replacement of electrolytes is warranted:

- Rapid rehydration may be needed following moderate to large fluid deficits incurred during exercise or other dehydrating activities (e.g., making weight).

- Replacement of large sodium losses may be needed during ultraendurance activities.

- Replacement of large electrolyte losses may be needed during exercise in certain individuals with high rates of sweat loss or high sweat content of electrolytes.

- Inability to consume everyday foods or a normal meal may limit potential to replace sodium during rehydration strategies. Many sport drinks (10-25 mmol/L sodium and 3-5 mmol/L potassium) may not address the replacement of large electrolyte losses during and after exercise.

- Oral rehydration solutions are recommended to treat or prevent dehydration associated with diarrhea and gastroenteritis in athletes.

Research Support

- Regarding postexercise rehydration, there is sound evidence that the replacement of electrolyte losses, particularly sodium, must occur before fluid balance is fully restored. In the absence of sodium replacement, replacement of fluid by the dehydrated athlete will lower plasma sodium levels and osmolality, decreasing thirst and increasing urine output despite only partial restoration of plasma volume (for review, see Shirreffs et al. 2004). Although sodium can be replaced via the consumption of high-sodium foods (e.g., bread, breakfast cereal, or other processed savory foods) or salt (sodium chloride) added to meals, it is sometimes beneficial to use specialized electrolyte-replacement supplements.

- The value of sodium and electrolyte replacement in reducing problems associated with large electrolyte losses from sweat is under discussion. In particular, the use of sodium supplements to reduce the risk of hyponatremia (low sodium concentrations) during ultraendurance events is unclear. Severe cases of hyponatremia are caused principally by "water intoxication," or overhydration, where the athlete consumes fluid at a rate that is substantially higher than actual sweat losses. Sodium replacement during exercise will not address this major risk factor for hyponatremia (see chapter 4, practical issue). The prevalence of hyponatremia not associated with hyperhydration, and its prevention by replacing large sodium losses during exercise with sodium supplements, requires further study. The prevention of cramps in susceptible athletes with sodium replacement is at present anecdotal (see chapter 10, research topic).

- Oral rehydration solutions are recommended in the treatment or prevention of dehydration associated with diarrhea and gastroenteritis.

Concerns Associated With Use

- There is no consensus regarding the value of sodium replacement during exercise.

- In some situations, salt supplementation during exercise may lead to gastrointestinal problems or cause further impairment of fluid balance.

- Increasing the sodium content of a drink generally reduces the drink palatability and may interfere with the voluntary consumption of fluid.

- The dietary guidelines for many countries promote a reduction in sodium and salt intake by the community, because of the link between salt intake and hypertension in susceptible people. Electrolyte replacement during and after sports may be considered as a special situation for a special subgroup of the population; however, general guidelines for healthy eating should not be overlooked.

Liquid Meal Supplements

Liquid meal supplements are available in the form of carbohydrate-rich, moderate-protein, low-fat powder for mixing with water or milk. They are also available in ready-to-drink form. These supplements provide a compact and easily prepared meal replacement or supplement. They are usually fortified to provide a substantial source of many vitamins, minerals, and essential amino acids (e.g., 25% recommended dietary intake in 250 ml serving).

Potential Situations for Use

- Liquid meal supplements are useful for athletes who need to increase energy intake without preparing or eating additional food or meals, such as athletes aiming to increase lean body mass, athletes coping with heavy training loads, and athletes undergoing growth spurts.

- These supplements provide substantial amounts of carbohydrate and protein (essential amino acids) and other micronutrients, making them useful as a postexercise recovery snack.

- Since they are a low-residue form of nutrition, these supplements can replace normal energy and nutrient intake while reducing gastrointestinal contents and body mass: Thus, they can replace one to three meals on the day before a weigh-in in weight-making sports. These supplements are also useful as a preevent meal for athletes with high risk of gastrointestinal upset during exercise.

- Liquid meal supplements provide a portable, nonperishable, and easily prepared meal or snack—providing energy, a balance of macronutrients, and a substantial source of micronutrients: Thus, they are useful for a traveling athlete who has minimal facilities for food preparation and storage, especially an athlete traveling to countries with inadequate food supply or problems with food hygiene.

Research Support

The use of liquid supplements to achieve sports nutrition goals is well supported.

Concerns Associated With Use

- Liquid meal supplements can often be overused, leading to inappropriate replacement of whole foods and overreliance on an expensive alternative. Food sources should always be considered as the first option for meals and snacks.

- The compact form of these supplements may lead to overconsumption of energy intake and unwanted weight gain by some athletes.

- A low-residue weight-making strategy may not be effective if athlete is already restricting dietary intake and has reduced gastrointestinal contents.

Sport Bars

Sport bars provide a compact source of carbohydrate and protein in a bar form. Typically, they are low in fat and fiber. Some are fortified with micronutrients (typically containing 25-50% recommended dietary intake of various vitamins and minerals per bar).

- Sport bars are a more concentrated form of carbohydrate than sport drinks and provide a substantial fuel boost when consumed during or after exercise.
- A solid form of carbohydrate intake may be useful to satisfy hunger during some forms of prolonged exercise (i.e., road cycling).
- Bars provide a compact and portable snack with balanced macronutrient content and a good source of micronutrients.

Potential Situations for Use

- Sport bars provide a compact fuel source during prolonged sessions of training or competition, especially when hunger is likely or it is impractical to carry substantial amounts of food.
- They are a nutrient-dense supplement providing energy and carbohydrate in a high-energy diet. They are useful for athletes undertaking a heavy training load, experiencing growth, or aiming to increase muscle mass.
- They provide a compact and portable source of carbohydrate, protein, and other nutrients for postexercise recovery. They are ideal for use where appetite is suppressed following exercise, access to food is limited postexercise, or the athlete has minimal time to eat between exercise sessions.
- They provide a compact, low-fiber source of carbohydrate; thus, they are useful as part of preevent meal for athletes at high risk of gastrointestinal problems during exercise and are useful in making-weight strategies as a low-residue snack.
- Bars are a convenient, portable, nonperishable snack providing energy, a balance of carbohydrate and protein, and micronutrients; thus they are useful for the athlete with a busy lifestyle and for a traveling athlete who has minimal facilities for food preparation and storage.

Research Support

- The use of sport bars to achieve sports nutrition goals is well supported.

Concerns Associated With Use

- Sport bars are often overused, leading to inappropriate replacement of whole foods and overreliance on expensive alternatives. Food sources should always be considered as the first option for meals and snacks.

- Fluid needs should also be considered during and after exercise.
- Athletes should be encouraged to practice using sport bars and to assess tolerance during training before using in the competition setting.
- Some sport bars are manufactured with higher-fat, lower-carbohydrate composition—especially to fit the Zone diet (40:30:30) energy ratio. There is no evidence to support performance benefits of this diet (see chapter 6: The Zone Diet, and table 4.f).

Sport Gels

Gels provide a highly concentrated source of carbohydrate (65-70%) in easily consumed and quickly digested gel form. They are substantially more concentrated in carbohydrate than sport drinks to provide a large fuel boost in a single serving. Some gels contain added electrolytes.

Potential Situations for Use

- Gels provide a compact fuel source for endurance sports lasting longer than 90 min, especially where it is impractical to carry large amounts of sport drinks (i.e., cycling, triathlon).
- Gels provide a compact fuel source for team sports athletes during breaks in play during extended training or competition sessions.
- Gels provide a compact and portable source of carbohydrate for postexercise recovery when regular foods are not tolerated by the athlete.
- Gels provide a low-fiber and compact preevent snack for athletes unable to tolerate regular foods and fluids.

Research Support
The use of sport gels to achieve sports nutrition goals is well supported.

Concerns Associated With Use

- Gels are a high-cost alternative to other suitable foods and fluids and should therefore be used only in specific situations for which they are most suited, rather than a general snack.
- Gastrointestinal intolerance may occur because of the concentrated carbohydrate load.
- Sport gels should always be consumed with adequate fluid to meet hydration needs.
- Athletes should practice use of gels and assess tolerance during training sessions if they are intended for use during competition.
- Gels may lead to overconsumption and overreliance on low-nutrient carbohydrate sources.
- Some gels contain other compounds such as medium-chain triglycerides, which may be poorly tolerated.

Multivitamin and Mineral Supplements

These supplements take the form of a broad-range, low-dose formulation of vitamins and minerals.

Potential Situations for Use

- These supplements can be used by athletes undertaking a prolonged period of travel, particularly to countries with an inadequate or otherwise limited food supply.
- They can be used by athletes undertaking a prolonged period of restricted energy intake (e.g., daily intakes below 8 MJ or 1,900 kcal for females or 10 MJ or 2,300 kcal for males for weight loss or weight maintenance.
- Multivitamin and mineral supplements are useful for athletes following a restricted dietary intake who are unable or unwilling to increase food range.
- They are useful for athletes undertaking heavy competition schedule, involving disruption to normal eating patterns.
- These supplements may be used to provide a placebo for athlete insisting on supplement use.

Research Support

- Athletes who restrict their total energy intake or dietary variety are at risk of an inadequate intake of vitamins and minerals.
- There is no evidence that supplementation with vitamins and minerals enhances performance except in cases where a preexisting deficiency exists.

Concerns

These supplements may provide a false sense of security to athletes who are otherwise eating poorly.

Antioxidant Vitamins C and E

A sudden increase in training stress leads to a temporary increase in the production of free oxygen radicals. Supplementation with antioxidant vitamins may help to reduce the oxidative damage until the body's antioxidant system adapts to the new challenge.

Potential Situations for Use

These antioxidants can be used for short-term supplementation for athletes undertaking a sudden increase in training stress or a shift to a more stressful environment (e.g., heat, altitude).

Research Support

There is no consistent evidence of performance enhancement following antioxidant supplement. Benefits may be subtle or short-lived.

Concerns

- Antioxidant systems are complex. There is a potential for antioxidant supplements to act as pro-oxidants if taken in excess.

- If adaptations to a training stimulus or other desirable physiological processes are achieved through pathways involving oxidative processes, antioxidant supplementation may reduce the effectiveness of the response.

Iron Supplement

Iron supplements are manufactured in a formulation providing ~100 mg of elemental iron per dose as ferrous gluconate or sulphate. Iron supplementation is a recommended therapy to treat iron deficiency: 100 mg/day taken on an empty stomach with vitamin C for 12 weeks until biochemical and hematological parameters improve.

Potential Situations for Use

Reduced iron status is a potential problem in some athletes whose dietary intake fails to meet iron requirements.

- Some athletes have a low intake of bioavailable iron because of poorly chosen vegetarian diets, chronic low-energy diets, and other dietary patterns that involve infrequent intake of red meat and inadequate substitution with other foods or combinations providing bioavailable iron.
- Some athletes have increased iron requirements: female athletes (menses), adolescent athletes undergoing significant growth spurts, pregnant athletes, and athletes adapting to altitude or heat training.
- Some athletes have increased iron losses because of gastrointestinal bleeding (e.g., ulcers, use of some anti-inflammatory drugs), excessive hemolysis caused by increased training stress (e.g., footstrike hemolysis in runners), and other blood losses (e.g., surgery, nosebleeds, contact sports).
- Iron supplementation may assist in the treatment or prevention of reduced iron status in athletes but should be considered part of a treatment package and taken under medical supervision.

Research Support

- Iron-deficiency anemia impairs exercise performance and adaptation.
- There is some evidence that female athletes who are not anemic but have low ferritin levels (<20 ng/ml) may show improvements in some performance-related parameters following iron supplementation.
- It is difficult to set ideal levels of hemoglobin and serum ferritin for optimal performance or levels that can diagnose suboptimal iron status. Typically, levels below 20 or 30 ng/ml are considered worthy of intervention. However, the individual history of the athlete and the presence of risk factors for reduced iron status should be considered in making a diagnosis (refer to chapter 5, reduced iron status in runners).

Concerns

- Excessive iron intake in some athletes may lead to hemochromatosis.
- Some iron preparations cause gastrointestinal upsets and constipation.
- Intravenous and intramuscular iron supplementation carries the extra risk of anaphylactic shock and problems involved with the use of needles.
- Iron supplementation per se does not deal with all the problems of eating patterns that are inadequate in energy and nutrients. Additional treatment and dietary counseling should be provided.

Calcium Supplement

Calcium is available in a formulation providing ~500 mg of elemental calcium in a dose as calcium gluconate.

Potential Situations for Use

Poor calcium balance may occur in individuals with inadequate calcium intake or with elevated calcium requirements.

- Low intake: Athletes who eat an inadequate energy intake or inadequate amounts of dairy and fortified soy products are at risk of an inadequate calcium intake.
- Calcium requirements are elevated by growth in children and adolescence (1,200 mg/day), pregnancy (1,200 mg/day), and breast-feeding (1,200 mg/day).
- Increased calcium intake may be needed to ensure calcium balance in female athletes with impaired menstrual status (1,500 mg/day).
- Calcium supplementation and intake of calcium-fortified foods (see chapter 13) may be needed to meet calcium intake goals in some individuals. Calcium supplementation should be used under medical supervision as part of an integrated program for bone health.

Research Support

- Inadequate calcium intake during key periods of lifecycle may lead to suboptimal bone status. See chapter 13 for more information.

Concerns Associated With Use

- Calcium supplementation does not guarantee bone status in absence of an adequate estrogen and progesterone status. Athletes with impaired menstrual status should receive appropriate attention to hormonal status and the dietary problems that underpin it.
- Athletes with disordered eating or eating disorders require significant treatment in addition to calcium supplementation. Inadequate energy and nutrient status are often difficult to correct without the cooperation of the athlete.

Creatine

Creatine is a naturally occurring compound found in large amounts in skeletal muscle as a result of dietary intake and endogenous synthesis from amino acids. Creatine monohydrate is the most common of creatine supplements.

- Muscle creatine content varies between individuals, perhaps related to gender, age, or fiber type (for review, see Hespel et al. 2001).
- The typical carnivorous diet provides approximately 2 g of creatine per day, but vegetarians have reduced body creatine stores, suggesting that endogenous production cannot totally compensate for the lack of dietary intake (Green et al. 1997). High dietary intakes temporarily suppress endogenous creatine production but increase muscle creatine and phosphocreatine content. Typical increase is ~20% up to a threshold of ~150-160 mmol/kg of dry weight muscle (Hespel et al. 2001; Hultman and Greenhaff 2000).
- There is considerable variability in response to creatine supplementation (for review, see Snow and Murphy 2003).
  - *Some individuals (perhaps 30% of the population) fail to increase muscle creatine content by a sufficiently large amount to affect exercise performance (Casey et al. 1996).*
  - *Response to creatine supplements may be related to initial creatine stores, with individuals with lowest levels often showing the greatest response. This may include vegetarians (Burke, Chilibeck, et al. 2003).*
  - *Individuals with preexisting stores of creatine close to threshold are unlikely to show additional benefit of creatine supplementation.*
- Creatine loading protocols have been well studied (for review, see Casey and Greenhaff 2000):
  - *Rapid loading may be achieved by 5 days of repeated doses (e.g., four 5 g doses) of creatine (Hultman et al. 1996).*
  - *A similar loading will occur over a longer period (28 days) with a slow loading protocol involving a daily dose of 3 g (Hultman et al. 1996).*
  - *Strategies to enhance creatine loading outcomes include co-ingestion with a substantial (50-100 g) amount of carbohydrate (Green et al. 1996) and exercise or training (Harris et al. 1992). These strategies may help all individuals to respond to creatine supplementation and reach the muscle creatine storage threshold.*
  - *Once the muscle creatine content has been saturated it will take at least 4 weeks to return to resting levels. A daily maintenance dose of 3 g will allow elevated levels to be sustained (Preen et al. 2003).*

- Phosphorylated creatine provides a number of important functions related to fuel supply in the muscle. The most well-known role is as an immediate and short-lived source of phosphate to regenerate adenosine triphosphate. The creatine phosphate system is the most important fuel source for sprints or bouts of high-intensity exercise lasting up to 10s.
- Creatine supplementation augments carbohydrate storage (Van Loon et al. 2004) and supercompensation (Robinson et al. 1999) in exercise muscle.

Potential Situations for Use

- Creatine supplementation may enhance the performance of a single high-intensity sprint or exercise bout, which is dependent on phosphocreatine stores.
- Creatine supplementation can enhance the performance of exercise involving repeated sprints or bouts of high-intensity exercise, separated by short recovery intervals. Such an exercise protocol is limited by resynthesis of phosphocreatine stores between bouts.
- Creatine can be used in a resistance training program to further increase lean body mass and strength.
- Creatine can be used in interval and sprint training programs.
- Creatine supplementation can be used during training and competition in sports involving intermittent work patterns (e.g., team and racket sports).
- Creatine can enhance the effectiveness of carbohydrate-loading program for endurance exercise.
- Enhancement of competition performance may be seen as a result of an acute loading protocol but also through chronic use to promote superior training adaptations.

Research Support

Various reviews and meta-analyses summarize the extensive creatine supplementation literature (Branch 2003; Greenhaff 2000; Hespel et al. 2001; Juhn and Tarnopolsky 1998a, 1998b; Kreider 1998). In general, the best supported use of creatine supplementation is for scenarios involving repeated sprints.

- Resistance training (see chapter 11: Strength and Power Sports, including table 11.c)
- Interval and sprint training (chapter 7: Sprinting and Jumping, including table 7.b)
- Team and racket sports (Tables 8.d, 9.d, and 10.c, chapter 10: research topic)
- There is no clear evidence for benefits to aerobic or endurance performance, although the potential benefits arising from enhanced glycogen storage have not been investigated. Conversely, the weight gain associated with creatine supplementation may cause a performance decrement in weight-sensitive

sports (chapter 5: Middle- and Long-Distance Running, table 5.e)
- Additional research is warranted using elite athletes and sport-specific tests including field studies.

Concerns Associated With Use

- Many athletes who use creatine either are unaware of correct supplementation protocols or persist in using unnecessarily high doses of creatine. Studies show that high doses of creatine do not further enhance creatine stores (Casey and Greenhaff 2000).
- An acute weight gain of 600 to 1,000 g is typically associated with loading and may represent water gain. This associated weight gain may be counterproductive to athletes competing in sports where power-to-weight ratio is a key factor in successful performance or those competing in weight-division sports.
- The long-term consequences of creatine use are unknown. There are anecdotal reports of an increased risk of muscle cramps, strains, and tears, but studies to date have not reported an increased risk of these events (see chapter 10: research topic). Creatine use in the doses presented here has not been seen to alter kidney function in otherwise healthy people.
- Creatine supplementation should be limited to well-developed athletes. Young athletes are able to make substantial gains in performance through maturation in age and training, without the need to expose themselves to the expense or small potential for long-term consequences of creatine use.

Bicarbonate and Citrate

High rates of anaerobic glycolysis by muscle during high-intensity exercise are associated with a build-up of lactate and hydrogen ions. When intracellular buffering capacity is exceeded, lactate and hydrogen ions diffuse into the extracellular space, perhaps aided by a positive pH gradient.

- It has long been known that alterations to blood pH change capacity for anaerobic glycolysis: Dietary strategies that decrease blood pH impair high-intensity exercise, whereas alkalotic therapies improve such performance (Dennig et al. 1931; Dill et al. 1932).
- Extracellular buffering capacity can be increased by loading with bicarbonate or citrate. These supplements may be taken in form of specialized sport supplements, as household products (e.g., bicarb soda), or as pharmaceutical urinary alkalinizers (McNaughton 2000).
- Typical doses for acute loading are 300 mg/kg bicarbonate and 300 to 500 mg/kg citrate, taken 1 to 2 hr before exercise. Buffering agents should be consumed with 1 to 2 L of water to reduce gastrointestinal problems attributable to osmotic diarrhea.

- A longer-term loading protocol with bicarbonate (500 mg·kg^{-1}·day^{-1}, spread over the day) may provide a more sustained increase in blood pH, with benefits being maintained for at least 1 day following the last bicarbonate dose (McNaughton et al. 2000; McNaughton and Thompson 2001). This protocol may be suited to

  - athletes who compete in a series of events spread over a couple of days (replacing the need to undertake multiple acute dose protocols), or

  - athletes who suffer gastrointestinal problems following intake of large doses of buffer agents (doses used in chronic protocol can be spread over the day and can be stopped the day before the athlete's event).

Potential Situations for Use

- An increase in extracellular buffering capacity may aid an athlete's capacity to produce power during sports or events limited by excessive buildup of hydrogen ions.

- Bicarbonate or citrate supplements can be used in high-intensity events lasting 1 to 7 min.

- These supplements can be used in sports involving repeated high-intensity sprints (e.g., team and racket sports).

- They can be used in prolonged high-intensity events lasting 30 to 60 min.

- Recent research suggests that chronic or repeated use of acute bicarbonate supplementation before interval training sessions can enhance training adaptations and improve subsequent performance of sustained high-intensity exercise.

Research Support

- A meta-analysis of 29 randomized, double-blind, crossover investigations of bicarbonate loading and exercise performance (Matson and Tran 1993) concluded that it has a moderate positive effect (weighted effect size of 0.44, meaning that the mean performance of the bicarbonate trial was 0.44 standard deviations better than the placebo trial). Overall, the relationship between increased blood alkalinity (increase in pH and bicarbonate) in bicarbonate trial and the performance outcome was weak. However, ergogenic effects were related to the level of metabolic acidosis achieved during the exercise, suggesting the importance of attaining a threshold pH gradient across the cell membrane from the combination of the accumulation of intracellular H$^+$ and the extracellular alkalosis.

- Performance outcomes vary between events and individuals. Few studies have been undertaken within an applied sports setting.

- The best supported use of bicarbonate or citrate loading is for events of 1 to 7 min of high-intensity exercise (see tables 5.d, 6.e, and 7.b).

- There is some evidence for benefits from bicarbonate loading to prolonged intermittent sprint protocols (see table 8.e) and prolonged high-intensity events (see tables 4.e and 5.d).

- There is new evidence that repeated use of bicarbonate loading before interval-based training sessions can increase training adaptations and enhance subsequent performance of sustained high-intensity exercise, at least when undertaken by moderately trained people (see table 6.e).

Concerns Associated With Use

- There have been reports of gastrointestinal distress following bicarbonate use

- Although the use of bicarbonate/citrate is not banned by anti-doping laws, it may cause acute changes in urinary pH. If an athlete is selected for a drug test, it may take hours for his or her urine to return to the pH ranges that are considered acceptable within sample collection protocols. The athlete may be required to wait at the Doping Control area until an accepetable sample is produced.

Caffeine

Caffeine occurs naturally in the leaves, nuts, and seeds of a number of plants. It enjoys social acceptance and widespread use around the world. Major dietary sources of caffeine, such as tea, coffee, chocolate, and cola drinks, typically provide 30 to 200 mg of caffeine per serving, whereas some nonprescription medications contain 100 to 200 mg of caffeine per tablet. The addition of caffeine (or guarana) to energy drinks, confectionary foods, and sport foods and supplements has increased the opportunities for athletes to consume caffeine, either as part of their everyday diet or for specific use as an ergogenic aid (see table 3.3). In January 1, 2004, caffeine was removed from the World Anti-Doping Agency (WADA) list of banned substances, allowing athletes who compete in sports that are compliant with the WADA code to consume caffeine, within their usual diets or for specific purposes of performance enhancement, without fear of sanctions. Caffeine has numerous actions on different body tissues. The actions may vary between individuals and include both positive and negative responses. Effects include the mobilization of fats from adipose tissue and the muscle cell, changes to muscle contractility, alterations to the central nervous system to change perceptions of effort or fatigue, stimulation of the release and activity of adrenaline, and effects on cardiac muscle. Recent evidence has changed perspective on two of the widely promoted effects of caffeine:

- That caffeine enhances endurance performance because it promotes an increase in the utilization of fat as an exercise fuel and spares the use of the limited muscle stores of glycogen. In fact, studies now show that the effect of caffeine on glycogen sparing during submaximal exercise is short-lived and inconsistent. (For reviews, see Graham 2001a and 2001b.)

- That caffeine-containing drinks have a diuretic effect and cause an athlete to become dehydrated. Caffeine-containing drinks such as tea, coffee, and cola drinks provide a significant source of fluid in the everyday diets of many people and any effect of caffeine on urine losses is minor, particularly in people who are habitual caffeine users. (For review, see Armstrong 2002.)

- Traditional protocols for the use of caffeine involve the intake of caffeine 1 hr before an exercise bout, in doses equivalent to ~6 mg/kg (e.g., 300-500 mg for a typical athlete). There is new evidence, at least from studies involving prolonged exercise lasting 60 min or longer, that beneficial effects from caffeine occur in the following cases:

- At small to moderate levels of intake (1-3 mg/kg of body weight or 50-200 mg of caffeine).

- When caffeine is taken at a variety of times (before or throughout exercise, or toward the end of exercise when the athlete is becoming fatigued.

- Without evidence of a dose–response relationship to caffeine; that is, performance benefits do *not* increase with increases in the caffeine dose.

Potential Situations for Use

- Caffeine has the potential to enhance the performance of a range of exercise protocols.

- Caffeine can be used during prolonged endurance or intermittent sports, including team sports, as a training aid or competition aid.

- Caffeine can be used before high-intensity events, as a training aid or competition aid.

- The mechanism underpinning performance benefits is unclear but is likely to involve alterations to the perception of effort or fatigue, as well as direct effects on the muscle.

Research Support

There is sound evidence that caffeine enhances endurance and provides a small but worthwhile enhancement of performance over a range of exercise protocols. These include the following:

- Short-duration, high-intensity events (1-5 min) (see tables 6.e and 7.b)

- Prolonged high-intensity events (20-60 min) (see tables 4.e and 5.d)

- Endurance events (≥90 min continuous exercise) tables 4.e and 5.d)

- Ultraendurance events (≥4 hr)

- Prolonged intermittent sprint events (team and racket sports) (see table 8.d)

- The effect on strength and power and sprints (10-20 sec) is unclear (see table 7.b).

- Further research is needed to define the range of caffeine intake protocols that provide performance enhancements and the range of sports

that may benefit from caffeine supplementation.

- Most studies of caffeine and performance have been undertaken in laboratories. Studies that investigate performance effects in elite athletes under field conditions or during real-life sports events are scarce and need to be undertaken before specific recommendations for caffeine supplementation protocols can be made.

Concerns Associated With Use

- Coffee is not an ideal source of caffeine for supplementation protocols because of the variability and unpredictability of the caffeine content of coffee drinks as served (Desbrow et al. in press). There is some evidence that other compounds in coffee may negate the ergogenic effect of caffeine (Graham et al. 1998), although another study showed that the previous intake of coffee does not negate the beneficial effects of larger amounts of caffeine taken just before exercise (McLellan and Bell 2004). Further research is needed on this issue, because in the real world, athletes often consume coffee before competing or training, either as part of their normal social and dietary patterns or as an intentional source of caffeine as an ergogenic aid (see table 3.3).

- It appears that current caffeine intake practices of athletes are ad hoc and unsystematic. Sport scientists observe that caffeine intake practices, both in social settings and in protocols deliberately undertaken to enhance training and competition performance, involve large or unmeasured doses or caffeine, a lack of awareness of the potential for side effects or negative outcomes from caffeine use, and a lack of awareness of emerging information about caffeine and sports performance.

- At higher levels of intake, caffeine has the potential to cause increases in heart rate, impairments or alterations of fine motor control and technique, and overarousal (interfering with recovery and sleep patterns). Impairment of technique may affect the performance of a number of sports, and overarousal may interfere with the ability to recover between training sessions or multiday competitions. These concerns add to the importance of finding the lowest effective dose of caffeine that can be used to achieve a performance enhancement.

- The efficacy of repeated doses of caffeine—for example, use for heats and finals, or multiple games in a tournament—also requires investigation. One study found that exercise endurance was enhanced in both a morning and an afternoon trial on the same day following repeated doses of caffeine. However, endurance was also enhanced in the afternoon trial when only a morning dose of caffeine was consumed (Bell and McLellan 2003).

- Caffeine may interact with other supplements and nutrients used by athletes (e.g., bicarbonate, cre-

Table 3.3 Caffeine Content of Common Foods and Drinks

Food or drink	Serving	Caffeine content (mg)
Instant coffee	250 ml cup	60 (12-169)[a]
Brewed coffee	250 ml cup	80 (40-110)[a]
Espresso or short black	1 serving	107 (25-214)[b]
Tea	250 ml cup	27 (9-51)[a]
Hot chocolate	250 ml cup	5-10
Chocolate bar—milk	60 g	5-15
Chocolate—dark	60 g	10-50
Viking chocolate bar	60 g	58
Coca-Cola	375 ml can	49
Pepsi Cola	375 ml can	40
Jolt soft drink	375 ml can	75
Red Bull energy drink	250 ml can	80
Red Eye Power energy drink	250 ml can	50
V energy drink	250 ml can	50
Smart Drink—Brain Fuel	250 ml can	80
Lift Plus energy drink	250 ml can	36
Lipovitan energy drink	250 ml can	50
Black Stallion energy drink	250 ml can	80
Powergel caffeinated sport gel (strawberry–banana and chocolate)	40 g sachet	25
Powergel double caffeinated gel (tangerine)	40 g sachet	50
Gu caffeinated sport gel (chocolate, vanilla, mixed berry, and orange burst	32 g sachet	20

The caffeine content of tea and coffee varies widely, depending on the brand, the way that the individual makes the beverage, and the size of the mug or cup. These values are for [a]a range of beverages as prepared by participants in a study or [b]a standard coffee from various commercial venues (Desbrow et al. in press). Some franchises (e.g., Starbucks) sell special brews that come in large volumes with extra-strong varieties of coffee. Some of these drinks can provide 500 to 1,000 mg of caffeine per serving.

Adapted from Australian Institute of Sport. www.ais.org.au/nutrition.

atine, carbohydrate), which needs to be explored in terms of performance outcomes and potential side effects.

- Although evidence of specific health problems is equivocal, long-term intake of large amounts of caffeine (>500 mg/day) is generally discouraged by health authorities.

Glycerol

Glycerol is a naturally occurring metabolite that provides the backbone of triglyceride (fat) molecules.

- When ingested, glycerol is rapidly absorbed and distributed throughout the body's compartments, until gradually excreted over the next 24 to 48 hr.
- Loading protocol is 1 to 1.5 g of glycerol per kilogram of body mass, consumed 2 hr preevent with a fluid load of 25 to 35 ml fluid per kilogram.
- Glycerol exerts a concentration or osmotic effect that allows the body to temporarily retain extra fluid that is consumed at the same time as the glycerol. Studies generally show that ~600 ml of fluid can be retained and is more effective than water loading alone.

Potential Situations for Use

- Glycerol can provide hyperhydration for an endurance athlete training or competing in hot humid conditions, where excessive fluid losses cannot be replaced sufficiently during the exercise.
- Glycerol can provide enhanced rehydration after weigh-in in weight-division or weight-restricted sports where dehydration has been used to make weight.

Research Support

- Studies on the effects on thermoregulation and performance have provided mixed results, but some studies have shown benefits to the performance of moderate- to high-intensity exercise performed in the heat by highly trained athletes (Anderson et al. 2001; Coutts et al. 2002; Hitchins et al. 1999). Details of these studies are provided in chapter 4; see table 4.e). Effectiveness may depend on environmental conditions and training and competition situations.

Concerns Associated With Use

- Some side effects are noted in individuals, including headaches and gastrointestinal problems, particularly when glycerol is consumed after a meal.
- Experimentation is required to ensure that performance is not impaired by additional body mass attributable to water loading.

Colostrum

Colostrum is a protein-rich substance secreted in breast milk in the first few days after a mother has given birth. Colostrum supplements are typically produced from bovine (cow) sources.

- Colostrum is rich in immunoglobulins and insulin-like growth factors (IGFs). Unlike the adult gut, the gut of a baby has "leaky" junctions that allow it to absorb proteins including immunoglobulins, thus developing the immunocompetence needed to survive outside the uterus.
- Colostrum supplementation is claimed to improve exercise performance and recovery and possibly improve body composition.
- The typical colostrum supplementation protocol used in most investigations involves an intake of 20 to 60 g of colostrum powder or liquid each day, and the literature indicates that at least 4 weeks of supplementation may be required to induce a benefit. However, some recent studies show benefits from using low colostrum doses (10-20 g/ day) in some athletes or situations.

Potential Situations for Use

- There is no indication of the potential situations or athletic populations that might benefit from colostrum supplementation.

- A mechanism by which colostrum supplementation benefits athletic performance remains speculative.

Research Support

- A modest number of studies have been conducted and published in peer-reviewed literature (Antonio et al. 2001; Brinkworth et al. 2002, 2004; Buckley et al. 2002, 2003; Coombes et al. 2002; Hofman et al. 2002; Kuipers et al. 2002; Mero et al. 1997, 2002, 2005; Shing et al. 2006). Details of these studies are presented in tables in the appendixes to chapters 4 through 8 and 11.
- Although these studies are well controlled and involve long-term supplementation with colostrum, they have been unable to show consistent or universal effects on athletic performance.
- Changes in body composition following colostrum supplementation are not consistent. Although one study reported an increase in lean body mass following a period of colostrum supplementation (Antonio et al. 2001), other studies found no changes in body mass or body composition (Hofman et al. 2002). A study that involved measurement of protein metabolism following a resistance training session found that colostrum supplementation failed to enhance net protein balance during recovery despite an increased plasma level of essential amino acids (Mero et al. 2005)
- A review of logbooks kept by participants in 8-week colostrum supplementation trials suggested that treatment resulted in fewer self-reported episodes of upper respiratory tract infections than reported by placebo-treated participants (Brinkworth and Buckley 2003). However, no difference in upper respiratory tract symptoms were found over 12 weeks of supplementation with placebo or colostrum in distance runners (Crooks et al. 2006). Colostrum supplementation has been reported to increase salivary immunoglobulin A in some (Crooks et al. 2006; Mero et al. 2002) but not all (Mero et al. 1997) studies.
- Although a few studies indicate that colostrum supplementation increases IGF-1 (Mero et al. 1997, 2002), other studies have failed to demonstrate this (Buckley et al. 2002; Kuipers et al. 2002).
- A mechanism by which colostrum supplementation benefits athletic performance remains speculative.

Concerns Associated With Use

- Colostrum supplementation is expensive. A colostrum supplementation protocol of 20 to 60 g/day typically costs $US20 to 50 per week. There is a need to investigate whether benefits can be achieved with smaller doses.
- Not all colostrum supplements are the same; even if some can be shown to provide benefits to athletic performance, this finding may not apply to all products.

β-Hydroxy β-methylbutyrate

β-hydroxy β-methylbutyrate (HMB) is a by-product of the essential amino acid leucine, proposed to influence muscle protein metabolism and cell membrane integrity. HMB is claimed to act as an anticatabolic agent, minimizing protein breakdown and the cellular damage that occurs with high-intensity exercise. It has been proposed that the anticatabolic effects sometimes seen associated with leucine feeding during times of stress are mediated by HMB. HMB is typically prescribed at a dose of 3 g/day in three divided doses of 1 g. Higher doses have been proven to be ineffective.

Potential Situations for Use

HMB supplementation is claimed to decrease protein breakdown associated with heavy training and in doing so enhance muscle size and strength development, promote fat loss, and attenuate exercise-induced muscle damage.

Research Support

- Several studies of HMB supplementation and resistance training have been reported in the peer-reviewed literature (Crowe et al. 2003; Gallagher et al. 2000; Hoffman et al. 2004; Jowko et al. 2001; Knitter et al. 2000; Kreider et al. 1999; Nissen et al. 1996; O'Connor and Crowe 2003; Paddon-Jones et al. 2001; Panton et al. 2000; Ransone et al. 2003; Slater et al. 2001). Indexes under investigation include changes in muscle strength, body composition, and muscle damage. Details of these studies are provided in the appendixes to chapters 4, 6, 8, 9, and 11.

- Interpretation of the data from the available literature is difficult because of limitations in assessment techniques and a lack of control over parameters likely to influence results (e.g., diet, training load, and gender).

- Most of the evidence supporting the use of HMB has been collected on previously untrained individuals. Extrapolation of this information to trained individuals should be viewed with caution because of natural training-induced adaptations (e.g., decrease in muscle protein breakdown associated with resistance training).

- One theory is that HMB supplementation might be most valuable in the early phases of a new training program or when previously untrained participants undertake resistance training, when it is able to reduce the large catabolic response or damage produced by unaccustomed exercise. However, once adaptation to training occurs, reducing the residual catabolism and damage response, HMB supplementation no longer provides a detectable benefit. This theory explains why HMB tends to produce favorable results in novice resistance trainers rather than well-trained participants and

why positive results are reported in shorter studies (i.e., 2-4 weeks) but not at the end of longer studies (i.e., 8 weeks).

- A recent meta-analysis of existing HMB supplementation studies found that the overall effect of supplementation is a small improvement in gain in muscle mass (effect size = 0.15) and strength (effect size = 0.19) when combined with resistance training (Nissen and Sharp 2003). This meta-analysis has received criticism because the studies emanate from only three different laboratories and may show experimental bias because of interdependence (Decombaz et al. 2003). Further research is needed.

Glutamine

Glutamine is an amino acid that provides an important fuel source for immune cells. It plays a major role in protein metabolism; in some circumstances it provides an antiproteolytic effect by offsetting the catabolic effects of glucocorticoid hormones.

- Studies in the early 1990s identified lowered plasma glutamine level as a marker of overtraining and fatigue in athletes, but a consensus has not yet been reached on how to best use this information.

- Glutamine supplementation is promoted as a nutritional supplement for athletes to maintain or boost immune function or to maintain muscle protein levels during periods of intensive training. It is claimed to prevent or lessen the severity of illness, particularly in susceptible athletes.

- Daily glutamine supplementation of 0.1 to 0.3 g/kg of body weight appears to be safe and shows no evidence of clinical toxicity after several weeks. Larger doses up to 0.6 $g\cdot kg^{-1}\cdot day^{-1}$ show no harmful effects after 5 days of administration in normal participants.

Potential Situations for Use

Glutamine can be used for prevention or clinical management of overtraining in susceptible athletes.

Research Support

- There is conflicting evidence about whether glutamine supplementation can attenuate postexercise decreases in plasma glutamine concentration.

- There is no conclusive evidence demonstrating that glutamine supplementation lowers incidence of illness in healthy athletes who consume adequate levels of protein.

- There is no evidence that chronic glutamine supplementation enhances the response to resistance training by reducing in protein breakdown (Candow et al. 2001; Falk et al. 2003; Lehmkuhl et al. 2003). Details of these studies are provided in the appendixes to chapters 7 and 11 (table 11.c).

Ribose

Ribose is a pentose (5 carbon sugar) naturally found in the diet. It provides the backbone of DNA, RNA, and adenine nucleotides (adenosine triphosphate, adenosine diphosphate, and adenosine monophosphate). The chemical production of ribose has become possible, and this product is now found in a number of commercial supplements, often in conjunction with creatine.

- The pentose phosphate pathway produces an intermediary phosphoribosyl pyrophosphate (PRPP), which participates in the synthesis or salvaging of adenosine triphosphate in the muscle cell. The synthesis of PRPP is thought to be a limiting step in this activity. It is proposed that ribose supplementation will bypass this limiting factor by increasing PRPP synthesis, thus enhancing the restoration of adenosine triphosphate levels in the cell.

- Clinical studies identify that some patients with ischemic heart disease have low PRPP levels. In such patients, ribose supplementation increases PRPP and improves cardiac function and exercise tolerance. This is clearly a situation in which PRPP is limiting.

Potential Situations for Use

- Repeated sprints of high-intensity exercise reduce the adenosine triphosphate and adenine nucleotide pool in the muscle cell by ~20%, which may persist for several days. In such a situation, ribose supplementation may be effective in enhancing de novo synthesis and recycling of these nucleotides, thus enhancing the recovery of the muscle adenosine triphosphate content.

- Supplementation protocols in recent studies typically involve daily doses of 10 to 20 g of ribose and have targeted athletes undertaking intermittent high-intensity exercise programs (weight training, interval training).

Research Support

- Several studies that have appeared in abstract form as conference presentations have reported favorable results following ribose supplementation in heavily training athletes. The brief form of these reports does not provide sufficient information to judge the quality of the study and the interpretation of results. Most of these studies have not appeared in full publication in peer-reviewed literature, although in many cases, several years have passed since the original presentation.

- Eight other studies have now been published in full in peer-reviewed journals. Details of these studies are provided in the appendixes to chapters 6, 7, and 11.

- One of these studies reported an improved outcome in the gains of a resistance training program when recreational level athletes consumed ribose supple-

ments, compared with a control group consuming a placebo (Van Gammeren et al. 2002).

- All other studies have failed to find a significant or consistent performance improvement in heavily training athletes who consumed ribose supplements, compared with a placebo trial (Berardi and Ziegenfuss 2003; Dunne et al. 2006; Falk et al. 2003; Hellsten et al. 2004; Kerksick et al. 2005; Kreider, Melton, Greenwood, et al. 2003; Op 't Eijnde et al. 2001). In fact, in one study, the group of rowers who received the placebo treatment (a small dose of dextrose) before and after training showed an enhanced improvement of their rowing performance at the end of 8 weeks compared with the rowers who received an equivalent amount of ribose (Dunne et al. 2006).

- In summary, there is no clear evidence to support benefits from ribose supplementation in well-trained athletes.

Concerns Associated With Use

- There are insufficient studies conducted over long time frames to allow discussion of health concerns associated with chronic intakes of large amounts of ribose, although oral intake of ribose is generally considered to be well tolerated.

- Ribose supplementation is expensive. At a recommended price of $70 for a 100 g supply, a daily dose of 10 to 20 g of ribose would cost $50 to $100 per week. It may take larger doses than this before benefits are seen.

Medium-Chain Triglycerides

Medium-chain triglycerides (MCTs) are fats composed of medium-chain fatty acids (MCFAs) with a chain length of 6 to 10 carbon molecules.

- MCTs are digested and metabolized differently than the long-chain fatty acids that make up most of our dietary fat intake.

- MCTs can be digested within the intestinal lumen with less need for bile and pancreatic juices than long-chain triglycerides.

- MCFAs are absorbed via the portal circulation.

- MCFAs can be taken up into the mitochondria without the need for carnitine-assisted transport.

- In clinical nutrition, MCT supplements derived from palm kernel and coconut oil are used as an energy supplement for patients who have various digestive or lipid metabolism disorders.

Potential Situations for Use

- MCTs are marketed as an easily absorbed and oxidized fuel source and a fat source that is less likely to deposit as body fat.

- MCTs could provide a fuel source during endurance and ultraendurance events that might spare glycogen and prolong the availability of endogenous carbohydrate stores. Co-ingestion of MCT with carbohydrate during prolonged exercise increases the rate of MCT oxidation, possibly by increasing its rate of absorption.

Research Support

- The role of MCTs as an energy in the general diet of athletes has not been well studied. Chronic intake was not shown to enhance substrate oxidation or performance (Misell et al. 2001). There is no information on effects on body fat deposition in athletes.

- The results of studies of MCT and carbohydrate during ultraendurance events are inconsistent. Table 4.f summarizes details of the available studies (Angus et al. 2000; Goedecke, Elmer-English, et al. 1999; Jeukendrup et al. 1998; Van Zyl et al. 1996; Vistisen et al. 2003). Results appear to depend on the amount of MCT that is ingested, the prevailing hormonal conditions, and the risk of gastrointestinal upsets.

- Studies in which the intake of large amounts of MCT raised plasma free fatty acid concentrations and allowed glycogen sparing, without substantial gastrointestinal side effects, have reported a performance benefit at the end of prolonged exercise (Van Zyl et al. 1996).

- Small intakes of MCTs that fail to change plasma free fatty acid content have no impact on metabolism and subsequent performance.

- Metabolic (and performance) benefits may be compromised when exercise is commenced with higher insulin levels, as is the case following a carbohydrate-rich preexercise meal (Angus et al. 2000; Goedecke, Elmer-English, et al. 1999).

- Underpinning the whole issue is the ability of participants to tolerate the substantial amount of MCT oils required to have a metabolic impact. The gastrointestinal tolerance of MCT is limited to a total intake of about 30 g, which would limit its fuel contribution to 3% to 7% of the total energy expenditure during typical ultraendurance events (Jeukendrup et al. 1995). In several studies, gastrointestinal upsets have impaired the performance of some (Jeukendrup et al. 1998) or most (Goedecke et al. 2005) participants.

- Differences in gastrointestinal tolerance between studies or within studies may reflect differences in the mean chain length of MCTs found in the supplements or increased tolerance in some athletes attributable to constant exposure to MCTs. The intensity and mode of exercise may also affect gastrointestinal symptoms.

Concerns Associated With Use

At intakes greater than 30 g, there is a high risk of gastrointestinal reactions that range in severity from insignificant

(Van Zyl et al. 1996) to performance limiting (Goedecke et al. 2005; Jeukendrup et al. 1998).

Chromium Picolinate

Chromium is an essential element, required in trace amounts. Dietary sources of chromium include yeast, nuts and legumes, some fruit and vegetables, chocolate, wine, and beer.

- Many countries have not set a recommended dietary intake for chromium; however, the U.S. Food and Nutrition Board has established an Estimated Safe and Adequate Daily Dietary Allowance (ESADDA) within the range of 50 to 200 µg/day (see Clarkson 1997).

- Dietary surveys often report the estimated chromium intake of many populations to be below this ESADDA; however, this may be an artifact of the lack of reliable food composition data for chromium. It has also been suggested that the ESADDA ranges for chromium have been set artificially high (for review, see Clarkson 1997).

- There is some evidence that daily training may increase urinary chromium losses, increasing chromium requirements and the risk of suboptimal chromium intakes. However, adaptations may also occur to improve absorption or retention of chromium in compensation (see Clarkson 1997). Athletes with restricted energy intakes are most at risk of low chromium intakes.

- Chromium supplements are available as nicotinate, chloride, and picolinate. Chromium picolinate is claimed to be the most biologically active form and is part of a patent held by the U.S. Department of Agriculture (Vincent 2003). It has become a popular supplement for weight loss, amassing annual sales of more than $US500 million (Vincent 2003).

- Typical chromium picolinate dosages are 200 to 400 µg/day.

Potential Situations for Use

Supplementation with chromium picolinate is claimed to increase muscle mass and reduce body fat by enhancing the disposal of glucose, amino acids, and fatty acids.

Research Support

- Claims for the efficacy of chromium picolinate have caused an interesting public debate between the patent holders and other trace element and mineral experts. This history is well documented by the review of Vincent (2003). The initial research that was used to publicize claims for chromium picolinate (Evans 1989) has been criticized for methodological flaws, such as lack of a control group, inadequate control of diet or training status, and the reliance on unreliable and insensitive methods of assessing body composition (Levafi 1993; Levafi et al. 1992).

- Several reviews of studies of the effects of chromium supplementation on body composition, in both obese participants and athletic populations, concluded that there is no clear evidence of changes to muscle mass or body fat levels above those achieved by training or dietary programs (Clarkson 1997; Lukaski 2001; Vincent 2003).
- There are few well-conducted studies involving acute (Davis et al. 2000) or chronic (Clancy et al. 1994; Hallmark et al. 1996; Hasten et al. 1992; Lukaski et al. 1996; Walker et al. 1998) supplementation with chromium in well-trained athletes. Details of these studies are provided in the appendixes to chapters 8 and 11.

Concerns Associated With Use

- Chromium potentially competes with trivalent iron for binding to transferrin, thus predisposing those with chronically high intakes of chromium to iron deficiency. Some (Lukaski et al. 1996), but not all (Campbell et al. 1997), studies have reported a reduction in iron status as a result of chromium picolinate supplementation.
- There is recent evidence that chromium picolinate probably causes oxidative damage of DNA, which warrants further research (Vincent 2003).

Coenzyme Q10

Coenzyme Q10, or ubiquinone, is a nonessential lipid-soluble nutrient found predominantly in animal foods and in low levels in plant foods. In the body it is located primarily in skeletal and cardiac muscle, inside the mitochondria.

- Coenzyme Q10 provides a link in the electron transport chain producing adenosine triphosphate and is part of the mitochondrial antioxidant defense system, preventing damage to DNA and cell membranes.
- Some cardiac and neuromuscular dysfunction is believed to result from coenzyme Q10 deficiency. Patients with ischemic heart disease often have low plasma coenzyme Q10 concentrations and improve their exercise capacity following coenzyme Q10 supplementation.
- The marketing campaigns for coenzyme Q10 supplement promote increased vigor and youthfulness as a benefit of their use.
- Typical dosage for supplementation is ~100 mg/day.

Potential Situations for Use

Coenzyme Q10 is claimed to enhance energy production and reduce the oxidative damage of exercise.

Research Support

- Peer-reviewed studies of coenzyme Q10 supplementation on exercise metabolism, oxidative damage caused by exercise, and performance are

summarized in the appendixes to chapters 4 and 5. Only one study has reported an ergogenic benefit of coenzyme Q10 on exercise performance; this study involved cross-country skiers (Ylikoski et al. 1997).

- By contrast, several studies have shown have shown evidence that coenzyme Q10 has an *ergolytic*, or negative, effect on high-intensity performance and training adaptations (Laaksonen et al. 1995; Malm et al. 1996, 1997). Data from these studies suggested that coenzyme Q10 supplementation does not increase muscle concentrations of Q10 and may *increase* the oxidative damage produced by high-intensity exercise in previously untrained participants as shown by increases in plasma creatine kinase in response to exercise (Malm et al. 1996). In these circumstances, coenzyme Q10 was believed to act as a pro-oxidant rather than an antioxidant. Training adaptations were impaired in healthy participants who undertook 5 days of high-intensity training while taking coenzyme Q10 supplements or in trained cyclists who undertook 6 weeks of supplementation, with the placebo group outperforming the coenzyme Q10 group at the end of the supplementation phase (Laaksonen et al. 1995; Malm et al. 1996, 1997).
- An increase in plasma Q10 concentrations in response to supplementation is not associated with an increase in Q10 concentrations in skeletal muscle or isolated skeletal muscle mitochondria (Svensson et al. 1999).
- Further work is required to investigate the effects of coenzyme Q10 supplementation on exercise performance and training.

Concerns Associated With Use

The issue of antioxidant supplementation is complex and as yet unsolved. There is evidence that supplementation with coenzyme Q10 can increase oxidative damage and impair the training response.

Pyruvate

Pyruvate is a 3-carbon carboxylic acid produced by the metabolism of glucose. It has two metabolic fates: (1) reduction to lactate in the cytosol or (2) oxidative decarboxylation to acetyl coenzyme A (CoA) by pyruvate dehydrogenase complex in the mitochondria.

- Two studies using sedentary participants reported that chronic supplementation (7 days) with large doses (100 g/day) of pyruvate and another 3-carbon metabolite, dihydroxyacetone (DHA), resulted in enhanced endurance in leg and arm ergometry protocols (Stanko, Robertson, Galbreath, et al. 1990; Stanko, Robertson, Spina, et al. 1990).
- Studies in animals and clinical situations have reported enhancement of fat loss with pyruvate and DHA supplementation; however, results are small

and hard to translate into a real-life setting (see Sukala 1998).

Potential Situations for Use

Marketing claims for pyruvate include enhancement of endurance performance and enhanced loss of body fat.

Research Support

- The marketing claims made for pyruvate supplements aimed at the weight loss market have been thoroughly reviewed and found to be unsupported hype (Sukala 1998).

- The available literature on pyruvate supplementation in athletic populations is scarce (Ebersole et al. 2000; Morrison et al. 2000; Stone et al. 1999; van Schuylenbergh et al. 2003) and does not support benefits to performance. Details of studies undertaken on athletes are summarized in the appendixes to chapters 4, 6, and 11.

Concerns Associated With Use

- The dosages used in the few studies reporting benefits in sedentary populations have been far larger than the manufacturer's recommended doses of commercially available products and have not provided DHA.

- Side effects reported from these large doses include significant gastrointestinal discomfort.

Inosine

Inosine is a nonessential nutrient with good dietary sources, including yeast and organ meats.

- Supplemental forms of inosine are available as a single chemical or as part of a multiagent formula targeting metabolic intermediaries.

- Suggested daily doses are 5,000 to 10,000 mg/day.

Potential Situations for Use

- Several theories have suggested mechanisms by which inosine supplementation could benefit exercise performance (for review, see Starling et al. 1996; Williams et al. 1990).

- Inosine is a precursor of the nucleotide inosine monophosphate (IMP) and could lead to an increase in adenosine triphosphate content.

- In vitro tests suggest that inosine may enhance the levels of 2,3-diphosphoglycerate in red blood cells, which theoretically could increase the release of oxygen into the muscle via a shift in the oxyhemoglobin curve.

- Inosine is believed to have vasodilatory effects and antioxidant properties.

Research Support

- The major support for inosine supplementation is testimonial, with reports from athletes, especially from Russian and Eastern European countries, and muscle-building magazines. One popular magazine, *Muscle and Fitness,* published an article describing a 6-week study of inosine supplementation on four trained athletes (Colgan 1988). The report claimed that the study was undertaken using a double-blind crossover design and found strength gains as a result of the supplementation. This study has not appeared in a peer-reviewed publication or in adequate detail to judge the validity of these claims. The athletes reported irritability and fatigue while taking the inosine supplements.

- Only four well-controlled studies of inosine supplementation in athletes have been published in the peer-reviewed literature. In one study, inosine was an ingredient in a multicompound ergogenic aid (CAPS) that failed to enhance performance of triathletes (Snider et al. 1992); see table 4.f.

- The three studies of isolated inosine supplementation all failed to find either favorable metabolic changes or performance benefits following inosine supplementation in well-trained participants (McNaughton, Dalton, and Tarr, et al. 1999; Starling et al. 1996; Williams et al. 1990). These studies are summarized in the appendixes to chapters 4, 5, and 7. There were no data to support any of the theoretical actions of inosine supplementation. Although muscle substrates were not directly measured in these studies, purported changes to adenosine triphosphate concentrations were unlikely to enhance exercise performance because adenosine triphosphate is not depleted by exercise, even at the point of fatigue.

- In fact, two studies reported that participants showed better performance of high-intensity tasks while on the placebo treatment than on the inosine trial, suggesting that inosine supplementation might actually impair the performance of high-intensity exercise (Starling et al. 1996; Williams et al. 1990). Potential mechanisms for exercise impairment include an increased formation of IMP in the muscle, either at rest or during exercise. High IMP concentrations have been found at the point of fatigue in many exercise studies; furthermore, IMP has been shown to inhibit adenosine triphosphatase activity (Sahlin 1992).

- Another possible mechanism of performance impairment is an increase in levels of uric acid, a product of inosine degradation. In three studies, 2 days of inosine supplementation did not change uric acid levels; however, 5 days and 10 days of intake doubled blood concentrations to levels above the normal range (McNaughton, Dalton, and Tarr, et al. 1999; Starling et al. 1996; Williams et al. 1990).

- Because there is a lack of evidence of performance benefits and the possibility of performance decrements and side effects, there is little to recommend the use of inosine supplements by athletes.

Concerns Associated With Use

- Chronic inosine supplementation may pose a health risk because high uric acid levels are implicated as a cause of gout.
- There is some evidence of performance impairment following inosine supplementation.

L-carnitine

Carnitine is a nonessential nutrient, found in dietary sources and manufactured in the liver and kidney from amino acid precursors (lysine and methionine). Most animal foods provide a dietary source of carnitine, but because of losses in cooking and preparation of foods, there are few data on the total content in the diet. Before the discovery of endogenous synthesis, the first reports on carnitine in the early 1900s described it as a vitamin (essential component of the diet).

- Carnitine is ingested or synthesized by humans in the l-isoform and is carried via the blood for storage, predominantly in the heart and skeletal muscle. Within these tissues, carnitine plays a number of roles related to fat and carbohydrate metabolism.
- Carnitine is a component of the enzymes carnitine palmityltransferase I (CPT-1), carnitine-palmityl-transferase II (CPT-II), and carnitine-acylcarnitine translocase (CAT), which are involved in the transportation of long-chain fatty acids (LCFAs) across the mitochondrial membrane to the site of their oxidation.
- During exercise, carnitine also plays the role of a "sink" for acetyl-CoA production. By converting this to acetyL-carnitine and CoA, carnitine helps to maintain CoA availability and to decrease the ratio of acetyl-CoA to CoA. When muscle carnitine activity is inadequate, as in the case of inborn errors of metabolism, individuals demonstrate lipid abnormalities and reduced exercise capacity. Carnitine supplementation is an established medical therapy for these conditions and helps to attenuate such symptoms.

Potential Situations for Use

- It has been suggested that carnitine supplementation might enhance fatty acid transport and oxidation.
  - *Carnitine is a popular component of supplements claimed to enhance the loss of body fat.*
  - *An increase in fatty acid oxidation during exercise could benefit endurance athletes if it resulted in a sparing of glycogen during events in which carbohydrate stores are otherwise limiting.*
- If carnitine supplementation could increase CoA availability, it might enhance flux through the citric acid cycle and enhance the activity of the enzyme pyruvate dehydrogenase, which is otherwise inhibited by high levels of acetyl-CoA. Increased oxidative metabolism of glucose could enhance high-intensity exercise that might otherwise be limited by excess lactate and hydrogen ion accumulation,

Research Support

Extensive reviews of carnitine function are available (Cerretelli and Marconi 1990; Clarkson 1992; Heinonen 1996; Wagenmakers 1991). They note that for carnitine supplementation to enhance exercise metabolism and performance, some of the following factors must occur:

- Heavy training must cause suboptimal levels of muscle carnitine.
- Carnitine supplementation must increase muscle carnitine content.
- Carnitine must be a limiting factor in fatty acid transport.
- Carnitine must be a limiting factor in pyruvate dehydrogenase activity or citric acid cycle flux levels.

However, the available evidence shows the following:

- Although studies have found an increase in plasma carnitine levels following carnitine supplementation of 1 to 6 g/day, muscle carnitine levels are not enhanced. However, a recent study showed that an increase in muscle carnitine uptake is possible with insulin stimulation and high plasma carnitine concentrations (Stephens et al. 2006); further research is required.
- Normal muscle carnitine levels appear to be adequate for maximal function of CPT-I and CPT-II.
- Pyruvate dehydrogenase is believed to be fully active within seconds of high-intensity exercise, and additional carnitine is unlikely to stimulate this activity further.

Studies that have investigated the effects of carnitine supplementation on exercise metabolism or performance have found little evidence of enhanced outcomes during submaximal or high-intensity exercise. Few studies have been undertaken on athletic populations; the results of available studies are summarized in the appendixes to chapters 4 through 6.

The effect of carnitine supplementation on body fat levels, although widely publicized in supplement advertising, has not been studied in athletic populations. A study on moderately obese sedentary females did not find evidence of enhanced loss of body fat with carnitine (Villani et al. 2000).

Concerns Associated With Use

Although studies of acute and long-term carnitine supplementation report that carnitine appears to be safe, this applies to L-carnitine preparations. It has been shown that D-carnitine causes depletion of L-carnitine in tissues, therefore creating a carnitine deficiency (Clarkson 1992). Athletes are advised to avoid commercial carnitine preparations that do not clearly specify that contents are >99% L-carnitine.

Ginseng and Other Herbal Tonics

There are several species of ginseng: American, Siberian, Korean, and Japanese (Bahrke and Morgan 1994). Although most of these ginsengs are related, belonging to the *Panax* species, Russian or Siberian ginseng is extracted from a different plant *(Eleutherococcus senticoccus)*.

- Ginseng has a long history as a health supplement. Ginseng has been used widely in herbal medicines of Asian cultures to cure fatigue, relieve pain and headaches, and improve mental function and vigor.

- Ginseng has been described by Eastern European scientists as an adaptogen, a substance purported to normalize physiology after exposure to a variety of stresses. An adaptogen is considered to exhibit a lack of specificity in its actions and can both reduce and increase a response that has been altered by a stressor. This theory is a philosophy of physiology or medicine different than traditional Western understanding.

- The root of the plants is considered the most valuable part, and a number of chemically similar steroid glycosides or saponin chemicals, known as ginsenosides, have been identified as active ingredients in ginsengs.

- The chemical composition of commercial supplement products is highly variable because of differences in the genetic nature of the plant source, variation in active ingredients with cultivation and season, differences in the methods of drying and curing, and differences in the process of supplement preparation. Some ginseng preparations also provide additional agents such as vitamins, minerals, or other herbal compounds.

- Several other herbal compounds with a history of use as medicine or tonics in other cultures have recently become available in supplements promoted to athletes. These include *Cordyceps sinensis,* a Chinese herb extracted from a mushroom, and *Rhodiola rosea,* popular in Asian and Eastern European medicine.

Potential Situations for Use

- Ginseng is claimed to reduce fatigue and improve aerobic conditioning, strength, mental alertness, and recovery.

- *Cordyceps* is claimed to increase vasodilation and facilitate the delivery of oxygen to the working tissue, whereas *Rhodiola* is said to stimulate the nervous system.

Research Support

- A number of studies of ginsengs and exercise performance have been published in non-English-language journals. These are generally ignored because of flaws in research design (failure to include a control or placebo group) or because of the absence of details of the study.

- A few studies have reported enhancement of physical exercise capacity or performance following chronic ginseng use by active populations (Liang et al. 2005; McNaughton et al. 1989; Pieralisi et al. 1991), but the majority have failed to detect an enhanced outcome (Allen et al. 1998; Dowling et al. 1996; Engels et al. 2001, 2003; Hsu et al. 2005; Morris et al. 1996).

- The available literature on supplementation with ginsengs or other herbal preparations in athletic populations is scarce and does not provide support for benefits to performance or recovery (Bahrke and Morgan 1994, 2000; Dowling et al. 1996; Goulet 2005). Data from studies on supplement studies on athletes involving ginsengs (Dowling et al. 1996; Ziemba et al. 1999) and other herbal preparations such as *Cordyceps sinensis* and *Rhodiola rosea* (Colson et al. 2005; de Bock et al. 2004; Earnest et al. 2004; Parcell et al. 2004) are summarized in the appendixes to chapters 4, 5, and 8.

- There is some support for claims that ginseng supplementation enhances well-being, recovery, or immune function (Hsu et al. 2005; Ziemba et al. 1999). However, other studies refute these findings (Engels et al. 2003; Gaffney et al. 2001).

Concerns Associated With Use

- The variability of the content of commercial ginseng supplements creates a major impediment to research. One study of 50 commercial ginseng preparations found that 44 products ranged in ginsenoside concentration from 1.9% to 9.0%, whereas six preparations failed to produce a detectable level of ginsenosides (Chong and Oberholzer 1988). Even if scientific evidence showed that ginseng could enhance exercise performance, athletes could not be certain of receiving the appropriate dose and type of active ingredients from all preparations in the commercially available range.

- Athletes should also be aware that herbal preparations are considered at higher risk of containing contaminants. Two separate studies have found commercial ginseng supplements to contain ephedrine, a stimulant in contravention to doping codes (Chong and Oberholzer 1988; Cui et al. 1994).

chapter 4

Road Cycling and the Triathlon

Our specific discussion of the nutritional challenges of competitive sports starts with the disciplines of triathlon and road cycling. These sports have been placed together because cycling is the longest component of a triathlon race and because competitive events in both sports can range from races of around 1 hr in duration to ultraendurance events of 6 to 10 hr. Although each sport has defining features, the physiological and nutritional requirements of specific races within each sport are variable—often being unique to each event.

Competition

Cycling enjoys a long history of organized competition, with famous events such as the Tour de France celebrating a century of races in 2003. Triathlon, on the other hand, is a relatively young sport, making its debut on the Olympic program at the 2000 Sydney Olympic Games. Nevertheless, both activities enjoy healthy participation rates at levels ranging from recreational to elite.

Road Cycling

Over the last century, men's road cycling has evolved into a professional sport dominated by sponsored trade teams whose individual members also compete for their national teams at World Championships (annually) and the Olympic Games (every 4 years). For female cyclists, the registration of professional trade teams is only a decade old, and the opportunities for a professional cycling career are fewer and less well rewarded (Martin et al. 2001). Competitive cycling at the international level is organized under the rules and conditions of the Union Cycliste Internationale (UCI), which recognizes a variety of race formats (see table 4.1) and awards an official scoring system of points for successful performance in sanctioned events.

Although this chapter will focus on elite-level cycling, the majority of cycling races around the world are organized by national, state, or collegiate cycling federations or clubs and are contested by subelite and serious amateur riders. Some mass participation races allow professional riders and recreational cyclists to compete in the same field, similar to the mixture of runners in Big City Marathon events. Some of these cycling events attract large fields—for example, the annual 105 km Cape Argus cycling tour in Cape Town, South Africa, restricts its race entries to 35,000 competitors.

The variety of common race formats found in competitive road cycling is summarized in table 4.1. The shortest races found in road cycling are the prologues, or brief time trials for individual riders, often held at the commencement of a stage race or tour. Finishing times for such races can be as little as 10 min. However, the duration of the individual time trial event on the program at the World Championships and Olympic Games is typically around 40 km ($\sim$60 min) for men and 20 km ($\sim$30 min) for women. There is a unique case where a time trial is conducted as distance completed in a specified time: The world record for 1 hr cycling is a well-recognized target for elite road cyclists, despite being completed on a cycling track or velodrome. The individual time trial represents a true test of the rider's cycling ability, requiring efficiency in technique and riding position and the ability to sustain high and relatively constant power outputs for the duration of the race. Analysis of the performance of elite time trial specialists shows that they are able to sustain exercise intensities near, or even slightly above, their lactate threshold, or onset of blood lactate accumulation, for 30 to 60 min (for review, see Mujika and Padilla 2001). For example, to set the best hour performance of 56.375 km on a nonstandard bike, English cyclist Chris Boardman produced an average power output of 442 W, equivalent to an oxygen uptake of $\sim$81 ml$\cdot$kg$^{-1}\cdot$min^{-1} or 90% of his $\dot{V}O_2$peak (Keen 1998).

Table 4.1 Characteristics of Typical Events Undertaken in Road Cycling and Triathlon

	Race format	Examples	Typical duration of race for elite competitors
CYCLING			
Single-day events	Mass-start road race	Paris-Roubaix, World Championship and Olympic Games road race	60-250 km (2-8 hr)
	Individual time trial	Time trial on World Championship and Olympic programs, 40 km time trial	20-35 km for women (30-50 min) 40-50 km for men (40-60 min)
Stage races	4-10 days with daily program including • mass-start road race, • individual time-trial, and • team time trial	Paris-Nice	Daily stages vary from prologue individual time trial (~15 km) to 250 km mass-start road race
Major tours	21-22 days with daily program including • mass-start road race, • individual time trial, and • team time trial	Tour de France, Giro D'Italia Vuelta a Espana	Daily stages vary from prologue individual time trial (~10 km) to 250 km mass-start road race Total racing time: 80-100 hr
TRIATHLON			
Sprint distance (ITU)	0.75 km swim, 20 km cycle, 5 km run		~1 hr
Olympic or standard distance (ITU)	1.5 km swim, 40 km cycle, 10 km run	Olympic race, World Championship race	1 hr 50 min to 2 hr (elite males); 2 hr to 2 hr 15 min (elite females)
Long distance (ITU)	4 km swim, 120 km cycle, 30 km run	World Championship race	5 hr 30 min to 6 hr (elite males); 6 hr 15 min to 7 hr (elite females)
Team event (ITU)	3 × (300 m swim, 7.8 km cycle, 2 km run)	World Championship race	
Half Ironman	1.9 km swim, 90 km cycle, 21.1 km run	World Championship race	4 hr elite males 4.5 hr elite females
Ironman	3.8 km swim, 180 km cycle, 42.2 km run (marathon)	Hawaiian Ironman World Championship	8-9 hr elite males 9-10.5 hr elite females 17 hr cut-off for age-group competitors

ITU = International Triathlon Union.

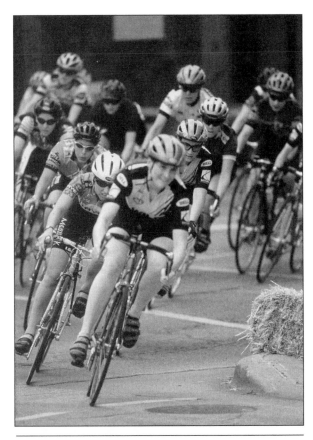

There are also many opportunities for recreational cyclists to take part in mass participation events including single-day races and multiday tours.

Mass-start road races, whether single events or stages within a tour, are conducted over a range of distances typically lasting 2 to 8 hr. Road races can be conducted on a loop course, but many courses cover the distance between two towns or landmarks. Criterium races, which involve multiple laps of a small loop circuit, are another popular road race format. Mass-start road races are characterized by lengthy periods of submaximal or aerobic work interspersed with periods of high-intensity activity. A number of factors cause road cycling to have this *stochastic* (intermittent and unpredictable) nature. Cycling intensity is affected by features of the race course such as climate, wind, hills, and road surface. The other important factor is race tactics. Drafting, or riding behind another cyclist or group of cyclists, reduces the energy cost of cycling by reducing the frontal area of drag or aerodynamic resistance of the following rider. As a result, the exercise intensities of cyclists riding within a large bunch or *peloton* can be quite modest—~150 W (Jeukendrup et al. 2000). However, power output data collected during actual races show multiple brief efforts at very high intensities and sustained periods of hard effort within the race, as the cyclists climb a hill, break away from a pack of riders, or sprint to the finish line. A professional cycling team generally contains a range of cyclists who excel at different specialties (e.g., time trial specialists, hill

climbers, or sprinters) or who are assigned different tasks within the race (e.g., *domestiques* who ride to support the team leader). As a result, the overall race performance of a cyclist is affected by both the type of course and his or her designated role within a team.

For elite competitors, the UCI calendar stretches from the early season stage races in January; through the major tours such as Giro D'Italia and the Tour de France, held in June and July; to the World Championships, typically held in October. World Cup (single-day) races are spread throughout this season. On average, professional cyclists may compete on 1 out of every 3 days during the competition season, for a total of ~100 days of racing each year. At subelite and serious amateur level, cyclists are more typically involved in a weekly schedule of club events or intercollegiate team racing, sometimes providing a summer and winter racing calendar.

Triathlon

Triathlons evolved during the mid- to late 1980s as a new endurance activity involving a multisport format. Initial events typically involved a swim–bike–run format, with the distance of each leg being determined by placing existing events in these disciplines in succession or by having competitors complete the distance between convenient landmarks in a series of different sporting activities. Variations on the triathlon format have included run–swim–run or run–bike–run races or the inclusion of canoe, mountain bike, or cross-country skiing legs in the race mix. In the 1990s, an international governing body, the International Triathlon Union (ITU), was created to promote the development and uniformity of the sport. By the turn of the millennium, progress encompassed a set of standard race distances (see table 4.1), the inclusion of the Olympic, or standard, triathlon race on the 2000 Sydney Olympic Games program, and a professional circuit and code of race rules for elite competitors. Although this chapter focuses mainly on the characteristics of ITU-sanctioned events, Ironman races organized by World Triathlon Corporation are also included because of the importance of the founding Hawaii Ironman race to the culture and challenge of triathlon.

Triathlon still involves a number of features that reflect its origin as a sport for all. Many events, even at the level of World Championships, include an elite or professional division as well as age-group races where subelite athletes compete against each other, grouped in 5-year age divisions. There are different race rules for the elite and age-group divisions in triathlon and different technical and tactical considerations for the separate legs of the triathlon compared with the individual sports from which they were derived. In the case of elite competitors, drafting is also permitted during the cycle leg of ITU triathlon races, whereas age-group triathletes and competitors in other races complete the cycle portion of the race as an individual time trial, maintaining a prescribed distance from other competitors. The cycling and running events within a triathlon also differ from their single-sport counterpart,

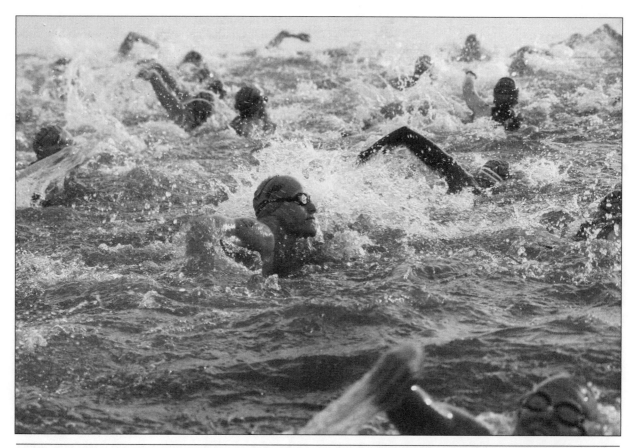

Unlike pool swimming, the swim leg of a triathlon may involve wet suits, currents and turbulence, and the opportunity to draft or streamline behind another competitor.

because the athlete undertakes these legs with a carryover effect of the preceding exercise activity.

Triathlon races can be divided into short (sprint and Olympic or standard) distance events, which involve 1 to 2.5 hr of activity for the best competitors, and the long (long-course and Ironman) events, which range from 4 to 10 hr for the race winners (see table 4.1). In the early years of triathlon, the best triathletes were often converts from the individual sports who were able to exploit their superior talent in one event into overall triathlon performance. Modern triathletes now require all-round expertise in each of the sporting disciplines and start dedicated preparation for a triathlon career at an early age. Team racing tactics between training partners or national team members are also becoming a feature of elite racing, especially when drafting during the cycle leg is allowed. Finally, fewer elite triathletes now compete successfully at the full range of triathlon distances, preferring to specialize in either short- or long-course racing.

The international race calendar provides a series of events including World Cup races, sponsored race series, and World Championships. Many countries also host a busy calendar of local events, allowing age-group competitors to race each weekend over the summer months if desired. Some races are specially targeted to school-age,

novice, or team competitors (a different athlete for each of the legs of the race). At the other end of the spectrum, races such as Ironman events require qualification in shorter or local races before entry to major events is offered.

Training

World-class professional riders typically cycle 25,000 to 35,000 km per year (Mujika and Padilla 2001), with much of their training being undertaken between events within the racing calendar or in the form of less important races and tours. The overwhelming majority of training is undertaken on the road, although wind-trainers and rollers allow specialized sessions to be undertaken, often indoors during winter months. Preseason and early season training is often spent trying to achieve specific physique goals—usually to reduce body mass and body fat levels. Riders typically organize their training and competition program to allow them to peak for one or several designated races or tours within the season, and the few observations of longitudinal responses of cyclists to such training suggest that it takes at least 4 to 5 years to develop a world-class cyclist, perhaps 2 to 6 years for a talented female cyclist and 4 to 8 for a talented male road cyclist (personal communication, David T. Martin, exercise physiologist, Australian Cycling Team).

Specialized training techniques or modified training programs, such as interval training or altitude training, have been shown to provide a small but worthwhile enhancement to the performance of elite cyclists. However, the benefits of racing as a form of training are also apparent, because professional cyclists improve their performance over the competitive season. Furthermore, the emerging data on power outputs achieved by cyclists during international level races suggest that racing presents a unique challenge that can only be replicated within the competition scenario (personal communication, David T. Martin, exercise physiologist, Australian Cycling team). With so much time being spent on the bike, elite cyclists rarely undertake any other type of training. One possible exception may be the relatively short periods of time in the preseason or while rehabilitating from injury when an elite cyclist may engage in limited resistance training, flexibility work, or other forms of aerobic activity.

At the serious club or collegiate level, cyclists generally undertake 300 to 600 km of training per week and may have greater opportunity to undertake specific training programs between their weekly or seasonal racing commitments than the elite cyclist on the racing circuit. Such training is undertaken not only to enhance the cyclist's physiology (e.g., improve aerobic capacity and shift lactate threshold) but also to improve riding technique and aerodynamic positioning.

Triathlon requires the athlete to master three separate sports. Triathletes undertake separate training session in each sport, often under a specialist coach, as well as training sessions that combine two or three of the activities, especially the combination of cycling and running. Typically, a triathlete will undertake two or even three separate training sessions per day, even in the case of the serious age-group competitor. Some training sessions are organized to achieve desirable changes in physique and physiology, such as a reduction in body fat or an increase in aerobic or anaerobic capacity. However, other sessions need to be dedicated to improvements in technique, especially in the highly technical sport of swimming. Despite an already busy training schedule, many triathletes undertake additional sessions of resistance training or flexibility work. Typically, the elite triathlete can expect to undertake 15 to 30 hours of training each week, whereas a serious age-group competitor may train 10 to 15 hr/week, increasing to more than 20 hr when preparing for a long-course race. According to the Web site of the Ironman race series (www. Ironmanlive.com), the typical competitor undertakes 7 months of preparation for an Ironman event, with a weekly training commitment ranging between 18 and 22 hr and achieving a mean volume of 11.3 km of swimming, 373 km of cycling, and 77 km of running.

There are various approaches to integrating the training and racing calendar in triathlon. Many elite competitors follow the international race circuit, which travels across the hemispheres to provide an almost year-round opportunity for competition. Such competitors race frequently, peri-odizing their training and competition programs to peak for important or designated events. Recreational triathletes may be limited to their local competition season during the warm-weather months, devoting winter months to training or engaging in cross-country running and cycling races. Some triathletes, particularly those focused on long-distance events, concentrate on heavier training volumes and a less frequent race program. For example, age-group competitors may find it difficult to schedule long rides and runs within the weekday work timetable, and their preparation for a long-distance race may require them to sacrifice weekends to such training rather than competing in the short-distance race calendar.

Physique and Physiology

The cyclist's success comes from generating power that is efficiently translated into movement against the rolling resistance of the road, aerodynamic resistance, and, in the case of uphill cycling, gravity. The striking physiological characteristics of elite road cyclists are a high aerobic capacity and the ability to sustain power outputs at a high fractional utilization of aerobic capacity (i.e., a high anaerobic capacity). Mujika and Padilla (2001) summarized the characteristics of a team of professional world-class male cyclists, reporting an average age of 26 years (range 20-33 years), height of 180 cm (160-190 cm), body mass of 69 kg (53-80 kg), and $\dot{V}O_2$max of 79 ml · kg^{-1} · min^{-1} (70-85 ml · kg^{-1} · min^{-1}). The reason for such variability is the specialization of riders according to the different challenges of a race (e.g., hill-climbing specialists, flat terrain riders, time trial riders, sprinters). Although all cyclists strive for low body fat levels to increase the power-to-mass relationship that assists general movement, body mass per se has a separate and major influence on uphill cycling because it determines gravity-dependent resistance. As a result, hill-riding specialists are smaller and lighter than other cyclists. Level-ground time trial specialists are typically larger and heavier than other cyclists, because a higher muscle mass can generate more power, and their lower body surface area to body mass relationship improves aerodynamic resistance. Although some of these characteristics are inherent to the genetically gifted athlete, most cyclists will strive through training and dietary manipulation to enhance muscle mass, body mass, and body fat level according to their desired specialty or need for all-round excellence.

Triathletes need to have a physique and physiological makeup suited to performance of swimming, cycling, and running. Selecting a mix of characteristics that are favorable for three different sports is an interesting challenge, because different factors may be important for each event and may vary according to the range of distances, course profiles, and race rules within each triathlon event. A high aerobic capacity is essential for the performance of all events within the triathlon. Physique characteristics might be expected to have more range—for example, upper-body muscle development is most evident in swimmers but is of minimal value and even detrimental to running performance. The degree to which body weight is supported varies markedly between swimming, cycling, and running, meaning that there is a range in the importance of power to weight to performance in each of these separate events. In the case of cycling and running, the importance of lightness and leanness to performance also varies with the terrain of a given event. A study of the morphological characteristics of triathletes from a variety of countries competing at a World Championship over the Olympic distance provided some insight into how these factors mix and match to create the ideal physique for triathlon. This study found that run time provided an important contribution to overall race outcome. Furthermore, a low level of body fat was the most important physique characteristic for overall race performance and was highly correlated with performance in each of the individual legs (Landers et al. 2000). Unfortunately, these data did not address the very important issue of whether leanness per se makes a triathlete faster or whether high-quality training makes a triathlete faster and also achieves leanness.

Lifestyle and Culture

Travel plays a large role in the lives of athletes at the elite level in both road cycling and triathlon. Professional athletes in these sports are likely to spend a large part of the competitive season traveling on the continental or international competition circuit. The dietary situation for cyclists in professional teams ranges over the racing season from self-catering (often with a team-provided *per diem* or daily allowance), to attending training camps with a catered menu, and finally to consuming meals within the infrastructure provided by the organizational bodies of large races or international competitions. Professional triathletes can also face a similar set of domestic arrangements. Challenges to good eating patterns include inadequate budgets, poor domestic skills, and a lack of familiarity with local foods and different eating customs in new countries. The athlete may suffer real or perceived hardship when foods that are important or part of his usual eating patterns are not available in the new environment. Fatigue and time management problems also interfere with the athlete's commitment to a well-organized eating program. Although the most highly paid and successful athletes are often well looked after by a support team, many junior and emerging athletes struggle with poor support to face the challenges of training and competing on the circuit.

Serious subelite road cyclists and triathletes face a different set of lifestyle challenges in combining a program of work or study with their training and competition goals. Training sessions, travel to local and national races, and the other requirements of a sporting life (e.g., medical appointments, massages) have to be squeezed in around school, college, or work commitments. Inadequate money and time often challenge good eating practices—it can be difficult to find the opportunities simply to *eat* adequate energy and fuel for a heavy exercise load in a busy day, let alone obtain and prepare the necessary food supplies. Creative solutions are needed to make the most of limited resources.

Triathlon and cycling both enjoy a strong cultural identity, which is spread at the most basic level via the written word (magazines), Internet, and the club scene. Bunch rides, group training sessions, and races all provide a meeting place for athletes to exchange ideas. At the elite level, particularly in cycling, the environment provided within the professional team is the major source of information and influence on nutritional practices. Some teams have a strong medical support group in which a doctor, an exercise physiologist, and occasionally a dietitian are the designated providers of expert nutrition advice. Team *soigneurs* carry out a range of duties on a cycle team, including first aid and massage, bike repairs, and manning the feed stations. Although they may not hold any professional qualifications, they play an important role on the ground and an even greater role in smaller teams that are unable to provide their riders with much professional sport science support. Soigneurs have a powerful influence in spreading information on dietary practices and supplement use. In general, speculation and word of mouth about the practices of other (successful) athletes carry a strong message.

Both triathletes and cyclists are quick to take up new ideas and copy practices they believe to be successful. The advantage of this culture is that it promotes and supports innovation. The disadvantage of this culture is that many athletes follow practices based on hearsay and hypothesis rather than sound scientific support. Indiscriminate use of supplements has become common among elite triathletes and cyclists. The risk of an inadvertent doping outcome is high in such cases, and such an outcome apparently has occurred in several cases involving prominent athletes. Intravenous use of supplements and nutrient preparations is another high-risk behavior sometimes in evidence and is especially dangerous when administered by people who are not medically trained. Fad weight loss practices, which range from ineffective to harmful, are also common. Of course, not all the practices that essentially develop at the coal-face of these sports are ineffective and based only on superstition or fashion. In some cases, scientists who undertake research on practices observed in triathlon and cycling merely confirm that the athletes were ahead of them in finding a new way to enhance performance. For example, cyclists and triathletes were drinking "defizzed" cola during the late stages of races long before scientists detected the performance benefit of this practice in a laboratory study (see Sport Foods and Supplements section). The situation in which sport scientists and athletes work together is likely to provide the optimal outcome for all.

Dietary Surveys

How do cyclists and triathletes eat to meet the nutritional needs of training and competition? The following section reviews the available information from dietary surveys conducted on high-level cyclists and triathletes. These results are discussed in light of the errors or bias that is introduced by dietary survey methodology.

Road Cyclists

Most of the available information on the dietary practices of serious road cyclists involves male riders ranging from national-level to world-class professionals. This information has been summarized in a table in the appendix to this chapter (table 4.e). Given the high energy expenditure of training, we would expect the most striking feature of the dietary patterns of road cyclists to be a high energy intake. Even with the likelihood of some underreporting, dietary surveys show that populations of serious cyclists report a high energy intake (daily intakes >250 kJ or 60 kcal per kilogram of body mass), and those with documentation of heaviest training loads report mean daily energy intakes >20 MJ (4,800 kcal) or 300 kJ (70 kcal) per kilogram (Garcia-Roves et al. 2000). Reported intakes that seem incongruously low (Johnson et al. 1985; Klepping et al. 1984) may reflect inadequate survey techniques, investigation during a period of weight loss, or a low training load. Information in these dietary surveys is typically insufficient to pinpoint which of these factors apply because few provide any independent measurement or substantial discussion of the accuracy or validity of their data. A recent exception is a study of energy balance during a 6-day preseason training camp undertaken by world-class professional cyclists (Vogt et al. 2005). In this study, cyclists reported a mean daily energy intake of ~13.5 MJ, which was estimated to cover only 70% of the estimated energy costs of training (~160 km per day for 5 days). However, the stated goal of this training camp was to reduce body mass in preparation for the competition season; in fact, a mean loss of 0.7 kg was reported over this period. In addition to having a general energy deficit over the day, cyclists were reported to consume minimal amounts of energy and carbohydrate during training sessions. Mean carbohydrate intake during a 5 hr training session was ~70 g; this falls short of the recommended 30 to 60 g/hr (American College of Sports Medicine 1996; Coyle 2004). In general, the ability to consume a high energy intake appears to be underpinned by an increase in the number of separate eating occasions each day. For example, some researchers found that their population of cyclists ate up to nine discrete meals and snacks each day (Johnson et al. 1985; Kirsch and Von Ameln 1981) or consumed almost 40% of total energy intake from snacks eaten between conventional meals (Van Erp-Baart et al. 1989a).

The apparent carbohydrate intake of high-level male cyclists during training periods is ~8 to 11 $g \cdot kg^{-1} \cdot day^{-1}$, which is within the range suggested to promote daily restoration of muscle glycogen concentrations (see table 1.2). The mean daily intakes of protein reported by male cyclists appear to meet or exceed any estimated increases in the protein needs of athletes undertaking a substantial training load (1.2-1.6 g/kg; see table 1.1). These outcomes are achieved largely as a by-product of high energy intakes, and we would expect the same to apply also to micronutrient intakes. In fact, studies that have included an estimation of vitamin and mineral intakes have all concluded that male cyclists report mean daily intakes in excess of recommended daily levels during training, even without taking into account the contribution of supplements (Garcia-Roves et al. 2000; Jensen et al. 1992; Johnson et al. 1985; Van Erp-Baart et al. 1989b). Of course, mean data may mask suboptimal intakes by some individuals within a group. Furthermore, dietary intake data are unable to measure true nutritional status of individuals or populations. Indeed, the adequacy of energy, macronutrient, and micronutrient intake can only be assessed for individuals and should consider a range of information including anthropometric, biochemical, hematological, and performance data (see chapter 2).

Fewer studies have been conducted of the training diets of high-level female road cyclists (see appendix, table 4.f). The lack of information and the poor detail about the characteristics of participants and study methodology make it difficult to make generalizations about the dietary habits of female cyclists during training. One exception, however, is the general observation that reported energy intakes of female cyclists are less than those reported by male cyclists, even when corrected for body mass. Whether this can be explained in terms of a lower training load, energy restriction to reduce body weight or fat, or an artifact of dietary survey methodology is uncertain. Observations from Martin et al. (2002) support both a relationship between energy intake and training load and the apparent potential for at least some female cyclists to underreport their true energy intake. In this study of the national Australian women's road cycling team, dietary intake and training energy expenditure were recorded during the racing season, with individual days of training during this period categorized as full training days or recovery days (light training). The results are presented in figure 4.1. A positive correlation between reported energy intake and training energy expenditure was found, with some cyclists showing patterns of dietary restraint on recovery days related to their desire to reduce body weight/body fat (Martin et al. 2002). A negative correlation was seen, however, between reported energy intake and body fat levels over all types of training (and racing). In other words, the cyclists with higher body fat levels reported lower energy intakes, corrected for body mass, than their leaner counterparts. Because there was no significant loss of body fat, signaling negative energy balance over the 70 days of the study, and because energy efficiency in female athletes may not fully account for this energy discrepancy (Horton et al. 1994), these findings suggest that cyclists with higher body fat levels were at risk of underreporting true energy intake.

The competition diets of cyclists are of interest from two separate angles. First, because professional cyclists may undertake 100 days of racing each season, food consumed during days of racing contributes significantly to the athlete's overall nutritional status and nutritional goals. This intake must continue to meet general needs for energy, protein, and macronutrients, even when the athlete's food choices are largely coming from race feeding stations and team hotels. Second, it is of interest to see how well the athlete is able to meet specific goals of competition eating, especially those related to carbohydrate and

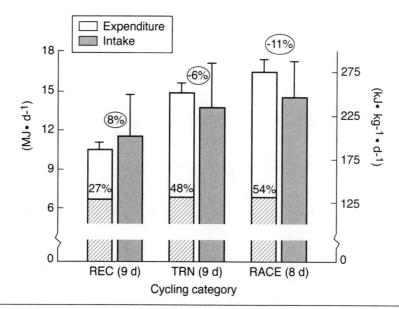

Figure 4.1   Reported energy intake (EI) and estimated total energy expenditure (TEE; mean ± SD) of elite female cyclists (n = 8) during day of recovery or light training (REC, 9 days), heavy training (TRN, 9 days), and racing (RACE, 8 days). Striped bars represent energy expended during sleep and noncycling activities. Energy expenditure during cycling is identified as a percentage of total daily energy expended above each striped bar. The difference between EI and TEE is presented as a percentage in a circle above each cycling category. Although EI was 8% higher than TEE during REC, EI was lower than TEE during TRN (–6%) and RACE (–11%).

Reprinted from Martin et al. 2002.

fluid replacement, before, during, and after the event. The data from dietary surveys of high-level male and female cyclists undertaken during periods of racing, including stage races, are summarized in table 4.g in the appendix to this chapter.

The most important nutritional consideration during many stage races is achieving adequate energy intake to match the extreme energy expenditure demands; for example, the Tour de France covers ~4,000 km over 21 days of racing. It appears that cyclists are successful in meeting this challenge because several studies have reported that typical changes in body mass over the duration of a Tour, representing depletion of body energy reserves, are minor (~1 kg loss) (Jeukendrup et al. 2000; Saris et al. 1989; Westerterp et al. 1986). Mean daily energy intake reported by cyclists in these stage races is 23 to 24 MJ (5,500-5,700 kcal) or ~350 kJ (~80 kcal) per kilogram. Two studies of energy balance during the Tour de France produced different outcomes. The first, using factorial methods to estimate total daily energy expenditure, reported close correlation between energy intake and expenditure, with matches occurring over 3 days as well as over the 3-week period (Saris et al. 1989). The authors noted that energy intake was at a high level of total digestive capacity. As a result, if an athlete were to fall behind with energy consumption, it would be impossible to eat in excess to correct the negative balance. Therefore, successful cyclists appear to focus on meeting energy needs daily. In the other study, doubly

labeled water (DLW) estimations of energy expenditure of cyclists undertaking the Tour de France produced values that were 13% to 35% greater than reported energy intakes (Westerterp et al. 1986). Because body composition was maintained throughout the study period, it is unlikely that energy expenditure exceeded intake by such substantial amounts. Therefore, this finding needs to be explained as an outcome of methodological problems—it is likely that both overestimation of energy expenditure by DLW and underestimation of true energy intake occurred.

Again, there is little information on the dietary practices of high-level female cyclists during competition. Martin and colleagues (2002) investigated race-day intakes during the domestic racing season of the Australian women's road team, which includes several of the top-ranked female cyclists in the world. The self-reported energy intakes of these cyclists were less than the body mass–adjusted energy intakes typically reported by male cyclists during racing (Martin et al. 2002). This finding is plausible, because road races for female cyclists typically involve shorter distances than men's road cycling races. There is no information about stage race practices of elite female cyclists, apart from one study detailing dietary intake of unspecified American cyclists undertaking a race involving 500 km of cycling over 11 days (Grandjean et al. 1992). This study found an even more modest energy intake in this group, which is plausible given the light racing load in this event. The female cyclists reported intakes of protein and micronutrients that generally met or exceeded relevant recommmended dietary intakes, with supplements providing additional amounts of these nutrients.

Three studies have compared the training and racing diets of the same group of cyclists: two groups of international-level road cyclists and a collegiate men's cycling team (Garcia-Roves et al. 2000; Jensen et al. 1992; Martin et al. 2002). Members of the Australian women's road cycling team reported consuming greater energy intake on days of racing and heavy training than on light training and recovery days. However, estimates of energy balance showed negative balance on the days of higher cycling energy expenditure, particularly during racing, countered by a positive energy balance on recovery days (see the highlight box on this page) (Martin et al. 2002). Increases in energy intake were achieved mostly by manipulation of carbohydrate intake—reported daily intakes of carbohydrate were 9.8 g/kg and 8.9 g/kg for racing and heavy training days, respectively, compared with 7.5 g/kg ($p <$ .05) on light training days. However, protein intake also changed between racing and training, being lower on racing and light training days ($\sim$2.2 g/kg) than heavy training days (2.5 g/kg, $p <$ .05). Suggested explanations for differences in energy and macronutrient intake between racing and training included underreporting of energy intake on recovery days, increased appetite on high-volume cycling days, the belief that more food is required or deserved during heavy training days, and the specific intake of energy-containing food and drinks on the bike during lengthy races and workouts (Martin et al. 2002).

Summary of Common Nutritional Issues Arising in Road Cycling and Triathlon

Physique Issues

- Desire to reduce body fat and body mass to enhance performance via enhanced power-to-mass relationship
- Risk of dietary extremism, disordered eating, and inadequate nutrition attributable to overemphasis on low body mass and body fat level

Training Issues

- High energy and carbohydrate requirements to meet a heavy training load
- Practical difficulties in consuming sufficient energy and carbohydrate intake in a busy day
- Recovery between training sessions (refueling, rehydration, repair, and adaptation)
- Adequate fuel and fluid intake during training sessions, including practice of race-day strategies
- Risk of low iron status, especially in female and vegetarian athletes, secondary to inadequate dietary intake and some increase in daily requirements
- Risk of menstrual disturbances in female athletes
- High level of interest in supplements and sport foods

Competition Issues

- Preparation of adequate fuel stores for race day: carbohydrate loading before endurance and ultradistance events (triathlon and selected cycling races)
- Preevent nutrition: topping up fuel and fluid levels without causing gastrointestinal discomfort during the race
- Consideration of caffeine use to enhance race performance
- Fuel and fluid replacement during race: strategies to suit race rules and culture (aid stations, feed zones, soigneurs, and team support crews)
- Stage racing (cycling): aggressive recovery between stages; meeting extreme needs for energy and carbohydrate daily
- Assurance that long-term nutrition needs (adequate intake of protein and micronutrients) are also met within competition eating, especially when race program extends for most of the year
- Travel: living on the race circuit

Garcia-Roves and colleagues (2000) collected weighed food inventories from six male cyclists from one of the world's top professional teams over 3 days of a training camp and 3 days of racing in the Tour de France. There were some limitations in the methodology used in this study—for example, the limited sample size and number of days of dietary assessment and the fact that the cyclists were in camp situation with regulated menus. However, this study found that during the race, cyclists reported an increase in energy intake (0.5 MJ or 1,200 kcal/day) and carbohydrate intake ($\sim$1 g $\cdot$ kg^{-1} $\cdot$ day^{-1}) without a change in fat intake, compared with the diets selected during the preceding training camp. Protein intake was also reported to increase during the race period (from $\sim$2.6 g/kg to 2.9 g $\cdot$ kg^{-1} $\cdot$ day^{-1}), perhaps attributable to an increased reliance on protein-rich drinks and sport supplements in the competition setting (Garcia-Roves et al. 2000).

Finally, a group of collegiate cyclists were studied during a period of training and over a weekend of racing (Jensen et al. 1992). This study found that the cyclists reported eating high carbohydrate intakes overall (9-10 g $\cdot$ kg^{-1} $\cdot$ day^{-1}), with intakes being greater on racing days attributable to an increased intake of fruit and bread and despite the reliance on restaurant eating.

Triathletes

Few studies have been undertaken on the dietary practices of elite and subelite triathletes during training, especially in females, and there are few recent studies that reflect the professionalism that has developed in the sport. Data from the available studies are summarized in the appendix to this chapter (table 4.g). Generally, studies of male triathletes conducted in the 1980s reported high intakes of energy (daily intakes > 250 kJ or 60 kcal/kg) and carbohydrate ($\sim$9 g $\cdot$ kg^{-1} $\cdot$ day^{-1}) by elite-level triathletes of the time, and two studies reported semivegetarian eating patterns (Brown and Herb 1990) or eating styles influenced by the low-fat high-carbohydrate Pritikin diet (Burke and Read 1987b). A high energy intake is expected given the training load (>19 hr/week) reported by triathletes in these studies. The exception to this finding is an investigation of triathletes undertaking the 1984 Hawaii Ironman event (Khoo et al. 1987). The study involved 30% of the total race field in this event, allowing it to provide a reasonable overview of dietary practices of these early ultraendurance triathletes. Although this issue is not discussed in the article, total energy intake reported by this group of triathletes seems incongruously low for the typical training loads of Ironman competitors. However, this may be explained by the survey instrument—a 3-day food record undertaken in the week leading up to the race—which may have been tainted by reduced food intake during the training taper. Other features of this study include commentary on supplement use by the triathletes, including megadoses of micronutrients and unusual dietary components, and apparent differences in the food choices of male and female triathletes. Whereas male triathletes reported frequent consumption of foods with a high energy density such as added fats, sugar, and ice cream, female athletes were more likely to consume fruits, vegetables, and whole-grain cereals. Further dietary surveys should be conducted on dietary intakes and food use patterns of triathletes, especially to reflect new practices and any differences between athletes focused on long-course and short-course training. Observations of nutritional practices during long-distance races are also important, and the few existing data are discussed in the following section.

Nutritional Issues and Challenges

The sidebar, "Summary of Common Nutritional Issues Arising in Road Cycling and Triathlon," summarizes common nutritional issues that arise in road cycling and triathlon as a result of programs to achieve and maintain optimal physique, support the training program, and optimize competition performance. Several of these issues are discussed in greater detail in this section of the book. Other issues, such as travel nutrition, are left to a more generic discussion in later chapters of the book.

Meeting Carbohydrate Requirements for Training

Carbohydrate is an important fuel for the training and racing performance of cyclists and triathletes. Guidelines for carbohydrate intake before, during, and after specific training sessions, as well as total daily intake, were presented in chapter 1 (see table 1.2). The superficial assessment of dietary patterns reported by high-level male cyclists suggests that they typically consume carbohydrate intakes of $\sim$8 to 11 g $\cdot$ kg^{-1} $\cdot$ day^{-1} (table 4.e), which would generally appear to address the need for daily restoration of muscle glycogen store. The same is likely to be true for male triathletes, but the typical carbohydrate intakes of female cyclists and triathletes are likely to be $\sim$10% to 20% less than that of their male counterparts. Although sports nutrition guidelines often suggest that a daily carbohydrate intake of 7 to 10 g/kg is sufficient for the everyday needs of most athletes, the prolonged daily training programs undertaken by some high-level cyclists and triathletes may necessitate higher carbohydrate intakes to meet the fuel needs of training and achieve optimal glycogen restoration between sessions. For example, well-trained cyclists undertaking 2 hr of training each day were found to have higher muscle glycogen stores after a week of consuming a diet providing 12 g of carbohydrate per kilogram body mass than when consuming the recommended intake of 10 g $\cdot$ kg^{-1} $\cdot$ day^{-1} (Coyle et al. 2001). Whether this contributes to better training performance and adaptation is still a source of debate (see research topic).

To optimize training performances, carbohydrate intake should be distributed over the day to provide fuel before and during the workouts and to recover afterward. One study of the daily eating patterns of high-level cyclists showed such a pattern: Cyclists were found to consume a substantial carbohydrate-rich breakfast before training and to aggressively consume carbohydrate-containing foods and drinks throughout training session (Garcia-Roves et al. 2000). Posttraining intake of carbohydrate to enhance recovery was also reported. However, this dietary survey was undertaken during a period of high-intensity training at a training camp, during which cyclists undertook eating patterns that mimicked their practices during stage races. How cyclists, and indeed triathletes, eat during more free-living and unsupervised training periods is unknown.

Neither dietary survey information nor general sports nutrition guidelines can fully address the adequacy of the refueling practices of cyclists or triathletes. In particular, these tools cannot assess the adequacy of dietary practices of the individual athlete. Guidelines should be considered as estimated ranges that can be fine-tuned for the individual athlete with more specific knowledge of her actual training program, past and present responses to training with various dietary strategies, and total energy budget. It is likely that some triathletes and cyclists fail to achieve adequate carbohydrate intake, either to provide fuel for specific training sessions or to restore glycogen content daily. Markers of this problem include poor performance and unnecessary fatigue in these individual training sessions or a general failure to achieve the expected outcomes of a period of training. These outcomes may occur separately or as part of a cluster of problems associated with restrained eating practices. This is discussed in greater detail in the next section.

A number of factors challenge an athlete's ability to achieve the high carbohydrate requirements of a heavy training program. These include restriction of total energy intake, inadequate practical nutrition skills or food composition knowledge, and a chaotic lifestyle and constant travel commitments. Diets specifically targeting a reduced carbohydrate intake wax and wane in popularity over time but are currently fashionable among some sports or athletic subgroups, either as a weight loss strategy or to achieve other purported claims of enhanced energy and performance. The Zone diet is discussed in more detail in chapter 6. The recently studied concept of "train low, compete high" in relation to glycogen stores (Hansen et al. 2005) has also encouraged coaches and athletes to consider that a low carbohydrate intake might enhance the outcome of training. Other limits to achieving carbohydrate intake goals can include inadequate carbohydrate in the background diet and food culture of the country of residence or poor availability of carbohydrate-rich foods and drinks in the athlete's immediate eating environment. The emphasis on bulky fiber-rich choices of carbohydrate foods can also limit total intake by overwhelming gastrointestinal comfort. Individual assessment, including assessment of training and competition performance, is needed to pinpoint and correct problems concerning optimal carbohydrate intake within the balance of total nutrition goals.

In some cases it may not be possible for the triathlete or cyclist to meet theoretical targets for carbohydrate intake at all times—for example, a female athlete who needs to restrict energy intake to reduce body mass may not be able to fully meet the carbohydrate requirements of her training program within a reduced energy budget. However, the athlete should identify the key training sessions or periods that are important for her long-term goals and ensure that she is well fueled for these sessions. In other words, carbohydrate intake may fluctuate over the training week and between training and racing according to the priority for loss of body fat or optimal performance. Dietary modifications that reverse suboptimal intakes of carbohydrate and energy may enhance performance. Frentsos and Baer (1997) reported that the self-chosen diets of six elite triathletes (two female and four male) provided intakes of energy ($\sim$140 kJ $\cdot$ kg^{-1} $\cdot$ day^{-1}) and carbohydrate ($\sim$5 g $\cdot$ kg^{-1} $\cdot$ day^{-1}) that were below recommended levels. After nutrition education, which included provision of an energy–nutrient supplement, these triathletes increased their apparent dietary intake to a daily intake of $\sim$240 kJ/kg and $\sim$9 g of carbohydrate/kg. Such dietary changes were associated with enhanced performance in a short-course race (Frentsos and Baer 1997).

Achieving Low Body Mass and Body Fat Levels

You had to become a slave to data, to performance indicators like pedal cadence, and power output measured in watts. You had to measure literally every heartbeat, and every morsel you ate, down to each spoonful of cereal. You had to be willing to look like a vampire, your body-fat hovering around three to four percent, if it made you faster. If you weighed too little, you wouldn't have the physical resources to generate enough speed. If you weighed too much, your body was a burden. It was a matter of power to weight.

Lance Armstrong, discussing the attention to detail required to race at optimal level in Every Second Counts

Maintaining a low level of body fat, and body mass per se, is the most highly desired physique goal in road cycling and triathlon. Although a low body fat level is associated with general success in these endurance sports, a light and very lean physique is especially important for hill climbing. The results of modeling studies and observations of physique differences between successful flat-terrain time trial riders and hill specialists show clearly that a reduction in body weight has a substantial effect on ability to cycle or run uphill. Curiously, there is little direct evidence of weight-loss practices in the peer-reviewed literature on road cycling. Martin and colleagues (2002) reported deliberate energy-restriction strategies in female endurance cyclists, with this being evident during days of light training designated as recovery days. In addition, Vogt et al. (2005) reported an energy deficit in the diets consumed by male professional cyclists at a 6-day preseason camp and an apparently conservative approach to carbohydrate consumption during training sessions; these measures were associated with a loss of 0.7 kg. These are the only studies to comment on this dietary interest.

In contrast, the culture of road cycling includes a strong focus on the achievement of extreme leanness. For example, an article in a popular cycling magazine cites the huge performance improvements of elite cyclists Indurain, Riis, Jonker, and Tafi resulting from their weight-loss achievements. This article praises the cyclist who went from "176 pounds and 8% body fat to 154 pounds and 3.5% body fat" and achieved an "emaciated" frame and "pipe-stem" arms (Matheny 1997, p. 58). Chris Boardman noted that he vigorously pursued loss of body mass in preparation for the Tour de France after his coach "computed what a loss of 1.5 kg would make over a typical hour-long climb of an average 8% gradient. The answer was 46 s on the climb, and overall on the tour, about seven minutes" (Boardman 2000, p. 46). Similarly, Lance Armstrong's autobiography claims that the chemotherapy used to treat his testicular cancer actually contributed to his Tour de France success, by causing a significant loss of body mass, including muscle mass, from his previous riding physique. "There was one unforeseen benefit of cancer: it had completely reshaped my body . . . now I was almost gaunt. . . . Eddy Merckx had been telling me to slim down for years, and now I understood why. . . . I had lost 15 pounds. It was all I needed" (Armstrong 2000, p. 224). Armstrong's coach also pointed to this weight loss during speculations about the factors underpinning his rider's miraculous comeback and dominance of the Tour de France: "Take 8 kg and add them to Lance on his finishing time at Alpe D'Huez, and if he maintained the same power output, he would have finished 3 min 47 seconds behind where he did finish. And that's only Alpe D'Huez" (Abt and Armstrong 2002, p. 18).

According to cycling magazines, already lean cyclists use a variety of strategies to further cut weight (Matheny 1997):

1.   Undertaking a hard 3 to 4 hr morning training in a fasted state ("promoting fat loss while training carbo-depleted")

2.   Consuming breakfast, a carbohydrate drink, during a 5 to 7 hr training session and then eating nothing after the postride carbohydrate-rich meal until next morning ("going to bed hungry to use fat stores during sleep")

3.   Suppressing appetite with diet drugs

4.   Undereating while riding a stage race—treating the race as training rather than an important competition and using the supervision of medical staff to ensure adherence to energy-restricted intake

Support for this last tactic is provided by the Tour de France diary of a cyclist who noted that his main race goal was to lose 4 kg and "come out at his ideal race weight" in preparation for specially targeted races at the end of the season (Fotheringham 1997). The cyclist described tactics of deliberate undereating after each day's stage and encouraging hunger, and he noted that designated weight loss during Tours was a common practice among cyclists outside the leading group, to supplement the conditioning achieved on training camps. Restriction of carbohydrate intake rather than energy per se—for example, not eating any carbohydrate-rich foods after 4 p.m.—is a currently popular but less drastic practice.

How can the published dietary surveys of cyclists and eating practices during stage races be reconciled with these anecdotal reports of extreme weight loss practices? It is possible that these practices are being underreported or concealed by cyclists. Or perhaps they are a recent phenomenon that has not yet been studied adequately, or perhaps they pertain to individuals whose results are masked within a group report. Alternatively, the existing research may not have used tools that are designed to collect this information. In any case, it appears that the present literature does not adequately address this issue, and research should be undertaken among road cyclists to document the prevalence, specific practices, and outcomes of weight-control behavior.

There is some official documentation that triathletes are also interested in achieving a light and very lean physique, including levels of body fat that are lower than is naturally achieved as a result of genetics and a high energy expenditure. A study of nearly 600 triathletes reported that the sport was susceptible to a high prevalence of disordered eating, based on self-reported evidence of preoccupation with food and weight at levels that are associated with subclinical eating disorders (DiGioacchino DeBate, et al. 2003). All study participants indicated dissatisfaction with their body mass and revealed attempts to lose weight by means of severe restriction of energy intake and food variety, excessive training, and the control of food intake based on strict dietary rules (DiGioacchino DeBate, et al. 2003).

Although low body fat and body mass are important characteristics for triathletes and cyclists, the pursuit of excessive leanness and very low body mass carries the potential risk of a variety of problems related to immediate and long-term health, performance, body image, and psychological well-being. It is difficult to predict which individual athletes will suffer such negative consequences, but factors that are likely to be important include the degree to which the athlete tries to reduce below his or her natural physique and the techniques and timing of the strategies used to achieve loss of mass and body fat. Penalties of unsound or extreme weight and fat loss measures are discussed in greater detail in chapter 5. The remainder of the discussion in this chapter covers ideas and strategies that may assist a cyclist or triathlete to reduce energy intake to achieve and maintain a light and lean physique without compromising health or performance.

Loss of body weight, principally from loss of body fat, should be achieved by a long-term program of daily energy deficit: in other words, by reducing energy intake, increasing energy expenditure, or both. Many different approaches can achieve this outcome, and athletes should consider seeking the expertise of a sports dietitian to help them develop a program that is tailor-made for their individual characteristics and goals. Table 4.2 summarizes the

Table 4.2 Ingredients for a Successful Weight or Fat Loss Program

Ingredient	Risks from too little	Risks from too much	Guidelines
A sustained daily energy deficit (energy intake less than energy expenditure)	• Very slow or absent results	• Insufficient energy to allow fuel needs to be met • Excessive loss of muscle mass rather than body fat	Strategy 1: Reduce usual eating patterns or increase energy expenditure (training) to create an energy deficit: • A daily energy deficit of 500 kcal (2,100 kJ) leads to a weekly loss of ~500 g of fat. • A daily energy deficit of 1,000 kcal (4,200 kJ) leads to a weekly loss of ~1 kg of fat. Strategy 2: Plan a new eating program, based on suggested level of minimal energy intake needed to support training program. Suggestions include • 30-35 kcal/kg LBM + energy cost of training.
Fuel (carbohydrate) intake to enable key training sessions to be successfully completed and to promote adequate recovery between sessions	• Inability to complete key training sessions • Inadequate adaptation to training program • Poor technique and concentration when fatigued, leading to bad technical habits and increase in risk of injury or accidents • Potential for increased loss of muscle mass (carbohydrate is "protein sparing"; inadequate carbohydrate status leads to greater loss of protein during exercise) • Additional stress on immune system and other hormonal systems (e.g., reproductive system)	• Excess fuel intake adds to can lead to inadequate energy deficit or even an energy surplus and weight gain • Note that many athletes overcompensate with carbohydrate intake during competition periods because of their fear of running out of fuel)	• Suggested guidelines for daily carbohydrate needs: • Minimal intake of light training program: ~3-5 g/kg • Minimal intake for moderate training program: ~5 g/kg • Minimal intake for heavy training program: ~7 g/kg • Intake for maximal glycogen storage: 10-12 g/kg • Special attention should be paid to carbohydrate intake before, during, and after workouts to balance fat loss vs. performance (see table 4.5)
Adequate intake of protein, vitamins, minerals, and other important food chemicals	• Interference with optimal health, function, and performance • Excessive loss of muscle mass rather than body fat	• Extra energy intake, which can lead to an energy surplus or inadequate carbohydrate intake	• Suggested guideline for protein intake during heavy training and racing while in moderate energy deficit: 1.4-1.6 g/kg. • Food plans should focus on nutrient-dense foods to maximize nutrient contribution from energy intake. • A broad-range multivitamin and mineral supplement may be warranted for long-term energy deficit.
Enjoyment of food and social eating occasions	• Denial of the psychological and emotional delights of eating, leading to personal and lifestyle imbalance • Overrestrictiveness, leading to binges	• Inability to achieve carbohydrate and nutrient needs within desired energy deficit; inadequate intakes or inability to achieve a sustained energy deficit	• Athletes should include some of their favorite foods and social eating opportunities in new plan to ensure that it can be sustained in the long term.

components of a fat loss or weight maintenance program that help to ensure an effective balance between attaining physique goals and maintaining performance and health. These characteristics can be found by remodeling existing eating habits or by designing a completely new meal plan based on a desirable energy and nutrient recipe. Many athletes like a prescribed eating plan and can apply their focus to achieving this for long periods. However, long-term adherence is best approached by recognizing that the athlete's existing eating habits have a certain appeal or practicality that will cause the athlete to gradually gravitate back to these patterns. Therefore, it is useful to assess the athlete's current or preferred diet, identify the factors that promote overeating, and provide solutions that will reduce or circumvent these problems (see table 4.3).

Cyclists and triathletes use a variety of strategies to use their training sessions (and even races) to promote weight loss. Table 4.4 summarizes common practices that are applied to training and energy intake, particularly carbohydrate intake, to promote loss of body fat. The principles of eating for fat loss are often in direct opposition to eating for optimal performance, and individual athletes vary in their response to each of these strategies. Therefore, each cyclist or triathlete should experiment to find her individual response to each strategy and determine how to fine-tune her eating to get the best results. Each athlete should discover, through experience and experimentation,

- what works to promote optimal performance—and is therefore used on race days, or for key training sessions;
- what works to promote fat loss—and is therefore used for less important training sessions (e.g., recovery sessions) and during periods designated for getting in shape; and
- what is the optimal balance between key training sessions and recovery and fat loss sessions.

Top cyclists and triathletes achieve their lean physique over a number of years of high-level training, and each individual athlete should concentrate on gradually optimizing his weight and body fat levels based on what seems a natural outcome of hard training and sensible eating. Many elite athletes are genetically blessed with a naturally lean physique and the ability to reduce body fat to even lower levels for targeted periods without unnecessary stress or penalties. The physique and body fat levels of these athletes will fluctuate over a small range throughout the preseason, racing season, and off-season. Large fluctuations are usually a sign of unnatural or extreme weight loss targets or inappropriate eating behaviors that swing between extreme restriction and binge eating.

Fueling Up for Competitive Events

Generally, events lasting longer than 90 min of continuous exercise challenge the athlete's muscle glycogen stores. This is hard to judge in a road cycling event where the actual intensity of the race may vary according to the tactics of the day and the terrain. It is also difficult to predict in the case of a triathlon where three individual modes of exercise (and, therefore, three sets of muscle groups) contribute to the overall event and where each leg of the race is undertaken at a lower workload than if the event was undertaken as an individual race. The triathlete and cyclist should prepare for each individual race in which they wish to perform well by at least normalizing muscle glycogen stores in the 12 to 36 hr leading up to the event. Opportunities for fueling will vary according to the sport and the athlete's program. For example, some cyclists compete in a race series or stage race where events are scheduled every day or couple of days. In other cases, triathletes or cyclists may want to continue to complete high-volume training right up to an event in view of their longer-term racing goals. In these situations there is little opportunity for an exercise taper to assist with glycogen restoration before each race session. Instead, the athlete should ensure that sufficient carbohydrate is consumed over the last 24 to 36 hr, and particularly after the last workout or race, to optimize refueling for the new event. In most road cycling races, there is ample opportunity to consume a substantial carbohydrate-rich meal on the morning of the event to replenish liver glycogen stores and further add to muscle glycogen content. Therefore, for some high-level cyclists, such race preparation is merely a fine-tuning of the daily eating routine in training.

Because single cycling races of >100 km and triathlons of half-Ironman length or greater are likely to result in considerable glycogen depletion, there may be merit in trying to supercompensate glycogen stores (carbohydrate load) before the event. A decision to undertake such a preparation will depend on the length of the race, the athlete's history of experiencing fatigue attributable to glycogen depletion in similar events, and the opportunity to enhance fuel availability by consuming carbohydrate in the preevent meal and during the event itself. The evolution of carbohydrate-loading protocols is examined in more detail in chapter 5. For most triathletes and cyclists, carbohydrate loading can be achieved over the 24 to 72 hr preevent via an appropriate exercise taper and focused attention on carbohydrate intake goals. For triathletes who are peaking for an important long-distance or Ironman race, carbohydrate loading is a dedicated activity to finish the preparation. However, mistakes are often made, particularly by subelite athletes, who can be caught up in the novelty and culture of a big race. Many athletes overtrain in the last days leading into the event. Other athletes do not have enough nutrition knowledge to guarantee that carbohydrate intake goals are met over these final days. Many athletes need to be properly educated on the latest principles and practice of the carbohydrate-loading protocol.

Many professional cycling and triathlon races have a mid-morning or afternoon start time, allowing competitors to fine-tune race fuel stores by eating a substantial carbohydrate-rich breakfast or brunch. In contrast, triathletes who compete in races starting between 7 and 9 am may be unable to eat such a large preevent meal, because of the early-morning start time or the increased

Table 4.3 Common Issues That Interfere With Success in Achieving Weight or Fat Loss Goals

Examples of causes	Examples of solutions
SIMPLY EATING TOO MUCH FOOD	
<ul><li>Having no concept of what is an appropriate amount of food.</li><li>Eating the same amount as other people (who have larger energy needs).</li><li>Allowing yourself to become very hungry—this usually leads to overeating.</li><li>All-you-can-eat or self-serve food service. Buffets tempt overeating and make it easy to lose track of total food intake.</li><li>Eating too fast. By the time you feel satisfied, you have eaten too much.</li><li>Being in constant contact with food during the day—losing tracks of snacks.</li><li>Mistaking fatigue from overtraining, lack of sleep, or dehydration as a lack of fuel and overcompensating with extra food.</li><li>Alcohol binges. Alcohol is a high-energy nutrient that reduces inhibitions about eating and promotes deposition of fat.</li><li>Failing to reduce food intake during exercise taper or inactivity.</li><li>Being overenthusiastic about "recovery eating." Post-workout snacks may address important nutritional goals; however, they are often in addition to the existing eating plan.</li></ul>	<ul><li>Have a plan of meals and snacks, tailored to meet your energy needs over the day. Don't worry about what other people are eating.</li><li>Get professional advice about appropriate portion control for various food types and how to exchange one food for another.</li><li>In a self-serve situation, plate your meal once. Don't go back for seconds.</li><li>Don't overrestrict or allow yourself to get too hungry—plan meals and snacks to keep the edge off hunger and prevent binges.</li><li>Use strategies to slow your rate of eating so that it takes longer to eat less; for example, make meals spicy or choose foods that are piping hot or served frozen.</li><li>Avoid buying jumbo sizes of foods, which encourage overeating. It isn't a bargain if you eat it all at once!</li><li>Be strategic with recovery nutrition. Rearrange meal schedules so that existing food intake is well timed to promote efficient recovery after workouts. If a postexercise snack is needed, choose nutritious foods and reorganize menus to take this into account.</li><li>Stay well hydrated to avoid fatigue associated with dehydration.</li><li>Avoid alcohol binges. Consider 1-2 glasses of alcohol as a treat to be built into your eating program.</li></ul>
EATING TOO MUCH FAT (FAT IS ENERGY DENSE)	
<ul><li>Hidden fats and oils in cooking—especially fried and deep-fried foods.</li><li>Hidden fats and oils in food preparation—especially dressings, sauces, and gravies.</li><li>Cream.</li><li>Thick butter or margarine spreads on bread.</li><li>Fatty cuts of meats.</li><li>High-fat dairy products.</li><li>Excessive use and large amounts of cheese.</li><li>Pastry (other than phyllo).</li><li>Nuts as snacks.</li><li>Desserts, cakes, Danish pastries, and rich desserts.</li><li>Full-fat ice cream.</li><li>Chocolate as more than a treat.</li><li>Thick spreads of peanut butter and chocolate spreads (e.g., Nutella).</li><li>Takeaways and fast foods.</li></ul>	<ul><li>Cook with minimum amounts of added fat—stir-fry in a wok with spray oil, microwave, grill, or steam. Choose monounsaturated oils.</li><li>Flavor foods with low-oil dressings, lemon or lime juice, balsamic vinegar, salsa, tomato sauce, or mustard.</li><li>Replace butter and margarine spreads with a scrape of avocado or mustard, salsa, or low-fat mayonnaise.</li><li>Make creamy sauces with evaporated nonfat milk.</li><li>Use reduced-fat cheese as a garnish rather than a thick layer.</li><li>Switch to low-fat milks and yogurts.</li><li>Choose lean cuts of meats, and trim all remaining fat.</li><li>Choose breads rather than pastry items at the bakery.</li><li>Use reduced-fat recipes for cakes and desserts, but keep the portion in check.</li><li>Budget for an appropriate number of treats each week—quality rather than quantity.</li></ul>

(continued)

Table 4.3 *(continued)*

Examples of causes	Examples of solutions
EATING TOO MANY ENERGY-DENSE, SATIETY-POOR FOODS[a]	

Examples of causes	Examples of solutions
Causes (in addition to excessive intake of fat): • Eating low-fat foods in large quantities (buckets of low-fat ice cream or frozen yogurt, jumbo low-fat muffins, family packs of 99% fat-free confectionery). • Failing to eat whole fruits, vegetables, and salad in adequate quantities—especially to balance out carbohydrate-dense foods (bread, rice, pasta, noodles). • Inadequate fiber intake. • Drinking juice or milk for fluid needs. • Using high-energy drinks (soft drinks, sport drinks, liquid meal supplements) outside training.	• Use vegetables and fruit to increase the volume (and reduce the energy density per mouthful) of meals and snacks. • Add thick salad fillings to sandwiches. • Increase the ratio of vegetables in recipes (e.g., in stir-fries, pasta sauces, pizza toppings). • Eat salad or add vegetables to the plate before serving meat and carbohydrate choices. • Eat fruit to finish a meal. • Choose fiber-rich versions of foods—whole-grain breads and cereals, whole fruits, and raw vegetables. • Eat fruit rather than drink juice. Allow one glass of juice daily. • Allow 3-4 servings of dairy foods each day, but avoid drinking milk for fluid needs. • Drink fluids to increase the volume of meals and snacks. However, apart from juice and dairy allowance, and drinks consumed for training and competition performance, stick to low-energy fluids (water, tea or coffee, plain mineral waters, or diet soft drink). • Combine protein and carbohydrate at meals or snacks to enhance total satiety value (e.g., nonfat milk hot chocolate and a slice of toast rather than 4 slices of toast). • Choose low glycemic index carbohydrate-rich foods (e.g., oat-based porridge or Bircher muesli instead of cornflake cereal).

Examples of causes	Examples of solutions
POOR EATING BEHAVIOR	

Examples of causes	Examples of solutions
• Having a chaotic lifestyle without an eating routine. • Having food within easy access for uncontrolled snacking. • Eating when bored or to fill in the gaps between activities. • "Being good" (restrictive) in the morning and then eating uncontrolled amounts of food in the evening. • "Being good" on weekdays allowing for binge eating on weekends. • Eating when upset. • Adding food to all social activities (e.g., popcorn at a movie, muffin while shopping). • Uncontrolled eating in partnership with alcohol binges. • Pretending that you are buying food "for later," or to share with others, when it is simply an opportunity for your own overeating.	• Eat planned meals or snacks and then put distance between yourself and food. • Chew gum or clean your teeth to prevent "picking" while preparing meals. • Deal with stressful issues rather than using food to deal with your emotions. • Have a list of enjoyable activities to fill in the gaps in the day. • Eat as a separate and focused activity. Treat other activities (e.g., watching a film, driving a car) in the same way. • Don't binge—eat and drink only while it is a relaxed and comfortable experience! • Stop considering not eating as "good." Restrictive eating usually ends up with a binge, so don't start the cycle.

[a]Satiety describes the feeling of being satisfied after eating. A high-satiety food keeps hunger away for a long time, whereas "satiety-poor" foods seem to disappear quickly.

Table 4.4   Strategies Used in Conjunction With Training Promote Loss of Body Fat

Strategy	Guidelines to achieve optimal performance	Change in guideline to promote fat loss	Advantages of using strategy to promote fat loss	Disadvantages of using strategy to promote fat loss
1. Undertaking extra training or cross-training to increase energy expenditure			• Contributes to the energy deficit needed to promote fat loss. • Keeps the athlete occupied and removed from food during the period of exercise.	• Increases the risk of injury and fatigue, thus interfering with primary workouts. • May cause severe hunger or a feeling of "virtue" leading to overeating after session—it is possible to eat more than the energy cost of the extra training, counteracting the original goal!
2. Undertaking morning training sessions in a fasted state	To enhance carbohydrate availability during the workout, consume foods and drinks to supply at least 1-4 g of carbohydrate per kilogram of body mass in the 1-4 hr before exercise.	Undertake morning training sessions before any food intake. Either • undertake an additional training session (45-60 min) before breakfast, or • begin the scheduled morning training session without consuming any energy-containing foods or drinks, and wait until 60-90 min into the session before consuming carbohydrate.	• Compared with exercise undertaken after a carbohydrate-rich snack or meal, exercise in a fasted state increases fat oxidation during the session, potentially promoting loss of body fat. • Potentially reduces total energy intake for the day by removing the preevent snack or meal.	• May cause severe hunger or a feeling of "virtue"—it is possible to overeat after the session, counteracting the original goal! • Increases the risk of fatigue and poor technique, interfering with the goal of the workout and increasing the risk of injury. An inability to complete the session may reduce total energy expenditure and the desired energy deficit. This effect can be counteracted by consuming carbohydrate during the session. • May increase protein breakdown during the session and cause greater stress on the immune system, leading to unwanted loss of muscle mass and an increased risk of illness.

(continued)

Table 4.4 (continued)

Strategy	Guidelines to achieve optimal performance	Change in guideline to promote fat loss	Advantages of using strategy to promote fat loss	Disadvantages of using strategy to promote fat loss
3. Undertaking workout with minimal or no carbohydrate intake during the session	Consume foods and drinks to supply at least 30-60 g of carbohydrate per hour during exercise. • Start intake at the beginning of a workout or even in the minutes before the race starts. • Ensure higher rates of intake as the session continues after 60 min. • Experiment to find the rate of carbohydrate intake for best performance.	• Drink water only during shorter or low-intensity sessions. • During longer or higher-intensity sessions, wait for 60-90 min before consuming any carbohydrate during the session. • Experiment to find the lowest possible carbohydrate intake that allows the session to be completed within training goals. • Ensure that hydration is well maintained even if refueling strategies are not as aggressive as race day.	• Exercise without carbohydrate intake is achieved with increased rates of fat oxidation, potentially promoting loss of body fat. Carbohydrate consumed during exercise (especially during the later stages of the workout) causes a much smaller change in exercise fuel use compared with carbohydrate consumed before exercise, so "savings" may be smaller than anticipated. • Potentially reduces total energy intake for the day by removing the energy cost of foods and drinks usually consumed during the workout, thus adding to the energy deficit needed to promote weight loss.	• May cause severe hunger leading to overeating after the session. A recent study reported that consuming carbohydrate during exercise caused participants to consume less energy at the next meal and the rest of the day, compared with control (water only during training) • Increases the risk of fatigue and poor technique, thus interfering with the goal of the workout and increasing the risk of injury. May even lead to inability to complete the session, thus reducing the total energy expenditure achieved toward the desired energy deficit. • May increase protein breakdown during the session and cause greater stress on the immune system, leading to unwanted loss of muscle mass and an increased risk of illness.
4. Waiting several hours after the workout before consuming carbohydrate or other food	To enhance recovery after the session, consume foods and drinks to supply at least 1 g of carbohydrate per kilogram of body mass in the 30-60 min after exercise, with normal meals resuming within the next hour. Choose nutrient-rich foods that also provide at least 10 g of high-quality protein.	Wait several hours after workout before consuming anything other than low-energy fluid. Look after rehydration needs only.	• Promotes additional fat oxidation after the session by remaining carbohydrate depleted. • Potentially reduces total energy intake for the day by removing the caloric cost of the postworkout recovery snack.	• May cause severe hunger leading to overeating when food is finally available. • Reduces effective recovery—interferes with refueling and optimal protein synthesis, thus generally interfering with the overall goals of the training program or directly reducing performance at the next workout. • May cause greater stress on the immune system, leading to an increased risk of illness.

risk of gastrointestinal discomfort that comes from eating large volumes of food before running. Each athlete should choose a preevent meal based on the individual goals of his or her race nutrition plan, the practical opportunities provided by the race schedule, and the lessons learned from previous races. Factors that might need to be taken into account are summarized in table 4.5.

Hydration Issues in Competition

In events lasting longer than 1 hr, the need and opportunity for intake of fluid and fuel during the race should be considered. Laboratory-based studies show clearly that endurance and performance are impaired when a participant is

dehydrated, especially in a hot environment. A fluid deficit of 1.7% body mass was sufficient to cause a detectable impairment in endurance in a high-intensity sprint following a 1 hr of laboratory-based cycling bout in hot (32°C) conditions (Walsh et al. 1994). Similarly, cyclists performed better in a laboratory time trial undertaken at the end of a 1 hr cycling bout when substantial fluid replacement was compared with a small fluid intake (Below et al. 1995). Chapter 1 indicated that as an athlete's fluid deficit increases, there is a continuously increasing deterioration in cardiovascular and thermoregulatory function, perception of effort, and work output. Skill and concentration are also impaired at moderate levels of dehydration, which could affect important aspects of cycling and triathlon races such

Table 4.5 Issues for the Preevent Meal in Cycling and Triathlon

Issue	Guidelines
Event is mid-morning to late afternoon.	There are opportunities to consume substantial amounts of carbohydrate-rich food on the morning of the event to enhance liver and muscle glycogen stores. Options include breakfast + preevent meal or snack or a large brunch; foods may be chosen from the athlete's usual carbohydrate-rich meal choices. The final meal timetable may depend on food availability, the need to travel or register at the race start, and personal choice regarding timing of final intake before competition.
Event is early in the morning.	The athlete can wake up 3 hr preevent to allow a larger breakfast or settle for a smaller, easily digested snack in the 1-2 hr preevent. Simple snacks include liquid meal supplements and fruit smoothies, sport bars and cereal bars, and ready-to-drink sport drinks or juices. Factors to consider include the importance of sleep, fuel needs, and the risk of gastrointestinal discomfort following food or fluids. If preevent intake fails to achieve preparation goals, the athlete should compensate with more aggressive refueling and rehydration tactics during the event.
There is overlap between preevent intake and intake during the race.	The combination of carbohydrate intake before and during a prolonged race is superior to the benefits from either strategy alone, although in most situations, intake during the event provides the greatest impact on performance. In practice, the athlete may not always achieve optimal nutrition for each situation. When one opportunity is missed or underused, greater emphasis on the other opportunity may help to compensate. For example, if heavy training or racing has been undertaken on the previous day, there may have been insufficient time and opportunity for complete restoration of muscle glycogen stores. In such a situation, the preevent meal can make a major contribution to fuel availability for the race. Alternatively, the athlete who has limited opportunity to refuel during a race should pay additional attention to the preevent meal or carbohydrate intake immediately before the race start.
There is greater risk of gastrointestinal discomfort during triathlon because of running leg.	Some athletes are at higher risk of gastrointestinal discomfort and upset. Risks appear to be greater in triathlon than cycling, because of the gastrointestinal impact of the running leg. Excessive intakes of fiber, fat, protein, and some sugars (lactose and fructose) in the preevent meal may increase the risk for some triathletes. Experimentation with the timing, volume, and food choices at the preevent meal may help to reduce the risk in susceptible athletes. Intake during the race (hyperosmotic drinks, intake of excessive amounts of fat and fiber) and moderate levels of dehydration should also be investigated.
Athlete is away from home and familiar food.	Cyclists and triathletes often compete away from their home bases, exposing themselves to a different food supply, reduced access to food, or an environment with poor food and water hygiene. It is useful for the athlete to bring a supply of foods from home to ensure the availability of suitable choices or favorite foods for the preevent meal. The preevent meal should be chosen from a menu with which the athlete is familiar and confident.
Other competitors have a different preevent meal.	There are many menu plans and food choices that may contribute to a suitable preevent preparation. Each athlete should have confidence in his or her own plan, based on successful practice in previous events. Nevertheless, it is useful to have some flexibility in case there are last-minute problems with food availability or changes to the start of the event.

as bike-handling skills and tactical decisions. Moderate to severe fluid deficits are associated with increased risks of gastrointestinal dysfunction and upset (Rehrer et al. 1990), impairing performance as well as interfering with any (late) attempt to rehydrate. Drinking to offset sweat losses and minimize the fluid deficit can reduce such physiological disturbances and may have other benefits such as reducing muscle glycogen use during prolonged cycling (Hargreaves et al. 1996).

In the field, it is often harder to see the negative effects of a fluid deficit. Several factors may hide or reduce the effects of dehydration during a cycle race or triathlon. Convective loss of heat attributable to wind and movement through the air is difficult to simulate in a laboratory setting; however, in the field it may provide assistance with thermoregulation (Saunders et al. 2005) to attenuate the effects of dehydration. Additionally, because the energy cost of cycling uphill or running on any terrain is correlated with body mass, the performance deficit associated with dehydration may be partially offset as the athlete becomes lighter. There are anecdotal reports that some top cyclists make a calculated decision not to fully rehydrate in some conditions—for example, allowing an acceptable level of dehydration to occur during a mountain stage to take advantage of a reduced body mass. A laboratory study investigated such voluntary dehydration on the ability of cyclists to ride their bikes up an 8% treadmill incline after 2 hr of cycling (Ebert et al. 2005). Trials were conducted in the heat ($\sim$30°C) with full rehydration or with low fluid intakes that allowed a loss of 2.1 kg (2.5% of body mass). Although a reduced body mass allowed cyclists to perform the hill climb at the same speed with a lower power output (308 ± 28 vs. 313 ± 28 W), endurance was reduced by $\sim$29%. Therefore, under laboratory conditions which attempted to simulate race issues, effects of dehydration appear to outweigh any physical advantages of weight loss. This balance needs to be tested in a field setting.

The gastrointestinal discomfort associated with the forced intake of the large amounts of fluid must also be taken into account. In moderate ambient conditions (20-21°C), forced replacement of sweat losses during a 1 hr laboratory cycling protocol did not enhance performance (McConell et al. 1997; Robinson et al. 1995) and in some cases impaired performance because of the discomfort of riding at such high intensities with a full gut (Robinson et al. 1995). An increased risk of gastrointestinal upset or discomfort is associated with drinking during high-intensity exercise, especially during running. Finally, in continuous sports like triathlon and cycling, there is often a time cost associated with consuming fluids, attributable to the need to slow down or move out of an optimally aerodynamic riding position to receive supplies from aid stations or handlers and then consume the drink. Therefore, in the real world, hydration plans for racing in triathlons and cycling events need to be practical and consider the big picture.

For racing at high intensities in hot conditions, it makes sense to plan for the minimum level of fluid deficit that can be practically achieved. This includes attention to fluid levels in the day and hours leading up to an event to ensure that the cyclist or triathlete is hydrated at the start of the event. Athletes may need to be aggressive with their fluid intake strategies to correct the dehydration associated with a previous training session or race, or they may need to adopt new daily drinking behaviors to accommodate a sudden exposure to a hot living environment. Even if the athlete is not aiming to fluid overload (discussed subsequently), there can be good reasons to have a substantial drink just before the start of a race. Effective rehydration during exercise depends on maximizing the rate of fluid delivery from the stomach to the intestine for absorption. One of the factors affecting gastric emptying is gastric distension attributable to the volume of stomach contents. Optimal delivery of fluid from the stomach can be achieved by starting exercise with a comfortable volume of fluid in the stomach and adopting a pattern of periodic fluid intake during the exercise designed to top up gastric contents as the gut empties (Noakes et al. 1991). Obviously, each athlete will need to experiment to determine the volume of fluid that will comfortably prime gastric emptying and in particular how this feels once exercise has commenced. However, as a general rule, most athletes can tolerate a fluid bolus of about 5 ml per kilogram of body mass (i.e., 300-400 ml) immediately before the event starts.

During the race, each athlete should use the available opportunities to drink as much as is practical, but less than the rate of sweat loss, to keep his or her fluid deficit to an acceptable level. There are few published data on typical sweat rates during cycling and triathlon races, and because of the variation in work rates and environment between and sometimes even within events, mean data may be a meaningless concept. Therefore, cyclists and triathletes are advised to gather their own data on sweat losses and overall fluid balance in a variety of training and race situations. This can be done by monitoring pre- and postexercise body mass and recording total fluid (and food) intake and any losses from urination over the session. This may help the athlete gauge the suitability of her hydration patterns and assess whether there may be a benefit in adopting a more aggressive approach. There is a wide range in voluntary fluid intakes during exercise among athletes, with people being categorized across a spectrum from "reluctant" to "avid" drinkers. However, it appears to be possible to improve the habits, skills, and gastrointestinal tolerance needed to increase habitual fluid intake during exercise, through practicing the intake of gradually larger volumes. These strategies should be considered by athletes who habitually achieve large fluid deficits during races. Equally, there are concerns that some individuals are capable of drinking at rates greater than their sweat losses under some conditions of sport, and these athletes should be counseled to adopt hydration practices that are less extreme.

The availability of fluids and the opportunity to drink vary between the sports and events within the sport. Even in the longest triathlons, fluid intake during the swim leg is unintentional; this leaves the cycle and run legs, and the transition to each, as the opportunities for refueling and rehydration. Most intake occurs during the cycle leg, because of its relative length and placement in the race order as well as the relative ease of consuming and tolerating fluid intake in comparison to the running leg (Kimber et al. 2002). In shorter triathlons, the top competitors often aim to drink in the early phase of the cycle leg, setting themselves up to run without interruption. As previously discussed, many take a calculated risk of allowing what they consider an acceptable degree of dehydration to occur under the conditions of the day. For non-elite participants who are out on the course for a longer time and with a greater priority on safety and enjoyment, the aim should be to make sensible use of the range of available drinking opportunities—neither overhydrating nor allowing large fluid deficits to accrue. Slower competitors have a lower overall sweat rate because of their lower work intensity, so it will be easier for them to drink at a rate that keeps pace with sweat losses (see practical issue).

Fluids are made available in most triathlons, and particularly mass participation events, from a network of aid stations in transition areas and appropriate parts of the cycle and run course. The frequency and placement of these aid stations vary according to the length of the course, the number of competitors, the ease of approach, and the expected environmental conditions of the race. Short races may provide only one station on each of the race legs and transition areas, whereas longer races have an intricate feed station network, usually associated with strategic splits in the race—for example, every 5 or 10 miles or 10 to 20 km in the bike leg and every 1 to 2 miles or 2 km in the run. This ensures, especially in long races held in extreme conditions such as the Hawaiian Ironman, that competitors do not have an unreasonably long period between opportunities to refuel, rehydrate, or seek help. Volunteers are usually placed at aid stations, particularly on the cycle leg, to hand out drink bottles (bidons) to passing competitors. There is greater opportunity for competitors to grab their own cups or drink bottles at aid stations during the run, although handlers can also help to streamline the process. Of course, triathletes can carry their own bidons on the cycle leg, and according to the duration of the race and the environmental conditions, they may have one to three bottle cages attached to the bike to carry the bidons. In longer races, empty bidons are discarded and replaced over the course of the race. In shorter events, the triathlete will usually aim to be self-sufficient for the whole race.

In the early rules of triathlon, the cycle leg was completed as an individual time trial, making an aerodynamic riding position of high importance. Special drinking devices were developed, such as the CamelBak and Bikestream, which allowed fluids to be stored in a bladder attached to a convenient site on the bike and provided by a drinking straw positioned within reach of the athlete's mouth as he assumed a racing position. Such drink devices, although creative, may be less important to competitors in a draft-permitted race where riding within the protection of a bunch provides more opportunity for drinking from conventional drink bottles. In fact, such devices may not be allowed under the race rules of elite competition. They are also less important in longer races, where triathletes need a greater supply of drinks and can afford to spend more time to ensure that their race intake is achieved. In longer races, some triathletes run with belts that are able to secure small water bottles with minimal impact on running speed or comfort; these athletes may believe that it is important either to be self-sufficient with supplies or to have self-paced access to fluid during the conditions of their event. They may also prefer the convenience of drinking from specially manufactured squeeze bottles than wrestling with spillage from open cups.

The culture and opportunities to drink fluids during a cycling race are different than those during the triathlon. Cyclists have the opportunity to carry their supplies using the bidon cages on their bike or the pockets in the back of their jersey. Feeding zones are set up in most races, with volunteer handlers or the professional team soigneurs handing out drinks and food supplies to their riders from these points. In professional races, team cars also follow the riders, and it is the job of the team domestique riders to get supplies from the car and ferry extra bottles to the designated leaders in the team. In most races, feeding zones and handouts are prohibited within a certain distance of the race start and finish and on technically dangerous parts of the course.

Many cyclists and triathletes undertake races in which significant dehydration is inevitable: where sweat rate is extremely high, when there is little opportunity to drink during the race, or when these factors are combined. In these situations, power outputs and sweat rates are high, and the top competitors are reluctant or unable to sacrifice time to allow significant intake of fluid. Some athletes have experimented with hyperhydration in the hours before the event to attempt to reduce the total fluid deficit incurred. Drinking extra fluid before exercise has been shown to increase total body water, expand plasma volume, and ultimately enhance performance in a subsequent exercise trial (Moroff and Bass 1980). Another study examined the effect of chronic periods of fluid overloading in moderately trained cyclists (Kristal-Boneh et al. 1995). Heat-acclimatized participants were required to double their usual fluid intake for a week, from a mean daily intake of 1,980 ml to 4,085 ml. This practice was found to reset normal fluid balance to retain an extra 600 ml of fluid. Several experimental trials in the heat found that superior hydration status increased heat tolerance, allowed maximal aerobic workload to be achieved at a lower heart rate, and improved performance in a cycling time trial. More work is needed to confirm these results, especially for elite competitors. However, they support the advice often given to athletes competing in a hot climate to increase their fluid intake over the days leading up to the event. Whether this advice merely ensures fluid balance rather than promoting fluid overload has not been adequately tested. Finally, a method of hyperhydration under current study involves the consumption of a small amount of glycerol (1-1.2 g/kg body mass) along with a large fluid bolus (25-35 ml/kg) in the hours before exercise. The results of studies using this protocol, which has been shown to increase body water by ~600 ml, are shown in appendix table 4.e, in the section on supplement use in cycling and triathlon.

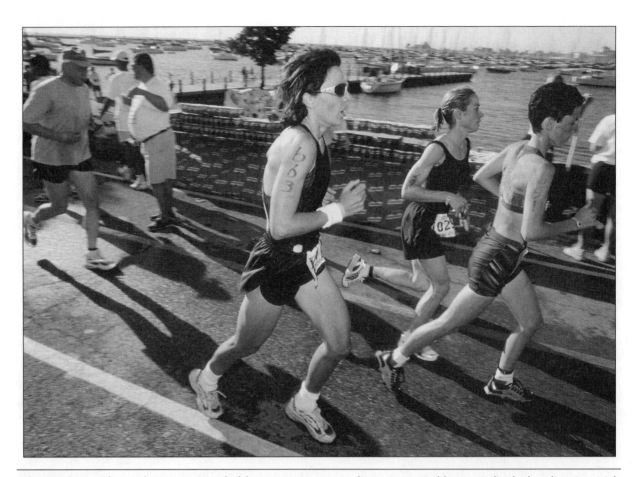

Substantial rates of sweat loss are expected of the top competitors in short-course triathlons or individual cycling time trials undertaken in hot weather.

There are some shortcomings and possible disadvantages to fluid overloading techniques. First, much of the fluid is excreted via urination, because the body has a well-developed system to regulate the volume and concentration of its fluid content both at rest and during exercise. Fluid overloading may have a detrimental effect on performance if it causes the significant interruption of having to urinate immediately before or in the early stages of the event. The discomfort and potential performance impairment caused by excess fluid in the gut have previously been discussed. In addition to any side effects of special protocols used to hyperhydrate before exercise (e.g., glycerol intake), the impact of any gain in body mass as a result of increased fluid retention might need to be taken into account, especially for athletes or courses where weight is a sensitive issue. Whether the small impairments in performance attributable to the increased energy cost of riding or running with a heavier body mass are more than offset by the improvement in fluid balance needs to be individually studied. Finally, if taken to extreme levels, excessive fluid intake may lead to hyponatremia, or "water intoxication." This situation is discussed further in relation to excessive drinking during exercise (see practical issue). Clearly, fluid overloading before an event is a strategy that needs to be researched before any more firm recommendations can

be made to athletes, and it should be undertaken under supervision.

Refueling During Events

If fatigue related to carbohydrate depletion occurs during a race, then the intake of carbohydrate during the event may prevent or delay the onset of this fatigue and enhance performance. Typically, events of greater than 90 min of continuous exercise are considered to benefit from strategies to enhance carbohydrate availability. However, the benefit from carbohydrate intake during any race will vary, depending on factors such as the fuel demands of the competition, environmental conditions, and the interaction with other strategies such as carbohydrate loading and preevent carbohydrate intake. In some studies of prolonged cycling, for example, a 100 km cycling time trial undertaken in the laboratory, no significant benefits to performance were observed when carbohydrate was fed during the bout (Madsen et al. 1996). On the other hand, carbohydrate intake by cyclists immediately before and during a laboratory-based time trial lasting about 1 hr produced a faster time (58.74 ± 0.52 min) compared with performance with a flavored placebo (60.15 ± 0.65 min) (Jeukendrup et al. 1997). These observations, which seem to be the opposite of the predicted responses, might be explained by a number of factors including the overall carbohydrate status of athletes, the amount of carbohydrate consumed, and, most important, the ability of the test protocol to detect small but worthwhile differences in performance.

Carbohydrate intake during exercise appears to enhance performance via a number of separate mechanisms. These include supplying an alternative fuel source when muscle glycogen content is depleted (Coyle et al. 1986), preventing the reduction in blood glucose content that might otherwise cause hypoglycemia (Coggan and Coyle 1987), and perhaps providing other benefits to the central nervous system mediated via perception of effort and muscle fiber recruitment. Although the oxidation of carbohydrate consumed during running bouts may help to spare glycogen utilization in at least some muscle fibers (Tsintzas, Williams, Boobis, et al. 1996) in the case of cyclists, glycogen sparing or net resynthesis of muscle glycogen may be limited to situations of intermittent high-intensity bouts (Yaspelkis et al. 1993) or low-intensity cycling (Kuipers et al. 1987). The beneficial effects of carbohydrate intake, at least in hot conditions, have been shown to be independent and additive to the performance enhancement that occurs with fluid replacement (Below et al. 1995). In the case of events lasting an hour or more, benefits appear to occur via stimulation of the brain and central nervous system to alter perceptions of fatigue or pacing. This is explored in more detail in chapter 5 (research topic).

The decision to consume carbohydrate during an event should be made by each athlete based on factors such as

- the duration and conditions of the event,
- history of fatigue and reduced performance in similar events or training simulation,
- general opportunities to maintain carbohydrate availability prior to the race, and
- available opportunities for during event refueling.

Many athletes want to identify the shortest event that might benefit from carbohydrate intake immediately before and during the race. In the case of single cycling events, several laboratory-based studies suggest that benefits may be seen in races of ~40 km or 1 hr duration (Below et al. 1995; Jeukendrup et al. 1997) but are absent for time trials of shorter duration (Palmer et al. 1998). In triathlon, a study of a simulated Olympic distance race found a worthwhile, but not statistically significant, enhancement of just over 1 min in run time and overall race time with the intake of a carbohydrate–electrolyte drink compared with placebo (Millard-Stafford et al. 1990). As is the case for balancing fluid replacement strategies against the time loss involved, the top athletes in the field often take a cautious view of carbohydrate replacement in short events. The decisions of subelite performers may be based on different priorities. In most cases, the intake of carbohydrate will not directly harm performance. Possible disadvantages include an unnecessary (but usually small) intake of energy for those who are weight sensitive and the possibility of gastrointestinal side effects when poor food or drink choices are made.

There are few situations where creative solutions can't be found to such problems if they exist. During events of up to 5 hr, a carbohydrate intake of 30 to 60 g/hr (hourly rate of ~0.5-1.0 g/kg of body mass) is generally suitable, and each athlete should experiment to find a feeding program that suits the needs and opportunities provided by her race.

The simplest way to refuel during cycling and triathlon events is to consume a carbohydrate–electrolyte sport drink (6-8% carbohydrate) according to the athlete's chosen fluid replacement plans. An hourly fluid intake of 500 to 800 ml, which is generally possible in most race situations, would also provide carbohydrate replacement of 30 to 65 g/hr. In their standard concentrations, sport drinks appear to have minimal impact on effective fluid delivery and rehydration goals. In fact, they may even assist fluid balance by encouraging a greater voluntary intake in comparison to water. However, in hot conditions, some athletes like to drink larger volumes of a diluted sport drink (3-4% concentration) to ensure optimal fluid intake and delivery. Another plan is to tailor-make drinks that gradually increase in concentration over the course of the race, giving priority to fluid delivery in the early phase of the race and increasing carbohydrate replacement as glycogen stores become depleted.

Cost, convenience, and flavor relief underpin the use of a range of other carbohydrate-containing drinks and foods during cycling and triathlon sessions. Table 4.6 provides specific comments about the features of various common choices. The advantages of foods, including special sport bars and gels, include compactness and portability as well as a change in flavor and texture during prolonged events. Foods and sport products can be carried in pockets in race jerseys or triathlon suits or in special pouches or belts strapped to the bike or the athlete. During the race, new supplies are picked up at aid stations or feed zones, with *musettes* (bags) containing a range of supplies being a familiar sight in professional cycling races. For cyclists who race 100 days a year, having a choice of refueling options, many of which provide a significant source of other nutrients, seems particularly useful. It also seems that athletes who compete in longer events (4-5 hr or more) self-select higher rates of carbohydrate intake during exercise than seen in shorter events—up to 1.5 g · kg⁻¹ · hr⁻¹ (~1.5 g/min). For example, a study of Tour de France cyclists reported mean carbohydrate intakes during daily stages of ~1.5 g · kg⁻¹ · hr⁻¹ (Saris et al. 1989). Meanwhile Ironman triathletes were seen to consume carbohydrate intakes of 1.5 and 1.2 g · kg⁻¹ · hr⁻¹ during the cycle leg for males and females, respectively, and 0.8 and 0.6 g · kg⁻¹ · hr⁻¹ in the run leg, for an overall race intake of ~ 1 g · kg⁻¹ · hr⁻¹ (Kimber et al. 2002). Although the use of concentrated gels or solid carbohydrate foods may increase the amount of carbohydrate that can be consumed, there may be a gender bias in race intake. In the Ironman study, females reported a greater intake of water and foods, whereas males apparently consumed a larger proportion of their carbohydrate from sweetened beverages (Kimber et al. 2002).

The peak rate of oxidation of exogenous carbohydrate during exercise from a range of single carbohydrate sources

Table 4.6   Drinks, Foods, and Sport Products Used to Provide Carbohydrate During Triathlon and Cycling Races

Product	Serving needed to provide 50 g of carbohydrate	Comments
Sport drink (carbo-hydrate–electrolyte drink)	600-800 ml of 6-8% drink	Simplest way to address fluid and carbohydrate needs simultaneously during events. Sodium content may increase voluntary intake of drink and help to address electrolyte losses from sweat. Standard concentration of 6-8% carbohydrate can be manipulated to increase priority of either carbohydrate or fluid depending on conditions. However, diluting beverages to a different concentration than their standard preparation may alter the taste profile so that it no longer maximizes voluntary intake.
Fruit juices, non-carbonated soft drinks	475-600 ml of 8-11% drink	Offer flavor relief and perhaps some cost savings. Often more concentrated than is considered ideal but can be converted into a "sport drink" by changing dilution and adding a half teaspoon (~3 g) of table salt per liter of drink. See notes for sport drinks on diluting beverages.
Soda and cola drinks	475 ml of 11% drink	More concentrated than sport drinks and contain little sodium. Offer flavor relief and, in the case of cola drinks, a small but apparently effective dose of caffeine. De-fizz before drinking.
Sport bars	1-1.5 × 60-75 g bar	Convenient and portable source of carbohydrate. Relatively nonperishable, although they may become sticky in hot weather. The most suitable bars are brands with a low-fat, high-carbohydrate composition; many also provide a reasonable source of protein and micronutrients. Other brands follow high-protein, or Zone (40:30:30 carbohydrate–fat–protein ratio) composition. One study has shown Zone bars to be less effective than high-carbohydrate sources as a race fuel for ultraendurance events (see table 4.f). As with all solid foods, the athlete should take care to meet fluid needs with a separate plan for drink intake.
Sport gels	2 × 45 g sachets	Convenient and portable source of carbohydrate that can be easily consumed from "quick-tear" packages or squeeze bottles and tubes. Some brands contain a small source of caffeine (e.g., 25-50 mg dose). The athlete should take care to meet fluid needs separately and should be aware of the reduced sodium content of some gels. May be used both on bike and run leg of a triathlon, because there is generally a low gastrointestinal impact as long as the athlete is well hydrated.
Bananas	2 medium	Popular fruit for bike. Convenient to peel and eat. Provides good source of carbohydrate. Although promoted as a source of potassium, it is not considered necessary to replace this electrolyte during exercise
Cereal bars and granola bars	~2 bars (30-35 g bars)	Convenient and portable source of carbohydrate. Relatively nonperishable, meaning that they will survive most environmental conditions. Fat and fiber content varies between brands, and some may be unsuitable for athletes with high risk of gastrointestinal problems
Sandwiches and rolls	1 medium (70 g) roll with tablespoon of jam; 1 round thin or 1.5 rounds thick sandwiches with jam; 1.5 medium or 2 small rolls with ham and cheese	Widely available and well-liked food on bike. Should be individually wrapped for portability. Depending on weather and taste preferences, sandwiches may have sweet (additional carbohydrate) or savory (protein) fillings. The athlete should look after fluid needs simultaneously. Fiber and fat content vary with choice of breads and fillings; some athletes may need to choose carefully to avoid gastrointestinal problems.
Cakes and cookies	1 large (80 g) or 4 small (20 g) cookies, 1 medium (110-120 g) muffin, 2 small (100 g) slices fruit cake	Well liked by cyclists. Increased portability when available in individually wrapped bags. Often high in fat, and some may be unsuitable for athletes with high risk of gastrointestinal problems. The athlete should look after fluid needs simultaneously.
Confectionery	60-70 g of sweets	Jelly babies and other jube-like sweets are popular and compact carbohydrate sources. Small portions allow "trickle feeding" of carbohydrate throughout a race. May be used both on bike and during run leg of a triathlon because there is generally a low gastrointestinal impact as long as the athlete is well hydrated.
Chocolate bars	1.5 × 60 g bar	Well-liked source of carbohydrate with high energy density. However, relatively high in fat and melts in hot weather. The athlete should look after fluid needs simultaneously.

is ~0.8 to 1.0 g/min (Jeukendrup and Jentjens 2000), although the intakes multiple sources of carbohydrates in the same drink achieve oxidation rates of 1 to 1.3 g/min (Jentjens, Achten, et al. 2004). Although the rate of carbohydrate intake needs to exceed oxidation rate, it is curious that reported rates of consumption of carbohydrate by some athletes in ultraendurance events appear to be so high. It is likely, in cases such as cycling stage races, that this intake is necessary to contribute to total energy and carbohydrate needs over the day. In fact, there is some evidence of net glycogen storage, at least in type II fibers, during the prolonged low-intensity cycling that might occur in the *peloton* (Kuipers et al. 1987). Presumably this would benefit sprint performance at the end of the stage. In the cycling leg in a triathlon, higher intakes of carbohydrate might be an outcome of the greater opportunities for feeding and the lower risk of gastrointestinal discomfort compared with running. Triathletes may use the cycling leg to consume well in excess of their carbohydrate requirements, thus preparing for a reduced rate of intake during the run. There is a need for more specific research on carbohydrate intake during ultraendurance events (>4-5 hr) to investigate possible benefits of these large intakes and the fate of carbohydrate in excess of the immediate fate of muscle oxidation. Kimber and colleagues (2002) reported that male triathletes showed an inverse relationship between carbohydrate intake during the run leg of the Ironman triathlon and time to complete this marathon, suggesting benefits from greater carbohydrate intakes.

Refueling practices must not interfere with fluid intakes and fluid balance. Laboratory studies have shown that during moderate-intensity cycling, solid and liquid forms of carbohydrate have similar effects on exercise metabolism and performance as long as total fluid intake is matched (Lugo et al. 1993; Robergs et al. 1998). Triathletes report a higher prevalence of gastrointestinal upsets and discomfort than is generally reported in cycling, with most of the symptoms occurring during the run section (Rehrer et al. 1992). The mode and intensity of exercise are contributors to such problems, but dietary factors may include dehydration, the intake of fat or fiber in foods consumed before and during the race, and hyperosmotic or concentrated drinks (Rehrer et al. 1990, 1992). Athletes who experience such problems will need to experiment with their choice of carbohydrate-containing foods and drinks.

Stage Races and Tours

It is challenging to maintain the large energy intakes required to meet energy expenditure during a prolonged stage race (24-25 MJ or 5,500-6,000 kcal per day), in the face of the limited time available for eating and the suppression of appetite after exhausting exercise. However, this challenge appears to be met by professional cyclists, with the help of support teams including medical and nutrition experts (Jeukendrup et al. 2000). Several studies have described the eating patterns of cyclists during the major cycling tours (Garcia-Roves et al. 1998, 2000; Saris et al. 1989). These surveys have reported on the spread of

energy and macronutrients over various meals or eating periods over the day as well as specific foods consumed at these times. Generally, studies report that cyclists follow a race-day pattern of a substantial, carbohydrate-rich breakfast, carbohydrate intake during the stage, and a postrace carbohydrate snack, as well as a dinner in the team or race hotel. Total daily carbohydrate intake reported by male cyclists during stage races appears to be ~12 to 13 g/kg body mass, reflecting the heavy fuel demands of this type of racing. Although total carbohydrate intakes during stage races have not changed substantially over the past decade, a possible shift in eating practices has been reported.

A 1989 study of the Tour de France (Saris et al. 1989) reported that cyclists consumed a substantial proportion of their daily energy and carbohydrate intake while cycling: 49% of total energy intake and ~60% of total carbohydrate intake were consumed during the race in the form of sport drinks, concentrated carbohydrate drinks, and sweet cakes. Carbohydrate was consumed at a rate of 94 g/hr (~1.4-1.5 g · kg^{-1} · hr^{-1}), along with a fluid intake of ~4.5 L during each day's stage. In contrast, Garcia-Roves and colleagues (1998) reported a different eating pattern in a study of cyclists undertaken a decade later. Although a similar total energy and fuel intake was achieved, cyclists reported a greater reliance on breakfast (prerace meal) and postexercise recovery meals (a substantial meal eaten 1 hr postrace and supper eaten 3-4 hr postrace) to provide energy and carbohydrate intake. Carbohydrate was consumed during the race at a lower rate of ~25 g/hr, and a lower rate of fluid replacement was also seen. These changes were suggested to result from more aggressive riding tactics, which prevent greater consumption of foods and drinks on the bike. Major carbohydrate sources consumed at meals in both studies included biscuits, cakes, confectionery, breads, pasta, rice, and sport foods. Whether this change in the spread of carbohydrate intake or fluid intake is a universal finding in current stage races is a topic that should be investigated. It is also important to determine whether such changes affect cycling performance or indeed whether other dietary patterns could achieve a better fit between practicality and performance. Further insight into the practicalities of eating during a stage race or tour is provided in the first practical issue in this chapter.

Sport Foods and Supplements

The use of supplements and sport foods is endemic in triathlon and cycling, particularly among top athletes. In chapter 3 we acknowledged that the lure of these products is understandable, given the considerable incentives and pressure to improve by the small margins that separate the winners and place-getters in sport. The lack of appropriate sport-specific studies, capable of investigating whether a product is worthwhile for a particular athlete, was also highlighted. This is an important area to be studied because, at best, supplements and sports foods have the potential to contribute to optimal nutrition and sport performance but at worst represent a waste of money and a risk of inadvertent doping outcomes. This chapter will finish with a summary of supplements and sport foods that appear to be of some value in road cycling and triathlon and a brief overview of research related to ergogenic aids and specific performance outcomes in these sports.

According to table 4.7, most of the available sport foods and some basic vitamin and mineral supplements have application to situations commonly faced by triathletes and cyclists. In such situations, the use of these products may help athletes to achieve various goals of sports nutrition. Among compounds considered to be ergogenic aids, caffeine has definite proof of performance benefits, with maximal effects being seen at low levels of intake. In fact, the observations made over the last decade of cyclists and triathletes drinking commercially available cola drinks during the latter stages of prolonged events spurred sport scientists to test the efficacy of the small amounts of caffeine on endurance performance (see figure 4.2). Figure

Table 4.7 Sport Foods and Supplements That Are of Likely Benefit to Cyclists and Triathletes

	Product	Comment
Use in achieving documented nutrition goals	Sport drinks	• Use to refuel and rehydrate during workouts and races and to rehydrate after the session. Contain some electrolytes to help replace sweat losses and increase voluntary intake of fluid.
	Sport gels	• Convenient and compact carbohydrate source for use during workouts and races.
	Sport bars	• Convenient and compact carbohydrate source for use during workouts and races. • Convenient, portable, and easy-to-consume source of carbohydrate, protein, and micronutrients for postexercise recovery.
	Liquid meal supplements	• Convenient, portable, and easy-to-consume source of carbohydrate, protein, and micronutrients for postexercise recovery. • Well-tolerated preevent meal that can be consumed to provide a source of carbohydrate quite close to the race start. • Convenient and compact source of energy and nutrients for the traveling athlete.
	Multivitamin and mineral supplements	• Supplemental source of micronutrients for traveling when food supply is not reliable. • Supplemental source of micronutrients during frequent racing program, when food program is focused on other goals (e.g., refueling) or reduced in variety and quality because of travel, budget, and practical restraints.
	Electrolyte supplements	• May provide source of sodium for supplement during long races, especially in individuals with heavy sweat and electrolyte losses. • Sodium supplement to assist with rehydration following moderate to severe exercise-induced dehydration.
	Iron supplements	• Supplemental form of iron for prevention and treatment of diagnosed cases of reduced iron deficiency. Should be taken under the supervision of a sports doctor or dietitian and in conjunction with dietary intervention.
	Calcium supplements	• Supplemental form of calcium for prevention and treatment of poor bone status when diet is unable to meet calcium requirements. Should be taken under the supervision of a sports doctor and dietitian and in conjunction with appropriate medical and dietary intervention
Documented ergogenic benefit	Caffeine	• Small to moderate doses (1-3 mg/kg BM) appear to be as effective as larger doses (5-6 mg/kg BM) in enhancing the performance of prolonged exercise. Further sport-specific studies are needed to investigate the range of triathlon and cycling races that might benefit from caffeine intake and the range of doses and consumption protocols (e.g., intake before, during, or toward the end) that are effective. May be consumed in cola and energy drinks or as an ingredient in some sport products (e.g., some gels). There is conflicting evidence over the efficacy of coffee as a source of caffeine, because it contains other chemicals that might negate the benefits.

	Product	Comment
Some potential for benefit	Glycerol for hyperhydration protocol	• May be useful when consumed (1-1.2 mg/kg) with large bolus of fluid (~20-25 ml/kg) before exercise to increase total body water content. This strategy might be useful to reduce overall fluid deficit in races undertaken in the heat in which large sweat losses cannot be practically replaced during the event—for example, cycling time trial or Olympic distance triathlon. Should be undertaken under the supervision of a sport scientist and with appropriate experimentation during training. • There is some, but not consistent, evidence that an increase in blood-buffering capacity might enhance the performance of short high-intensity events of 30-60 min duration (e.g., cycling time trials or sprint triathlons). Typical dose to raise extracellular pH is 300 mg/kg BM bicarbonate or 500 mg/kg BM citrate 1-2 hr prerace. Further field studies are needed with high-level athletes to confirm benefits. Risk of gastrointestinal problems should be noted, especially in combination with high-intensity running, but appear to be reduced by taking dose with large volumes of fluid (1-2 L). The risk of gastrointestinal upsets should be assessed especially in triathlon, because of the generally higher prevalence of gastrointestinal problems in running. Longer-term bicarbonate loading (5 days @ 500 mg/kg/day in split doses) have also been investigated and may be useful for events carried out over several days or for athletes who suffer from gastrointestinal discomfort following a single dose of bicarbonate. There is also recent evidence that chronic bicarbonate loading during training (loading immediately before interval training) may enhance training adaptations and the subsequent performance of sustained high-intensity exercise.

BM = body mass.

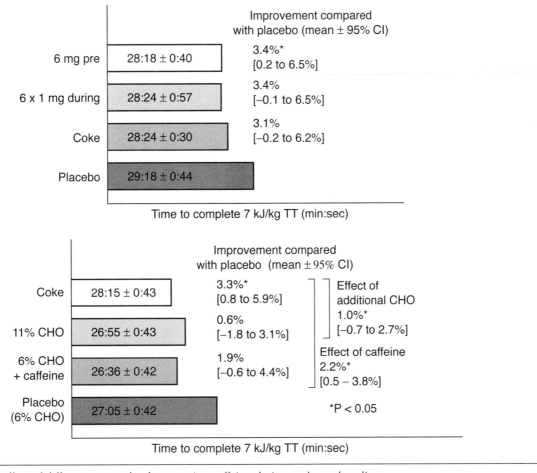

Figure 4.2 Effect of different protocols of consuming caffeine during prolonged cycling.

* = P<0.05

4.2 is about the caffeine study and should go here. Other products that offer the potential of enhancing performance for some aspects of triathlon or cycling performance are glycerol and bicarbonate or citrate. The literature on which these conclusions were made is presented in the appendix to this chapter (table 4.e).

A much larger number of the purported ergogenic aids used by cyclists and triathletes are unlikely to offer real performance advantages. This group includes creatine, carnitine, β-hydroxyl β-methylbutyrate (HMB), medium-chain triglycerides, coenzyme Q10, pyruvate, amino acids consumed during exercise, antioxidant vitamins, and some herbal products. Table 4.f in the appendix summarizes the scientific literature on the use of these products for cycling and triathlon and the conclusions made by this author on the likelihood that they would be of true value in these sports. For the most part, the studies selected for review in tables 4.e and 4.f involve trained cyclists and triathletes and an exercise protocol that has relevance to performance of real-life events. On selected occasions, studies involving recreational cyclists have been included for their historical value or because of an interesting characteristic of the study protocol. In the case of coenzyme Q10, data from recreational athletes show evidence of a detriment to performance or failure to adapt to training (Laaksonen et al. 1995; Malm et al. 1996, 1997). The scarcity of well-controlled studies on many supplements and sport foods, particularly involving elite athletes and females, necessitates some guesswork about the likelihood that a particular product would be either valuable or of low priority. The interpretation of the available data was undertaken with some empathy for what is a worthwhile change in performance in a typical cycling or triathlon race.

Finally, in many cases, particular (proposed) ergogenic compounds that are used by athletes in these sports, and reviewed in chapter 3, have not been tested in a cycling- or triathlon-specific protocol and no further comments can be made about these products. The reader is therefore referred to the general conclusions reached in chapter 3.

RESEARCH TOPIC

Do High-Carbohydrate Diets Really Benefit Training Adaptation and Performance? Issues of Terminology and Detecting Performance Changes

Official guidelines for athletes have been unanimous in their recommendation of high carbohydrate intakes in the everyday or training diet, based on the perceived benefits of promoting optimal recovery of muscle glycogen stores between training sessions (American College of Sports Medicine et al. 2000; Devlin and Williams 1991; Ekblom and Williams 1994; International Olympic Committee 2004; Maughan and Horton 1995). However, such advice has received criticism from both outside and within sport science circles. For example, in the Wolffe Memorial Lecture presented by South African sports medicine expert professor Tim Noakes to the American College of Sports Medicine in 1996 (Noakes 1997), carbohydrate intake guidelines were identified as one of five key paradigms in sport science that need to be revisited. Professor Noakes argued that the position that all endurance athletes should ingest diets rich in carbohydrate could be refuted by at least two sources of information. First, he asserted that "despite the recent intrusion of sports nutritionists dedicated to the promotion of high carbohydrate diets," athletes do not eat such carbohydrate-rich diets in training and have not increased their carbohydrate intake over the past 50 years. Presumably, if it were advantageous to athletic performance, we might expect athletes to follow this advice. Second, he summarized that the present literature fails to provide clear support for the benefits of chronic high carbohydrate intakes on training adaptations and performance of athletes undertaking intensive daily workouts. Are these claims justified?

We undertook a large review of the published dietary surveys of serious athletes (Burke, Cox, et al. 2001). This review found that the mean values for their reported daily

Research Priorities

Further research is needed to better understand the current practices of top cyclists and triathletes and to investigate various dietary strategies that can contribute to successful performance in various types of events. Areas that are of high priority for sport-specific research include the following:

- Validation of dietary survey techniques in cyclists and triathletes
- Nutrition practices of high-level triathletes and female road cyclists during training and racing
- Weight control beliefs and practices of male and female road cyclists
- Current hydration and fuel intake practices of cyclists and triathletes during single events, ultraendurance races, and stage races and whether these contribute to optimal performance
- Use of supplements and sport foods by cyclists and triathletes and their specific benefit to performance in various events in these sports

carbohydrate intake of athletes were ~50% to 55% of total energy intake (see table 4.8). This is compared with early sports nutrition guidelines that athletes should consume diets providing at least 55% of energy from carbohydrate (Maughan and Horton 1995) or 60% to 65% of energy from carbohydrate (American Dietetic Association 1993). In the case of endurance athletes, carbohydrate intake recommendations have been set variously at >60% of energy (Ekblom and Williams 1994) and 65% to 70% of dietary energy (American Dietetic Association 1993). At first glance it appears that the real-life dietary patterns of athletes fall dramatically short of the expert guidelines. However, this mismatch can be largely explained as a result of confusion arising from the terminology used to make these recommendations.

Although nutrition guidelines for the community have expressed recommendation for carbohydrate intake as a proportion of total dietary energy intake (percentage energy), the athlete's requirement for carbohydrate can be more specifically targeted to the fuel needs of his or her training or competition program. These estimates of carbohydrate requirement should be expressed relative to the body mass of the athlete, to roughly account for the size of the muscle mass that must be fueled. Newer sports nutrition guidelines, including the recommendations presented in chapter 1, are presented in this way (American College of Sports Medicine et al. 2000; Burke, Kiens, et al. 2004). Suggested target ranges for carbohydrate intake, although still recognized as being estimated figures, have been set at 5 to 7 g/kg body mass per day during moderate training loads and 7 to 12 $g \cdot kg^{-1} \cdot day^{-1}$ for prolonged training. The summary of dietary surveys of athletes published from 1990 to 2000 (table 4.8) shows mean values of reported daily carbohydrate intake of 7.6 and 5.8 g/kg for male endurance and nonendurance athletes and 5.7 and 4.6 g/kg for their female counterparts. This suggests the daily carbohydrate intakes of the typical male athlete fall within target ranges for fuel needs, particularly if these figures are adjusted for

the expected feature of underreporting on dietary records. Of course, these mean estimates do not guarantee that all groups of athletes or specific athletes meet these recommended intakes or indeed that they meet their actual fuel requirements. Such determinations can only be made on an individual basis. Female athletes appear to be at a higher risk of carbohydrate intakes below these ranges, largely as a result of lower energy intakes.

One disadvantage of using percentage of energy terminology to provide advice to athletes about their carbohydrate needs is that it is not practical or user friendly to people with a simple knowledge of nutrition. How can athletes tell if a meal or their day's intake provides a carbohydrate target of 60% of energy? To convert existing information from food labels and food composition into this form requires some expertise and mathematical skill. Most important, however, our review of dietary surveys of athletes provides clear evidence that the two methods of describing carbohydrate intake are not interchangeable. Among groups of male athletes, we found evidence of a loose but positive correlation between reported intakes of carbohydrate (g/kg) and the energy contributed by carbohydrate in the diet (Burke, Cox, et al. 2001). In other words, male athletes who change their eating patterns to increase the energy contribution of carbohydrate in their diets are likely to increase their carbohydrate intake per kilogram of body mass. Nevertheless, the correlation was too low to guarantee that a particular target for grams of carbohydrate intake based on specific fuel needs translates into a certain percentage of dietary energy. Furthermore, in the case of female endurance athletes, the correlation between the carbohydrate–energy ratio and total carbohydrate intake (g per kilogram of body mass) was minimal. This is because of the confounding issue of restricted energy intake in some individuals or groups. These athletes may consume 70% to 75% of total energy from carbohydrate in an energy-restricted diet (meet old guidelines) but still only achieve 3 to 4 g of carbohydrate per kilogram of body mass (fall below

Table 4.8 Self-Reported Intakes of Serious Athletes

Group	Energy intake (MJ)	Energy (kJ/kg BM)	Carbohydrate (g/kg BM)	Carbohydrate (% of energy intake)	Recommended carbohydrate intake ($g \cdot kg^{-1} \cdot day^{-1}$)
NON-ENDURANCE ATHLETES					
Males (n = 313)	14.13	183	5.8	52	5-7
Females (n = 163)	7.56	135	4.6	54	5-7
ENDURANCE ATHLETES					
Males (n = 377)	15.13	227	7.6	56	7-12
Females (n = 213)	9.42	172	5.7	55	7-12

BM = body mass.

Data are the weighted means of daily intakes from dietary surveys reported 1991-2000 (Burke, Cox, et al. 2001). From Burke et al. 2001.

fuel-based targets). We concluded that it was meaningless to assess or recommend carbohydrate intake based on energy percentages. This recommendation was included in the guidelines (Burke, Kiens, et al. 2004) underpinning the 2003 consensus statement by the International Olympic Committee on nutrition for athletes (International Olympic Committee 2004).

The most important criticism of the recommendation for high carbohydrate intakes lies with the failure of longitudinal studies to show consistent benefits to training adaptations and performance from such eating practices compared with moderate-carbohydrate diets (see table 4.g). Although there is good evidence of superior recovery of muscle glycogen with a higher carbohydrate intake, only two of the available studies show a clear enhancement of training outcomes (Achten et al. 2004; Simonsen et al. 1991). The most recent of these studies creates considerable interest with its finding that a higher carbohydrate intake was able to reduce, but not entirely prevent, the overreaching syndrome that can occur when a period of intensified training is undertaken (Achten et al. 2004).

It is curious that benefits from high-carbohydrate eating have not been a universal outcome from training studies. Several methodological issues are important, including the overlap between what is considered a moderate- and high-carbohydrate diet in various studies. In studies where moderate-carbohydrate diets appeared to provide sufficient fuel to meet training requirements, additional benefit would not be expected from higher carbohydrate intakes. Another important issue is whether sufficient time was allowed for differences in the training responses of athletes to lead to significant differences in the study performance outcome. After all, studies on tapering and reduced training show that the performance of some types of exercise may be maintained for up to 3 weeks, despite a reduced training stimulus (Mujika and Padilla 2000a, 2000b). Finally, the protocol used to measure performance in studies should receive scrutiny to see if is sufficiently reliable to detect small but real improvements that would be significant to a competitive athlete (Hopkins et al. 1999).

One possible conclusion from the available studies of chronic dietary patterns and exercise performance is that athletes can adapt to the lower muscle glycogen store resulting from moderate carbohydrate intake such that it does not impair training or competition outcomes. However, no study shows that moderate carbohydrate intake promotes superior training adaptations and performance compared with higher carbohydrate diets. A recent well-publicized study with an ingenious design involved untrained participants who undertook a 10-week program of "one leg" cycling (Hansen et al. 2005). The participants consumed a high-carbohydrate diet so that both legs received the same fuel. However, one leg did a block of training every day, while the other did the same number of blocks of training in a pattern of two sessions in a row on one day followed by a rest day. The leg that trained twice a day appeared to gain better endurance and adaptations than the leg that completed daily training sessions. The authors suggested that exercise undertaken with low glycogen levels (i.e., as achieved in the second training session of a day) achieved a greater training stimulus, and proposed that athletes should "train low" and "compete high" in relation to their glycogen levels. This is an interesting outcome that needs to be investigated in a more sports-related context, using already trained athletes and a conventional exercise protocol that can measure performance changes. However, there is an important caveat to the popular interpretation that the Hansen study supports a low-carbohydrate diet in training. Since participants in this study consumed high-carbohydrate diets, the "twice-a-day" trained leg presumably undertook their alternate training sessions with well-stocked glycogen stores after a rest day and a good chance to fuel. This periodization of training, which means that some sessions are undertaken "fresh", while others are undertaken in a more fatigued or depleted state, is a hallmark of the training programs of most elite endurance athletes. This is likely to balance the optimization of training stimulus with the ability to train hard and maintain health. This is a different concept to a prolonged period of restricted carbohydrate intake, which exposes the muscle and other body systems to constant deprivation of this fuel.

Clearly, further research needs to be undertaken, using specialized and rigorous protocols, to better examine the issue of chronic carbohydrate intake in heavily training athletes. Because such studies require painstaking control over a long duration, it is not surprising that there are few in the literature.

It is interesting to return to the argument expressed earlier, that we should look to elite athletes to provide a model of what is ideal nutrition, because they would self-select, or have access to information promoting, the diet that would best enhance their performance. There are several factors against accepting the proposal that the world's best athletes must be consuming an ideal diet as well as the specific idea that the reported carbohydrate intakes of athletes recorded in the available dietary surveys are optimal. First, in real life we observe that sports people use a mixture of science, superstition, circumstance, and popular belief in all aspects of their preparation. Trial and error is a slow and inexact teacher and may not lead the athlete to optimal practice in all areas. Because nutrition plays an important but *facilitating* role in sport performance, it is likely that some athletes are successful in spite of, as well as because of, their dietary practices. Second, although dietary surveys presented throughout this book have included some top competitors within their samples, the dietary intakes of most of the world's best athletes remain unknown. For example, little is known of the nutritional practices of the Kenyan and Ethiopian runners who dominate middle and distance running, although some report that the native diet is heavily focused on carbohydrate-rich grains (Onywera et al. 2004; Tanser 1997). Finally, dietary surveys do not have the power to test the effect of dietary intake on performance. Descriptive studies may, within reason, identify a range of carbohydrate intakes within and across groups; however, they are not able to test how much this contributes to the performance of individuals or groups. Although we may like to look to top athletes as role models, we must accept the caveat that many may not achieve optimal nutrition practices.

In summary, the real or apparent failure of athletes to achieve the daily carbohydrate intakes recommended by sports nutritionists does not necessarily invalidate the benefits of meeting such guidelines. These recommendations are based on plentiful evidence that strategies that enhance carbohydrate availability also enhance endurance and performance during a single session of exercise. Although the literature fails to provide clear support that long-term high-carbohydrate intakes enhance the training adaptations and performances of endurance athletes, there is a challenge for sport scientists to undertake well-controlled studies that will better test this hypothesis.

RESEARCH TOPIC

Adaptation to High-Fat Diets in Endurance and Ultraendurance Athletes

One of the characteristics of well-trained athletes, and an outcome of an endurance training program, is an enhanced ability to oxidize fat during submaximal exercise. This adaptation is useful, given the relatively large fat stores found in even the leanest of athletes. This includes the significant levels of fat found inside the muscle (intramuscular triglyceride or IMTG) as well as blood lipids and body fat stored in adipose tissue. In most people, these fat stores would be capable of fueling moderate-intensity exercise lasting at least several days in duration! By contrast, carbohydrate stores in the blood and muscle are only sufficient to fuel 1 to 2 hr of submaximal exercise, and the depletion of these stores is associated with fatigue and impairment of exercise capacity.

Generally, the nutritional strategies used in endurance sports focus on increasing the availability of body carbohydrate stores—for example, carbohydrate loading, or consuming carbohydrates before or throughout an event. An alternative angle for performance enhancement would be to find a fuel source to replace muscle glycogen and slow its rate of use during exercise. The considerable supply of body fat provides such a possibility, and strategies such as fasting, supplementation with carnitine and caffeine, preexercise intake of high-fat meals, and intake of medium-chain triglyceride fats during exercise have been attempted in the hope of enhancing rates of fat utilization during exercise (for review, see Helge 2000). The protocol receiving the greatest attention recently is a high-fat, low-carbohydrate diet, in the expectation that the muscle will adapt to this diet by up-regulating its capacity for fat utilization.

Fat Loading

The immediate effect of short-term (1-3 day) exposure to high-fat, low-carbohydrate eating is to lower resting muscle glycogen stores. Predictably, this impairs an athlete's ability to perform prolonged exercise by causing premature glycogen depletion. However, longer periods (>7 days) on such a diet cause metabolic adaptations that enhance fat oxidation during exercise and compensate for the reduced carbohydrate availability. It has been suggested that such "fat loading" strategies might enhance the performance of endurance and ultraendurance athletes by making them better able to tap into body fat stores. Adaptations may occur in the form of up-regulation of the enzymes involved in transport and metabolism of fats in the muscle as well as enhanced storage and restoration of IMTG stores. Studies that have examined this theory are summarized in table 4.h. Although the overall support for fat loading is not strong, these studies have provided some interesting findings.

One outcome has been the apparent potential for individual responses—for example, results in the same study can range from a large positive outcome to small negative change (Phinney et al. 1983). In addition, some authors have claimed that fat adaptation produced a sparing of muscle glycogen—a lower rate of muscle glycogen contribution—during submaximal exercise (Lambert et al. 1994; Phinney et al. 1983). However, participants in these studies *started* the bout with low glycogen stores, a factor that in itself reduces the rate of glycogen utilization during exercise. True glycogen sparing can only be proved if participants start each exercise protocol with similar muscle stores. Finally, one study tracked fuel metabolism during exercise at 5-day intervals and found that the major adaptations to the high-fat diet occurred within the first 5 days (Goedecke, Christie, et al. 1999). This suggests that athletes can achieve metabolic adaptations without having to undergo radical dietary change for lengthy periods. Such extreme diets not only are hard for the layman to construct but in the long term may be associated with impaired training outcomes as well as health complications. For example, previously sedentary individuals have followed high-fat or high-carbohydrate diets for periods ranging from 4 to 7 weeks while taking up aerobic exercise (Helge et al. 1996, 1998). Although participants appeared to adapt well to training on both diets at 4 weeks (Helge et al. 1998), in the 7 week study, the participants on the high-fat treatment showed poorer endurance than the high-carbohydrate group at the end of this period (Helge et al. 1996). Endurance capacity was enhanced but not fully made up by switching the high-fat group to a glycogen-restoring diet for 1 week, suggesting that long-term exposure to high-fat diets may cause some residual impairment of the training adaptation. Therefore, if high-fat diets are to be valuable to athletes, exposure must be limited to a practical and useful period.

Dietary Periodization

Recent studies have extended the interest in fat adaptation strategies into a dietary periodization model for well-trained athletes—optimizing muscle fat utilization with the minimal necessary exposure to a high-fat diet and then trying to refuel muscle glycogen stores without washing out the enhanced capacity for fat oxidation. In this way, an athlete could be prepared for an event with optimized availability of both fat and carbohydrate fuel substrates. Table 4.i provides an overview of such studies.

Three studies undertaken at the Australian Institute of Sport compared the results of a week of high-carbohydrate eating with 5 to 6 days of a high-fat diet followed by 1 day of a high-carbohydrate diet in highly trained triathletes and cyclists (Burke et al. 2000, 2002; Carey et al. 2001). The high-fat diet depleted muscle glycogen, whereas stores were maintained while participants undertook daily training on the high-carbohydrate diet. The final day of rest and high carbohydrate intake equally restored—in fact, supercompensated—muscle glycogen concentrations, regardless of the preceding diet. Various exercise options were tested at the end of this dietary preparation, each involving a steady-state phase to investigate metabolism followed by a time trial to measure performance. The conditions are summarized in Table 4.i and include endurance exercise (2.5 hr) with and without extra carbohydrate immediately before and during the exercise trial and ultraendurance exercise (5 hr) with carbohydrate support.

In each of our studies, participants reported symptoms of lethargy, mild headaches, and fatigue during the high-fat treatment phase. All participants had trouble completing at least one of their programmed training sessions, complaining of either an increased perception of effort or difficulty maintaining the desired training pace. These generalized symptoms appeared to decrease as the week progressed. During the exercise bout at the end of the week, the fat-adaptation treatment was associated with substantially higher rates of fat utilization and lower rates of carbohydrate oxidation. We were able to determine that the reduction in carbohydrate use was almost entirely accounted for by a sparing of muscle glycogen stores and that the difference in carbohydrate use was maintained even during the trial where additional carbohydrate was consumed during exercise. Thus, the high-fat diet caused powerful metabolic adaptations that persisted and were independent of body carbohydrate availability. We did not determine the source of the additional fat oxidized during the exercise.

Despite these seemingly favorable metabolic adaptations, we failed to detect benefits to the performance of endurance and ultraendurance exercise protocols, although another group reported an enhancement of the performance of a 3 hr cycling task using a similar dietary preparation (Lambert et al. 2001). The only other study of ultraendurance and fat-adaptation and glycogen restoration strategies also failed to find significant performance differences in a 100 km time trial undertaken within the 5 to 6 hr protocol, compared with the outcomes on a pretreatment trial (Rowlands and Hopkins 2002). In reviewing these findings (Burke and Hawley 2002), we attempted to explain why such dramatic metabolic changes might fail to transfer into a clear performance outcomes. We suggested that sport scientists often fail to detect small changes in performance that might be worthwhile in real-life sport and that group results might be skewed by existence of "responders" and "nonresponders" to fat adaptation strategies (Burke et al.

2000; Phinney et al. 1983). We also hypothesized that what we initially viewed as glycogen sparing during exercise might, conversely, be a down-regulation of carbohydrate metabolism or glycogen impairment. Our recent work has supported this last idea; we found that our fat adaptation and carbohydrate restoration protocol was associated with a reduction in the activity of pyruvate dehydrogenase at rest and during exercise (Stellingwerff et al. 2006). This outcome would impair rates of glycogenolysis at a time when muscle carbohydrate requirements are high.

A study by Havemann and colleagues (2006) appeared to put all these results into perspective. This study applied our fat adaptation and carbohydrate restoration model to a laboratory-based cycling protocol (100 km) that involves several features of a real-life race: self-pacing and the interspersing of high-intensity bouts of cycling with more moderate-intensity segments. The results showed that there was little effect of the dietary strategy on the overall race outcome but that the cyclists suffered an impairment of their ability to undertake the 1 km sprints throughout the race. Many people see endurance and ultraendurance sports as events only involving submaximal exercise, hence the interest in increasing fat utilization and conserving limited endogenous carbohydrate stores. However, the strategic activities that occur in such sports—the breakaway, the surge during an uphill stage, or the sprint to the finish line—are all dependent on the athlete's ability to work at high intensities that are carbohydrate dependent. The emerging story is that fat adaptation strategies cause the significant penalty of impairing this critical ability.

There may be some extreme and unconventional events in which performance requires only a prolonged ability to work at low intensities. Athletes in these events might still like to tinker with fat adaptation strategies. In addition, scientists may want to continue to explore this model to understand the intricacies of the regulation of metabolism during exercise. However, for the typical range of endurance and ultraendurance events in which athletes still need a top gear, there seems no justification to recommend fat adaptation and glycogen restoration strategies. Athletes in these events would be contemplating a protocol that is difficult and sometimes unpleasant to complete, and they would also be playing with the possibility of sabotaging their efforts.

PRACTICAL ISSUE

Ironman Eating

The Ironman race in Hawaii has come a long way since 1978, when 15 men lined up for the first time in Oahu to do the island's three endurance events back to back (the Waikiki Roughwater swim of 2.4 miles or 3.8 km, the Around Oahu Bike race of 112 miles or 180 km, and the Honolulu marathon of 26 miles 385 yards or 42.2 km). The race started from a wager to see which of the traditional competitors of each individual event was the fittest athlete overall. Gordon Haller won the event in a time of 11 hr

46 min 58 s (11:46:58). The race continued as an annual event and in February 1982 attracted popular attention via a sports program on U.S. mainstream television. Millions of viewers saw the leading female, Julie Moss, come within sight of the finish line, suffering from what appeared to be a severe combination of dehydration, carbohydrate depletion, and gastrointestinal distress. She staggered and fell continuously, oblivious to the crew of people amassing around her. Finally as she lay prostrate within yards of the finish, the second female competitor ran past her to claim victory. Julie eventually crawled on her hands and knees to complete the event. This race promised a variety of things to the people who would come to swell its ranks (including the author of this book), from personal challenge to extreme athletic performance.

The Hawaii Ironman race, which celebrated its 25th anniversary in 2003, is now the world championship of an international series of professional races. The field is now limited to ~1,500 competitors in both elite (professional) and age-group categories, with competitors qualifying for their place through a range of events, including the series of International Ironman and half Ironman races, many of which also require prequalification. Although Ironman races are conducted over the same distances, the Hawaiian race offers particular physiological and nutritional challenges because of the extreme winds and heat (30-34°C, 90% humidity) in the lava fields over which most of it is conducted. The course records now stand at 8:4:8 for men (Luc van Lierde, 1996) and 8:55:25 for women (Paula Newby-Fraser, 1992).

In the early years of the event, the recognized nutritional challenges of race hydration and refueling were managed by personal handlers and a couple of feed stations offering the opportunity for competitors to pick up their own "special needs bag." Out of concern for the medical risks involved with severe dehydration, competitors of the first races were weighed prerace and at various check-in points along the route. Those who accrued a body mass deficit beyond a level judged to be critical were to be removed from the race. Gradually, as the event increased in numbers and professionalism, the race directors assembled a network of aid stations and an intricate support team, including an army of volunteers to staff these feed stations. According to the race Web site (www.ironmanlive.com), during each race these volunteers hand out 200,000 cups and 30,000 bike bidons, containing 100,000 gallons of sport drinks, water, cola drinks, and soup. The Ironman medical team, although it has long since stopped monitoring body masses of every competitor, provides support from various medical stations and tents on the course. Over the years, it has hosted a number of medical and scientific studies on race competitors.

Aid stations in the Ironman race are placed at the transition areas and at intervals of ~5 miles and ~1 mile on the bike and run courses, respectively. When I competed in Hawaii from 1985 to 1989, aid stations provided a range of foods (chocolate chip cookies, bananas, orange quarters, guava jelly sandwiches) and drinks (sport drinks, water, cola drinks, and chicken noodle soup). In the days before aerodynamic handlebars and bike shoes with lock-in pedal systems, competitors were provided with generic advice, such as "eat and drink as much as you can" and "alternate between drinking water and sport drinks." Most of our information came from fellow competitors or from books written by successful competitors such as Dave Scott, Scott Tinley, and Sally Edwards.

Today's Ironman menu reflects the progress in food technology and marketing skills of the sports nutrition industry, as well as the increase in sports nutrition knowledge. Although everyday foods and drinks are still available and provide a welcome flavor change en route, most triathletes refuel using specialized sport products such as sport drinks, gels, and bars. Race nutrition advice is now more specialized and specific, with a range of sources of credible information from sport scientists and sports dietitians being available in books, on Web sites, and by personal consultation. There is a prevailing attitude toward aggressive refueling strategies, especially on the bike, with hourly targets often set at 1 to 1.2 g of carbohydrate per kilogram of body mass. Race intake may change in amount and choice toward the end of the bike leg and during the run because of the increased risk of gastrointestinal discomfort and the reduced opportunities to consume foods and drinks while on foot. Despite this, it appears to be possible to meet an hourly carbohydrate intake of 0.6 to 1.0 g/kg body mass. It is hoped that better nutrition practices have contributed to the faster race times of modern Ironmen, but it is likely that a wider pool of competitors and better equipment and training techniques have made the major impact. Still, it is interesting that some of the original Ironman champions, such as Dave Scott, Scott Tinley, Mark Allen, and even Julie Moss, have continued to come back to the race over time. In 1994, Dave Scott, at age 40, finished the race in second place in a time of 8:24:32. This was almost exactly an hour faster than his winning race time in 1980 of 9:24:33 at 26 years of age.

It is a tribute to the preparation of Ironman triathletes and the race organizers that ~90% of the race field successfully completes the race each year within the time limit of 17 hr. Despite the knowledge and experience available, however, there have been a number of dramatic race collapses by top competitors over the years, including Paula Newby-Fraser in 1995 and Chris Legh in 1997. High levels of dehydration (>3% loss of body mass as fluid) are associated with a reduction in gastric emptying and an increased risk of gastrointestinal disturbances. It is difficult to correct this situation because forced intake of fluid and carbohydrate can lead to gastric discomfort and upset (creating more loss of fluid and electrolytes) rather than effective rehydration and refueling. It is hard to hide from the effects of inadequate fluid and fuel status, gastrointestinal upsets, or a combination of the two in the extreme heat or over the extreme distances of Ironman Hawaii. Butt there are also case studies that show that too much intake can cause problems—not just intake that is too little or too late

Recently, the Ironman has helped to draw attention to one of the controversial areas of sports nutrition and sports medicine: hyponatremia occurring in association with exercise. Over the past decade the medical teams associated with mass-participation marathons and ultradistance races such as Ironman races and ultramarathons have noted that a significant proportion of finishers or collapsed athletes who present to their service areas have a reduced blood sodium level. Some of these triathletes are severely below the normal sodium range of 135 to 150 mmol/L (e.g., <130 mmol/L) and present with symptoms including confusion, convulsions, collapse, and coma. Several deaths in ultraendurance events and marathons have been attributable to encephalopathy or other outcomes of this severe hyponatremia. Different theories have been proposed to explain the occurrence of hyponatremia in prolonged exercise events, and the debate between different experts in the field and the medical directors of various races has been loud and bitter.

On one side are experts such as professor Tim Noakes, with clinical experiences from the Comrades (90 km) marathon in South Africa and the South African Ironman triathlon, and Dr. Dale Speedy, with clinical experience from the New Zealand Ironman. These races are held in more temperate conditions than the Hawaiian race. According to their theories, the cause of hyponatremia is water intoxication, caused by athletes consuming excessive amounts of fluid during exercise, in volumes greater than their sweat rates and the body's capacity for urine excretion. Hallmarks of this theory would be evidence of consumption of large amounts of any fluid and an increase in body mass over the course of the event. Advice to prevent this problem rests with education to avoid overhydration before and during prolonged exercise.

However, an alternative viewpoint was promoted by medical team members of the Hawaii Ironman race, Drs. Bob Laird, Doug Hiller, and Mary O'Toole. In their clinical experiences, hyponatremia can also be associated with dehydration. They postulated that hyponatremia could occur because of losses of large amounts of fluid and sodium via sweat, followed by partial replacement of fluids and minimal replacement of salt. Prevention of this problem involves continuation of hydration practices before and during the race, with the use of fluids containing sodium, such as sport drinks, rather than low-sodium beverages such as juices, water, and cola drinks. Salt tablets or electrolyte supplements that could be added to drinks might further reduce the risk of problems with athletes identified as "high sodium losers."

A number of published studies on Ironman triathletes have provided data that has helped our current understanding of hyponatremia to evolve:

- During the 1996 New Zealand Ironman race, 95 triathletes who presented for medical care after the race (17% of the race field) were compared with 169 athletes who did not seek help but had body mass recorded pre- and postrace. Both groups showed a reduction in body mass postrace (mean = 2.5% and 2.9% body mass for medical service attendees and nonattendees, respectively). Dehydration accounted for 26% of primary diagnoses, whereas hyponatre-

mia accounted for 9% of diagnoses but four out of five admissions to the hospital. There was an inverse relationship between postrace sodium concentrations and percentage change in body mass. One hyponatremic athlete (Na = 130 mmol/L) reported consuming 16 L of fluid over the race and gained 2.5 kg (Speedy et al. 1997).

- Pre- and postrace body mass and race sodium concentrations were monitored in 330 finishers from the 660 athletes entered in the 1997 New Zealand Ironman race. An inverse relationship was noted between postrace plasma concentrations of sodium and percentage change in body mass, and women were noted to have lower race sodium levels and a smaller loss of body mass over the race than male competitors. Eighteen percent of these finishers (58 athletes) were hyponatremic: 47 with mild and 11 with severe (Na < 130 mmol/L) disturbances. Among the "severe" group, body mass changes ranged from –2.4% to 5%, with eight athletes either gaining or maintaining body mass over the race. By contrast, body mass changes in the "mild" group were more variable (–9.25% to 2.2%). Thus, although mild hyponatremia can be associated with both under- and overhydration, severe symptomatic cases are mostly associated with fluid overload (Speedy et al. 1999).

- All entrants in the 2000 South Africa Ironman race were monitored pre- and postrace. Body mass at the start of the race was significantly correlated with total finish time, run time, and bike time (lighter athletes were faster). Change in body mass was unrelated to postrace rectal temperature or marathon time but negatively related to postrace sodium concentrations. Less than 1% of participants were hyponatremic (Sharwood et al. 2002).

- Eighteen participants were monitored prospectively during the 1997 New Zealand Ironman race. Mean change in body mass over the race was –2.5%, with median reported hourly fluid intakes of 889 ml on the bike and 632 ml during the run. Median values for calculated fluid losses were 808 ml/hr for the bike and 1,021 ml/hr for the marathon. Plasma volume increased over the race (median = 11%), with an inverse relationship between changes in plasma sodium concentrations and body mass. Five participants developed hyponatremia (Speedy, Noakes, Kimber, et al. 2001).

- The 650 starters in the 1998 New Zealand Ironman race received an education program on appropriate fluid intake practices and a reduced number of aid stations. Dehydration was diagnosed in 12% of the 117 athletes seeking medical attention after the race. Four of the 117 received care for symptomatic hyponatremia compared with 25 from 114 in the previous year's race. Mean change in body mass among 1998 athletes was –3.1% compared with

–2.6% for 1997 race (Speedy, Rogers, Noakes, Thompson, et al. 2000).

- Seven hospitalized hyponatremic athletes from the 1997 New Zealand Ironman were monitored during overnight recovery and compared with 11 race finishers with sodium levels within normal ranges. Hyponatremic athletes were smaller and reported less weight loss over the race (–0.5% vs. –4.4%). During recovery, participants excreted a fluid excess of 1,346 ml and decreased plasma volume by ~6%, whereas controls showed a fluid deficit of ~520 ml and a 1% increase in plasma volume. Estimated median sodium deficit was similar between groups (88 vs. 38 mmol/L) (Speedy, Rogers, Noakes, Wright, et al. 2000).

- Voluntary fluid overload at rest was monitored in six athletes who experienced symptomatic hyponatremia during the 1997 New Zealand Ironman and six other (normal) finishers from the same race. All participants consumed 3.4 L of fluid over 2 hr with five participants and four controls developing hyponatremia. There were no differences between groups in relation to serum or urine electrolytes or urine production. Maximal rates of urine production fell behind the rate of fluid intake, and serum sodium decreased in an inverse correlation with change in body mass. The authors did not detect any unique pathophysiological characteristic to explain why some athletes develop hyponatremia in response to fluid overload (Speedy, Noakes, Boswell, et al. 2001). Although several studies have concluded that concentrations of renal hormones such as antidiuretic hormone were not outside normal ranges in participants who developed hyponatremia, it is now recognized that such levels are inappropriate for the prevailing plasma and urine osmolality (Hew-Butler et al. 2005).

- Thirty-eight competitors in the South African Ironman were given salt tablets to provide ~700 mg/hr sodium during the race. Salt consumers were then matched to a control group who didn't receive salt, according to change in body mass over the race and prerace sodium levels. The salt group recorded a mean loss of 3.3 kg and significantly increased serum sodium concentrations. When participants were matched for body mass changes, salt intake was associated with trend for higher postrace sodium concentrations. When matched for prerace sodium, salt consumers had a significantly smaller body mass loss during the race (–4.3% vs. –5.1%). Salt intake was associated with a reduction in loss of body mass but did not significantly influence serum sodium levels more than fluid replacement alone. No participants in either group developed hyponatremia. Salt supplementation was not necessary in this group of athletes who apparently only partially replaced fluid and other losses during the race, as indicated by loss of body mass (Speedy et al. 2002).

- 114 triathletes from an initial pool of 145 volunteers completed an intervention during the South African Ironman race. These athletes were provided either with salt tablets (n = 53) or placebo tablets (n = 61) and asked to take these ad libitum during the race, with a recommended intake of 1-4 per hour. Each group was found to take ~15 tablets over the race, which in the case of the treatment group provided a mean intake of 3.6 g of sodium. The average weight change over the race was ~3 kg in each group or ~3.7% of body mass, and the mean finishing time for groups was similar (~12 h 40 min). There was no difference in plasma sodium concentrations over the race in either group. All subjects retained plasma sodium levels within normal ranges except for one participant in the placebo group who gained weight over the race and required medical treatment for symptomatic hyponatremia (Hew-Butler et al. 2006).

Further research is needed to investigate the prevalence and causes of hyponatremia under hotter conditions such as in the Hawaii Ironman Triathlon and the role of sodium loss or replacement under conditions of greater rates of sweat loss. Field studies need to be undertaken and interpreted with care, with consideration of protocols to examine prerace and postrace hydration status. For example, although it is convenient to recruit and collect information from participants at prerace activities in the days before the race, this can sometimes lead to differences in the techniques or instruments used to record "pre" and "post" data. The selection of the most meaningful time point to collect baseline data is important—the athlete's body mass and hydration status will differ between the week, the day, or the moments immediately before the race start if she has carbohydrate loaded or fluid loaded. Randomized controlled trials also need to be undertaken to investigate the issues identified in field studies. In the meantime, it appears that hyponatremia can be associated with both underhydration and overhydration but that fluid overload is the most important risk factor for the development of serious and symptomatic cases (Almond et al. 2005; Noakes et al. 2005). Case histories of those who have developed dangerous problems involving hospitalization and occasionally death have reported fluid intakes during exercise that are excessive and even bizarre. However, other factors may also contribute including large salt losses from "salty sweaters" (Montain et al. 2006) and inadequate suppression of antidiuretic hormone (Noakes et al. 2005).

Clearly there is a need for endurance and ultraendurance athletes to have advice on fluid intake that is individualized to both the conditions of the race and their personal sweat losses. Advice to all race competitors should now include warnings about the problem of overdrinking. This might be based on individual rates of sweat loss or perhaps the setting of an upper limit on fluid intake over long periods. Elite triathletes who exercise at high intensities (high sweat rates and poor opportunity to drink large amounts of fluid) are at low risk of such problems, but education strategies need to be targeted at slow competitors who combine low rates of sweat loss with ample opportunities to drink large amounts of fluid as they stop at race aid stations. Female competitors seem to be at greater risk of problems, perhaps because they tend to be slower than their male counterparts, sweat at lower rates, and are more likely to be conscientious in listening to messages to drink to stay well hydrated or drink as much as you can. The value of sodium replacement during a race is unclear. Studies show that it has little effect on preventing the hyponatremia involved with fluid overload (Almond et al. 2005; Speedy et al. 2002). However, large sodium losses by "salty sweaters" have been shown by mathematical modeling to lead to low plasma sodium concentrations (Montain et al. 2006), and the addition of sodium to exercise fluids can attenuate the decrease in plasma sodium levels seen with sodium-free fluids when fluid intake is less than sweat losses (Vrijens and Rehrer 1999). Further research is needed to ascertain the role of sodium replacement in reducing the risk of hyponatremia associated with dehydration.

PRACTICAL ISSUE

Feeding the Tour de France Cyclist: Interview With Exercise Physiologist and Sports Nutrition Specialist Dr. Asker Jeukendrup

Asker, how long have you been working with the Dutch Rabobank cycling team and how did you become involved?

I have been working with the Rabobank cycling team since 1996. Holland had gone from being one of the leading cycling countries to being a fairly insignificant country in the early 1990s. The Rabobank cycling team was introduced in 1996 to give Dutch cycling a boost and a chance to get back to the top. At that time I was finishing my PhD at Maastricht University and was still an active cyclist myself. Because of earlier links of the team director with Maastricht University (Theo de Rooy, one of the team directors, was a cyclist participating in Wim Saris' Tour de France study in 1988), they started to talk to me about the possibility of getting some scientific input in this new cycling plan, which was designed to educate and train young riders to become professional cyclists.

How does the team regard the Tour in terms of nutrition? Is it just another stage race, or are there special considerations and strategies that are unique to this event?

The Tour de France is certainly not just another race; it is one of the hardest physical challenges, and the riders know that there is more competition in the Tour de France than in any other race. That, in combination with the fact that the Tour lasts 3 weeks, makes nutrition even more important. Although the principles are very much the same as after 1-day races or other stage races, various problems are associated with the fact that this race is so long. For example, gastrointestinal problems may occur during the latter part of the race, and it is also difficult to keep the food attractive.

Do cyclists undertake special nutrition strategies in preparation for the Tour—for example, weeks before and then days before it starts?

Most of the riders will race until the week before the Tour de France, and their dietary pattern will be determined by these races. Some of these last races are quite hard, and although riders will try to start the Tour de France at a certain body weight and composition, in reality it is difficult to make major adjustments to their diet when racing is this hard. The days before they may stock up on some carbohydrate, but on day 1, the prologue is only a few kilometers, and for that day it is not necessary to supercompensate.

Studies that have monitored energy needs during the Tour report a mean daily energy expenditure of about 24,000 kJ. It is also suggested that it would be impossible to make up a significant energy deficit if a cyclist fell behind with his eating. How are the cyclists made aware of how much energy or carbohydrate they need to eat each day?

Yes, energy expenditures (and intakes) can be as high as 36 MJ. Of course, eating such quantities can be very problematic, especially when you are exhausted, when your hunger feelings have disappeared, when you have been eating the same food every day for 2 weeks, and when your gastrointestinal system is not functioning optimally. Whether it is impossible to make up an energy deficit probably depends on the cause of this deficit. If it is caused by gastrointestinal disturbances, it is indeed very unlikely that a cyclist will recover and make up for the deficit. However, in the absence of gastrointestinal problems, it is not impossible to make up such deficits. Cyclists usually know from experience and from monitoring their weight how much they have to eat to prevent major energy deficits. They practice this not only in the Tour de France but in fact almost all year long. Most cyclists will have 90 to 100 race days a year, and some even more, so there is plenty of time to practice and to make mistakes.

Can you describe the eating patterns over a typical day on the Tour, say on a 200 km stage? How do the cyclists distribute their energy intake over the day, and what kind of foods and drinks would be consumed at each eating occasion over a day—breakfast, on the ride, after the ride, dinner?

Three hours before the race the riders will eat a fairly substantial breakfast, consisting of bread, muesli, cornflakes, and some fruit, with coffee, milk, and orange juice. Sometimes when stages are very long a plate of pasta or rice is consumed, often without sauce, something I have often called functional eating. On the bike they consume small cakes, small white rolls with jam, and energy bars and they drink 2% to 8% carbohydrate solutions, depending on the weather conditions. Often they also consume cola drinks and water. The advantage of water is of course that it can also be used as a cooling aid. After the race they will typically consume a carbohydrate drink with some protein or drink a carbohydrate solution with a ham sandwich (after hot stages, drinking is usually preferred). Back in the hotel they will snack on fruit, energy bars, and cakes until dinner. Dinner is when they eat the largest amounts. It is amazing how much these relatively small and lean guys (average weight is about 70 kg and their body fat is typically 5-8%) can eat. Plates of pasta or rice provide a large amount of the daily energy intake. Often this is accompanied by some chicken, white fish, or red meat. The quality of this meal is entirely dependent on what the hotels provide; sometimes the food is well prepared but often the meals are overcooked and not very tasty. In the evening there is still time to eat smaller amounts of sweets, cake, and fruit before the riders go to sleep.

Dutch researchers who studied cyclists riding in the Tour in the late 1980s reported that the cyclists consumed as much as 50% of the day's total energy intake and 60% of their carbohydrate from foods and drinks consumed on the bike. However, a decade later, Spanish researchers suggested that the patterns had changed and aggressive riding tactics made it impossible to consume substantial amounts while riding. What are your observations and thoughts about eating on the bike in the Tour?

The energy intake on the bike is certainly smaller than 50%. Studies have also demonstrated that only about 1,000 kJ of energy can be oxidized every hour in the form of ingested carbohydrate. That would mean only 5,000 kJ during a 5 hr stage of the 24,000 kJ they have to consume daily. In the Spanish study you are referring to, the energy intake in the form of carbohydrate on the bike was very low (about 250 kJ/hr), and even with the aggressive riding of modern cycling, it should be possible to increase this somewhat. We advise the riders usually to maintain a carbohydrate intake equivalent to 1,000 kJ/hr, and often they are successful in doing so.

Do you have any figures for typical sweat losses on the bike? What would the extremes of the ranges be, taking into account the extremes in weather and workloads (intensity × duration) for each stage? How well do the cyclists rehydrate during each stage, and do you often need to use aggressive poststage rehydration strategies?

Sweat losses can easily amount up to 3 L/hr. Fortunately this is not the sweat rate for the entire stage and may only

apply to the final part of the race or parts where the racing is very hard and aggressive. In several races we have measured body weight losses, and these are typically 1 to 4 kg or 1.5% to 6% of body weight. There are enormous individual differences, with some riders who almost never lose any weight and some who lose a lot of weight despite drinking relatively large amounts.

Have you experimented with special sport foods, drinks, and supplements for stage racing? What types of products are useful?

Efficacy of products is always difficult to establish in the field. It is a lot easier to make such measurements in the lab, and even in the most controlled conditions it is often impossible to detect differences that could be very relevant in competition. Nevertheless, we usually take the approach that what is proven in well-controlled lab conditions should also work in the field. As such, we are now experimenting with drinks that contain carbohydrate mixtures that result in higher oxidation rates than conventional sport drinks, and this seems to be of benefit. More energy can be consumed on the bike, and these drinks also seem to cause less gastrointestinal distress. People who are interested in these carbohydrate mixtures should read the series of publications from our lab!* Until they do, the Rabobank cyclists can benefit from this potential advantage.

Although the typical person might think it sounds like fun, it must become a chore to eat your way through so much food day after day for the 3 weeks of the Tour. Do you have different strategies across different phases of the Tour to deal with the food boredom or gastrointestinal distress that must eventuate?

This is probably the biggest challenge. The problem is that carbohydrate foods are bulky and rather dry, and there is no real way around that. What we have attempted to do is to provide the riders with additional carbohydrate sources that are more attractive. It is often an enormous treat for the riders to receive fresh pancakes in their hotel rooms, in addition to the bowls of rice and plates of spaghetti. We have also tried sweets, marshmallows, gummy bears, and wine gums (this year the team took 9 kg of wine gums to the Tour). These tactics seem to have been adopted now by many other teams.

Finally, if consuming the carbohydrate is really difficult, hidden carbohydrates may be a solution. It is possible to add maltodextrins to tea, coffee, and several other foods without changing the taste. For these amazing athletes, eating is sometimes as much a challenge as the racing itself.

*Publications from Dr. Jeukendrup's laboratory include Jentjens, Achten, et al. 2004; Jentjens and Jeukendrup 2005.

chapter 5

Middle- and Long-Distance Running

Running might appear to be the least complicated of sports, requiring the athlete to simply propel himself or herself, one foot in front of another, over a predetermined distance. However, there are obviously more challenges and complexity to running than meets the eye—the first man to run a marathon apparently died soon afterward! In this chapter we consider middle- and long-distance running events ranging from 800 m to the marathon. These events place significant demands on both the anaerobic and aerobic power systems and, as the duration of the event becomes longer, on the body's fuel stores. Nutrition has a key role in both the training and competition phases, and sport scientists have taken an interest in studying and writing about many of the nutritional concerns of runners. The running boom in the 1970s and 1980s provided the first opportunity for the science of sports nutrition to reach the attention of the masses. Today, millions of recreational runners seek strategies to enhance their performance, simply for the satisfaction of achieving a personal best.

Competition

The International Association of Athletics Federations (IAAF), previously known as the International Amateur Athletic Federation, is the international governing body for events classified into track and field, road running, cross country, and racewalking. Middle-distance and distance running events fall directly within the first three categories of competition, and common races undertaken in modern times are summarized in table 5.1. The 20 km and 50 km racewalking events are not specifically discussed in this chapter; however, these technical events share many of the nutritional characteristics of distance running. Although the official events contested at IAAF-sanctioned events such as World Championships, Olympic Games, or the Golden League and Grand Prix meets are limited in number, there are many variations on these distances that exist historically or at other levels of competition—both for serious runners (e.g., National Collegiate Athletic Association [NCAA] track-and-field or cross-country competitions) or recreational participants (e.g., community fun runs). Running events can be conducted over a variety of surfaces and terrains—from indoor to outdoors and from flat and specially engineered tracks to community roads and even hilly or muddy fields.

According to competition, events may be run as a single race—for example, a community fun run, a Big City Marathon, or an event at an NCAA meet or the Golden League or Grand Prix program. Alternatively, a series of heats, semifinals, and finals are used to decide the eventual winner of the 800 to 10,000 events on the Olympic Games and World Championship programs. Therefore, although on some occasions the runner must prepare for a single race, in other events a successful competitor must sustain performance for two to three races over 3 to 5 days. Even where athletes compete in single events, they may be part of a circuit or race series that requires competition every 3 to 14 days. Such is the nature of competition on the lucrative professional circuit in Europe, at meets within the NCAA season, or in the cross-country schedule for club athletes. In general, the main competition for track and field occurs in summer, whereas cross country has a winter season. Most road races attracting large fields of both elite and community-based participants are scheduled over the warmer months from spring to late autumn. The schedule of Big City Marathons, which includes races in Boston, Chicago, New York, London, and Paris, extends from April to November. Although there are limits on the size of the race fields in these events, the number of participants can range from 15,000 to 35,000.

Middle- and long-distance races require the sustained production of high rates of energy production, with the typical contribution of anaerobic and aerobic energy systems varying according to the speed and duration of the race (see table 5.2). Of course, such figures represent the typical energy consideration *averaged* over the entire race and don't take into account the change in contribution of the energy systems over time or as a result of changes in conditions within a race (e.g., wind, terrain, elevation) and race tactics (surging, drafting behind another competitor, kicking at the race finish). Middle-distance races require a high capacity for anaerobic metabolism; for example, elite 5,000 m runners run at a pace close to their $\dot{V}O_2$max for ~13 min. Aerobic metabolism accounts for the great majority of the energy cost of long-distance events, especially half-marathon and marathon races. However, there are critical times in these races requiring

Table 5.1   Typical Middle- and Long-Distance Running Events

	Middle distance	Distance events
Track program	800 m	10,000 m
	1,500 m	Marathon
	Mile	
	3,000 m	
	Steeplechase (2,000 and 3,000 m)	
	5,000 m	
Road running	Mile (occasionally organized as celebrity event)	Fun runs (typically 5-15 km)
		Half-marathon (21.1 km)
		Marathon (42.195 km)
		Ekiden relay (6 runners complete total of 42.195 km)
Cross country		Local and club events typically 3-12 km
		NCAA program: 5-8 km females and 8-10 km men
		World Championship program: 4 and 8 km females, 4 and 12 km males

Table 5.2   Energy Systems and Race Performance in Middle- and Long-Distance Running Events

Event	Current world record or world best performance (hr:min)	Percentage contribution from aerobic metabolism to total energy cost of race	Percentage contribution from anaerobic metabolism to total energy cost of race
800 m	1:41.11 (M) Wilson Kipketer 1:53.28 (F) Jarmila Kratochvilová	60	40
1,500 m	3:26.00 (M) Hicham El Guerrouj 3:50.46 (F) Yunxia Qu	80	20
5,000 m	12:37.35 (M) Kenenisa Bekele 14:24.53 (F) Meseret Defar	95	5
10,0000	26:17.53 (M) Kenenisa Bekele 29:31.78 (F) Junxia Wang	97	3
Marathon (42.2 km)	2:04:55 (M) Paul Tergat 2:15:25 (F) Paula Radcliffe	>99	<1

Adapted from Maughan 2000.

anaerobic effort—for example, a surge, a hill, or a sprint finish—that may be the ultimate factor in determining the order of race finishers. The factors that limit performance vary between events, according to the duration and environment of the race. Because many of these factors—such as fluid balance, the availability of carbohydrate fuel, and even the disturbance to acid-base status arising from anaerobic glycolysis—can be manipulated by dietary strategies, nutrition is an important component of the athlete's preparation for competition.

The elite level of middle- and long-distance running, particularly in males, is dominated by African runners: Kenyan and Ethiopian competitors dominate events such as cross-country running, the steeplechase, the 10,000 m, and the marathon, whereas athletes from Northern Africa are the outstanding competitors in 1,500 to 10,000 m events. Most middle- and long-distance runners increase their competitive race distances as they grow older, with many long-distance runners remaining competitive at world-class level at 35 to 40 years of age.

Training

There is currently much debate among athletes, coaches, and exercise physiologists regarding the specific training techniques that best promote the physiological and biomechanical attributes underpinning enhanced running performance. For example, many coaches steadfastly believe that performance in most running events can only be improved by extremely high volumes of training. Although such debate is likely to continue, there are some common threads to modern training techniques. The components of the physical preparation for the middle- and long-distance runner include (Hawley 2000)

- Prolonged involvement in sport since early age
- Year-round training (3-4 hr/day) and competition, with only short (2-4 weeks) breaks for active recovery between seasons
- Periodization of the year into macrocycles of conditioning phase, transition and competition preparation phase, competition, and recovery
- A "hard–easy" approach to the microcycles of training within the week or each phase
- A high volume of aerobic conditioning throughout the year (100 km/week for middle distance, 150 to 200 km/week for long distance.
- Prolonged (>2 hr) steady-state aerobic workouts performed as a single, continuous training session
- Speed work, performed at velocities or power outputs that are faster than planned competition pace and effort
- High-volume, low-intensity resistance training in the noncompetitive phase (especially for the middle-distance runner)

- Sustained race-pace workouts or pace training (i.e., interval training)
- Use of time trials over intermediate distances to assess fitness and pace judgment
- Stretching and mobility exercises
- Peaking or tapering before major competitions

Specialized training techniques such as altitude training and heat acclimatization before competition in a hot environment are also often undertaken. Altitude training is a popular training technique among coaches and athletes, particularly since the emergence of the dominance of black African runners who come from a background of high-altitude living. However, it remains a controversial area, with coaches and scientists still arguing over the merits of periods in a hypoxic (lower oxygen) environment with the aim of achieving physiological adaptation that translate into enhanced performance at sea level. There are several approaches to altitude training for runners who usually reside at low altitudes. The traditional protocol is short-term (3-4 weeks), continual exposure to altitudes of 2,000 to 3,000 m, although a variation on this technique is to intersperse several intermittent periods (1-2 weeks) with quality training at sea level. The latest developments in altitude training include protocols based on "living high and training low"—sleeping at altitude to incur the desired physiological adaptations, but training at a lower environment to allow the session to be undertaken at full capacity. "Nitrogen houses," specialized rooms in which a hypoxic environment is created by increasing the nitrogen content of the circulating air, have been developed to make the live high, train low program practical, if not expensive. These and other altitude-simulation facilities, such as altitude tents, make it possible for the athlete to sleep overnight at altitude and then train under her normal conditions by day.

Physique and Physiology

Successful middle-distance and distance runners are renowned for a high maximal aerobic capacity ($\geq$70-80 ml $\cdot$ kg^{-1} $\cdot$ min^{-1} for males and $\geq$60-70 ml $\cdot$ kg^{-1} $\cdot$ min^{-1} for females), the ability to work for long periods at a high fractional utilization of this capacity, and an economical running style. Their defining physical features are a light build with a low level of subcutaneous body fat. Consideration of the body power-to-weight ratio has become a mantra in all sports where the athlete is required to move his or her own body mass. Whereas sprinters emphasize the power side of the balance, weight becomes more important at the distance end of the spectrum. Body mass determines the total energy cost of running, whereas body fat signifies dead weight that must be transported over the ground. Clearly, low levels of both total mass and fat mass would assist fast and economical movement. There is also some evidence that elite runners carry particularly low levels of body fat on their lower limbs (Legaz and Eston 2005).

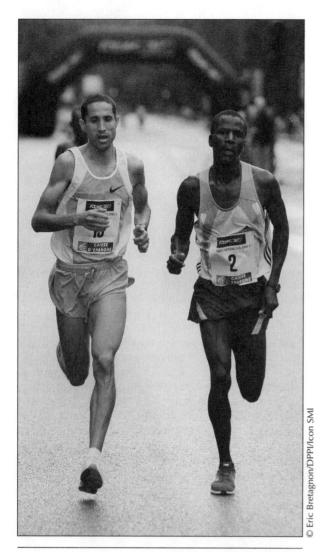

© Eric Bretagnon/DPPI/Icon SMI

Low levels of both total mass and fat mass become even more important when the event involves long distances or movements against gravity (e.g., running up hills in a road or cross-country race or jumping over the barriers in a steeplechase). Because upper-body musculature is unimportant for running performance, elite runners typically exhibit minimal evidence of muscle development in their arms and upper torso.

Middle-distance runners tend to be taller than their long-distance counterparts—longer legs assist with the stride length needed for speed.

Although there is variability in the size of long-distance runners, many of the world's top competitors have a small and compact physique—typified by the winner of the 1996 Atlanta Olympic men's marathon, South African Josia Thugwane (~45 kg), or Japanese female marathon runner Mizuki Noguchi (~39 kg), who won in the heat of the Athens 2004 Olympics. It has been postulated that a small physique offers thermoregulatory advantages for dis-

tance events run in the heat, both by reducing the absolute amount of heat that is produced (smaller muscle mass) and by achieving a more efficient dissipation of heat generated by the body (enhanced ratio of surface area to volume). This hypothesis has been both been modeled (Dennis and Noakes 1999) and tested in the laboratory (Marino et al. 2000). Dennis and Noakes (1999) calculated theoretical rates of heat production from running speed and rates of heat exchange in various environmental conditions for marathon runners ranging from 45 to 75 kg. According to their calculations, at a temperature of 35°C and 60% relative humidity, a 45 kg runner running a marathon at 2 hr 13 min pace (19.1 km/hr) could maintain thermal balance by evaporating ~1.5 to 1.6 L of sweat per hour to dissipate ~1,000 W of heat. Under the same ambient conditions and heat dissipation characteristics, a 75 kg runner would have to slow down to a pace of 12.2 km/hr (3 hr 28 min marathon) to maintain thermal balance.

Laboratory testing of highly trained distance runners, ranging from 55 to 90 kg, over a variety of environmental temperatures (15, 25, and 35°C) with 60% relative humidity and constant wind speed, showed that the increase in rectal temperatures and indexes of heat storage in runners was highly correlated with body mass at the highest ambient temperature (Marino et al. 2000). Furthermore, body mass affected heat production and running speed during an 8 km time trial. The authors concluded that because lighter runners store less heat at the same running speed, they are able to run farther or faster before reaching a limiting core temperature and enjoy an advantage in conditions where heat dissipation mechanisms are at their limit.

Although very low levels of body fat are a striking feature of successful middle- and long-distance runners, it is hard to distinguish whether this is a critical factor in determining successful performance, the outcome of the high training volumes needed for successful performance, or a combination of both factors. Nevertheless, many distance runners are convinced that they must achieve minimum body fat levels per se, even if this means reducing body fat levels below what seems the natural or healthy level for their bodies. This seems particularly true for female runners, because the natural levels of body fat across the female population (15-25% body mass) are higher than the levels (5-12% of body mass) that seem *de rigueur* for distance runners. Many individuals or racial groups are naturally predisposed to low body fat levels or to carry less penalty from attempts to achieve and maintain such low levels. Furthermore, some runners vary their body fat levels over a season so that very low levels are achieved only for a specific and short time. Although the acute loss of body fat and body mass may produce some immediate benefits to running performance through simple changes in the physics of running, when it is achieved by unsound measures or with considerable effort to work against naturally defended body fat levels, the long-term consequences will impair health and performance. These problems are discussed in greater detail in subsequent sections of this chapter.

Lifestyle and Culture

After a run in the morning, they'd start the day with Percy's prescription for breakfast: raw oatmeal mixed with dried fruit, nuts, wheat germ and chopped bananas. Before any of the boys knew it was called muesli (or granola), they were chomping away on it from giant bowls, served dry: there was no flood of milk. Percy was a strong believer in letting the teeth do the work, like primitive man—real men didn't eat mushy food anyway. He also believed that taking fluids with meals upset the natural action of the digestive juices of the stomach, which was why water was banned from the table, and tea and coffee forbidden for some hours afterwards.

The dietary philosophies of Percy Cerutty,
coach of Australian Herb Elliot,
1960s world record holder and Olympic Gold medalist, undefeated over the mile (Sims 2003, p. 193)

Runners from many eras have believed that diet played an important role in their training preparation and competition performances. Furthermore, throughout the ages, many prominent runners and their coaches have believed that a strict approach to eating was required to achieve their nutritional goals. Just as these runners made a commitment to a punishing training program, many practiced a dietary zeal and restrictiveness that might be considered, in hindsight, to be dietary extremism if not disordered eating. It is understandable that the perfectionism and the exceptional drive that push individual athletes to outstanding performances are also likely to drive them to make dietary changes beyond the level that could be considered necessary or useful. Among modern-day runners, the issue most likely to produce extreme dietary patterns is the pursuit of a low body mass and body fat levels. Clearly there is a need to promote a new culture within middle- and long-distance running: to accept the value of balance and moderation and to embrace individuality and the long-term perspective.

Runners have also earned a considerable reputation for adopting new sport science information and new eating styles. Carbohydrate loading, developed by Scandinavian scientists in the late 1960s, was quickly embraced by marathon runners at all levels. Similarly, the proposed benefit of caffeine intake before endurance events was reported in scientific journals in the early- to mid-1970s, followed closely by articles in running magazines. Throughout the running boom of that period, it was common to see runners drinking black coffee from flasks as they milled around the start line doing their prerace activities. Pritikin eating was the popular diet of the late 1970s and 1980s, and runners embraced it with such enthusiasm that a separate book was written on the Pritikin diet for runners.

The literature on running and sport science has been devoured by runners of all calibers. Magazines such as *Runner's World* have had a long history of reaching international audiences, and there are now many Web sites devoted to running. Prominent sport scientists who have enjoyed their own running pursuits—professors Tim Noakes, Dave Costill, and Ron Maughan—have written widely for the educated lay audience. Professor Noakes' book, *Lore of Running*, is considered the ultimate reference.

Dietary Surveys

Dietary surveys undertaken on serious middle- and long-distance runners range from data collected on runners at the 1948 Olympic Games to investigations of the eating patterns of contemporary runners. Data from the available studies, excluding those on groups of runners who were identified as suffering from eating disorders, are summarized in tables 5.a and 5.b in the appendix to this chapter. Many of the runners captured in the available surveys are clearly not elite, typically undertaking 50 to 100 km/week in training. However, recent surveys of elite Kenyan runners provide information of special interest (Fudge et al. 2006; Onywera et al. 2004). These studies are discussed in more detail subsequently.

The self-reported energy intake from the available dietary surveys of male distance runners shows a typical daily energy intake of ~12 to 16 MJ (2,850-3,800 kcal), equivalent to ~200 to 240 kJ or 48 to 57 kcal per kilogram of body mass. The expected absolute energy requirements of female runners should be ~20% to 30% less than their male counterparts, principally to take into account their smaller size, although a smaller training volume is also likely. However, the available surveys of female runners (table 5.b) are striking in suggesting typical energy intakes below this, often in the order 6 to 9 MJ (1,400-2,100 kcal) per day. The reported energy intakes of some individuals and groups of female runners are sometimes less than what would be expected to cover the energy cost of the athlete's training, let alone basal energy needs (Barr 1987). The issue of the apparent energy discrepancy reported by many runners, particularly females, is covered in the second research topic in this chapter.

The typical daily carbohydrate intake of male runners involved in these dietary surveys appears to be ~7 to 8 g/kg BM; such intakes fall with the range of carbohydrate intakes promoted for optimal daily refueling (see chapter 1). Protein intakes in these runners are typically greater than 1.5 g/kg BM per day, with mean values reported by some groups exceeding $2 \text{ g} \cdot \text{kg}^{-1} \cdot \text{day}^{-1}$. Such intakes are easily able to meet any increases in protein requirement resulting from heavy training, should these occur (see table 1.2). Reported intakes of micronutrients, where these have been estimated, exceed typical recommended dietary levels. Of course, these studies cannot make conclusions about whether these runners meet their dietary needs and goals, either as a group or as individuals within a group.

Summary of Common Nutritional Issues Arising in Middle- and Long-Distance Running

Physique Issues

- Desire to reduce body fat and body mass to enhance performance via enhanced power to mass relationship
- Risk of dietary extremism, disordered eating, and inadequate nutrition attributable to overemphasis on low body mass and body fat level

Training Issues

- High energy and carbohydrate requirements to meet a heavy training load
- Recovery between training sessions (refueling, rehydration, repair, and adaptation)
- Adequate fuel and fluid intake during training sessions, including practice of race-day strategies
- Compromise in achieving fuel requirements, and adequate intake of protein and micronutrients when energy intake is restricted to achieve body mass and body fat goals
- Risk of low iron status, especially in female athletes and vegetarian eaters, secondary to inadequate dietary intake and some increase in daily requirements
- Risk of menstrual disturbances in female athletes secondary to energy drain
- Risk of gastrointestinal disturbances and discomfort during prolonged or high-intensity running sessions

Competition

- Preparation of adequate fuel stores for race day: carbohydrate loading before marathons
- Preevent nutrition: topping up fuel and fluid levels without causing gastrointestinal discomfort during the race
- Distance running: fuel and fluid replacement during races longer than 30 min: consideration of need and opportunities for intake at aid stations
- Middle-distance running: consideration of citrate or bicarbonate loading before races to enhance buffering capacity and race performance
- Middle and distance running: consideration of caffeine use to enhance race performance
- Travel: traveling to major competitions and on race circuit

The summary of the reported dietary intakes of female runners paints a less positive picture. Many studies report that mean intakes of the group, or significant proportions of individual members within a group, fail to meet sport-related guidelines for carbohydrate and population guidelines for micronutrients. These findings are clearly linked to the lower energy intakes reported in these studies of female runners, which make it difficult to consume energy-containing macronutrients in adequate amounts or enough of the foods containing key micronutrients. Again, it is important to note that such dietary surveys cannot diagnose nutrient deficiencies or a failure to meet sports nutrition goals, especially at the level of individual athletes. However, the more that reported intakes fall below recommended guidelines, the greater is the risk of real inadequacies. Of course, reported dietary intakes need to be interpreted with an understanding of the limitations of dietary survey methodology, including the real possibil-

ity that athletes are underreporting true intake on dietary surveys (see research topic).

The literature on dietary habits practiced in most sports is marred by the scarcity of information from the world's best athletes—in the case of distance running, the Kenyan and Ethiopian runners. These Africans are known to train exceptionally hard, come from rural backgrounds often at moderate altitudes, and have a culture of supporting their families and extended families on the proceeds of an international running career. Two recent studies have tracked elite male Kenyan runners from the Kalenjin ethnic group, which has dominated distance running over the past 15 years (see table 5.a). Dietary studies conducted during training camps reported energy intakes that seemed inadequate for estimated energy expenditure (Fudge et al. 2006)—although in one study, the energy deficit appeared to be deliberate and explains the lean physiques for which these athletes are noted (Onywera et al. 2004).

Other features included a high carbohydrate intake (~10 $g \cdot kg^{-1} \cdot day^{-1}$ accounting for ~70% of dietary energy), low fat intake (~15% of energy), and adequate protein (~1.5 $g \cdot kg^{-1} \cdot day^{-1}$). Although fuel intake was considered optimal in terms of amount and timing of intake (within an hour of training), no fluid was consumed during training and the reported daily intake of drinks was modest (2.3 L/day). Food consumption patterns included a limited food variety with reliance on food from vegetable sources; staples such as milk, sugar, bread, rice, potatoes, legumes, cabbage, porridge, and maize meal accounted for nearly 90% of total energy intake (Onywera et al. 2004).

How these athletes eat when they join the international running circuit, especially for the long periods when they are based in the Northern Hemisphere, is another matter that should be considered. An unpublished report prepared by 2004 world cross-country champion, Benita Johnson, from interviews conducted with a group of elite London-based Kenyan runners, also describes simplistic eating patterns based on traditional eating styles, using foods such as maize meal, flown in from Kenya. "Their fridge and cupboards are almost bare, containing only essentials—loaves of bread, oranges, Kenyan tea leaves (chai), chicken or beef, milk (full cream), and olive oil for cooking." She describes the following essential components of the Kenyan diet: ugali (thick maize meal porridge eaten at least once a day and often served with chicken or beef and potatoes), chapatti bread (made from flour, oil, and water and cooked in a frying pan), chai tea (Kenyan green tea, served with sugar and full-cream milk), toasted white bread, potatoes, and olive oil (for cooking). The runners reported that they rarely ate restaurant or takeaway foods ("London is so expensive. . . . I cannot waste my money on eating out as that money could go a long way being spent in my country") and did not believe in the need for supplements ("You cannot buy vitamin and mineral tablets in Kenya anyway; many Kenyans wouldn't have even heard of a multivitamin tablet") (Johnson 2002). It would be valuable to conduct further in-depth studies on the eating practices of these athletes.

Nutritional Issues and Challenges

The goal of training is to prepare the runner to perform at her best during major competitions. Whatever the event, nutrition plays a substantial role in the achievement of various factors that will see a runner take the starting line in the best possible form. Everyday eating patterns must supply runners with the fuel and nutrients needed to optimize their performance during training sessions and to recover quickly afterward. The runner must also eat to stay in good health and in good shape. Special strategies of food and fluid intake before, during, and after a workout may help to reduce fatigue and enhance performance. These will often be important in the competition setting but must be practiced and fine-tuned during training so that successful strategies can be identified.

The highlight box summarizes common nutritional issues that arise in middle- and long-distance road running as a result of issues related to optimal physique, training, and optimizing competition performance. Several of these issues are discussed in greater detail in this section of the book. Other issues, such as weight loss and choosing an appropriate preevent meal, were covered in the previous chapter, whereas other challenges such as eating while traveling are left to later chapters of the book.

Energy Restriction and Disordered Eating

When Alison Outram and Lucy Hasell ran their way into Great Britain's Junior women's cross country teams in 1995 and 1996, it should have marked the start of two promising international careers. . . . Just months later, both girls were admitted to specialist eating-disorder units in different parts of the country. . . . "I kept up running internationally for as long as I could, until I saw a specialist who told me and my parents that I might only have one week left to live" says Outram. Her teammate Hasell, was sent to a Somerset clinic where she was only allowed out of bed if she was in a wheelchair. "At that weight, those were the bounds that were considered radically safe for me," Hasell says, "although a few months earlier, at exactly the same weight, I had been running for Britain." . . . "I ran in one Great Britain team which consisted of six runners and a reserve. Of those seven, I know that as many as five were suffering from some kind of eating disorder, including me" says Outram.

Peta Bee "Starved of a Chance," Runner's World, July 1997, pp. 48-51

If success relies on the athlete carrying his or her own body mass over 42 km or over the hills of a cross-country course, then a light and lean body is clearly desirable. This is good news for runners whose genetic backgrounds have predisposed them to small and lean frames. But it can leave other runners with naturally larger frames or higher levels of adiposity trying to whittle themselves down to an unnatural size and level of body fat in order to be competitive. Although many male runners eat and train specifically to reduce their body fat and racing weight, the battle for body fat and weight control is most usually identified as a female problem. This may be because females generally need to push their body characteristics further from their natural shape than male runners to achieve the leanness that is considered ideal; however, they are also likely to incur greater penalties as a result. Many become focused on body shape per se instead of their long-term health and performance. Most do not see that a balance or compromise may be required.

The pressure to achieve a theoretically ideal shape comes from many directions, including coaches, the media, the culture of the sport, the observations of others, and the individual's inner drive to be perfect. There are many examples of female runners who have experienced great success in the first years of becoming serious about their sport. A sudden increase in the training load, accompanied by a significant loss of body weight, is duly rewarded by improved performances. However, this is then followed by the frustrations of injuries and illnesses, as the athlete struggles to maintain or recapture an unnaturally low level of body fat via a punishing volume of training and restricted eating. The illusion that this is the key to success pushes the athlete into a cycle of patchy performances interspersed with injury. Some athletes develop frank medical or psychiatric problems such as eating disorders, osteopenia (impaired bone density), and chronic menstrual dysfunction. More develop subclinical versions of these problems. The highlight box on this page summarizes the theoretical problems that can be associated with efforts to achieve an unnaturally low weight and body fat level.

The problem of eating disorders in runners is both topical and emotive among athletes, coaches, and sport scientists. There is at least circumstantial evidence that athletes are at higher risk of developing eating disorders than is the general population and that the highest risk occurs in sports in which a low body mass and body fat level are essential. Several surveys have identified female distance runners as a particularly vulnerable group or at least have identified high rates of eating disorders among groups of female runners (Brownell et al. 1988; Clark et al. 1988; Weight and Noakes 1987). The relationship between

a sport and the prevalence of eating disorders is complex and may include the following factors:

• Successful athletes demonstrate some of the personality characteristics that are considered high risk for the development of eating disorders in the general population (viz. perfectionism, dedication, narrow focus). These characteristics are praised when applied to training achievements.

• Some sports place athletes within an environment where there is considerable pressure to achieve low levels of body fat and body mass and where there are rewards or positive reinforcement for those who achieve weight or fat loss. On occasion, the culture of the sport may condone and even romanticize weight control behaviors that should really be considered disordered eating.

• Individuals who already suffer from disordered eating problems may be drawn to a sport in which their practices can be camouflaged, at least temporarily. They may be able to pass off restrained and unusual dietary practices, a focus on weight loss although already thin, and excessive exercise as part of the lifestyle of being involved in such a sport.

The true prevalence of eating disorders among runners or other athletes is unknown. The research in this area is confused by differences in the definitions of eating disorders and by different methods for diagnosis and assessment. The criteria by which clinical diagnoses of the eating disorders are made—anorexia nervosa, bulimia nervosa, and eating disorder not otherwise specified (American Psychiatric Association 1994)—are quite rigid and require professional assessment (see chapter 13, practical issue). Many athletes

Problems That May Occur As a Result of Attempts to Reduce Body Weight and Body Fat to Unnaturally Low Levels

Problems Arising From Low Body Fat Level Per Se

• Impaired thermoregulation; heightened sense of feeling cold and increased risk of hypothermia in cold environments attributable to lack of insulation
• Lack of padding on buttocks and thighs leading to discomfort and bruising when in prolonged contact with hard surfaces
• Risk of reduced cushioning of internal organs if involved in acute contact injury

Problems Arising From Methods Used to Reduce Body Fat Levels

• Increased risk of injury resulting from overtraining
• Hormonal imbalances including impairment of menstrual cycling in females, resulting from energy drain—low available energy supply
• Fatigue or inability to complete training because of inadequate intake of carbohydrate fuel
• Increased risk of illness resulting from suppression of immune system (inadequate intakes of energy, carbohydrate, protein, and perhaps some micronutrients)
• Inadequate intake of protein and micronutrients in energy-restricted diet leading to suboptimal performance and body function
• Increased risk of disordered eating and eating disorders; unnecessary food-related stress

with disordered eating fail to fulfill these criteria. Most of the standard questionnaires developed to predict the risk of eating disorders in general population, such as the Eating Attitudes Test (EAT) (Garner and Garfinkel 1979) and Eating Disorder Inventory (EDI) (Garner et al. 1984), appear to underestimate the true prevalence of disordered eating in athletes. These tools have been criticized because their constructs may not be appropriate or valid for athletes. Most important, because these questionnaires are transparent—that is, they ask the athlete directly about disordered eating behavior—the athlete may try to hide the occurrence of true problems and provide false answers. Self-reports must always be treated with caution, particularly when the issue is sensitive. Follow-up from two studies in which athletes were assessed for eating disorders using the EAT or EDI inventories showed the frailty of these assessment tools (Wilmore 1991). In the first study of 110 athletes from a range of sports, no athlete was found to score in the disordered eating range of the EAT survey instrument. However, during the subsequent 2-year period, 18 of these athletes received either inpatient or outpatient treatment for eating disorders. In the second study of 14 nationally ranked American female distance runners, the EDI identified only three athletes as having possible but not clear eating disorders. Later, two of these three and a further five runners required inpatient or outpatient treatment for eating disorders.

Athletes who have problems with eating and body image are variously described as suffering from "anorexia athletica" (Sundgot-Borgen 2000), disordered eating, or subclinical eating disorders, where these problems lie on the continuum between the normality of healthy eating and a positive self-image and a diagnosis of an eating disorder according to the rigid diagnostic criteria of the *Diagnostic and Statistical Manual of Mental Disorders* (fourth edition). At all levels these problems will interfere with the health, performance, and happiness of the athlete. There are warning signs that can indicate disordered eating. Athletes, coaches, sport scientists, and medical professionals, as well as parents, should be made aware of these signs. Early diagnosis of the problem is likely to be important in determining the success of therapy and the degree to which significant side effects and health problems are experienced by an athlete. Chapter 13 (practical issue) provides greater discussion of these issues.

Runners should be encouraged to set realistic weight and body fat goals; these are specific to each runner and must be judged by trial and error over a period of time. Ideal weight and body fat targets should be set in terms of ranges and should consider measures of long-term health and performance rather than short-term benefits alone. In addition, runners should be able to achieve their targets while eating a diet that is adequate in energy and nutrients and free of unreasonable levels of food-related stress. Further discussion on dietary strategies to assist with loss of weight and body fat can be found in the section titled Achieving Low Body Mass and Body Fat Levels in chapter 4, including practical information summarized in tables 4.2, 4.3 and 4.4 on pages 83-88. The advice of a sports dietitian is valuable in helping runners to set realistic goals regarding loss of body fat and weight as well as sound eating practices that encompass all their nutritional goals.

Menstrual Disturbances

For more than 30 years there have been reports of disturbances to the normal menstrual function of female athletes, with many of these reports involving female runners (Barrow and Saha 1988; Kaiserauer et al. 1989; Lutter and Cushman 1982; Marcus et al. 1985; Shangold and Levine 1982). The exact prevalence of this problem is unknown and varies between athletic groups; however, studies report that between 1% and 44% of female athletes experience amenorrhea at any given time, compared with an incidence of 2% to 5% in the general female community (Otis et al. 1997). Part of the problem in collecting accurate figures of the true prevalence of menstrual disturbances lies with the variation in definitions of such disorders. However, the general definitions of amenorrhea are as follows (Otis et al. 1997):

- Primary amenorrhea: absence of menstruation in a girl by age 16
- Secondary amenorrhea: absence of three of more consecutive cycles after menarche

Of course, other forms of menstrual disturbance also occur with irregular menses (oligomenorrhea), altered luteal phase, and anovulatory cycles. Exercise-associated amenorrhea is hypothalamic in origin and results in decreased production of ovarian hormones and low concentrations of estrogens (Otis et al. 1997). Factors that may be implicated in the etiology of menstrual disturbances in athletes are discussed in the first research topic in chapter 13.

The earliest reports considered the cessation of a regular menstrual cycle to be a benign and reversible condition, based on the fact that it did not seem to have long-term consequences to fertility and reproductive outcomes. Indeed, many runners still see the cessation of menses to be a convenience and a benchmark or reward for heavy training or reduced levels of body fat. However, during the mid-1980s, evidence of a more sinister outcome of disturbed menstrual status became apparent, with reports of reduced bone density in groups of amenorrheic runners (Cann et al. 1984; Drinkwater et al. 1984; Marcus et al. 1985). Because low concentrations of ovarian hormones, as seen in postmenopausal women and women with premature ovarian failure, are associated with bone loss, it is not surprising that female athletes with menstrual disturbances are at risk of reduced bone mass (Kerr et al. 2006). This can occur as a result of increased rates of bone loss as well as failure to optimize bone accretion during adolescence and early adulthood. Not all amenorrheic athletes develop low bone mass or bone loss at all regional body sites.

Bone homeostasis is a complex situation, with continual remodeling occurring under the influence of factors such as mechanical loading on the bone, hormonal environment, and calcium homeostasis (Kerr et al. 2006). Bone health in amenorrheic athletes is dependent on a number of factors including the length and severity of menstrual dysfunction, bone mineral density before the onset of amenorrhea, the type of skeletal bone loading undertaken during athletic activity, nutritional status, and genetic components (Otis et al. 1997). This issue is covered in more detail in the section titled Bone Status and Calcium Balance in chapter 13.

The problems associated with low bone mass in female athletes, particularly runners, lie not only with the risk of a premature onset or osteoporosis but also with the immediate problem of stress fractures. These partial or complete bone fractures result from the bone's inability to withstand repetitive, subthreshold stress. Stress fractures represent an accumulation of microdamage in excess of the bone's capacity to repair and remodel, and risk factors for their development include increased bone load or stress, decreased bone strength, and interference with bone repair (Brukner and Bennell 1997). A review of the literature shows that stress fractures are more common in athletes with past or current menstrual disturbances, with a relative risk loading of two to four times that experienced by eumenorrheic groups (Brukner et al. 1999). Recurrent or chronic stress fractures can prevent the athlete from competing at important times and interfere with her ability to undertake the training volume necessary for high level performance. Many athletes have had promising careers ended by this injury pattern.

The coexistence and interrelatedness of this cluster of problems in female athletes led to the identification of a syndrome called the female athlete triad (Otis et al. 1997). As previously discussed (chapter 1), its components were initially identified as the clinically frank problems of eating disorders, amenorrhea, and osteopenia. The more recent revision of the triad considers that each component involves a spectrum and that each female must continually consider her position along the axes of energy supply, menstrual health, and bone health (Loucks and Nattiv 2005). This change recognizes both the benefits of earlier attention and treatment and the likelihood that negative outcomes occur at a much earlier stage than previously considered. An important message is that female runners who suffer from disordered eating or restricted energy intake, menstrual disorders, and impaired bone health should seek early and expert intervention. Treatment is likely to require the teamwork of a sports physician, endocrinologist, physiologist, coach, sports dietitian, and sport psychologist as well as the athlete and her family. The complexity of the issues involved should not be simplified, and each case should be treated on an individualized basis. There is some likelihood that male runners who suffer from restrained eating practices and overtraining may also encounter some problems with altered hormone status or low bone density. Further study of this issue is needed.

Reduced Iron Status

As we have seen in the previous section, an effective way to promote awareness of a new issue in sport is to create a syndrome. One disadvantage of this approach is that it can lead to overdiagnosis or an oversimplified approach to treatment. Such is the case of iron deficiency in sport.

Middle- and long-distance runners were one of the first groups of athletes targeted as being at high risk of iron deficiency, following early observations of changes in their hematological characteristics with the onset of training (Yoshimura 1970). Early studies showed that runners experienced a decrease in hemoglobin after commencing or increasing high-volume training, a characteristic that seemed unfavorable for the performance of events reliant on the delivery of oxygen to working muscles (Brotherhood et al. 1975). This phenomenon was called *sports anemia*. It was later found to be an artifact of the increase in blood volume that accompanies heavy aerobic exercise, and it was also found neither to contribute to performance impairment nor to respond to iron supplementation (Brotherhood et al. 1975; Magnusson et al. 1984). Nevertheless, the attention drawn to the iron status of runners and other athletes continued to develop over the next decades as the role of iron in various exercise-related functions was recognized and new indexes of iron status, such as serum ferritin, became commonly available. The prevailing attitude among many athletes, coaches, sports physicians, and sport scientists during the 1980s was that endurance athletes, particularly middle- and long-distance runners, needed to take active steps to deal with a high risk of iron deficiency. When screenings or individual assessments were undertaken, the target levels for serum ferritin were often set well above those of normal population standards, to provide a safety margin. Iron supplementation through tablets, and less frequently through intramuscular injection, was standard practice for many athletes. Because oral iron supplements are available over the counter, athletes often self-medicated as a precaution against developing iron deficiency or as a treatment of suspected problems. In many cases no medical assessments were undertaken to confirm the existence of a real problem. Rather, the symptoms of tiredness or suboptimal training were considered sufficient to initiate such a treatment. Since then, our appreciation of new issues in the iron status of athletes has produced a more cautious and individualized approach.

About 3 to 5 g of iron is found in the body in three main pools: storage iron (ferritin and hemosiderin found predominantly in the spleen, liver, and bone marrow), transport iron (transported through the plasma and extravascular fluids by the carrier, transferrin), and oxygen transport iron (within the active centers of hemoglobin in the erythrocyte and myoglobin in the muscle). The majority of iron in the body is carefully recycled, with iron from destroyed erythrocytes being salvaged for storage or reincorporation into new reticulocytes. Iron status is a result of the balance between the small amounts of dietary iron that are absorbed each day and small iron losses from skin, sweat, and the gastrointestinal and urinary tracts. Factors involved in an imbalance or drain of iron are summarized in chapter 1, goal 3. An important consideration is that, apart from blood loss, there is no mechanism to remove excess iron from the body. Important functions of iron and iron-related compounds in the body related to exercise are as follows:

- As a transporter of oxygen in the blood (hemoglobin) and muscle (myoglobin)
- As a component of enzyme systems such as the electron transport chain, ribonucleotide reductase (required for the production of DNA), catalase, and succinate dehydrogenase
- As a catalyst in the production of free oxygen radical species

Further information on iron metabolism can be found in reviews by Deakin (2006) and Eichner (2000).

Whereas a small percentage of the population (usually male) suffers from hemochromatosis or iron overload disease, whereby excessive amounts of iron are absorbed and deposited in major organs, the more common problem with iron status in the general community is iron depletion. The depletion of the body's iron stores is thought to progress through a number of stages with different functional and diagnostic criteria (see Deakin 2006). At the end stage of iron-deficiency anemia, there is inadequate iron available in the bone marrow for the normal manufacture of hemoglobin and erythrocytes. Interference with oxygen transport and enzyme function leads to clinical symptoms associated with the impairment of muscle metabolism, brain metabolism, immunity, and temperature control. Such a status clearly interferes with optimal training and competition performance.

Finding the true prevalence of problematic iron depletion in runners and other athletes is dependent on answering the following questions:

1. Can reference standards for biochemical and hematological parameters that are used to diagnose the stages of iron deficiency in normal populations be applied to athletes?
2. At what stage of iron depletion are impairments to exercise performance observed?
3. What is optimal iron status for an athlete, particularly an endurance athlete?

The most contentious and badly interpreted issue concerning the iron status of athletes is the effect of reduced iron status, in the absence of anemia, on performance. Generally it is assumed that serum ferritin levels reflect the total storage of ferritin iron in the body. Low serum ferritin levels have become synonymous with reduced iron status, and the effect on performance has been investigated mostly by studying the effects of iron supplementation on the performance of athletes with low ferritin levels. Reviews of the literature have concluded that the evidence is unclear that iron depletion, in the absence of anemia, impairs the performance of a single exercise task or that iron supplementation enhances the performance of athletes with moderately low serum ferritin but normal hemoglobin levels (Fogelholm 1995). This literature includes a number of studies on female runners (Klingshirn et al. 1992; Newhouse et al. 1989; Powell and Tucker 1991) in which iron-depleted but nonanemic participants received iron supplementation or placebo treatments for periods of 2 to 8 weeks. In each

study, there was no difference in performance changes between supplementation and placebo treatments, even when supplementation increased in serum ferritin levels (Klingshirn et al. 1992; Newhouse et al. 1989). In two other studies of female runners, a performance improvement was seen after iron supplementation in participants with low ferritin levels in apparent contradiction to these results. However, participants in these studies also experienced an increase in hemoglobin levels in response to the therapy, suggesting that the participants had suboptimal hemoglobin levels before the supplementation (Lamanca and Haymes 1993; Schoene et al. 1983).

There are several criticisms of the available studies of iron supplementation in iron-depleted groups. These include the failure to implement a standardized or recognized iron supplementation program, differences in the cutoff values considered as low and adequate for serum ferritin, and the mixing of participants with varying levels of ferritin within treatment groups. On the other hand, studies have investigated the effect of iron status on single protocols of exercise, failing to address the complaint commonly made by athletes with reduced iron stores that they fail to *recover* between a series of competition or training sessions. A recent study (Brownlie et al. 2004), which exposed previously untrained participants with nonanemic iron depletion to a 4-week training program, found that those who had evidence of a tissue iron deficiency (based on abnormal serum transferrin receptor concentrations) had an impaired adaptation to this training compared with a similar group who received iron supplements. By contrast, iron supplementation did not affect endurance cycling performance at the end of the training program in the iron-depleted group who were not tissue iron-depleted.

Despite much publicity about iron depletion problems in athletes, it is likely that the true prevalence of iron-deficiency anemia in runners and other groups is not greater than the occurrence in the general population. According to one review (Haymes 1998), the prevalence of anemia reported among groups of athletes ranges from 0% to 12.5%, whereas low ferritin levels might be expected in 0% to 44% of an athletic group. However, because many studies lack control groups for comparison and use different cutoff values to designate low or suboptimal levels, it is hard to gain an overview of the true problem. Another review in which only studies with control groups were included (Fogelholm 1995) found that the reported prevalence of iron deficiency anemia was quite low (<3%) and was similar between athletes and untrained individuals. Meanwhile, the pooled mean prevalence of low serum ferritin was 37% (range 13-50%) in male and female athletes and 23% (10-46%) in controls. The highest prevalence of low ferritin levels was seen in endurance sports, and among female and adolescent athletes, irrespective of the type of sport and intensity of training (Fogelholm 1995).

In summary, low iron status does occur among athletes and can be problematic for performance, but it occurs for essentially the same reason that it occurs in the general population: a lower than desirable intake of high bioavailability iron. Iron requirements may be increased in some athletes because of increased gastrointestinal or hemolytic iron losses. Distance runners are likely to be at the high end of these losses. However, the most important risk factor is still the low-energy or low-iron diet. Females, vegetarian eaters, and those following diets with restricted quantity and variety are at highest risk. The management and prevention of iron deficiency require professional diagnosis from a variety of clinical, hematological, dietary, and medical data and often involve teamwork among sports medicine and nutrition experts. Sports medicine professionals need to be reminded to consider nonsporting issues in the development of iron deficiency—for example, iron loss secondary to ulcers or malignancies. Occasionally medical problems are overlooked and a simple sports nutrition explanation is assumed. The consequences of such a misdiagnosis can be severe.

Hematological and biochemical tests that are routinely measured to indicate iron status should be cautiously applied to athletic populations because various issues related to exercise can alter these parameters, both to falsely elevate or to decrease the measures. For example, hemodilution (resulting from the plasma volume expansion with increased aerobic exercise) and hemoconcentration (caused by dehydration associated with exercise) can both occur in athletes, providing false decreases or increases in concentrations of plasma constituents. Because ferritin is an acute phase reactant, infection and inflammation are likely to elevate serum ferritin levels independently from iron status. Most of these parameters are also subject to diurnal fluctuations and other physiological variations. Therefore, blood tests should be collected in a way that minimizes interference from these issues—for example, taken after a rest day to avoid acute phase increases in ferritin or taken after ensuring that the athlete is well hydrated. The results should also be interpreted with consideration of these issues.

In athletic populations, ferritin levels below 30 to 35 ng/ml (Nielsen and Nachtigall 1998) are generally marked for further consideration or review. A good comparison is the established iron status history of the individual, because it can provide information on recent changes and the range in changes that might be considered normal and problematic.

Other hematological and biochemical tests are becoming available to add further clarity to the assessment of iron status. These include the measurement of serum transferrin receptors (which are increased in response to reduced iron status to assist in the transport of iron from the blood to tissues) and the characteristics of reticulocytes. However, these tests are not routinely available in all laboratories and need to be studied carefully in relation to iron status in athletes. Finally, support for an assessment of low iron status assessment, and in particular a substantial reduction in blood parameters of iron status, can often be found by looking for the presence of risk factors for iron drain or negative iron balance (see chapter 1, goal 3).

Oral iron supplements provide part of the usual therapy recommended to treat iron deficiency and anemia. Most authorities recommend that such therapy should be prescribed on a case-by-case basis, as part of a treatment plan involving strategies to reduce or prevent unusual iron losses and dietary counseling to maximize the intake of bioavailable iron (Deakin 2006; Nielsen and Nachtigall 1998). The recognized therapy is a daily dose of 100 mg of elemental iron (~500 mg of ferrous sulfate), taken on an empty stomach. Many people also consume a vitamin C supplement or juice to enhance the absorption of this organic iron. Typically, a 3-month period of supplementation is needed to restore depleted iron stores (Nielsen and Nachtigall 1998). In some cases, when it is not possible to enhance dietary iron intake sufficiently, iron supplementation is continued at a lower dose, or as a one- to twice-weekly intake to prevent ongoing iron drain. Although iron supplements are available as over-the-counter medications, there are dangers in self-prescription as a tonic or long-term supplementation in the absence of medical follow-up (see the highlight box on this page).

A rapid reversal of iron depletion and increase in iron stores can be achieved via intramuscular injections of iron. This is sometimes provided in cases of extreme iron depletion that carry a significant penalty to the individual involved or where oral iron intake is not tolerated. However, in some athletic circles it has become popular as a more high-tech method of supplementation and is even used in cases where iron deficiency has not been character-

Risks and Side Effects Associated With Routine Iron Supplementation, Particularly Self-Medication Practices

- Gastrointestinal side effects from oral supplements
- Iron overload (hemochromatosis) in susceptible people, especially males
- Interference with absorption of other minerals (e.g., zinc and copper)
- Anaphylactic shock arising from iron injections
- Failure to treat other causes of fatigue (e.g., inadequate sleep, overtraining, fuel depletion)
- Failure to enhance other nutritional adequacies (e.g., inadequate intake of carbohydrate or other minerals)
- Failure to consider causes of iron drain that might need medical treatment (e.g., ulcers, malignancies)

ized. A recent study (Dawson et al. 2006) showed a course of iron injections (5×2 ml over 10 days) to be associated with a faster and higher increase in serum ferritin in previously iron-depleted females than 30 days of a daily iron tablet. However, both groups had achieved a mean ferritin concentrations above 30 ng/ml by the end of the treatment period. Since changes in performance were not measured in this study, we do not know if the intramuscular iron therapy offered any real benefits above oral iron supplementation. Because iron injections carry a risk of anaphylactic shock as well as iron overload, they should not be regarded as a benign therapy. Iron injections will not increase hemoglobin levels or other iron parameters in people who are not otherwise suboptimal in iron status (Ashenden et al. 1998).

Dietary interventions to reverse or prevent a further decline in iron status involve strategies to increase total iron intake as well as to increase the bioavailability of dietary iron. The importance of this latter factor may not always be appreciated by athletes. In one study of female runners (Snyder et al. 1989), subpopulations who described themselves as meat eaters and those who rarely consumed red meat reported similar amounts of dietary intake of iron estimated from food records. However, analysis of the likely bioavailability of this iron, based on food iron sources and meal combinations, found that non–meat eaters had a substantially lower score for absorbable iron intake. This explained the lower iron status of this group, because they were matched for other important factors such as training volume and pregnancy history. Dietary strategies to increase iron bioavailability are summarized in table 5.3 and should be integrated with eating patterns and food choices that meet the runner's other nutrition goals. This often requires the special expertise of a sports dietitian.

Carbohydrate Needs for Optimal Training and Recovery Between Races

In most major championships, competition in events ranging from 800 to 10,000 m races is conducted as a series of heats and finals. Depending on the competition program, a runner may be required to compete in a number of events over a day or days. Even where runners compete in a weekly competition (e.g., cross-country season or Grand Prix series), optimal recovery is desired to allow the runner to undertake training between races. Outside the competitive season, the training schedules of most serious runners involve multiple daily workouts, which in the case of elite runners add to a weekly volume of 100 to 200 km. The carbohydrate demands of quality or race-pace sessions or interval workouts are particularly high. The value of achieving rapid recovery of muscle fuel stores between sessions should be considered, particularly in view of the likelihood that runners with restricted energy intakes fail to achieve carbohydrate intakes that meet the guidelines suggested for optimal daily resynthesis of glycogen.

A number of studies have examined acute recovery from a single running bout. Several studies have reported that muscle glycogen concentrations do not completely recover over 24 to 48 hr following a very strenuous running session (e.g., marathon) or unaccustomed eccentric loading, despite the intake of a plentiful carbohydrate supply (Asp et al. 1997; Blom et al. 1987; Sherman et al. 1983). It is hard to account for these findings other than to note disruption to muscle cell function resulting from unaccustomed muscle damage. However, an increase in total carbohydrate intake in the first 24 hr of recovery (Doyle et al. 1993) or a greater recovery time (up to 7 days) may be required to fully replace muscle glycogen stores following a running session of unaccustomed intensity, duration, or eccentric work. Nevertheless, consuming a high-carbohydrate diet appears to benefit the performance of a single bout of prolonged exercise or the recovery between two bouts of exercise. For example, Fallowfield and Williams (1993) followed two matched groups of runners who completed two treadmill runs at 70% $\dot{V}O_2max$, 24 hr apart. On the first occasion, which was preceded by a moderate-carbohydrate diet ($\sim$6 $g \cdot kg^{-1} \cdot day^{-1}$), participants ran for 90 min or until fatigue. In recovery for the second run, the groups either continued a moderate carbohydrate intake or consumed an isocaloric high-carbohydrate diet ($\sim$9 $g \cdot kg^{-1} \cdot day^{-1}$). In the second bout, in which participants were required to run to fatigue, run times of the moderate carbohydrate group were shorter than in the first bout, whereas the high-carbohydrate runners were able to match their first performance, showing restoration of running capacity between sessions. Although muscle glycogen concentrations were not monitored in this study, it was assumed that the higher carbohydrate intake allowed greater recovery of fuel stores between sessions.

Logically, benefits from enhancing the acute recovery between sessions should translate over time into better training adaptations and long-term performance gains. However, as discussed in chapter 4 (research topic), evidence that high-carbohydrate diets promote superior training outcomes compared with moderate intakes of carbohydrate is curiously unclear. The literature includes three training studies involving runners, with two of these studies finding that a higher carbohydrate training diet was beneficial to long-term performance (Achten et al. 2004; Kirwan et al. 1988). Kirwan and colleagues (1988) used a crossover design to compare running economy in 10 well-trained runners who increased their training by 150% for 5 days, while consuming either a high (8 $g \cdot kg^{-1} \cdot day^{-1}$) or moderate (4 $g \cdot kg^{-1} \cdot day^{-1}$) intake of carbohydrate. Runners experienced a gradual decline in muscle glycogen concentrations over the week in both dietary treatments, but fuel stores were better preserved with the higher-carbohydrate diet. At the end of the 5 days, treadmill testing revealed a reduced running economy at two different running speeds with the moderate-carbohydrate diet compared with the higher-carbohydrate treatment. Contrasting outcomes were found by Sherman and colleagues (1993), who followed two groups of well-trained runners over 7 days of training; the runners consumed diets providing daily carbohydrate intakes of 5 g/kg (gradually reduced muscle glycogen levels)

Table 5.3 Dietary Strategies to Increase Intake of Bioavailable Iron

Guideline	Practical examples		
Consume enough energy to allow nutrient goals to be met. Avoid chronic periods of energy restriction and severe weight loss.	Be aware that it is difficult to meet recommended dietary intakes for iron when consuming a diet providing less than 1,500-2,000 kcal (6.3-8.4 MJ) per day		
Include sources of bioavailable heme iron regularly at meals, both to provide a source of well-absorbed iron and, via the presence of a "meat factor," to enhance the absorption of nonheme iron from these and other foods consumed at the same meal. • Include small amounts of lean red meats in meals at least 3-4 times each week. • Consider shellfish or liver (e.g., pâté) as an alternative to red meat. • Add chicken and pork meats and dark cuts of fish at other meals to provide a reasonable source of iron and to enhance iron absorption at the meal. • Choose ways to add meats to a high-carbohydrate meal—for example, sandwich with roast beef, pasta with bolognaise sauce, lamb kebabs with rice, beef stir-fry with vegetables and noodles. • Choose lean cuts of meats and trim of all fat and skin. Cook using low-fat methods, which involve no added fat or small amounts of polyunsaturated and monounsaturated oils.	**Heme sources of iron (animal foods)**		
	Liver	100 g (cooked weight)	11.0 mg
	Liver pâté	40 g (2 tbsp)	2-3 mg
	Lean steak	100 g (cooked weight)	4.0 mg
	Bolognaise sauce	100 g (1/2 cup)	
	Chicken (dark meat)	100 g (cooked weight)	1.2 mg
	Fish	100 g (cooked weight)	0.6-1.4 mg
	Oysters	100 g (10)	3.9 mg
	Salmon	100 g (small tin)	1.5 mg
Include foods that are good sources of nonheme iron at most meals, especially meals at which heme sources are not eaten. • Use cereal foods that are iron-fortified (e.g., many commercial breakfast cereals). • Include iron-rich foods such as whole-grain cereals, dried fruit, legumes, eggs, nuts and seeds, and green leafy vegetables in meals and recipes. • Note that many of these foods assist the athlete to meet carbohydrate intake goals. • Note that animal food sources contain nonheme iron in addition to heme iron.	**Sources of nonheme iron:**		
	Eggs	100 g (2 small)	2.0
	Breakfast cereal (fortified)	30 g (1 cup)	2.5 mg
	Whole-grain bread	60 g (2 slices)	1.4 mg
	Spinach (cooked)	145 g (1 cup)	4.4 mg
	Kidney beans or lentils (cooked)	100 g (2/3 cup)	2.5 mg
	Tofu	100 g	1.9 mg
	Sultanas	50 g	0.9 mg
	Dried apricots	50 g	2.0 mg
	Almonds	50 g	2.1 mg
Mix and match foods at meals so that factors that enhance iron absorption are present when nonheme iron provides the major source of iron or where factors that inhibit iron absorption are also present: • Ascorbic acid (vitamin C) • Other food acids such as citric acid • Meat factor	Examples of food matches: • Breakfast cereal eaten with citrus fruits, berries, or tropical fruits (fresh fruits or juices) • Omelet with tomato and parsley • Chili con carne: kidney beans with lean beef • Dried fruit and nuts with fresh citrus, berry, or tropical fruits • Salad added to whole-grain bread sandwich		

Guideline	Practical examples
Reduce the impact of food factors that inhibit iron absorption from sources eaten at the same meal: • Phytates (whole-grain cereal) • Tannin (tea, coffee) • Calcium • Peptides from soy products	Strategies include these: • Divide meals into those with a iron-focus and those in which iron intake isn't the priority. • Counteract inhibition factors by adding factors that enhance iron absorption at the same meal. • Consume foods containing vitamin C and other food acids at meals containing phytates (e.g., milk on breakfast cereal), counteracted with citrus fruits, berries, or tropical fruits (fresh fruits or juices). • Avoid adding bran to meals (e.g., unprocessed bran to cereal mixes) • Consume tea and coffee, if taken strong, between meals rather than with meals.

or 10 g/kg (maintained muscle glycogen concentrations). At the end of this period, the runners undertook two treadmill runs to exhaustion at 80% $\dot{V}O_2$ max with a short recovery interval at the end of a training session. There were no differences in run times between groups.

The final study exposed well-trained runners to 7 days of intensified training supported by both moderate- (5.4 $g \cdot kg^{-1} \cdot day^{-1}$) and high- (8.5 $g \cdot kg^{-1} \cdot day^{-1}$) carbohydrate diets (Achten et al. 2004). During the 11 days of investigation on each dietary treatment, runners undertook a series of monitored training sessions involving either a submaximal preload followed by an 8 km time trial on a treadmill or an outdoor 16 km time trial. Muscle glycogen utilization decreased during submaximal running on the moderate-carbohydrate diet, and there was a decline in time trial performances in both types of sessions. However, the high-carbohydrate treatment was associated with less impairment of running performance, signified by a smaller decrease in 8 km time trial performance and maintenance of 16 km performances. The authors concluded that a high-carbohydrate diet reduced symptoms of overreaching in runners during intensified training compared with a moderate-carbohydrate diet but could not prevent it entirely.

Although it appears sensible to advise runners to consume carbohydrate intakes that promote recovery of muscle glycogen stores between training sessions and races, the direct association with enhanced performance is complex and multifactorial. Such a recommendation may be unfeasible or unwelcome for many female runners whose priority to achieve and maintain low body mass and body fat levels requires a restricted energy intake and, by association, a carbohydrate intake that fails to meet the targets suggested for optimal daily glycogen storage (e.g., 7-10 $g \cdot kg^{-1} \cdot day^{-1}$). Advice for these runners should take into account the detrimental outcomes from chronic situations of energy drain and unreasonable body physique goals and should encourage a greater intake of energy and carbohydrate than many presently appear to achieve. There are anecdotal observations from some female runners that such changes are associated with better training consistency and long-term performance, even when body fat levels are higher than previously desired. However, for most female runners, moderate energy restriction is still likely to limit daily carbohydrate intakes to ~5 to 7 $g \cdot kg^{-1} \cdot day^{-1}$. Many

female runners seek a compromise by periodizing their nutrition goals and dietary carbohydrates intakes over the season, so that lower intakes and physique goals are the priority of training periods, whereas greater carbohydrate intakes are allowed during competition preparation and recovery to maximize glycogen stores.

Fueling Up for Competition

Middle-distance and long-distance events involve running intensities that require high rates of carbohydrate oxidation, and preparation for such races should ensure that muscle carbohydrate stores are matched to the anticipated fuel needs of the event. In shorter events (800-1,500 m), the main limitation to performance is the disturbance in acid-base balance, which results from high rates of anaerobic glycolysis, rather than substrate depletion. Of course, an adequate supply of muscle glycogen is needed for such races, and runners should avoid training and dietary strategies that would cause them to commence a race with depleted muscle glycogen stores. There is even some evidence that supercompensation of muscle glycogen levels may enhance the capacity for high-intensity workloads, although it is not clear whether this results from an accompanying alkalosis or from reduction of glycogen depletion from specific muscle fiber pools (Maughan and Greenhaff 1991). However, for middle-distance events and distance events of 5,000 m through the half-marathon, it is usually suggested that substrate needs can be meet by normalizing muscle carbohydrate stores before the race. In the absence of muscle damage, such fueling up can be achieved with 24 hr of a relative exercise taper and a carbohydrate intake of 7 to 12 g/kg BM.

In races of longer duration fueled by moderate to high rates of carbohydrate oxidation, the muscle's carbohydrate requirement is greater than its normal storage capacity. The depletion of muscle glycogen stores is associated with a feeling of fatigue and the necessity to reduce race pace. Similarly, the nutritional strategy devised to counter the depletion of muscle glycogen stores during an event—carbohydrate loading or glycogen supercompensation—was first popularized by marathon runners because of its clear application to improving exercise endurance and performance over this race.

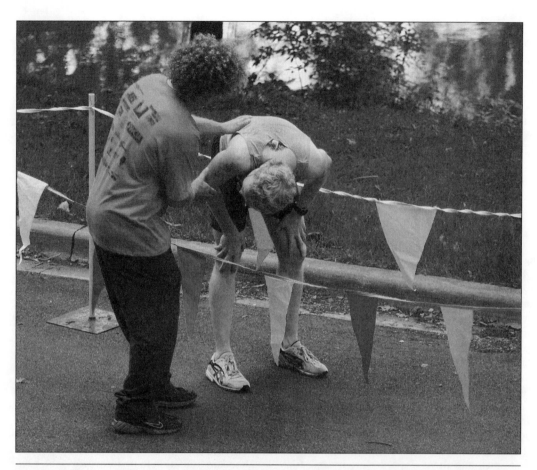

Depletion of muscle glycogen stores occurs so predictably during the later stages of a marathon that the term *hitting the wall* that emanated from the experiences of marathon runners has become so well known that it is now part of everyday jargon.

The term *carbohydrate loading* is used in the general population to describe anything from fueling up for an endurance event like the marathon to rationalizing a food binge of great quantity and dubious quality. Strictly speaking, carbohydrate loading refers to practices that aim to maximize or supercompensate muscle glycogen stores before a competitive event that would otherwise deplete these fuel reserves. Carbohydrate loading protocols may elevate muscle glycogen stores to ~250 mmol/kg of wet weight (ww), or up to twice the concentration of the resting muscle. Since the 1930s it has been recognized that high carbohydrate intakes enhance the capacity of the muscle to undertake prolonged submaximal exercise (Christensen and Hansen 1939). Carbohydrate-loading protocols were an outcome of studies undertaken in the late 1960s by Scandinavian sport scientists who used percutaneous biopsy techniques to examine fuel utilization and enzyme activities in the muscle in response to exercise and recovery. In a series of studies (Ahlborg et al. 1967; Bergstrom et al. 1967; Bergstrom and Hultman 1966; Hermansen et al. 1967), these researchers found that the capacity for prolonged moderate-intensity exercise was determined by preexercise stores of muscle glycogen. Several days of a low-carbohydrate diet depleted muscle glycogen stores and reduced cycling endurance compared with a normal diet of moderate carbohydrate intake. However, the subsequent intake of a high-carbohydrate intake over several days caused a supercompensation of glycogen stores and prolonged cycling time to exhaustion. A clever research design involving one-leg cycling showed that glycogen supercompensation was localized to the muscle that had been previously depleted, and studies identified the activity of glycogen synthase enzyme as an important factor in glycogen synthesis (Bergstrom and Hultman 1966). These pioneering studies produced the classic 7-day model of carbohydrate loading, involving a 3- to 4-day depletion phase of hard training and low carbohydrate intake followed by a 3- to 4-day loading phase of high carbohydrate intake and exercise taper. Early field studies of prolonged running events showed that this strategy enhanced sport performance, not by allowing the athlete to run faster but by prolonging the time that race pace could be maintained (Karlsson and Saltin 1971). Carbohydrate-loading practices were taken up first by competitive marathon runners and later by recreational runners who joined the running boom in the 1970s and 1980s.

The classical studies were undertaken on healthy but essentially untrained men. Later studies using well-trained participants were able to develop a modified version of this carbohydrate-loading strategy. Sherman and colleagues (1981) showed that the muscle from well-trained runners was able to supercompensate its glycogen stores without the necessity of a severe depletion or glycogen stripping phase. The runners in that study elevated their muscle glycogen stores with 3 days of taper and high carbohydrate intake, regardless of whether this was preceded by a depletion phase or a more typical diet and training preparation (see figure 5.1). For well-trained athletes at least, carbohydrate loading was positioned as an extension of fueling-up strategies (rest and high carbohydrate intake) over ~3 days. The modified carbohydrate loading protocol was offered as a more practical strategy for competition preparation, avoiding the fatigue and complexity of extreme diet and training requirements associated with the previous depletion phase.

More recent examinations of carbohydrate-loading strategies have focused on the time course of glycogen storage, with one study investigating muscle glycogen concentrations after 1 and 3 days of rest and a high carbohydrate intake (10 g/kg BM) in well-trained male athletes (Bussau et al. 2002). This study found that after 1 day, muscle glycogen content increased significantly from preloading levels of ~90 mmol/kg ww to values of ~180 mmol/kg ww. Thereafter, glycogen levels remained stable despite another 2 days of rest and carbohydrate intake. The authors concluded that a 24 hr period of physical inactivity and a high carbohydrate intake was sufficient for trained athletes to maximize muscle glycogen levels; this strategy represented an improved 1-day carbohydrate loading protocol. However, the rates of glycogen storage achieved in this study were not abnormally high compared with other literature

values (90 mmol/kg ww in the 24 hr period of observation) and that participants in this study undertook their last training session on the day before the loading protocol officially started, thus explaining the high preloading glycogen values. In essence, the study provides a midpoint to the glycogen storage figure provided by the study of Sherman (figure 5.1) and shows that the supercompensation is not linear and may not require a full 72 hr period in rested participants. Therefore, rather than promoting a unique strategy for carbohydrate loading, this study suggested that optimal refueling is probably achieved within 36 to 48 hr of the last exercise session, at least when the athlete rests and consumes adequate carbohydrate intake.

Supercompensated levels of muscle glycogen persist with subsequent rest and carbohydrate intake until an exercise bout is undertaken (Goforth et al. 1997). However, only recently has there been investigation of an athlete's ability to repeat glycogen supercompensation protocols. Well-trained cyclists who undertook two consecutive periods of exercise depletion followed by 48 hr of high carbohydrate intake (12 g · kg^{-1} · day^{-1}) and rest were found to elevate glycogen stores above resting levels on the first occasion but not the next (McInerny et al. 2005). Further studies are needed to confirm this finding and determine why glycogen storage is attenuated with repeated carbohydrate loading.

Most studies of glycogen storage have been conducted with male participants, with the assumption that the results also apply to females. However, Tarnopolsky and colleagues (1995) reported that female athletes failed to supercompensate muscle glycogen stores compared with male participants and failed to show a performance benefit following this dietary strategy. It is difficult to undertake gender comparison studies because of problems in matching males and females for important parameters such as

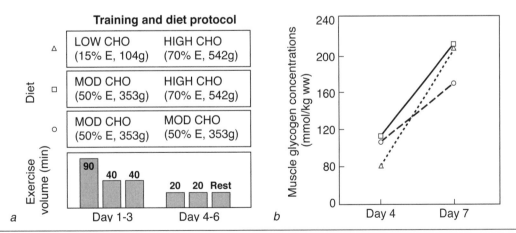

Figure 5.1 *(a)* Trained runners undertook 3 × 6-day dietary protocols in conjunction with a gradual taper in training: 6 days of a moderate carbohydrate (CHO) intake, 3 days of a low CHO intake followed by 3 days of high CHO intake (classical loading), and 3 days of moderate CHO intake followed by 3 days of high CHO intake. *(b)* In trained muscle, the modified loading protocol was associated with supercompensation of muscle glycogen stores on day 7, similar to that achieved by the classical protocol, which involved a strict depletion phase.

Reprinted from Sherman et al. 1981.

aerobic capacity (relative vs. absolute values). Furthermore, studies of carbohydrate loading in females can be criticized for the intake of relatively smaller amounts of dietary carbohydrate and restricted energy intakes. Indeed, when female athletes are provided with sufficient energy and carbohydrate intake, they are able to achieve a significant increase in glycogen storage, similar to that seen in a male population (see figure 5.2) (Tarnopolsky et al. 2001).

Gender differences in substrate utilization and storage are still being investigated and explained (for review, see Tarnopolsky 1999). There is some evidence that the menstrual status of female athletes affects glycogen storage, with greater storage occurring during the luteal phase rather than the follicular phase (Hackney 1990; Nicklas et al. 1989). With this in mind, a carbohydrate-loading study using a modified protocol was undertaken with well-trained female athletes who were in the luteal phase of their menstrual cycle (Walker et al. 2000). This program achieved a 13% increase in muscle glycogen stores compared with storage on a moderate carbohydrate intake and increased time to exhaustion during submaximal cycling. This study showed that when sufficient carbohydrate is consumed in a favorable hormonal environment, female athletes can increase their glycogen stores and improve exercise endurance (Walker et al. 2000). However, although male participants were not included in this study to allow a direct comparison, the researchers noted that the supercompensation achieved by the females was of a lower magnitude than commonly reported in studies of male athletes. By contrast, other studies have shown that protocols involving 3 to 4 days of high carbohydrate intake (9-12 g/kg BM per day)

and rest produced similar increases in muscle glycogen in male and female participants (James et al. 2001; Tarnopolsky et al. 2001). However, not all studies have shown that such increases in glycogen storage lead to a significant performance enhancement in trained female runners (Andrews et al. 2003; Paul et al. 2001) or cyclists (Paul et al. 2001) Of course, these outcomes may be an issue of the type of performance protocol chosen and whether it was long enough to benefit from additional muscle glycogen stores or sensitive enough to allow the detection of small but worthwhile improvements in performance. Thus, the existence and practical significance of physiological limitations to glycogen storage in female athletes remain to be further investigated. In the meantime, it is likely that the main challenge related to carbohydrate-loading practices of females is the practical issue of consuming adequate carbohydrate and energy intake.

Theoretically, carbohydrate loading can enhance performance in sporting events that would otherwise be limited by glycogen depletion. The results of studies of carbohydrate loading and running include failure to find detectable benefits in well-trained runners on 10 km treadmill running (Pitsiladis et al. 1996), a 20.9 km race on an indoor track (Sherman et al. 1981), and a 25 km treadmill run (Sullo et al. 1998). By contrast, carbohydrate loading has been shown to enhance overall performance of a 30 km cross country run (Karlsson and Saltin 1971), a 30 km treadmill run in trained men (Williams et al. 1992), and a 25 km treadmill run in moderately trained men (Sullo et al. 1998). Where these performance enhancements were found, carbohydrate loading was associated not with an increase in

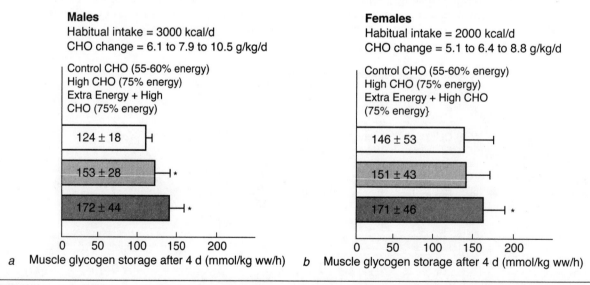

Figure 5.2 Trained male and female participants followed various diets for 4 days in conjunction with rest. *(a)* Increasing the percentage of carbohydrate (CHO) from 55% to 75% of total energy within habitual energy intakes caused an increase in muscle glycogen stores in males but not in females. *(b)* Only when total energy intake was increased and total carbohydrate intake was substantially increased (~9-10 g·kg⁻¹·day⁻¹) did females show a similar response to males in supercompensating muscle glycogen stores.

* = P<0.05.

Adapted from Tarnopolsky et al., 2001.

overall running speed but with maintenance of race pace during the last part of the run compared with the control trial or control group. Even when carbohydrate loading did not cause a statistically significant enhancement of total 30 km running time, participants were found to run faster over the last 5 km than in a control trial (Williams et al. 1992). Therefore, runners should consider carbohydrate loading protocols for races of 30 km and longer.

Fluid and Fuel Intake

The detrimental effects of severe levels of heat stress and dehydration in distance running events have been well publicized through the spectacular collapses of runners in high-profile events—for example, Dorando Pietri in the 1908 Olympic Games marathon, Jim Peters in the 1954 Vancouver Empire Games marathon, and Gabrielle Andersen-Scheiss in the first Olympic marathon for women in the 1984 Los Angeles Games. The risk of hyperthermia is greater during exercise in hot and humid conditions and greater for the fastest runners because of their greater rate of heat production. Over the years, many of the major events in distance running such as the Olympic Games or World Championships have been held in hot climates and have drawn attention to the problems of heat stress during running. In such conditions, a slower pace should be adopted to reduce the rate of heat production. Smaller runners have an advantage over larger competitors because the smaller runners have better heat dissipation characteristics attributable to a lower rate of heat production and a relatively greater surface area from which to dissipate it (see "Physique and Physiology" section in this chapter).

Dehydration adds an overlay to heat stress because the reduction in blood volume that accompanies the accruing body fluid deficit reduces circulatory flow to the skin for convective cooling and for the evaporation of sweat. This causes a greater increase in body temperature. Dehydration reduces the performance of prolonged exercise by increasing cardiovascular stress, increasing the perception of effort and the risk of impaired gastrointestinal function and discomfort, and reducing concentration and mental function (Sawka and Pandolf 1990). These effects increase with the size of the fluid deficit and the temperature of the environment and have prompted the development of education strategies to assist the runner to keep dehydration tolerable levels during workouts and races of greater than 30 to 40 mins (see the first practical issue for an account of the history of such education messages and fluid intake practices). Sweat losses during running vary between runners and events, according to body size, gender, state of acclimatization, pace, and environmental conditions. The tools available for the prediction of sweat losses during running provide general estimations for rates of sweat loss during running within the range of 600 to 2,000 ml/hr (Barr and Costill 1989).

In modern distance running events, especially road races, the intake of fluid (and other race supplies) by runners is achieved by drinking supplies from aid stations provided by the race organizers. In large community-participation events, a generic supply of water, sport drinks, and sponges is provided, although elite competitors are usually provided with opportunities to supply their own race beverages at specially marked tables. Studies of voluntary fluid intakes of runners during longer distance events generally show a fluid intake of 300 to 600 ml/hr, replacing less than 50% of sweat losses during events (Noakes et al. 1988). Anecdotal reports about fluid intake by the top runners in the fields of marathons suggest even lower intakes—200 ml/hr (Noakes 2002). In addition, few runners routinely consume fluids in substantial amounts during training sessions.

There are a variety of reasons for conservative drinking behaviors in runners. The lack of intake during training may reflect the lack of access to fluids—particularly specially prepared fluids such as sport drinks—at typical training venues. Even when fluids are available during races, some runners are reluctant drinkers because of the loss of time in obtaining fluids at aid stations and in drinking these fluids and risk of gastrointestinal discomfort or upset. There is some evidence to suggest that such practical issues impede fluid intake in running; a study of triathletes found that the rate of intake of fluid during the running leg of the race was significantly lower than that achieved during the cycle leg (Kimber et al. 2002). Finally, because the energy of running decreases with a reduction in body mass, the performance deficit associated with dehydration may be partially offset as the athlete becomes lighter by failing to replace all of her sweat losses. This hypothesis needs to be tested in a scientific manner. Nevertheless, it is probable that some top runners make a calculated decision to allow dehydration to occur in some conditions. This implies a lack of knowledge of the predominantly laboratory-based studies that show performance benefits associated with more aggressive fluid and carbohydrate replacement or the belief that these benefits do not cross over into the field.

Many runners could likely benefit by updating their knowledge and practice of fluid and fuel intake, both in training and during races. By drinking during training, and experimenting with the use of sport drinks during longer sessions, runners should come to better appreciate the real benefits of these strategies. Practice may also help athletes to learn the skills and tolerance for drinking on the run, improving their potential for superior strategies on race days. Leaders in the race will need to find a well-considered balance between promoting fluid and fuel intake versus spending time at aid stations and attenuating loss of body mass. For those who are in the main part of the field, and whose aim is to finish the race to their best ability and enjoyment, there should be greater emphasis on better replacement of fluid and fuel needs.

Recent events in distance running and other exercise activities (e.g., military exercises) have drawn attention to a new dimension of this concept of better replacement of fluid and fuel needs during prolonged exercise. The death of a female participant in the 2002 Boston marathon from hyponatremic encephalopathy related to excessive fluid consumption (Smith 2002) provides one example of the need to provide careful advice on drinking practices during running. Previously, it has been assumed that runners will sweat at rates that are far in excess of their practical ability to consume fluids during the session. In most situations this appears to be the case, and many runners can be encouraged to make better use of opportunities for fluid and carbohydrate intake during longer races, especially in hot environments. However, mass-participation events have seen a growth in the percentage of recreational runners for whom finishing the event is a goal and who appear to be less talented, less well trained, or both (Noakes 2002). Noakes provided a comparison of the New York Marathon from 1978 (8,600 competitors) and 2001 (23,600 competitors). In the earlier race, nearly 10% of the race field finished in less than 3 hr, with 7% of competitors taking greater than 5 hr to complete the course. More than 20 years later, despite advances in sport science and training methods and faster times for the race leaders, the median race time for the marathon had increased by more than 60 min with 2.4% competitors finishing in less than 3 hr and 23% in more than 5 hr (Noakes 2002).

It has been proposed that the increased participation of "back of the pack" runners who exercise at slow intensities with low sweat rates, yet use a network of aid stations to drink as much as possible, is at least circumstantially linked with the increasing number of reports of hyponatremia in ultradistance sports. Indeed, a study of 488 runners from the Boston marathon found that 13% experienced hyponatremia at race finish (0.6% at a critical level), with hyponatremia being associated with substantial weight gain, consumption of fluids every mile, a race time >4 hr, female sex, and low body mass index (Almond et al. 2005). It is important to educate runners, particularly of recreational caliber, that they should not drink in excess of their rate of sweat loss. The issue of hyponatremia is covered in greater detail in chapter 4, practical issue.

Runners and other athletes are often advised to monitor changes in body mass over an exercise session to provide an estimate of total sweat losses and the success of current fluid intake practices in replacing these during the event or workout. The use of this information to adjust fluid intake practices according to the individual's typical sweat rates under given conditions is potentially better than drinking to a plan based on arbitrary and generic advice. However, certain caveats need to be put in place. First, it must be recognized that during events of prolonged moderate- to high-intensity exercise, changes in body mass do not provide a true representation of the fluid deficit that needs to be replaced. For example, some part of the weight change involves the oxidation of fuels (carbohydrate and fat stores), which causes the production of metabolic water. In addition, the liberation of the water bound with muscle glycogen stores, especially in the carbohydrate-loaded marathon runner, presumably adds to total available water stores without changing body mass. Unless the runner voids both before and after the session and monitors body mass nude and dried, the mass of urine in the bladder and sweat trapped in hair and clothing will lead to an underestimation of the fluid deficit. A study of female distance runners who completed a 30 km run found that the simple measurement of body mass changes in hot (30°C) conditions, corrected only for fluid intake

during the run, achieved a mean estimation of total sweat loss that was close to actual sweat loss (Cheuvront et al. 2002). The small overestimation of sweat losses produced by this method (1.13 vs. 1.07 L/hr; 6% overestimation) was further improved by correcting for urine losses (<1% overestimation). However, in a cool environment (14°C), this simple field measurement significantly overestimated the mean value for total sweat losses (0.88 vs. 0.70 L/hr; 31% overestimation) even with the correction for urine losses (14% overestimation).

In summary, it is unlikely that any detriment will occur during prolonged sessions of running if a small fluid deficit is allowed to accrue—for example, to have the runner aim for a drink intake that replaces a maximum of 80% of the typical changes in body mass seen in similar sessions or to allow for a 1% to 2% (~1 kg) loss of body mass over the session. For the majority of faster runners, such outcomes will still require proactive strategies for fluid replacement, and, of course, all fluid intake plans need to be tailored to avoid gastrointestinal discomfort from excessive intake (Daries et al. 2000). By contrast, slower runners should be warned against overestimating sweat needs and fluid losses and cautioned against excessive fluid intakes.

The use of carbohydrate–electrolyte drinks (sport drinks) during races of 60 min or longer provides the runner with the potential to replace fluid and carbohydrate simultaneously, with the option of altering the carbohydrate concentration of the drink (typically 4-8% or 4-8 g/100 ml), according to the priority of rehydration or refueling in a particular event. Chapter 4 provides an overview of other carbohydrate sources consumed during endurance sports (see table 4.7); however, distance runners are generally limited by gastrointestinal concerns to confectionery and sports gels as alternative forms of carbohydrate replacement. The benefits of carbohydrate intake during prolonged sessions of exercise (>90 min of exercise) are well documented (Coombes and Hamilton 2000; Hargreaves 1999), with reports dating back to the Boston marathon in the 1920s that the consumption of sweets during the race prevented the occurrence of symptoms of hypoglycemia and enhanced the performance of runners (Gordon et al. 1925; Levine et al. 1924). More recent studies involving prolonged running protocols in which an enhancement of performance was found with carbohydrate ingestion include a 40 km outdoor run in the heat (Millard-Stafford et al. 1992), a 30 km road run (Tsintzas, Liu, et al. 1993), a marathon run on a treadmill (Tsintzas et al. 1995), and a ~2 hr treadmill protocol to exhaustion at 70% $\dot{V}O_2$max (Tsintzas, Williams, Wilson, et al. 1996). The generally accepted mechanisms of performance enhancement from carbohydrate ingestion during prolonged exercise include prevention of hypoglycemia, sparing of liver glycogen, and provision of an additional muscle fuel substrate (Hargreaves 1999). However, in the case of running, there is some evidence of muscle glycogen sparing, at least in selected fibers (Tsintzas, Williams, Boobis, et al. 1996; Tsintzas, Liu, et al. 1993).

Whether consuming carbohydrate during shorter distance events such as the half-marathon is beneficial is unclear (see research topic), with the potential mechanism of any performance enhancements being attributable to effects on the central nervous system rather than provision of muscle fuel. Although most studies of this nature have been undertaken with cycling protocols, one study involving a 15 km treadmill run in a hot environment found an improvement in speed over the last, self-paced portion of the run when carbohydrate was ingested immediately before and during the run compared with a placebo trial (Millard-Stafford et al. 1997). By contrast, carbohydrate intake during an 18 km run failed to enhance performance of a large group of runners or the fastest runners in the group compared with water (van Nieuwenhoven et al. 2005). Whether an aggressive intake of carbohydrate is worthwhile and practical for world-class runners who run at speeds of ~20 km/hr is another issue. One investigation reported that the intake of a concentrated carbohydrate product (sport gel) by highly trained distance runners was associated with a slower running time in a half-marathon in individuals who experienced gastrointestinal discomfort (Burke et al. 2005).Overall, the effect of the carbohydrate gel on performance was trivial, but it caused a statistically significant but clinically unimportant increase in the time taken to run through feed zones. Further studies are needed.

Gastrointestinal Problems

Gastrointestinal discomfort and upset can interfere with the performance and enjoyment of exercise for many athletes.

Although the exact prevalence of problems that can occur in both the upper and lower gastrointestinal tract is not well known, it appears likely that running is a high-risk sport for these events. Other risk factors for the development of these problems were outlined in chapter 1, goal 16, and included exercise at high intensities (e.g., race pace), being relatively unfit or unaccustomed to the required exercise, moderate to severe levels of dehydration, and the consumption of certain foods and fluids before and during the exercise session. Females appear to be at higher risk of gastrointestinal problems than males, and exercise seems to exacerbate underlying or preexisting gut problems. Some problems such as reflux, flatulence, abdominal pain, and bloating may present as a nuisance rather than an impediment to exercise. Nevertheless, other problems such as diarrhea and vomiting not only directly interfere with performance but threaten the athlete's ability to follow or benefit from his race plan for fluid and carbohydrate intake.

Persistent and severe gastrointestinal problems need to be immediately referred to a sports physician and perhaps a gastroenterologist (for review, see Fallon 2006). With appropriate treatment, including medication where necessary, the athlete who suffers from problems such as celiac disease, gastritis or ulcers, ulcerative colitis, and irritable bowel disease will be able to resume an appropriate exercise plan. Problems such as gastrointestinal bleeding should be immediately referred for attention and diagnosis, because there are often underlying pathologies that benefit from early diagnosis as well as exercise-related causes. Dietary

Nutrition Guidelines for Minimizing Exercise-Related Gastrointestinal Symptoms During Running and Other Exercise

- Athletes who suffer from gastrointestinal reflux during exercise should identify their response to potentially offending foods (e.g., fatty and spicy foods, alcohol, caffeine, and chocolate), especially when consumed on the day or hours preceding exercise.

- Athletes who suffer from diarrhea during exercise should experiment to see if any of the following high-risk foods or nutrients, when consumed in the hours before exercise, increase the risk or severity of this problem: caffeine, high-fiber foods, lactose-rich foods (e.g., milk, ice cream), fructose-rich foods (fruits and fruit juices), excessive intake of protein-rich and fatty foods.

- The risk of diarrhea and bowel upsets may be reduced by ensuring that the last solid food is eaten at least 3 hr preexercise: Liquid meals may offer an alternative way to provide preevent nutrition.

- A low-residue diet on the evening or day before important events may reduce the risk of diarrhea and bowel upsets.

- During exercise, the athlete should remain well hydrated: Often complaints about gastrointestinal upsets following the intake of fluids during the event are attributable to moderate to severe dehydration and thus the delay in drinking, rather than to the fluid per se.

- Athletes at risk of gastrointestinal problems should experiment with dilute solution of carbohydrate drinks (2-4% concentration of carbohydrate) and gradually increase carbohydrate content as tolerated when there is a priority to refuel during the event.

- High-fiber foods (e.g., some cereal bars, breads, and fruit), concentrated carbohydrate drinks, and caffeine may also increase the risk of gastrointestinal problems when consumed during exercise, and the athlete should experiment with such items in training before using in an important event.

guidelines for minimizing the risk or severity of exercise-related gastrointestinal symptoms are summarized in the highlight box on page 129.

Sport Foods and Supplements

Most middle- and long-distance runners, even at a recreational level, are consumers of sport foods and supplements. Some of these products are specially designed to help a runner meet specific needs for energy and nutrients, including fluid and carbohydrate, in situations where everyday foods are not practical to eat (see the highlight box on this page). This is particularly relevant for intake immediately before, during, or after exercise. These supplements can be shown to improve performance when they allow runners to achieve their sports nutrition guidelines. However, they are more expensive than normal foods, a consideration that must be balanced against the convenience they provide (see table 5.d in appendix). Other supplements that may be of value to a runner are micronutrient preparations that are used to treat or prevent a vitamin or mineral deficiency, as directed by a sports nutrition expert.

As is the case for most sports, nutritional ergogenic aids—products that promise a direct and supraphysiological benefit to sports performance—are the supplements that most seem to fascinate runners. In general, these supplements have been poorly tested or have failed to live up to their claims when rigorous testing has been undertaken on middle- and long-distance running performance. Exceptions to this are caffeine and bicarbonate, each of which may enhance the performance of certain runners or certain events under specific conditions (see table 5.c in appendix). Caffeine in particular has a special role and history of use in running; the results of early studies of caffeine and endurance performance were quickly popularized by articles in running magazines, making a prerace caffeine (coffee) intake a regular practice at marathon events. The benefits of other potentially useful supplements such as glycerol and creatine have not been clearly demonstrated in middle-distance and distance running (see table 5.e in appendix) but merit further research. The reader should also read the research related to these supplements presented in chapters 4 and 6, because there may be some crossover between benefits seen in other sports with shared characteristics. Finally, the claims made in support of the majority of other supplements and compounds marketed as ergogenic aids are not supported by scientific research (table 5.a). Of course, more research is needed, using rigorous control and carefully chosen protocols to test the claims for most products. In many cases, particular (proposed) ergogenic compounds that are used by middle-distance and distance runners, and reviewed in chapter 3, have not been tested in an appropriate protocol and no further comments can be made about these products. The reader is therefore referred to the general conclusions reached in chapter 3.

Runners should seek expert advice about potentially valuable supplements and sport foods to ensure that the appropriate conditions of use apply to their situation and that they are aware of the optimal timing and doses of use. In many cases, there is a lack of event-specific research, and the runner may need through trial and error to refine the practice that gives him or her the greatest benefits. At best, the unsupported nutritional ergogenic aids offer a placebo to runners. However, the downside includes the waste of considerable amounts of money, inadvertent doping, or health problems caused by contamination of products. In most cases, runners would be better rewarded by directing their resources and interest to a more credible area of sport performance, such as better equipment, improved training techniques, or advice about nutrition or psychological preparation.

Research Priorities

Areas that are of high priority for sport-specific research include the following:

- Validation of dietary survey techniques in runners, especially to investigate the phenomenon of energy discrepancies in athletes with apparently restricted energy intakes
- Nutrition practices of high-level runners during training and racing
- Weight control beliefs and practices of male and female runners
- Energy drain and menstrual disturbances in females and the potential for similar problems in male athletes (e.g., lowered testosterone concentrations)
- Optimal iron status for runners and other endurance athletes; sensitive markers for problematic changes in iron status
- Current hydration and fuel intake practices of runners including preparation for events and intake during longer events
- Use of supplements and sport foods by runners and their specific benefit to performance in various events

Table 5.4 Sport Foods and Supplements That Are of Likely Benefit to Middle- and Long-Distance Runners

	Product	Comment
Use in achieving documented nutrition goals	Sport drinks	• Use to refuel and rehydrate during prolonged workouts (middle-distance and distance runners) and races (distance runners) and to rehydrate after the session. Contain some electrolytes to help replace sweat losses and increase voluntary intake of fluid.
	Sport gels	• Convenient and compact carbohydrate source that can be carried for use during prolonged workouts and distance races (half-marathon and above).
	Sport bars	• Convenient, portable, and easy-to-consume source of carbohydrate, protein, and micronutrients for prerace meal or postexercise recovery.
	Liquid meal supplements	• Convenient, portable, and easy-to-consume source of carbohydrate, protein, and micronutrients for postexercise recovery. • Well-tolerated preevent meal that can be consumed to provide a source of carbohydrate quite close to the race start; seems to be better tolerated than solid food by some athletes with high risk of gastrointestinal problems. • Convenient and compact source of energy and nutrients for the traveling athlete.
	Multivitamin and mineral supplements	• Supplemental source of micronutrients for traveling when food supply is not reliable. • Supplemental source of micronutrients during prolonged periods of energy restriction.
	Iron supplements	• Supplemental form of iron for prevention and treatment of diagnosed cases of reduced iron deficiency. Should be taken under the supervision of a sports doctor or dietitian and in conjunction with dietary intervention.
	Calcium supplements	• Supplemental form of calcium for prevention and treatment of poor bone status when diet is unable to meet calcium requirements. Should be taken under the supervision of a sports doctor and dietitian and in conjunction with appropriate medical and dietary intervention.
Strong potential for ergogenic benefit	Bicarbonate or citrate loading	• There is reasonable evidence to support the benefits to middle-distance running events (800 and 1,500 m) of bicarbonate or citrate loading to reduce blood pH and enhance extracellular buffering capacity. Typical doses are 300 mg/kg BM bicarbonate or 500 mg/kg BM citrate, taken 1-2 hr preevent. The risk of gastrointestinal upsets should be assessed but may be reduced by the intake of large amounts of fluid with the citrate or bicarbonate dose. Further field studies are needed with high-level athletes to confirm benefits. Track runners who intend to load for a series of events over a day or consecutive days (e.g., heats and finals) should experiment with a lower dose for the second or subsequent races in view of residual increase in buffering capacity from earlier doses. Alternatively, a chronic protocol of bicarbonate loading (500 $mg \cdot kg^{-1} \cdot day^{-1}$ for 5 days spread into a series of doses over the day) may allow a more sustained increase in blood buffering capacity. There is recent evidence that chronic bicarbonate loading (loading prior to each session of interval training) may enhance training adaptations and the ability to perform sustained high-intensity exercise. It may also allow the athlete to train harder.
	Caffeine	• Caffeine appears to enhance the performance of prolonged high-intensity exercise or endurance events and may be of benefits to middle- and long-distance running events. Small to moderate doses (1-3 mg/kg BM) appear to be as effective as larger doses (5-6 mg/kg BM) in enhancing the performance of prolonged exercise. Further sport-specific studies are needed to investigate the range of running events that might benefit from caffeine intake and the range of doses and consumption protocols (e.g., intake before, during, or toward the end of prolonged events) that are effective. May be consumed in cola and energy drinks or as an ingredient in some sport products (e.g., some gels). There is conflicting evidence over the efficacy of coffee as a source of caffeine because it contains other chemicals that might negate the benefits.

BM = body mass.

131

RESEARCH TOPIC

Does Carbohydrate Replacement Also Enhance the Performance of Sports Lasting 1 hr?

Depending on the environment, a well-trained athlete can sustain a workload of ~75% to 85% of $\dot{V}O_2$max or just below the onset of blood lactate accumulation for around 60 min. Events of this duration in sport include a 40 to 50 km time trial or the 1 hr time trial in cycling, the half-marathon in running, and a sprint triathlon. Traditionally, sport scientists have believed that the (normalized) muscle glycogen stores of the trained athlete are sufficient to support the fuel needs of such events. After all, several studies have shown that an increase in muscle glycogen stores via carbohydrate loading protocols does not improve performance in field studies or laboratory protocols of this duration (Hawley, Palmer, et al. 1997; Sherman et al. 1981). On this basis, supplying additional carbohydrate immediately before or during an event lasting 60 min would not be expected to improve performance, at least by any mechanism that involved glycogen sparing or provision of an additional fuel substrate in the face of glycogen depletion. Because blood glucose concentrations are usually maintained or even slightly elevated by exercise around these intensities, it is also unlikely that carbohydrate intake during a 60 min race would provide an advantage in terms of preventing or reversing hypoglycemia. Typically, performance in these events is thought to be limited by other factors—for example, in the case of exercise undertaken in hot conditions, thermoregulatory factors.

It is therefore puzzling to see a growing body of literature reporting performance benefits from carbohydrate supplementation during high-intensity exercise lasting around an hour. Studies that have investigated such protocols in trained participants are summarized in the highlight box on this page and include studies of both running and cycling protocols and both hot and cool environments. Although some studies failed to detect performance enhancements from carbohydrate intake within the event (Burke et al. 2005; Desbrow et al. 2004; Kovacs et al. 1998), the majority of studies are supportive of benefits (Anantaraman et al. 1995; Below et al. 1995; Carter et al. 2003; Jeukendrup et al. 1997; Millard-Stafford et al. 1997; Nikolopoulos et al. 2004). The features of these studies are summarized in table 5.a in the appendix.

Two theories involving the brain and central nervous system have been suggested to explain the benefits of carbohydrate ingestion during these exercise activities (Carter et al. 2003):

- Slightly higher blood glucose concentrations may influence the sites affecting motivation, pacing, and motor output in the central nervous system or higher brain center.

- Carbohydrate intake may directly stimulate receptors and nerve endings in the mouth and gastrointestinal tract that communicate to the hypothalamus and other brain centers.

Several studies have attempted to distinguish between these theories. In the first investigation, cyclists undertook a time trial lasting about 1 hr with or without a protocol to achieve slightly elevated blood glucose levels without stimulating mouth and gut receptors (Carter, Jeukendrup, Mann, et al. 2004). Specifically, intravenous delivery of carbohydrate at a rate of 1 g/min was undertaken during a cycling time trial. This intervention increased blood glucose levels compared with a saline infusion and contributed 14% of total carbohydrate oxidized (~27 g) during the workout. Despite an increased availability of plasma glucose for oxidation, there was no change in total carbohydrate oxidation and no enhancement of the performance of the set amount of work (61.20 ± 1.82 vs. 61.37 ± 1.9 min, not significant) (Carter, Jeukendrup, Mann, et al. 2004).

The second study involved cyclists undertaking a 1 hr time trial on two occasions, with the use of a mouth rinse as every 12.5% of the work was completed (Carter, Jeukendrup, and Jones 2004). On one occasion, the mouth rinse was a 6.4% carbohydrate drink, whereas a flavored placebo drink was consumed on the other occasion. Although the mouth rinse was not swallowed during either trial, the carbohydrate trial was associated with an increased power output and faster performance time than the placebo trial (59.57 ± 1.5 vs. 61.37 ± 1.56 min, $p < .01$). The 3% enhancement of performance was similar to that seen in similar protocols in which carbohydrate drinks are consumed in comparison to a placebo solution (Jeukendrup et al. 1997). It was suggested that rinsing with the carbohydrate drink triggered carbohydrate receptors in the oral cavity, leading to stimulation of areas in the brain associated with motivation or pacing. This apparently allowed the cyclists to complete the time trial at a higher work output but with a similar sense of pacing and perceived effort. Such an intriguing possibility warrants further investigation.

Finally, surface electromyogram (EMG) activity was monitored in leg muscles in a study that found a strong trend (13% improvement) in endurance when carbohydrate was consumed during a protocol involving cycling at 85% $\dot{V}O_2$max (Nikolopoulos et al. 2004). Carbohydrate intake was associated with a reduction in EMG activity toward the latter part of the trial and at the point of fatigue. This suggests that carbohydrate intake changes afferent sensory input and that a neural control mechanism (a "governor") may be responsible for reducing or limiting exercise capacity. These authors suggested that different regulators may be involved in terminating constant power exercise (endurance) versus those than regulate effort during a self-paced time trial (performance). Further investigation of the possibility for performance enhancement with carbohydrate intake during high-intensity exercise is warranted.

RESEARCH TOPIC

Energy Efficiency: Do Some Female Distance Runners Really Consume Such Low Energy Intakes Yet Run 100 km a Week?

A striking feature of many of the dietary surveys of female athletes is the low level of energy intake reported by many groups and individuals. Distance runners seem to have attracted the most attention in this regard. In a number of surveys, reported daily energy intakes of the group average around 6,000 to 8,000 kJ or 1,500 to 2,000 kcal (Beidleman et al. 1995; Deuster et al. 1986; Drinkwater et al. 1984; Kaiserauer et al. 1989; Mulligan and Butterfield 1990; Myerson et al. 1991). These lower values are roughly equivalent to the basal metabolic needs of these women and would certainly not supply sufficient additional energy to fuel a demanding training program in the range of 60 to 200 km/week. In addition to these dietary surveys, most sports nutrition practitioners and weight loss counselors are familiar with challenging situations involving athletes who claim that they can't reduce their weight or body fat levels despite "hardly eating anything." Several factors may explain apparently low energy intakes of female athletes, particularly distance runners.

- **Active period of loss of body mass or body fat.** It is possible that most of the dietary surveys of female athletes have captured data on groups who are in an active phase of deliberately restricting energy intake to reduce body fat levels and are therefore in negative energy balance. This would appear to be an unlikely explanation, however, because in many studies, participants either are described as being weight stable or did not appear to change body mass or composition over the duration of the survey.

- **Artifact of dietary survey methodology.** It is possible that the dietary surveys of female athletes represent an underreporting of the true energy intake of these athletes. Errors occurring in self-reported food diaries, commonly used in athletic surveys, were discussed in chapter 2 (research topic) and include these:

  ○ The athlete alters her dietary intake during the period of recording so that it fails to reflect her usual intake. This is often attributable to the inconvenience of recording.

  ○ The athlete inaccurately records her dietary intake to improve the perception of what she is eating (i.e., she underestimates or omits to record her intake of foods seen as undesirable or falsely reports the intake of foods seen as desirable).

  ○ The athlete makes errors of quantification or description in recording her food intake.

  ○ According to the review in chapter 2, the bias of such errors is to underreport true energy intake—generally by ~20%. However, individuals who are overfat or dissatisfied with their body mass and body image generally underreport to an even greater extent.

- **Energy efficiency.** There is much anecdotal support for the theory that some athletes are energy efficient—that they can balance their basal metabolic needs and the energy cost of eating and exercise at a level that is substantially lower than their expected energy requirements. It is possible that some components of total energy expenditure (TEE) are reduced in some groups or individuals—for example, a lower physical activity outside training or a reduced resting metabolic rate (RMR). In the case of females, studies frequently report that female distance runners with menstrual disturbances maintain energy balance on a lower reported energy intake than regularly menstruating runners who are matched for training volume (Barr 1987). Lebenstedt and colleagues (1999) studied female runners and triathletes whose menstrual function was determined by assessing salivary progesterone levels to classify them into normal function (12 periods per year) or menstrual disturbances (9 or fewer periods per year). Although the reported energy intakes and activity levels of these two groups were not different, the women with menstrual disturbances had a significantly lower RMR and reported significantly higher scores on a test of restrained eating. Another study found that amenorrheic runners had a significantly lower RMR than eumenorrheic runners and inactive controls, with their reported energy intakes being similar to the inactive controls despite higher activity levels (Myerson et al. 1991). These last two studies show that differences in reported dietary intakes between groups cannot be entirely explained as results of survey artifacts and that women with menstrual disturbances may exhibit energy efficiency, as either a cause or an effect of menstrual dysfunction. The issue of the energy drain and menstrual disturbances are discussed in more detail in chapter 13, first research topic.

There is additional research evidence both to support and to contradict the theory of energy efficiency. Evidence supporting energy efficiency was found in a group of male endurance athletes, classified as either low energy intake or adequate energy intake (Thompson et al. 1993). The low energy eating athletes (n = 12) reported the consumption of a daily energy intake that was ~6,150 kJ or 1,490 kcal less than the adequate energy group (n = 11), whereas the activity levels of both groups were similar. Despite these differences in apparent energy intake, both groups had been weight stable for at least 2 years and had similar levels of fat-free mass. RMR was found to be significantly lower (p < .05) in the low energy intake group compared with the adequate energy intake groups, providing one mechanism to explain lower energy requirements. However, there was no difference in the thermic effect of a meal.

In a more comprehensive study of this phenomenon, the same group studied a group of male endurance athletes who were selected on the basis of being adequate (n = 4) and low energy consumers (n = 6) from comprehensive 7-day diet and activity records (Thompson et al. 1995). These records verified a substantial mismatch between estimated energy intake (food diaries) and expenditure (factorial methods) of the low-energy group (see table 5.5). When these athletes were studied for 24 hr in a respiratory chamber, the low energy consuming group was found to have significantly lower values for daily TEE, RMR, and spontaneous physical activity or daily fidgeting than the control group—confirming lower sedentary energy expenditure. It is likely that the lower spontaneous movement of the low energy consuming group would be amplified in a free-living situation. Although the energy cost of training was not measured in this study because of the constraints of the metabolic chamber, it is possible that this also differed between groups. The thermic effect of food would also be expected to be lower in the low-energy consumers, as a result of the smaller amount of food consumed in a day. However, even these measured and hypothesized differences between groups did not entirely account for the energy discrepancy, pointing to additional underreporting in the food records of the low energy consuming group.

Data disputing the severity of energy efficiency can be found in a study of nine female distance runners (Edwards et al. 1993). Mean reported daily energy intake of the group (7-day food records) accounted for only 68% of expenditure (doubly labeled water), although athletes were apparently weight stable during the study period. Among individual runners, the daily energy discrepancy ranged from 431 kJ (4% of TEE and within measurement error) to an unlikely 8,041 kJ (58% of TEE). Although this may have been supportive of a true energy discrepancy, the authors noted that reported energy intake was inversely correlated with TEE and body mass. Other evidence showed that the heaviest runners suffered from dissatisfaction and disturbances of their body image and were most likely to underreport on food diaries.

Several other sophisticated energy balance studies have also been carried out on athletes, with the finding of substantial discrepancies between reported energy intakes and energy requirements among female athletes in weight-conscious sports (Beidleman et al. 1995; Edwards et al. 1993; Fogelholm et al. 1995; Schulz et al. 1992) without showing any support for metabolic efficiencies. In addition, some studies have been able to directly show that athletes reduce their food intake while recording dietary surveys (Schulz et al. 1992). Of course, it is important that any study of metabolic rates in female athletes control for the presence and the stage of the menstrual cycle, because these factors are known to change RMR (Barr et al. 1995; Lebenstedt et al. 1999). Not all studies have included such control.

Researchers and practitioners should be cautious in interpreting the results of self-reported assessments of dietary intake. The widespread underestimation of true energy intake adds to the mystery of the apparent discrepancies in energy requirements and energy balance among athletes. Until better dietary assessment tools are available, this problem will prevent a true understanding of the consequences of restrained eating practices in general and will interfere with the management of individual athletes.

Table 5.5   Differences in Energy Intake and Energy Expenditure of Male Endurance Athletes Self-Selected As "Low Energy" or "Adequate Energy" Consumers

	Low energy group (n = 6)	Adequate energy group (n = 4)
DATA FROM FOOD AND ACTIVITY RECORDS DURING FREE-LIVING PERIOD		
Mean daily energy intake	11.9 ± 3.2 MJ[a]	18.9 ± 4.5 MJ
Total daily energy expenditure	18.2 ± 2.7 MJ	17.8 ± 1.1 MJ
Daily energy balance	−6.4 ± 2.2 MJ[a]	1.1 ± 3.8 MJ
DATA FROM 24 HR IN RESPIRATORY CHAMBER		
24 hr energy expenditure	8,498 ± 561 kJ[a]	9,360 ± 548 kJ
Resting energy expenditure	6,903 ± 419[a]	7,426 ± 400 kJ
Spontaneous physical activity	65 ± 20 min[a]	108 ± 34 min
	657 ± 251 kJ[a]	933 ± 155 kJ

[a]Significantly different than adequate energy group.

Data from Thompson et al. 1995.

PRACTICAL ISSUE

The Changing Face of Guidelines for Fluid and Carbohydrate Ingestion During Distance Running

Don't take any nourishment before going 17 or 18 miles. If you do you will not go the distance. Don't get into the habit of eating or drinking in a marathon race: some prominent runners do, but it is not beneficial.

J.E. Sullivan, from a 1909 book on marathon running (Sullivan, 1909, p. 39)

Fluids and foods consumed during the marathon at the 1928 Olympic Games in Amsterdam by 10 runners from a variety of countries: Nil (2 runners), 1 egg (1 runner), lemonade with added sucrose (2 Japanese runners), tea (2 runners), cocoa (1 runner), milk (1 runner), tea and grapefruit (1 runner).

Study of the nutritional habits of athletes at 1928 Olympic Games (Best and Partridge 1930)

If the eating of candy during a race was encouraged by Athletic Organizations, it seems possible that new records might be achieved in very long-distance running.

From a 1936 textbook on exercise (Grace Eggleton 1936, p. 153)

In those days it was quite fashionable not to drink (during a distance running event) until one absolutely had to. After a race runners would recount with pride "I only had a drink after 30 or 40 km." To run a complete marathon without any fluid replacement was regarded as the ultimate aim of most runners, and a test of their fitness.

Jackie Meckler, champion distance and ultradistance runner in the 1940s to 1960s, cited in Noakes (2003a, p. 199)

Aid stations are allowed in distance running events only after 15 km, and water is the only provision permitted.

1953 International Amateur Athletics Federation (IAAF) guidelines for distance running, Rule no. 165.5, cited in Noakes (2003a, p. 200)

Rules prohibiting the administration of fluids during the first 10 kilometers of a marathon race should be amended to permit fluid ingestion at frequent intervals along the race course. . . . It is the responsibility of the race sponsors to provide fluids which contain small amounts of sugar (less than 2.5%) and electrolytes. . . . The addition of even small amounts of sugar can drastically impair the rate of gastric emptying.

During exercise in the heat, carbohydrate supplementation is of secondary importance and the sugar content of oral feedings should be minimized.

1975 position statement on prevention of heat injuries during distance running (American College of Sports Medicine. 1975, p. vii)

An adequate supply of water should be available before the race and every 2-3 km during the race. . . . Aid stations should be stocked with enough fluid (cool water is the optimum) for each runner to have 300-360 ml at each aid station. The runner is encouraged to drink 100-200 ml of fluid at each aid station, every 2-3 km.

1987 position statement on prevention of thermal injuries during distance running (American College of Sports Medicine 1987, p. 529)

Slow runners (running at 10 km per hour and drinking 100 ml at aid stations 3 km apart) will receive 330 ml each hour, whereas fast runners (running at 20 km per hour, and drinking 200 ml each 2 km) will receive 2000 ml per hour.

Scientists Ed Coyle and Dr. Scott Montain commenting that a literal interpretation of the 1987 ACSM guidelines is neither practical nor useful (Coyle and Montain 1992, p. S325)

During intense exercise lasting longer than 1h, it is recommended that carbohydrates be ingested at a rate of 30-60g per hour to maintain oxidation of carbohydrates and delay fatigue. This rate of carbohydrate intake can be achieved without compromising fluid delivery by drinking 600-1200 ml/hr of solutions containing 4-8% carbohydrates.

1996 position stand on exercise and fluid replacement (American College of Sports Medicine 1996, p. i)

There is no evidence that athletes must drink "the maximal amount that is tolerable" to optimize performance and prevent medical consequences. . . . To protect all exercisers from this preventable condition (fatal hyponatremia), rational and evidence based advice must be provided. In particular, exercise must be warned that the overconsumption of fluid (either water or sports drink) before, during or after exercise is unnecessary and can have a potentially fatal outcome.

Professor Tim Noakes, in an editorial in the 2003 British Medical Journal (Noakes 2003b, p. 113)

The release of new guidelines for fluid replacement during exercise by the American College of Sports Medicine (ACSM 2007) and the Updated Fluid Recommendation from the

International Marathon Medical Directors Association [IMMDA] (Hew-Butler et al. 2006) provides an opportunity to examine the evolution of recommendations over time. History has seen considerable changes to the guidelines and practice of fluid intake during running. As illustrated in the quotes at the beginning of this section, early advice to runners ranged from extreme avoidance of drinking to the intake of small fluid volumes. Over the years, the debate has concerned the choice of beverages as well as the terminology used to provide guidelines for the volume of fluid intake that runners should consume. The science of sports nutrition has evolved over the past 40 years and continues to evolve with new studies and new techniques. Position statements, even when made by experts, can only make guidelines based on the knowledge of the day. Expert statements are generally prepared by consensus and, as such, represent a conservative view that the authors believe can be substantiated by research. Therefore, guidelines may be considered state of the art at the time of their release but may need to be altered over time in view of new information or the recognition that a more practical education message is needed. This evolution is well demonstrated by changes in the position stands of the American College of Sports Medicine on fluid intakes during exercise over the past 3 decades.

Excerpts from the statements of the 1970s and early 1980s show that the primary focus was to promote rehydration by athletes during endurance events. In fact, the first guidelines targeted the rules of the International Amateur Athletic Federation, which had previously prevented race organizers from providing fluids during the first 10 km of distance races and either directly prevented or discouraged competitors from drinking substantial amounts of fluids during competition. During the 1970s, most studies of fluid intake during exercise were based on techniques that emphasized the inhibitory effect of solutes in fluid on gastric emptying. Therefore, recommendations for exercise fluids promoted drinks with a low solute content (water or dilute solutions of carbohydrate). The 1975 guidelines can now be seen as proactive in terms of fluid needs but conservative in view of the accumulating data from studies showing the benefits of consuming carbohydrate during prolonged exercise. Even when the guidelines were rewritten in 1985, the priority of hydration over refueling was retained despite even greater amounts of evidence supporting performance enhancement with carbohydrate intake. Again the emphasis was on combating dehydration by promoting fluid intake during distance events, and it was considered helpful to provide athletes with examples of the volumes of fluid that should be consumed during a race. In hindsight it is easy to show that rigid recommendations have little practical relevance to the range of runners who compete in a variety of events.

In addition to expanding its focus to a range of sports and exercise activities instead of distance running, the 1996 position stand on exercise and fluid replacement was updated in two important ways. First, it recognized that substantial amounts of carbohydrate and fluid can be simultaneously replaced during exercise and that refueling

provides a performance benefit across a range of exercise activities. This change in thinking was supported by newer studies of gastric emptying and hydration status showing that more concentrated carbohydrate drinks (4-8%) can be consumed during exercise without compromising fluid needs. Other studies show that benefits of carbohydrate intake are now recognized to extend beyond the traditional setting of prolonged endurance exercise to intermittent team games and even high-intensity activities lasting about 1 hr (see research topic).

The other change was to replace blanket recommendations for fluid intake during exercise. Recommendations for a certain volume and timing of fluid intake during exercise do not take into account the myriad factors that govern fluid needs and fluid intake practices across sports. Newer guidelines recognize that each athlete needs to consider issues in his or her sport such as individual sweat rates, access to fluid, opportunities to drink, and risk of gastrointestinal discomfort when organizing a plan of fluid intake. Ideally, athletes should be assisted to assess the needs and opportunities for fluid and carbohydrate intake in their sport and to devise their own plans. The need for an individualized approach to fluid intake during exercise is a key recommendation of the recent ACSM and IMMDA guidelines on hydration during exercise (ACSM 2006; Hew-Butler et al. 2006).

In terms of optimal hydration, athletes are advised to consume fluids to keep pace with sweat losses or at least 80% of the change in body mass over the session. However, in most competition and training situations, athletes are limited to drinking what is practical rather than to replace fluid losses. This appears to be 300 to 800 ml of fluid per hour in most running events, volumes that are well below sweat rates of many runners. Even where drinks are made available to runners at aid stations during an event, several practical factors govern total fluid consumption. Because drinking during races occurs literally on the run, each runner must balance her intake against the possibility of gastrointestinal discomfort or upset as well as the time lost in slowing down to approach an aid station and to consume the fluid. Most top runners appear to consider the trade-off to be greater than the benefits. This may be because they are unlikely to perceive small but significant performance benefits with better hydration, but it must also include the possibility that benefits seen in the laboratory are not always translated into performance enhancement in the field. Of course, top runners are highly influenced by tactical considerations—minimizing the time lost at aid stations or opportunities for competitors to break away. By contrast, better hydration strategies are usually possible and are recommended for recreational runners for whom safety and enjoyment are the key priorities.

The most recent piece in the evolving picture of fluid guidelines is the recognition that better hydration practices must include warnings for an upper limit on fluid intake recommendations for exercise. The vast majority of observations of fluid intake practices during running have shown a mismatch between fluid intake and sweat losses during the session, with a gradual fluid deficit and loss of body mass accruing over the session. This has caused experts to concentrate on encouraging runners to increase fluid intakes during running, at least within practical constraints, to better match their estimated sweat losses. However, the apparent increase in reported cases of hyponatremia caused by fluid overload occurring during endurance and ultraendurance sports has highlighted a different situation occurring in the case of runners at the back of the pack. It appears that at least some slower runners have overinterpreted messages to consume fluids in volumes of as much as is practical and drink fluids in amounts that are excessive, or at least in excess of their low rates of sweat loss. For these reasons, new guidelines for fluid intakes during running and other exercise must include special warnings to athletes that fluid intakes should not exceed sweat losses and that the athlete should not show an increase in body mass over the course of a race or training session.

The form of this new advice remains a topic of debate. Some scientists, notably professor Tim Noakes, argue that athletes should be encouraged to drink to the dictates of thirst with the advantages of drinking to minimize any fluid deficits being overrated (Noakes 2003b). Others, such as this author, have both a greater belief in the benefits of hydration during exercise (ACSM 2007) and a concern that thirst-based advice is vague and potentially open to the same misunderstanding as the guidelines it seeks to replace. This is particularly relevant in Western societies in which issues of overconsumption present the greatest nutrition problems and in which commonly available portion sizes of foods and drinks are so large that they override any sense of hunger, thirst, or need. On this basis, it seems reasonable to promote education messages and strategies that teach athletes to become familiar with their usual rate of sweat loss and to develop fluid intake plans that are relevant and practical. The evolution of these messages and their impact on the behavior of athletes will be studied with interest.

PRACTICAL ISSUE
The Changing Face of Carbohydrate Loading

The original carbohydrate-loading protocol was probably one of the first modern sports nutrition strategies to receive widespread publicity. It had all the ingredients of a good story—scientists using a special technique to directly study a muscle, evidence of a benefit to athletic performance—as well as good timing. The first studies hit scientific journals in the late 1960s and early 1970s and included a field investigation showing that the increase in muscle glycogen stores achieved by this technique led to enhanced performance of a 32 km running race (Karlsson and Saltin 1971). In this study, the carbohydrate-loader runners achieved a better running time, not by running faster but by being able to maintain their race pace better in the latter stages of the run.

Carbohydrate loading was first used in a competitive situation by a dominant British distance runner, Ron Hill,

at the European Championship marathon in Athens in 1969. The race was noticed because it featured a spectacular reversal of performance by Hill, who was well behind the race leader, Gaston Roelants of Belgium, at 20 miles, but ran strongly in the later stages of the race to win comfortably in a time of 2 hr 16 min 48 s. Hill was one of the athletes favored to win the marathon at the 1972 Olympic Games in Munich, but his carbohydrate-loading preparation was disrupted by the terrorist activities that caused the race to be rescheduled. Hill practiced a strict form of carbohydrate loading, with an extreme depletion phase consisting of a long hard run followed by 3 days of training on a diet that was almost carbohydrate-free. He then switched to 3 days of reduced training on a very high carbohydrate diet. His regimen had already started by the time the race was rescheduled to a day later, and in the confusion of the altered timetable he underperformed to finish sixth. Nevertheless, the dietary strategy received publicity especially during the emerging boom of distance running and population marathons during the 1970s and 1980s. It quickly became entrenched in the folklore and practice of the marathon as a means to prevent the runner from hitting the wall—that is, experiencing the overwhelming fatigue that would otherwise occur at the 20 to 22 mile or 32 to 38 km mark of the marathon as a result of depleted muscle fuel stores.

The initial carbohydrate-loading protocol was essentially developed on untrained men (the Swedish researchers themselves) and required a depletion phase of heavy exercise and low-carbohydrate diet to activate the glycogen synthase enzyme and stimulate subsequent supercompensation of muscle glycogen stores. In fact, glycogen supercompensation was limited to the muscles that had previously been depleted. The role of the depletion in achieving the subsequent increase in muscle glycogen and other possible metabolic benefits during a marathon run is still being debated within both scientific and athletic circles. A strict depletion phase carries the disadvantages of causing severe fatigue and perhaps an increased risk of injury while continuing to train in a fuel-depleted state. It also adds to the length of the preparation, which may not be practical in some of the situations in which carbohydrate loading might be useful.

> The diet makes you feel like death warmed up. You have no energy at all, you're really in heaps of trouble. . . . I could feel myself getting more tired and exhausted and run down. I was absolutely gone. . . . It's the toughest thing about a marathon. I've enjoyed marathons a lot more since I've stopped doing it.
>
> *Steve Moneghetti, winner of Berlin, Tokyo, and Commonwealth Games marathons, on his depleting experiences before carbohydrate loading (Howley and Moneghetti 1997, p. 133)*

Personally I don't carbo load (with a depletion). One of the principal reasons is that the hectic schedule of professional racing doesn't give me enough of a break to methodically carbo load. While top marathoners rarely race more than two world-class marathons a year, I'm racing approximately once every three days. The depletion phase puts too much stress on the body to be practical. I think it's the kind of stress a top cyclist can do without.

Greg LeMond, three-time winner of the Tour de France

It is interesting to note that some world-class runners still include a strict depletion phase in their carbohydrate practices, even though contemporary guidelines for sports nutrition declare it to be unnecessary for well-trained athletes. This may reflect a cautious culture in running where modern athletes believe they must duplicate the practices of earlier successful runners. Alternatively, it may be because most distance runners only race over the marathon distance once or twice each year, preventing them from having opportunities to experiment with different versions of the technique to see which is most successful. Finally, interest in fat adaptation techniques (see chapter 4, second research topic) includes the theory that the depletion phase of low-carbohydrate high-fat eating might achieve other physiological adaptations in the well-trained muscle to allow it to perform in the subsequent race with an enhanced glycogen-sparing capacity. Recent research has failed to support the benefits of such fat adaptation; instead, there is accumulating evidence that it might impair the athlete's capacity for high-intensity (carbohydrate-dependent) exercise (Burke and Kiens 2006). Therefore, this depletion phase cannot be recommended.

Despite the general recognition of the principles and application of carbohydrate-loading techniques, it is uncertain whether all runners have sufficient practical knowledge to achieve the training and nutritional strategies involved. Many athletes do not have the opportunity or discipline to organize a suitable race taper that will allow glycogen to store optimally over the last days before the event. Recreational runners and obsessive exercisers often find the lure of one last hit out hard to resist, when they are unaware of the importance of the taper. One study investigated the eating practices of 76 runners who had declared their intention to carbohydrate load for a marathon, over the 3 days before the event (Burke and Read 1987a). Although the runners reported a good knowledge of the scientific principles of carbohydrate loading, the food intakes of many runners during the loading days revealed carbohydrate intakes that were well below the daily targets of 7 to 12 g/kg that are considered necessary for optimal glycogen synthesis. Specific food choices and eating patterns revealed the following problems:

- Some runners interpreted carbohydrate loading as eating large meals based on junk food choices. Their choice of takeaway and fast foods, confectionery, and dessert items often led to high intakes of fat rather than carbohydrate.

- Some runners continued to consume large amounts of foods that were protein-rich (e.g., meats) and fiber-rich but low in carbohydrate (e.g., salads and most vegetables), possibly displacing carbohydrate-rich foods from meals and snacks. Because there are gastrointestinal limits to the total amount of food that can be eaten each day, it appears that some runners did not realize that they must reduce their

Carbohydrate Loading Considerations

Situations Suitable for Carbohydrate Loading

- Event involves exercise of greater than 90 min continuous or additive duration.
- In previous events, athlete has experienced feeling of overwhelming fatigue and "no fuel."
- Sport allows athlete to devote 2 to 3 days to tapered exercise and high carbohydrate intake prior to event.
- There are no contraindications to high carbohydrate intake.
- The athlete's usual diet provides a carbohydrate intake of less than 7 to 10 g/kg, so that specific dietary changes are needed to ensure that glycogen storage is optimized before the event.

Situations Unsuitable for Carbohydrate Loading

- Event involves exercise of less than 60 to 90 min continuous or additive duration.
- Training or competition calendar does not provide opportunity for 2 to 3 days of tapered exercise.
- Athlete has unstable diabetes, hyperlipidemias, or other medical conditions in which a high carbohydrate intake is contraindicated.
- Athlete competes in a sport that has weight divisions or is weight sensitive, and he can't afford gain in body mass (~1-2 kg) associated with storage of additional glycogen and water in muscle.

intake of carbohydrate-poor foods to allow for substantial amounts of carbohydrate-rich foods to be consumed.

- Some runners continued to consume "diet" and "no added sugar" versions of foods and drinks, failing to recognize the value of sugar as a compact carbohydrate source. It appears that these runners cannot reconcile a short-term nutritional goal (e.g., a specific increase in carbohydrate intake for muscle fuel) within their daily "healthy" eating practices or their restricted energy intakes.

Such a study should be repeated to see if the education messages focused on specific issues of sports nutrition and the increase in specialized sports foods available to contemporary runners have increased their likelihood of achieving nutritional targets for carbohydrate loading. Examples of a carbohydrate-loading menu that achieves a carbohydrate intake of ~10 g/kg for a 65 kg male runner and 50 kg female runner are provided in table 5.6, as well as a summary of the situations in which carbohydrate loading may be an appropriate competition strategy (see the highlight box on page 138).

Table 5.6   A Carbohydrate-Loading Menu Providing Carbohydrate Intakes of ~10 $g \cdot kg^{-1} \cdot day^{-1}$ for a 65 kg Male Runner and 50 kg Female Runner Before a Race (Day 4)

Day	65 kg male runner (~650 g/day carbohydrate)	50 kg female runner (~500 g/day carbohydrate)
Day 1 The menu focuses on the carbohydrate-rich foods; other foods can be added to balance the meal. An exercise taper should accompany this menu to optimize muscle glycogen storage. It is possible that glycogen supercompensation can be achieved by 2 days of such a diet, at least in well-trained runners who can arrange a suitable exercise taper.	Breakfast: 2 cups of flake cereal + cup milk + banana 250 ml of sweetened fruit juice Snack: 500 ml bottle soft drink 2 slices of thick toast + jam Lunch: 2 large bread rolls with fillings 200 g of flavored yogurt Snack: Coffee scroll or muffin 250 ml of sweetened fruit juice Dinner: 3 cups of cooked pasta + 3/4 cup sauce 2 cups of gelatin dessert Snack: 2 crumpets and honey 250 ml of sweetened fruit juice	Breakfast: 2 cups of flake cereal + cup milk + banana 250 ml of sweetened juice Snack: 500 ml bottle soft drink Lunch: 1 large bread roll with fillings 200 g of flavored yogurt Snack: 2 slices of toast + jam 250 ml of sweetened fruit juice Dinner: 2 cups of cooked pasta + 1/2 cup sauce 2 cups of gelatin dessert Snack: 250 ml of sweetened fruit juice 2 crumpets and honey
Day 2	Breakfast: 2 cups of flake cereal + cup milk + cup of sweetened canned fruit 250 ml of sweetened fruit juice Snack: 500 ml fruit smoothie Lunch: 3 stack pancake + syrup + 2 scoops ice cream 500 ml soft drink Snack: 100 g of dried fruit 250 ml of sweetened fruit juice Dinner: 3 cups of rice dish (e.g., fried rice, risotto) Snack: 2 cups of fruit salad + 2 scoops of ice cream	Breakfast: 2 cups of flake cereal + cup milk + cup sweetened canned fruit 250 ml of sweetened fruit juice Snack: 500 ml fruit smoothie Lunch: 2 stack pancake + syrup + 2 scoops ice cream 500 ml soft drink Snack 50 g of dried fruit 250 ml of sweetened fruit juice Dinner: 2 cups of rice dish (e.g., fried rice, risotto) Snack: 1 cup of fruit salad + scoop ice cream
Day 3 Many runners like to increase the focus on low-fiber and low-residue eating on the day before a race, allowing them to reach the start line feeling "light" rather than with gastrointestinal fullness.	Breakfast: 2 cups of cereal (low fiber) + cup milk + banana 250 ml of sweetened fruit juice Lunch: 4 white crumpets + jam Dinner: 2 cups of white pasta + small amount of sauce Over day 1 L of liquid meal drink or 1 L of sport drink + 3 sport gels 200 g of jelly confectionery	Breakfast: 2 cups of cereal (low fiber) + cup milk + banana 250 ml of sweetened fruit juice Lunch: 2 white crumpets + jam Dinner: 1.5 cups of white pasta + small amount of sauce Over day 1 L of liquid meal drink or 1 L of sport drink + 3 sport gels 200 g of jelly confectionery

Athletes of differing sizes should scale this intake up or down according to their body mass.

chapter 6

Swimming and Rowing

Swimming and rowing both involve prolonged training sessions that are typical of an endurance sport. Yet competition is conducted over significantly briefer duration compared with other endurance sports: The majority of swimming events last less than 2 min for elite competitors, and the longest pool race take 14 to 18 min for the top finishers. Similarly, elite crews and scullers typically take 5 to 8 min to complete their events over a 2,000 m course. The very large volumes of training in the programs of rowers and swimmers continue to provoke discussion and disagreement among coaches and scientists. A shared characteristic of these sports, often put forward in support of the high training volumes, is the importance of technique in performance. Both sports require large power outputs to be produced in a highly coordinated and specific pattern. Considerable practice is necessary for athletes to acquire the feel or fine technique for these sports. The consequence is that the nutritional concerns of rowers and swimmers involve an amalgam of challenges. During the training phase, these athletes share the priorities of endurance athletes, whereas in the competition setting, the issues are more related to brief duration events.

Competition

Competition in swimming and rowing involves a range of different events in which athletes practice different techniques of movement—for example, sweep or sculling events in rowing or the four different strokes of swimming. Rowing and swimming also commonly involve a program where a series of heats, semifinals or repechages, and finals are used to determine the overall winner of an event.

Swimming

At the international level, competitive swimming is organized under the rules of La Federation Internationale de Natation (FINA), which is also responsible for diving, synchronized swimming, and water polo. Swimming includes events in four separate strokes (freestyle, butterfly, backstroke, and breaststroke) as well as the individual medley (same swimmer undertakes all strokes) and relays. Within swimming circles, races are typically divided into sprint (50-100 m), middle-distance (200-400 m), and distance events (800-1,500 m), although this distinction differs from the physiologically based definitions applied to other sports. For example, the shortest sprint in swimming has a duration of >20 s, whereas the world records for distance events are 7 to 8 min and 14 to 16 min for 800 and 1,500 m, respectively (see table 6.1). Therefore, competitive swimming is characterized by high rates of energy turnover, with relative priority on high-energy phosphates and anaerobic glycolysis for sprint events and aerobic glycolysis for the distance events. High levels of blood lactate (12-20 mmol/L in elite males; lower levels in females) are often observed at the end of races, particularly 100 to 400 m events, with likely limitations to performance resulting from disturbances of intracellular pH.

FINA events are swum in both long-course (50 m pool) and short-course (25 m pool) formats, with long-course swimming being better recognized and included on the Olympic program. The long-course program for key international meets currently stands as an 8-day meet with both morning and evening sessions and a total of 26 and 32 events for Olympics and World Championships, respectively (see table 6.1). Typically, 400 m events and relays involve heats (morning) and finals (evening) on the same day, whereas events of 50 to 200 m are conducted as heats and semifinals (same day) and finals (following evening). The distance events of 800 and 1,500 m freestyle involve a morning heat and finals on the evening of the following day. As a result of the elongated competition program and the trend to specialize in a few events, it is becoming less common for an elite swimmer to compete in more than two events at any single session. Nevertheless, the race programs of exceptional swimmers such as

Table 6.1   Events on the International Program for Swimming and Rowing

Sport	Events	Times for world class competitors (min:s)
Swimming 26 events on Olympic program, 32 events at World Championships	50 m • Freestyle, backstroke,[a] breaststroke,[a] butterfly[a]	0:21-0:32
	100 m • Freestyle, backstroke, breaststroke, butterfly	0:47-0:68
	200 m • Freestyle, backstroke, breaststroke, butterfly, individual medley	1:44-2:26
	400 m • Freestyle, individual medley	3:40-4:48
	800 m • Freestyle[b]	7:39-8:40
	1,500 m • Freestyle[c]	14:34-17:30
	Relays • 4 × 100 m freestyle, 4 × 100 m medley, 4 × 200 m freestyle	3:15-8:00
Rowing 14 classes on Olympic program, 24 classes at World Championships	Sculling (2 oars per rower) • Single	6:36-7:10
	• Double (2 rowers)	6:04-6:40
	• Quad (4 rowers)	5:37-6:15
	• Lightweight single[a]	6:47-7:20
	• Lightweight double	6:10-6:5
	• Lightweight quad[a]	5:45-6:35
	Sweep (1 oar per rower) • Pair (2 rowers)	6:14-6:55
	• Four (4 rowers)[c]	5:41-6:30
	• Coxed eights (8 rowers plus coxswain)	5:41-6:00
	• Coxed pair[d]	6:42
	• Coxed four[d]	5:58
	• Lightweight pair[a]	6:29-7:20
	• Lightweight four[c,d]	5:45
	• Lightweight coxed eights[a,d]	5:20

[a]Not on Olympic program; [b]Olympic program only includes this event for women; [c]Olympic program only includes this event for men; [d]World Championship program only includes this event for men

Michael Phelps and Ian Thorpe may require competition on 6 to 7 days of the 8-day program, with two or three races on some evening sessions (semifinal of one event, final of another event, and a relay leg). FINA-sanctioned events also include World Cups and Grand Prix series where a short program may be swum over 1 to 3 days and may involve timed finals as well as the heats and finals format. At the elite level, swimmers typically organize their competition program to peak for one or two international meets per year (plus the qualification trials that most countries hold to select their national teams). However, in recent years, it has become more common for swimmers to seek opportunities to race more frequently throughout the training season, at international World Cup and Grand Prix series as well as collegiate, state, and nationally organized events.

In the United States, swimming is an important sport within the National Collegiate Athletic Association (NCAA) program. Events are typically swum in yards rather than meters, except for competition in an Olympic year, and involve short-course (25 yd) and long-course (50 yd) formats. A common race format in NCAA swimming is the series of dual, triangular, or quadrangular meets, where swimming teams from a number of schools compete for points over a truncated race program lasting 1 to 2 days. Around the world, swimming competition is organized through schools and clubs, with divisions for age-group and open swimming. In shorter swim meets and carnivals, talented swimmers may undertake a number of races in close succession, although the rules of some competitions, including the NCAA, limit the number of events that each competitor may enter on the same program.

It can take years to develop the technical skills of swimming, and swimmers traditionally start training at a young age. However, an unusual feature of elite level swimming is the reasonably regular emergence of outstanding athletes who achieve world-class performances at ages as young as 14 years. Until recently, elite swimming careers finished as athletes reached their early 20s. However, improved

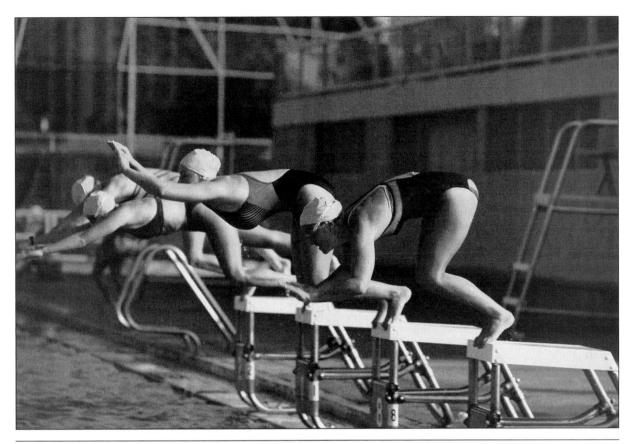

A thriving masters swimming program offers competitive opportunities for older swimmers.

funding and rewards for swimming performance have encouraged modern swimmers to extend their careers for another decade. In fact, the list of World Champions from the 2003 Barcelona meet included Jenny Thompson, Inge de Bruijn, and Alexandre Popov, swimmers from three different countries aged in their 30s. Popov achieved the outstanding result of winning the high-profile 50 m and 100 m freestyle events—a repetition of the feat he achieved 11 years earlier at the 1992 Barcelona Olympic Games.

Rowing

Federation Internationale des Societies d'Aviron (FISA), the international governing body of rowing, is the oldest international sport federation in the Olympic movement. The standard international rowing event is conducted over a 2,000 m course, with classes being divided according to gender, the number of rowers in the boat (1, 2, 4, or 8), the absence or presence of a coxswain to steer the boat and direct the rhythm of the oar-strokes, and the method of use of oars. In sweep competition, also known as crew, each rower has a single large oar while a sculling boat is powered by rowers who use two shorter oars simultaneously on each side of the boat. At the international level of rowing there is a separate weight category division for lightweight rowers (see chapter 12).

The major international competitions for rowing are the Olympic Games and the annual World Championships. However, there are many other international- and national-level regattas and World Cup events conducted around the world, providing high-level competition over the summer rowing season. Although rowing has been included on the Olympic program since the beginning of the modern era in 1896, women's rowing was only introduced in 1976, followed by lightweight rowing in 1996. Boat classes represented on the Olympic (14 classes) and World Championship (24 classes) programs are summarized in table 6.1. Separate national and international competitions exist for different age groups including the senior B competition (under 23 years), youth and juniors (under 18 years), and masters rowing (>27 years and following retirement from open rowing). At other levels of rowing competition there are some variations on the 2,000 m race distance, with examples including the legendary boat race between Cambridge and Oxford universities, which has been conducted annually on the Thames River since 1829, over a 6 km course. Rowing continues to be an important sporting program at many colleges and universities around the world. In the United States, the annual race between crews from Yale and Harvard Universities dates back more than 150 years.

High-level competitions in rowing are generally held as multiday regattas, with the duration ranging from 3-day World Cup events to the week-long program of the Olympics and World Championships. Events are completed as a series of heats or preliminaries, repechages for additional qualification, semifinals, and finals. At high-level competition, a crew may need to race three to four times over 4 to 7 days before final outcomes are decided. It is rare for international-level rowers to compete in more than one boat; however, at lower-level competition, some rowers may compete in a number of races on the program, sometimes even on the same day.

The 2,000 m rowing event, typically completed by elite rowers in 5.5 to 8 min, is characterized by an unusual but apparently effective pacing strategy. During the first minute of the race, rowers achieve their highest power outputs and stroke ratings, slowing in the middle of the race apart from brief strategic moves to maintain competitiveness, and finishing the last minute with an increase in power and ratings (Hagerman 1994). This seemingly uneconomical pacing strategy appears to be chosen in part to overcome the initial inertia of the stationary boat and in part to keep in contact with the leading crews in the race. This pattern requires an average power output equivalent to $\dot{V}O_2$max to be sustained for most of the race, despite a substantial anaerobiosis. Overall, the aerobic–anaerobic contributions to fuel utilization during the race are about 70-80%:20-30%. High blood concentrations of lactate are observed at the end of the race and include values of 15 to 22 mmol/L for males and 10 to 20 mmol/L for females (Hagerman 1994).

Training

The training programs undertaken by elite swimmers are typically based on the practices and experiences of successful coaches rather than scientific evidence of superior performance outcomes. A high-volume program is common, with swimmers undertaking 9 to 12 pool sessions a week, typically completing one or two workouts of 1.5 to 3 hr each day, and amassing a total weekly volume of 30 to 70 km. The pool workout consists of aerobic warm-up and cool-downs, drills to improve technique and practice race strategies (e.g., starts and turns), and interval sets with repeated bouts of swimming over varying intensities, duration, and recovery periods. Although the ratios vary between swimmers according to their event specialty, and over the phases of the training season, the overall outcome is ~40% of training at intensities less than 80% $\dot{V}O_2$max, 40% to 60% at intensities of ~80% $\dot{V}O_2$max, and less than 5% at >100% $\dot{V}O_2$max or event-specific race pace (Troup et al. 1994). The training year is divided into phases with weekly microcycles within the longer macrocycles of training, a gradual shift in emphasis from conditioning, and race intensity preparation and a defined taper before competition.

Dryland sessions built into the training program include stretching and flexibility work as well as specific resistance training (typically two or three sessions per week), which has been demonstrated to increase muscle protein synthesis (Tipton et al. 1996). Other forms of cross-training such as running and cycling are undertaken by some swimmers, particularly during the early conditioning phase of the season or as a means to achieve weight control or loss of body fat. In total, the elite swimmer may spend 20 to 30 hr/week in training, with the commitment to daily training commencing in age-group swimmers as young as 10 years. One argument for the high volumes of training undertaken by swimmers is the need to develop an efficient technique or feel for the water. However, other coaches have experimented with different approaches to the preparation of successful swimmers, including lower training volumes, more race-pace or event-specific swimming, and a greater focus on resistance training.

The contemporary training practices of high-level rowers also favor high-volume programs, featuring on-water sessions, the use of rowing ergometers, specific resistance training programs, and cross-training such as running and cycling. The elite rower typically undertakes two, and sometimes three, training sessions per day to develop each of the separate characteristics of skill, aerobic and anaerobic endurance, and muscular power. Sessions are usually described in terms of the desired work intensity of the main pieces and their stress on various energy systems. Training is periodized within microcycles and macrocycles built into the program. The early part of preparation is spent on aerobic conditioning and specific power-based resistance training. Where weather or availability of water space limits on-water training, there is a greater emphasis on dryland and ergometer training. As the competitive season approaches, there is an increase in the intensity of aerobic training and in the ratio of anaerobic exercise. Throughout the summer competitive season, rowers undertake a mixture of aerobic and anaerobic training according to the need to peak for competition. As is the case for swimmers, most world-class rowers have a limited off-season, usually lasting 3 to 4 weeks. Altitude training is a common feature in the programs of many elite rowers and swimmers.

Physique and Physiology

Success in swimming and rowing relies on the production of large power outputs with highly coordinated and efficient technique. Swimmers and rowers have a high absolute aerobic capacity, although when expressed per kilogram of a muscular body mass, this is lower than other endurance athletes. Typically, rowers and swimmers are taller, stronger, and heavier than their sedentary counterparts or other endurance-trained athletes, with some studies showing an increase in the mean height and lean body mass of elite competitors over the past decades and a difference between competition winners and nonfinalists (Hagerman 1994; Troup et al. 1994).

The biomechanical requirements of rowing favor athletes with long levers (long limb lengths) and a large muscle mass that is capable of producing high power outputs over a sustained period. Of course, physique factors need to be combined with good on-water technique and, in the case of crews, strong team cohesiveness. An official study of the anthropometry of rowers from 30 countries at the Sydney 2000 Olympic Games reported mean heights and body mass of 76.6 kg and 181 cm for females and 94.3 kg and 194 cm for males (Kerr et al. 2007).

Swimmers, particularly sprinters, are characterized by a lengthy frame and long arms and a high level of muscularity in legs and upper body. An official study of the anthropometry of swimmers at the 1991 World Championships in Perth, Australia, reported mean heights and body mass of 171.5 cm and 63.1 kg for females and 183.8 cm and 78.4 kg for males (Carter and Ackland 1994). There appear to be some differences in the physical characteristics of swimmers in different events, with distance swimmers and breaststroke swimmers tending to be smaller (shorter and with lower body mass) than sprinters and backstroke specialists.

Swimming and rowing are weight-supported events. Although the athletes move their own body mass, they are supported by the buoyancy of water or by the boat, reducing the penalty or energy cost involved in this movement. As a result, although rowers and swimmers are leaner than their sedentary counterparts, they are heavier and have typically carried higher body fat levels than other endurance-trained athletes. The training programs of rowers and swimmers are associated with an increase in lean body mass and a loss of body fat over the season (Petersen et al. 2006; Pyne et al. 2006). Over recent times, however, the typical body fat levels of elite swimmers and rowers have gradually decreased, with the achievement of low levels of body fat becoming a major issue in swimming. This has occurred without empirical evidence to show that body fat level is an important determinant of swimming performance. In fact, one study that investigated the correlation between swimming performance and the physical characteristics of a large group of female swimmers reported that body fatness (measured by densitometry) was a relatively unimportant predictor of competition performance (Stager et al. 1984). Rather, lean body mass was a better predictor of swimming ability. It is sometimes argued that a certain level of body fat is useful for the swimmer, enhancing buoyancy and body position in the water, or providing rounded body surfaces that have more favorable drag characteristics than angular protrusions.

Although it would be valuable to undertake more cross-sectional studies of performance and physique in swimming, the limitations of such data must be acknowledged. Such studies can only look for relationships between variables and outcomes and say nothing about individuals within a group or whether correlations are cause and effect or accidental. For example, in the case of observations of the extreme leanness of certain elite swimmers, it is hard to distinguish between the effects of body fat levels on performance per se and the influence of the high-volume training or dietary commitment that was needed to achieve such a physique. It is likely that each swimmer has a range of desirable physical characteristics within which he or she trains and performs well. It would take a sophisticated longitudinal study in which body fat levels were manipulated over a broad range to assess exactly how wide these tolerance levels on ideal body fat ranges are. The present cultural environment of swimming places enormous pressure on female swimmers to be lean. Although scientists argue against setting a single strict standard for body fat across a group, many coaches do not heed this advice. The existence of eating disorders, poor body image, and generally restricted eating among female swimmers is noted and will be discussed in a later section of this chapter.

Lifestyle and Culture

The high training volumes undertaken by rowers and swimmers lead to considerable lifestyle challenges. This commitment may begin when the athlete is young, and it must be juggled within the school and family timetables. Early-morning training schedules are a ritual of each sport—necessitated by school or work schedules, the availability of pool or water space, and the desire to provide recovery time between the two main workouts in a day. Meals are often eaten on the run, and the family meal schedule often needs to be planned around the training and transport needs of school-age athletes. Many athletes find it difficult to assume responsibility for their food intake as they move from home to an independent living situation or even the collegiate or institute dining hall. The developing swimmer or rower often finds conflict between achieving the nutritional goals of his or her sport while facing the special nutritional, social, and emotional issues of adolescence and early adulthood.

Dietary Surveys

The available literature on dietary practices of serious swimmers includes studies of the habitual training diets of swimmers of collegiate, national, and international level from a variety of countries (see tables 6.a and 6.b in the appendix to this chapter). Because few investigations have been undertaken over the past decade, it is uncertain whether these surveys fully capture contemporary dietary practices. For example, author Barry Sears has claimed in his books *Enter the Zone* and *Mastering the Zone* that gold medalists from 1992 and 1996 American Olympic swimming teams were devotees of his Zone diet (Sears 1995, 1997). Because these diets are a potential departure from the usual or recommended intakes of energy and macronutrients, it is of interest to confirm these claims. There are

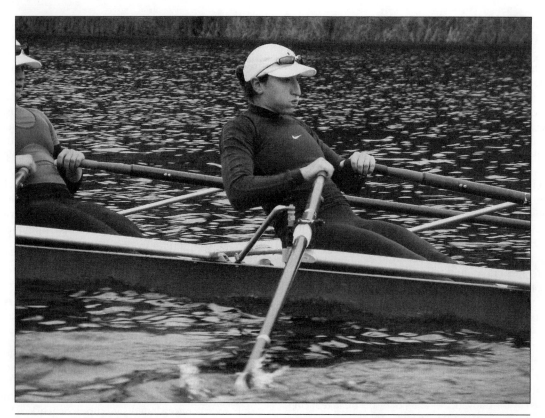

Older swimmers and rowers often combine their sport with collegiate scholarships or university studies, continuing the demanding lifestyle.

relatively few studies of the reported dietary practices of serious rowers, with available studies being summarized in table 6.c.

Swimmers

Given the typical training programs undertaken by swimmers and their high levels of lean body mass, we would expect reported energy intakes to be high both in absolute terms and relative to body mass. This appears to be the case for male swimmers, with most studies reporting daily energy intakes of 15 to 20 MJ (4,000-5,000 kcal) or >200 kJ/kg body mass (>48 kcal/kg). Other studies that have monitored energy balance have found that male swimmers typically report intakes that are commensurate with the estimated energy expenditure for that phase of their training (Van Handel et al. 1984) and can adjust energy intakes to cope with an increase in training volume. For example, interventions to substantially increase training volumes in two studies of male collegiate swimmers were associated with appropriate increases in mean intakes of energy and carbohydrate (Barr and Costill 1992; Costill, Flynn, et al. 1988). Typically, carbohydrate intakes reported by male swimmers appear to be ~6 to 8 g · kg^{-1} · day^{-1} and protein intakes in the range of 1.5 to 2.0 g · kg^{-1} · day^{-1}.

Some studies of energy balance in female swimmers report intakes that are close to estimates of energy requirements. For example, female swimmers undertaking 14 to

18 hr a week of training were reported to consume a daily energy intake of 2,470 kcal in comparison to an estimated energy expenditure of 2,675 kcal/day (Vallieres et al. 1989). However, appropriate energy intake does not appear to be a universal finding of all investigations, with Van Handel and coworkers (1984) reporting that female swimmers differed from their male teammates by reporting energy intakes that were substantially lower than anticipated. In a study of female national-level swimmers undertaking a daily training load of 17.5 km, measured energy expenditure measured via doubly labeled water techniques was 23.4 MJ/day, whereas estimated energy intake was 13.1 MJ, accounting for ~57% of total energy expenditure (Trappe et al. 1997). In general, the typical daily energy intakes reported by female swimmers are ~8 to 11 MJ (2,000-2,600 kcal) or ~140 to 170 kJ/kg (33-40 kcal/kg). The apparently lower energy intakes of female swimmers in comparison with their male counterparts may reflect underreporting, restricted energy intake to achieve fat loss goals, or lower training expenditures. Typical daily intakes of carbohydrate (4.5-6 g/kg body mass) and protein (1.3-1.8 g/day) are proportionally lower than those reported by male swimmers, although if related to lean body mass these differences are reduced.

Studies of micronutrient consumption reported by swimmers have found that intakes of vitamins and minerals meet country-specific dietary recommendations, for both males (Barr 1989; Berning et al. 1991; Van Handel et al. 1984) and females (Barr 1989, 1991; Berning et al. 1991; Vallieres et al. 1989; Van Handel et al. 1984). However, several studies of groups of female swimmers have reported intakes of iron (Vallieres et al. 1989; Van Handel et al. 1984) or calcium (Barr 1991) that were less than the recommended levels. In these cases, low intakes of minerals were explained by the apparently low energy intake by these female swimmers, because the nutrient densities of food choices were similar between males and females.

Rowers

There is a paucity of research on the nutritional practices of rowers, particularly contemporary studies of high-level athletes. As for swimmers, we would expect to see high intakes of energy and carbohydrate, both in absolute terms and relative to body mass. Such energy intakes would normally allow protein and micronutrients to be consumed at levels that easily meet guidelines for athletes. The lack of data to confirm these expectations prevents further discussion of the dietary practices of these rowers. Future research is eagerly welcomed.

Nutritional Issues and Challenges

The intensive training programs undertaken by rowers and swimmers require attention to nutrition strategies that fuel and promote recovery from each session, achieve optimal levels of lean body mass and body fat, and meet all micronutrient needs. Major alterations in energy expenditure that occur between various phases of the competitive calendar (high volume training, taper, and the off-season) require an adjustment of food intake. Special strategies of food and fluid intake before, during, and after exercise are particularly appropriate for workouts, although competition eating strategies must also ensure that the athlete is well fueled and hydrated for each race. Recovery between races will be important for most competition situations. Several of these issues, summarized in the highlight box on this page, are discussed in greater detail in this section of the book. Other issues, such as travel nutrition, are left to later chapters.

Common Nutritional Issues Arising in Swimming and Rowing

Physique Issues

- Desire to increase muscle mass and strength through specific resistance training program
- Desire to achieve and maintain generally low body fat levels to optimize power-to-mass relationship
- Swimmers: changes in physique during adolescence
- Female swimmers: difficulty achieving and maintaining acceptably low body mass and body fat levels, especially postadolescence; risk of dietary extremism and disordered eating resulting from frustration with weight control

Training Issues

- High energy and carbohydrate requirements to meet a heavy training load and growth needs during adolescence or active gain of muscle mass
- Practical difficulties in consuming sufficient energy and carbohydrate intake in a busy day
- Aggressive recovery needed between training sessions (refueling, rehydration, repair, and adaptation)
- Adequate protein intake to meet increased requirements resulting from heavy training and to promote gain in muscle mass and strength in response to resistance training
- Adequate fuel and fluid intake during training sessions
- Consideration of creatine loading to enhance response to resistance and interval training

Competition

- Swimming: adjusting energy intake during taper to prevent excessive gain of weight and body fat
- Preparation of adequate fuel stores for race day: fueling for multiday regattas and competition meets
- Postrace recovery between events, or between heats, semifinals, and finals
- Consideration of bicarbonate or citrate loading before events lasting 2 to 8 min
- Consideration of caffeine use to enhance race performance
- Travel: traveling to major competitions and on race circuit

Training and Growth

Energy expenditure is increased by high levels of lean body mass, growth (including the response to a resistance training program), and a high-volume training program. In some swimmers and rowers, these three factors coexist to create very large energy demands—for example, the male swimmer or rower who faces an increase in training commitment during periods of adolescent growth spurts. Some (Barr and Costill 1992; Costill, Flynn, et al. 1988) but not all (Costill, Flynn, et al. 1988) athletes with high energy requirements are able to find strategies to meet such demands and, in the case of high training volumes, an adequate carbohydrate supply to fuel the workouts. This achievement is important to allow growth and to maximize the adaptations to training, including the success of specific weight training programs. However, other rowers and swimmers struggle to meet their requirements. Eating opportunities can be limited by a busy timetable, poor access to food over the day, or the gastrointestinal discomfort associated with eating meals that are too large or too close to training sessions. The challenges and solutions for addressing high energy demands are discussed in more detail in the first practical issue in this chapter. Specific issues related to meeting fuel requirements, either day to day or in response to acute needs of a workout, are discussed in subsequent sections.

In addition to coping with large energy needs, many swimmers and rowers have to adjust to rapidly changing energy needs. This can occur because of fluctuations in growth patterns or changes in training volume. The energy requirements of competition are considerably less than those of the training programs typically undertaken by most rowers and swimmers, and in the case of swimmers, the final phase of competition preparation is marked by a substantial taper in training volume. Many swimmers, particularly females, find it difficult to adjust their food intake to suit the lower energy needs of the taper or off-season. A longitudinal study (Almeras et al. 1997) tracked energy balance in a group of six elite female swimmers over a 13-month period, which included training, taper, and the off-season. During the season, the swimmers reported a mean intake of ~10.5 MJ (2,500 kcal) per day, ranging from 9.2 to 11.1 MJ over the period during which their weekly mileage was 18.8 hr/week (range = 10-35 hr). However, energy intake was significantly lower than the daily energy expenditure of 12 to 13 MJ (2,860-3,100 kcal), estimated from activity records and a method using relationships between heart rate and $\dot{V}O_2$. A 2-month period of detraining at the end of the season was associated with a mean increase in body mass of 4.8 kg, which included a gain of 4.3 kg of fat mass. The estimated energy cost of this fat gain was 170 MJ or ~2.8 MJ/day (670 kcal/day), similar to the energy cost of training normally undertaken by the swimmers. This suggests that they were unable to voluntarily adjust energy intake.

Many swimmers and rowers gain body fat during the off-season, suggesting a substantial reduction in activity levels in the absence of an organized training program.

Further study needs to be undertaken to determine whether the mismatch in energy intake results from to the failure of appetite to adjust to lower energy needs, difficulty in changing habitual eating practices, or a liberalization of the athlete's dietary choices during postseason celebrations and activities. This information could be of practical use to many elite swimmers and rowers who want to limit the extent to which they become deconditioned during breaks between competitive seasons.

Adolescents

The training programs undertaken by high-school-age swimmers and, to a lesser extent, rowers are typically greater than those undertaken by high-school-age athletes in most other sports. In fact, many swimmers reach world-class performance level while in their teenage years. The commitment to high-level and high-volume training exposes the young athlete to special nutritional requirements. These training-related requirements are superimposed on the nutritional requirements of adolescence as well as the social and cultural issues related to food that develop in this age group. The convergence of these issues can provide a challenge for the athlete, parent, and coach.

The onset of puberty is associated with major and rapidly occurring changes in size, shape, and body composition for both male and female athletes. Growth spurts increase energy requirements, and a high-energy diet is required to fuel both the daily training program and deposition of new tissue. For male athletes, adolescence is associated with a substantial increase in muscle mass under the influence of testosterone, with a decline in body fat levels occurring according to the balance between energy intake and requirements. Females experience a converse change—substantial deposition of body fat and a smaller increase in muscle mass. The increase in body fat is influenced both by female sex hormones and by the reversal of higher energy requirements as height velocity begins to decrease. Of course, the new dietary patterns associated with adolescence can exacerbate the trends seen in both sexes. For males, the programmed changes in physique accompanying adolescence are generally favorable for the performance of sports such as rowing and swimming. However, for females, the increase in body fat and change in body shape can interfere with optimal performance and create concern for the athlete. This can be exacerbated by other issues being experienced by the adolescent female—renegotiation of relationships with authority figures such as parents and coaches and problems associated with poor body image and self-esteem.

The eating patterns of adolescents reflect a number of new influences, including the growing independence from family, an increase in peer influence, and assumption of responsibility for food intake within a number of new commitments and duties. Distinctive eating habits associated with adolescence include skipped meals, unusual food choices at meals, increased snacking, and increased reliance on takeaway and convenience foods. Gender differences in food intake become apparent during adolescence, with females becoming more aware of dietary issues and the nutritional content of foods as well as undertaking dieting behaviors to reduce body mass and body fat levels.

For many adolescent male swimmers and rowers, the chief nutritional concern is to achieve adequate energy intake. High energy requirements, irregular eating patterns, a busy timetable, and poor nutritional knowledge can all challenge the athlete's ability achieve this fundamental goal (see practical issue). Although a high energy intake generally allows an athlete to meet goals for most macronutrients and micronutrients, the irregular and often chaotic eating patterns of many adolescents prevent them from consuming key nutrients at strategic times (e.g., recovery eating) or lead them to consume suboptimal intakes of micronutrients because of reliance on energy-dense but nutrient-poor convenience foods. Although protein needs are increased during adolescence, protein does not appear to be an "at-risk" nutrient, because dietary surveys of adolescent swimmers report daily intakes that are above 2.0 g/kg body mass in the case of male swimmers (Almeras et al. 1997; Barr 1989; Berning et al. 1991; Van Erp-Baart et al. 1989a) and, even in the case of females with lower relative energy intakes, above 1.5 g/kg body mass (Almeras et al. 1997; Barr 1989; Berning et al. 1991).

The micronutrients most likely to be at risk of suboptimal intakes appear to be minerals, particularly iron. Iron requirements are increased not only by growth and the onset of menstruation in females but also by a small increase in iron loss resulting from the training process. Although iron losses from exercise-related hemolysis are generally associated with contact and foot-strike sports (Eichner 1995), one study reported observed signs of a mild effort-induced hemolysis after competitive endurance swimming as shown by reduced haptoglobin concentrations (Selby and Eichner 1986). Other aspects of a swimmer's training may also have an impact on iron needs; for example, altitude training has been shown to draw on the iron reserves of male swimmers (Roberts and Smith 1992). In general, however, male swimmers report intakes of iron and other minerals that are in excess of country-specific daily recommendations (Barr 1989; Berning et al. 1991; Van Handel et al. 1984). In fact, longitudinal studies of male swimmers over a competitive season have failed to find evidence of a reduction in parameters of mineral status, including iron (Lukaski et al. 1990) and copper and zinc (Lukaski et al. 1990). The situation for female swimmers is conflicting, with some studies reporting apparent intakes of iron and other minerals in excess of daily recommendations (Barr 1989, 1991; Berning et al. 1991; Vallieres et al. 1989; Van Handel et al. 1984) and others reporting intakes below these guidelines in a significant proportion of participants (Barr 1989, 1991; Berning et al. 1991; Tilgner and Schiller 1989; Vallieres et al. 1989; Van Handel et al. 1984). Restricted energy intakes, fad diets, and poorly chosen vegetarian eating practices are implicated in suboptimal intakes of iron; many adolescent females undertake experimentation with these dietary behaviors.

Routine iron supplementation is not recommended for any athlete (see chapter 5); indeed, some studies have failed to show changes in iron status in a group of female swimmers over the course of the competitive season (Lukaski et al. 1990). In one study, although iron status of swimmers appeared to improve slightly over a 16-week training program, half of the group had serum ferritin levels below 12 ng/ml at the end of the season (Petersen et al. 2006). Nevertheless, there was no relationship between performance and iron status in this group. Other studies of female swimmers have reported that low ferritin levels were correlated with low dietary intakes of iron (Vallieres et al. 1989) or that a moderate-dose (Brigham et al. 1993) or high-dose (Walsh and McNaughton 1989) iron supplement was needed to prevent a decline in iron status over the course of the swimming season. Therefore, it seems reasonable to undertake individualized risk assessment and screening of the iron status of female swimmers and rowers, particularly those practicing dieting behaviors.

Body Weight, Body Fat, and the Female Swimmer

In diaries she kept from 1971-74, Gould reveals the pressure she felt, which led to her retirement from international swimming at the age of 16 . . . there was the constant pressure over her weight and eating habits. "One thing about my diet, yes I am 11 lb overweight" Gould's diaries of the time reveal. "I ate incorrectly (muffins, chocolate, lollies, chips) because I felt unloved." Later Gould prayed for help to lose weight: "Lord I really need you. I know that you have helped me already, but if you can just help me to take off this weight I can be much more effective in glorifying you."

From an article on Australian swimmer Shane Gould (winner of five medals at the 1972 Munich Olympic Games, one-time holder of all world records in freestyle swimming for women) (Chynoweth 2001, p. 12).

I feel good, and at my current weight, I feel I have never trained better. . . . But my coach wants me (to lose weight) . . . because that's what I weighed last year when I set the world record. . . . He reminds me of my weight a lot, and I have to train differently than I would like. . . . After our afternoon workout, which lasts about 2 hours, most people on the team work out in the weight room. This is what I feel I need. Instead, I have to run to lose the weight.

Discussion between American female swimmer (Olympic gold medalist and world-record holder) and psychiatrist Kelly Brownell (Brownell et al. 1992, p. 5)

Gain of body fat, whether during adolescence or during off-season, is a source of concern for many female swimmers and their coaches. Although some deposition of body fat is an inevitable consequence of adolescence, an excessive amount or rate of increase is generally associated with a reduction in performance. This is understandable given the sudden change in fluid dynamics and biomechanics caused by such a drastic alteration in body shape, composition, and mass. However, in the real-life settings in which these problems occur, it is hard to differentiate the purely physical and biomechanical changes from the effects of interrupted training or poor eating patterns that are inevitably part of the landscape.

Even though swimming is not generally considered a sport in which low levels of body fat are a primary determinant of performance, many swimming coaches rate weight and body fat levels of their athletes as an issue of concern or importance. In addition, there is both research and anecdotal evidence of a worrying prevalence of weight control phobias among female swimmers. These include disordered eating or pathogenic weight loss behaviors including skipping meals or fasting, use of saunas, vomiting, and use of diet pills (Benson 1991; Dummer et al. 1987; Taub and Benson 1992). In a study of Spanish female athletes, swimmers recorded higher scores on an eating disorders questionnaire than most other athletic groups, including distance runners (Toro et al. 2005). More than half the respondents in a large survey of elite female swimmers reported that their coaches regularly measured body mass at training sessions or told them to lose weight (Benson 1991). This survey also reported that most swimmers responded in negative ways to punitive measures used to restrict their body weight (e.g., removing privileges such as team travel or swimming rights, restricting the swimmers' food intake or snacks). Such behavior was labeled by the authors as indicating "insensitivity and misdirected guidance." In the survey of Spanish athletes, pressure exerted by the coach was associated with a high risk of symptoms of bulimia (Toro et al. 2005). Conversely, in another survey, swimmers were found to hold misconceptions about their real weight and body fat levels, but coaches were rated by swimmers as being a less important source of information about their weight than parents, peers, or other people (Dummer et al. 1987).

It is now recognized that a risk factor for the development of disordered eating among athletes is the necessity to wear figure-revealing or skimpy sport clothing (Otis et al. 1997). The constant display of a changing body shape is a particularly stressful activity for the adolescent female swimmer with self-esteem and body image problems. Indeed, an association between eating disorder risks and the requirement to exhibit their bodies in public was identified in the female swimmers studied by Toro and colleagues (2005). Therefore, a complex array of factors contribute to the pressure felt by many female swimmers regarding weight and body fat levels.

Although there is no single or simple way to solve all problems related to this issue, several useful strategies can be identified. First, recognize that it takes years for a young swimmer to develop her ideal body physique (Pyne et al. 2006). Sport scientists and coaches should identify a *range* of levels of body mass and fat that correspond to optimal health and performance for each swimmer, including changes in physical characteristics accompanying adoles-

cence, maturation in age and training, and even the phases of the competitive season. This can be identified by monitoring performance and changes in mass and body fat over a period of time. At times, some swimmers may need to lose body fat to fall within their ideal range, particularly after an injury or a break from training. Other swimmers may need guidance to deal with the change in their physique and nutritional requirements during puberty. However, rather than providing a stressful or punitive environment with regard to weight control, the coach should direct the swimmer to receive expert nutrition advice and then provide support for such a program. Strategies that may be useful to assist in weight reduction and loss of body fat in the athlete undertaking high-volume training are discussed in more detail in chapter 4. In the case of young swimmers, counseling regarding family eating patterns or activities to help the swimmer develop her own domestic skills and practical nutrition knowledge may be valuable. Finally, early intervention and expert psychological counseling should be sought for athletes who are experiencing troubles with body image and self-esteem.

Refueling and Rehydration Strategies During Workouts

Although competitive events in rowing and swimming involve sustained high-intensity workloads, the brief duration of a single race is unlikely to be associated with levels of fluid loss or fuel depletion that are limiting for performance. There are exceptions to this principle, for example, lightweight rowers who dehydrate and restrict their food intake in order to make weight and then compete in a hot environment (see chapter 12), and swimmers or rowers who are involved in a series of races over a short time period with inadequate time or opportunity for recovery between. By contrast, training sessions are undertaken at moderate and high intensities over prolonged periods—factors that cause high sweat losses and high rates of glycogen utilization. As a result, strategies to replace fluid and carbohydrate during exercise are appropriate to the training situation but may not be appreciated by athletes who perceive that they participate in a sprint-based sport. Other obstacles to refueling and rehydration strategies immediately before or during workouts are summarized in the highlight box on page 151.

There are relatively few investigations of the fluid and fuel needs of swimmers and rowers during training sessions, the typical voluntary intakes of fluid and carbohydrate by the athletes, or the effects of hydration and fueling practices on the short-term or long-term outcomes of the training process. Studies that have examined fluid balance during real-life rowing or swimming training sessions are summarized in table 6.d. This literature includes a fluid balance study that monitored all the on-water sessions undertaken by two groups of well-trained rowers over a week of training in different climates. The results showed mean sweat rates of ~2 L/hr for males and 1,400 ml/hr for females when workouts lasting 90 to 120 min were carried

Common Obstacles to Fluid and Food Intake Before and During Training Sessions Undertaken by Rowers and Swimmers

Intake Before Sessions

- It is often impractical to consume substantial amounts of food or drink before the early-morning training sessions (starting between 4:30 and 6 am) that are typically undertaken by swimmers and some rowers.

- For collegiate athletes or others living in boarding accommodation with fixed dining facilities, it is often difficult to get access to suitable foods before early-morning sessions, especially at outdoor venues such as lakes and rivers.

- The horizontal position undertaken in swimming, and the crouch position undertaken at the start or catch phase of the rowing stroke, can increase the risk of gastric reflux in susceptible athletes, limiting their ability to tolerate substantial amounts of fluids or food before or during a workout.

The prolonged high-intensity nature of many workouts, especially test sets or race pieces, exacerbates this problem and can also lead to nausea in some athletes. Many athletes are therefore reluctant consumers of fluids or foods before or during such workouts.

Intake During Sessions

- It is impractical to consume fluids or foods while directly engaged in swimming or rowing activities. Therefore, athletes are limited to refueling and rehydrating during breaks in the session—between interval sets in swimming or pieces in rowing. The coach must organize the session to provide appropriate breaks.

- Food or drink supplies for rowing sessions must typically be carried in the boat. There is often a practical limit to the amounts that can be carried.

- Because they are already wet, swimmers are generally unaware of their sweat losses in the pool.

They may be unaware of significant losses during sessions undertaken at sustained high intensities or in warm environments (heated indoor pool or outdoor pool in summer; pool temperature higher than usual) and without these visual cues of sweat loss fail to realize the need for fluid intake during and after the session.

out in hot conditions (Burke 1995). The same training program undertaken by a matched group of rowers under cool conditions caused an average hourly sweat loss of 1,200 and 800 ml/hr, respectively. The rowers were aware of the need to consume fluid during training, but total fluid intake was limited by the need for the rowers to carry their own supplies out on the boat and by the need to stop rowing in order to drink. A number of rowers incurred fluid deficits of at least 2% of body mass per session, even under cool conditions. Practical issues in improving fluid intake include organizing sufficient drink breaks between pieces in the session and having adequate supplies on the boat or with the coach. Of course, gastrointestinal discomfort may limit total fluid intake during rowing workouts involving high-intensity pieces.

Before the results of swimming studies are discussed, we must acknowledge that the methodologies involved in most fluid balance studies (viz. measurement of changes in body mass and the mass of drink bottles over the session, with an attempt to account for urine losses) have unique limitations when applied to aquatic sports:

- Larger discrepancies in weight measurements resulting from residual fluid on the skin, hair, and clothing that is more difficult to towel-dry in a standardized way.

- Failure to account for water absorbed through the skin.

- Failure to account for water accidentally swallowed from the pool in fluid intake calculations. Although there is no practical way to measure water accidentally swallowed from the pool, it is likely that it occurs and is greatest when water is more turbulent (e.g,. high-intensity sets) and in certain strokes (e.g., backstroke).

- Failure to account for all urine losses (e.g., undeclared urine losses that take place in the pool). There is no practical way to uncover how often such unreported urine losses might occur; however, it is worth noting that urine losses during a swimming session can be significant. For example, among swimmers who left a workout for a restroom visit in one study, the weight changes pre- and postvisits ranged from 100 to 1,200 g per swimmer per session (Cox et al. 2002).

In addition, aquatic sports offer greater opportunities for conductive and convective losses of body heat than do land-based sports, reducing the role of evaporative cooling in thermoregulation while swimming. However, data collected using different methodologies confirm the potential for substantial sweat losses while exercising in water. A study using deuterium oxide (labeled water) found that daily water turnover in young swimmers (mean training volume ~6 km/day) was nearly 2 L/day greater than in an age-matched group of sedentary controls (Leiper and Maughan 2004). The authors attributed these differences to nonrenal losses, presumably sweat losses during and after training sessions. Therefore, although there is greater potential for errors in estimating fluid losses and intakes during swimming and other aquatic sports, we can expect swimmers to incur fluid losses during workouts.

The largest data set on fluid balance during swimming was collected from members of the Australian National Swimming Team during a 3-week training camp during the taper phase before a major international swim meet (Cox et al. 2002). Data were collected from 13 separate training sessions in an indoor pool and included 295 separate observations. Workouts with a mean distance of ~4 km were designated as "aerobic," "anaerobic threshold," "maximal oxygen consumption," and "race pace or speed work" by coaches according to the nature of the main set of the session. On average, sweat losses were estimated at ~365 ml/hr and ~415 ml/hr for female and male swimmers, respectively, with sweat losses being greater during the anaerobic threshold sessions than the predominantly aerobic workouts.

This study also found substantial differences in the fluid intakes of individual swimmers, ranging from 0 to 2,140 ml/session for males and 0 to 1,140 ml/session for females. In 17% of the sessions undertaken by males, more than 1,000 ml was consumed, whereas an intake of this volume was observed in only 1% of measurements made on female swimmers. Males typically consumed sufficient fluid to replace or even exceed their estimated sweat losses in a session, a situation that is regarded as unusual in land-based sports. Only in anaerobic threshold sessions, which were associated with lower intakes of fluid as well as higher sweat rates, was there any overall mismatch in mean estimates of fluid balance. Whether voluntary drinking practices observed in this study were driven by the swimmers' belief in a need for fluid replacement or by carbohydrate replacement from a sport drink is uncertain. Regardless, practices probably represent the best-case scenario for real-life field conditions—the swimmers were highly motivated to drink during training, it was compulsory to keep a drink bottle on pool deck during the session, and a supply of cool sport drinks was provided. Other swimmers may not be as well motivated or provided with opportunities to refuel and rehydrate during the session; these swimmers and the reluctant drinkers in the present group might benefit from better fluid practices during training. Indeed, other investigations summarized in table 6.d report a range in estimations of sweat loss during swimming sessions from ~450 to 1,600 ml/hr but lower fluid intakes. Fluid intakes of swimmers in one study were considered inadequate because the overall loss of 2.5% body mass over the 3 hr session was associated with an increase in rectal temperature (Soler et al. 2003).

There are few data on the effects of fluid intake on rowing or swimming performance, either in training or during competition. Dehydration and rowing performance have been examined in the case of lightweight rowing practices to make weight (see chapter 12), but these results need to be interpreted in light of the food restriction practices that typically accompany dehydration techniques. One investigation (Maresh et al. 2001) provides some insight into the effect of fluid intake on swimming by examining the effect of moderate hyperhydration, achieved by 2 days of increased fluid intake (2 L/day), on performance of a 200 yd time trial by collegiate swimmers. This intervention, which increased body mass by a mean of 0.5 kg, was undertaken to counteract the large reductions in plasma volume that occur during swimming as a result of the fluid shift from the vasculature to interstitial and intracellular compartments. Although there was no reduction in plasma volume reduction or any significant differences in time trial performance between the two treatments, a correlation between changes in performance and changes in body mass achieved by the hyperhydration was noted, suggesting the importance of adequate hydration in swim performance.

Interval training in swimming is characterized by high rates of carbohydrate oxidation and substantial depletion of glycogen content in the deltoid muscles of well-trained swimmers (Costill, Hinrichs, et al. 1988). Similar demands on carbohydrate reserves are expected during rowing training, attributable to the interaction of the moderate- and high-intensity workloads and the prolonged duration of workouts. Therefore, strategies that increase carbohydrate availability during workouts, preventing or delaying the depletion of body carbohydrate stores, might be expected to enhance training performance. These effects might be seen in terms of better maintenance of muscle workloads as well reduced central or neuromuscular fatigue—an interaction that is important in sports involving coordinated technique and fine motor control.

One study has compared the acute effect of small changes in dietary carbohydrate intake on metabolism and performance during typical swimming test sets undertaken by well-trained swimmers (Reilly and Woodbridge 1999). The workouts included 200 yd swims at submaximal and maximal swimming velocities, as well as time trials over 100, 200, and 400 yd. The dietary conditions imposed over the 3 days before each trial involved a normal mixed diet and a 10% increase or reduction of carbohydrate intake. Reduction in carbohydrate intake was associated with impaired 400 yd swimming performance, whereas the elevation of carbohydrate improved performance of 100 and 400 yd time trials. The modest dietary manipulations shifted the relationship between swimming velocity and blood lactate response; this observation is important because this relationship is traditionally monitored over a training cycle as a sign of the training response (a lower lactate level for a given swimming speed is considered to indicate a positive training effect). These results do not undermine the general relationship between fast swimming performances in competition and high levels of lactate production, but they show the limitations of using lactate monitoring without dietary control as an indicator of training performance and prescription.

The effect of carbohydrate intake immediately before a swimming workout was investigated in a study of triathletes undertaking a 4,000 m time trial (Smith et al. 2002). The swim, undertaken after 48 hr of standard diet and training and an overnight fast, was preceded by a placebo drink or a carbohydrate drink providing 0.5 g/kg carbohydrate either 35 min or 5 min beforehand. There was a trend to a faster swim time with the glucose feeding (2.5% improvement, range = 24 s to 5 min); however, this difference failed to reach statistical significance. Although this study does not mimic the conditions of the typical interval-based sessions undertaken by swimmers, it supports a potential benefit from carbohydrate intake associated with early morning workouts and allays general fears of detrimental outcomes related to carbohydrate intake during the half hour before exercise. Another study of carbohydrate intake (1 g/kg body mass) during an interval training session (~6 km or 2 hr) by collegiate swimmers also failed to find an overall improvement in training performance of the group, as monitored by mean times during a 10 × 100 yd test set at the end of the session (O'Sullivan et al. 1994). However, compared with the placebo trial, carbohydrate ingestion prevented a decline in blood glucose concentrations in two participants and was associated with better performances in these swimmers.

Apart from direct enhancement of training performance, other advantages may accrue when nutritional support is provided during a workout. Prolonged and high-intensity exercise is associated with perturbations to the immune system (Gleeson et al. 2001). Disturbed immune function may occur through two principal mechanisms related to low carbohydrate intake: direct immunosuppression attributable to the depletion of glucose, a key substrate for the high metabolic needs of immune cells, and indirect impairment via increased concentration of stress hormones (Gleeson et al. 2001). Some (Henson et al. 1999; Nehlsen-Cannarella et al. 1997) but not all (Bishop et al. 1999; Henson et al. 2000) studies have reported that there is less disturbance to immune system parameters during the postexercise period when carbohydrate is consumed during prolonged exercise than when the athlete is deprived of carbohydrate. However, the ideal study in which chronic carbohydrate support during training is shown to correlate with reduced frequency or severity of illness in athletes is yet to be undertaken. Notwithstanding these limitations, the current literature suggests that good health and protection of the immune system may be a secondary but substantial benefit of carbohydrate intake during training. Finally, a study of elite swimmers reported that the consumption of sport drink during workouts during a phase of intensive training was associated with lower plasma concentrations of enzymes creatine kinase and lactate dehydrogenase than when water was consumed (Cade et al. 1991). The reduction in the postexercise increase in these enzymes, considered in this study to be an index of muscle damage, was attributed to a reduction in exercise-induced muscle catabolism secondary to the sustained available of muscle carbohydrate supply.

Further studies should investigate the benefits of strategies to promote carbohydrate availability during training sessions on short-term and long-term training outcomes. Such studies should aim to monitor small changes in performance, such as changes in technique, as well as functional changes to the immune response to exercise such as a reduction in days of sickness over the training year. In the meantime, the present literature suggests that there are possible benefits, and few disadvantages, to strategies that support adequate fuel status during training.

Eating for Recovery

An aggressive approach to recovery is needed to tackle the high-volume training schedules of elite swimmers and rowers and the short periods between multiple workouts in a day. The second research topic and practical issue in this chapter provide a more detailed discussion of postexercise recovery, including the restoration of the fluid and fuel deficits accrued during a workout and the promotion of protein synthesis to repair muscle damage and achieve the adaptations arising from the training stimulus. Although studies can measure the achievement of physiological markers of recovery, it would take patience and large resources to conduct an investigation that can detect whether better recovery translates into better long-term training adaptations and performance. This issue has been best examined in relation to refueling (chapter 4, research topic). Given the high fuel requirements of the training programs of swimmers and rowers, these athletes have often been chosen for studies of the effect of moderate- versus high-carbohydrate diets on training outcomes.

A sudden increase in training volume over a 10-day period was found to produce differing effects in a squad of collegiate swimmers; some members (n = 8) appeared to tolerate the intervention, whereas a subgroup (n = 4) failed to adapt (Costill, Flynn, et al. 1988). The discriminating feature of swimmers who complained of muscle fatigue, irritability, and an inability to finish some workouts was a failure to increase total energy and carbohydrate intake in response to the increased training. Whereas swimmers who automatically matched their new fuel demands with a greater carbohydrate intake (8.2 g/kg body mass) maintained muscle glycogen stores, the "failed" swimmers reported a carbohydrate intake of 5.3 g/kg and showed a gradual decline in muscle glycogen levels over the training week. At the end of the intervention, the squad undertook a performance battery including measurement of maximal power (swim bench), 2 × 25 yd freestyle swim with 2 to 3 min recovery interval, $\dot{V}O_2$max in pool, and swimming efficiency at submaximal pace. There were no differences from baseline measurements and between groups, except for a reduction in swimming efficiency in the subgroup with the moderate carbohydrate intakes. Because muscle glycogen content is unlikely to be a limiting factor in the performance of a sprint race, it is not surprising that competition performance was unchanged after the 10-day study. However, we might speculate that a longer duration of poor training would eventually diminish the adaptations achieved and impair race performance.

A more conventional crossover intervention was undertaken by another group of male collegiate swimmers, who completed a 9-day training block while consuming an energy-matched diet with a daily carbohydrate intake of either 6.5 or 12.1 g/kg body mass (Lamb et al. 1990). The swimmers completed two training sessions per day involving intervals over variety of distances, together with timed 1,500 m and 3,000 m swims during afternoon sessions during last 5 days of each intervention. This study did not measure the effect of these dietary interventions on muscle glycogen stores but found no differences between dietary treatments in mean swimming times over a range of distances. There are several ways to interpret these results: Either the moderate-carbohydrate diet was sufficient to fuel the training program of the swimmers, the swimmers were able to adapt to less than optimal refueling, or the performance measurements were inadequate to detect differences between the diets that might ultimately become important.

Finally, collegiate rowers were divided into two matched groups to complete a 4-week training program on energy-matched diets providing either 5 or 10 g/kg body mass of carbohydrate per day (Simonsen et al. 1991). Monitoring of muscle glycogen content showed that rowers in the moderate-carbohydrate group were able to maintain muscle carbohydrate stores, whereas the high-carbohydrate diet promoted an increase in stores over the duration of the study. Training performances were monitored throughout the 4 weeks, with the rowers undertaking 3 × 2,500 m rowing ergometer time trials with an 8 min recovery interval at the evening workout on days 1, 3, and 5 of each week. In the moderate-carbohydrate group, power outputs during the ergometer rowing time trials were maintained over the 4 weeks, leading to an overall improvement of 1.6% at end of the training block. Meanwhile, the high-carbohydrate group showed an improvement in time trial power outputs over same time frame of 10.7%, which was significantly different by the final week. This study provides evidence that a higher carbohydrate intake supports superior training adaptations and performance in highly trained athletes undertaking a heavy training program, and it suggests that several weeks may be needed before these differences become detectable.

Guidelines for enhancing recovery after a demanding training session are well founded in terms of acute measurements of fluid and fuel stores. However, it is more difficult to monitor the outcomes of these strategies in terms of long-term changes in training adaptations and performance. The strongest evidence of benefits appears to come from studies that are undertaken on athletes with the highest training demands and that are conducted over longer time periods, and the results of further studies are eagerly awaited. In the meantime, it appears prudent for athletes such as rowers and swimmers to take an aggressive approach to recovery between sessions undertaken within the same day and during phases of high-volume training.

The Zone Diet and Swimmers

The Zone diet made its first public appearance in the mid-1990s via some articles in popular American swimming magazines (Whitten 1993a, 1993b). The articles provided testimonials from coaches from the Stanford swimming team that recent successes of their swimmers were associated with a new nutrition program developed by Dr. Barry Sears. It was claimed that the diet, described as a low-energy program based on a 40:30:30 energy ratio (carbohydrate–protein–fat), was taken up by the members of the squad, leading to six swimmers qualifying for the U.S. Olympic team and winning eight gold medals at the 1992 Barcelona Olympic Games. In his later books on the Zone diet (Sears 1995, 1997), Barry Sears claimed credit for eight more gold medals by U.S. swimmers at the Atlanta Games. It is therefore not hard to understand that the Zone diet is often discussed in swimming circles.

There is no research evidence to support the claims of enhanced performance, better control of body fat, and superior health with the Zone diet. In fact, the only study of the Zone diet involving 7 days of adherence to the diet by moderately trained males reported a reduction in body mass (attributable to reduced energy intake) over the week but also a reduction in treadmill running time to exhaustion at 80% $\dot{V}O_2$max (Jarvis et al. 2002). There is also no corroborating evidence from the Stanford swim team that they adhered to the diet, although the individual swimmers are well known for their competitive success. Clearly, there is a need for well-controlled investigations of the Zone diet and athletic performance to test the basis of these anecdotal stories. However, there are several difficulties to unraveling the tale, including the challenge of pinpointing exactly what the Zone diet is, especially when applied to high-level athletes. The popular press often refers to the Zone diet as high protein or low carbohydrate, and the 40:30:30 energy ratio label is generally used to summarize the basic Zone philosophy. However, an examination of the principles and recommended practice, even as described by Barry Sears himself, reveals a number of areas of confusion. According to the book *Enter the Zone* (Sears 1995), the Zone diet is distinguished by the following features:

• The Zone diet is followed by consuming a "Zone favorable" meal or snack at least every 5 hr during the day, to set insulin ratios for the next period.

• The central principle of the Zone diet comes from setting protein requirements according to lean body mass and activity level. The prescribed protein intake ranges from 0.5 g/lb (1.1 g/kg) of lean body mass for an inactive person to a maximum of 1.0 g/lb (2.2 g/kg) of lean body mass for people undertaking very high activity levels (heavy resistance training and twice-daily training sessions). For a lean swimmer or runner in heavy training (eg., male with 8-10% body fat and female with 12-20% body fat), this recommendation translates to a daily protein intake of ~2 g/kg body mass (males) and ~1.8 to 1.9 g/kg body mass (females). For the sedentary population, the recommendation equates to ~0.8 to 1.0 g/kg body mass for a person carrying body fat levels of 10% to 25%. These baseline values are not different than those in the dietary guidelines recommended by expert panels of most countries—that is, they do not promote a high protein intake. The higher protein recommendations for athletes in heavy training are at the high end of the range suggested by exercise scientists, but they appear similar to the self-chosen diets reported by current athletes, at least when in energy balance. Therefore, the Zone diet does not advocate higher protein intakes than the conventional dietary guidelines or as found in typical Western eating patterns. A major recommendation, however, is that protein should be spread out over the day in a series of meals and snacks.

• The next principle of the Zone diet is that carbohydrate intake should be matched to protein intake in a ratio of 4:3 and that carbohydrate intake should be spread out over the day and with the focus on low glycemic index choices. Typically, this sets carbohydrate intakes at low to moderate levels ranging from ~1 to 1.5 g/kg body mass in sedentary individuals to 2 to 3 g/kg body mass in highly active people. This is a major departure from sports nutrition guidelines that promote a carbohydrate intake more closely tied to the muscle fuel costs of training and competition activities.

• A sleight of hand that is typical of many weight loss diets is the Zone promise that you don't need to worry about the amounts of food you eat—rather, "you can eat all you like." In fact, the Zone diet is a self-declared low-energy, or calorie-restricted, diet. However, the energy restriction is hidden inside the prescription of food into fat, carbohydrate, and protein blocks each day. Simply speaking, protein intake—which typically stays at the recommended intakes that most people habitually achieve—is switched from providing around 12% to 18% of total dietary energy intake (typical Western diet) to the new mark of 30% of energy intake (Zone diet). In other words, the individual continues to eat the same amount of protein, but total dietary energy intake is halved around it. Carbohydrate is pruned to take up 40% of the reduced energy consumption, leaving fat intake to make up the remaining 30% of energy. By way of example, the strict Zone diet prescription has been constructed for three individuals—the author of this book, an elite female swimmer, and an elite male rower (see column 2 of table 6.2). This table illustrates that the Zone diet prescribes an energy intake well below the energy requirements of all participants. Clearly, if the Zone diet is followed strictly, it will allow the body to tap into body fat stores just as any other food plan achieving an energy deficit.

To the best of my knowledge, the prescription of the Zone diet to an athlete with high energy needs has not been clearly spelled out in any of Dr. Sears' books or other writings. There are two different approaches that an athlete could take to increase his energy intake to meet his actual energy needs.

1.   One approach is to multiply the 40:30:30 ratio to the higher energy needs of the athlete. This approach has been followed in the examples of our three athletes (see column 3, table 6.2). However, this approach would result in much larger intakes of protein than recommended by the Zone book.

2.   The other approach is to maintain protein (and carbohydrate) intakes at the core Zone principle and increase fat intake to meet additional energy needs. Although this strategy is not properly described in any of the Zone books, it appears to be the principle favored by Sears. For example, the advertising jacket on Zone books proclaims "athletes perform better on a high fat diet." In addition, in a reply to a summary on the Zone diet published in the peer-reviewed journal *Sports Medicine* (Cheuvront 1999), Dr. Sears said, "elite athletes must add significant amounts of extra fat (and primarily monounsaturated fat) to their diet. This is to maintain their percentage body fat in an appropriate range suitable for the needs of their particular sport" (Sears 2000, p. 289). The final column of table 6.2 shows the outcome of applying this strategy to our sample athletes. According to these calculations, fat intake would increase to ~65% of total energy intake. This is similar to the high-fat diets that have been trialed for short- and long-term adaptation periods in athletes. These diets have not provided benefits to training or performance and, in fact, have been associated with an impaired ability to use carbohydrate and perform at high-intensity work rates (see chapter 4, research issue).

The final aspect of the Zone diet philosophy, at least according to the initial books, is that supplementation with vitamins and minerals other than vitamin E is unnecessary (Sears 1995). However, according to a recent interview with Barry Sears, supplementation with pharmaceutical-grade fish oil should be undertaken (Whitten 2002). The rationale and evidence for benefits from this practice are not explained.

There is a need for the Zone diet to be clearly explained for high-energy consumers and for well-controlled studies of this diet to be undertaken in athletes. In the meantime, most dietitians and nutritionists who have assessed the dietary intake of people who claim to be following the Zone diet will confirm that it includes a wide variety of eating practices and interpretations. Some individuals studiously count food blocks, others avoid certain carbohydrate-rich foods totally or in combination with others, and some people simply buy "Zone"-endorsed foods such as bars and powders and add these to their existing diets. In real life, and particularly over the long term, people do not adhere closely to rigid dietary rules or eating plans. Rather they gradually adopt a plan based on their interpretation of the original diet or a compromise between the dietary rules and their preferred or practical food choices. Therefore, in addition to the lack of scientific investigations of athletic performance following diets such as the Zone, it is uncertain whether free-living athletes who provide testimonials about their experiences on such dietary programs are actually following the principles on which these programs are based.

Table 6.2   Calculations for the Zone Diet Applied to Athletes

Participant	Basic Zone diet, with energy restrictions as prescribed in 1995 book: • Protein = 0.5-1.0 g per kg LBM according to activity level (=30% total energy intake) • Carbohydrate = 40% of energy • Fat = 30% energy	Zone diet modified for athletes, achieving predicted energy requirements with 40:30:30 energy ratio of carbohydrate, protein, and fat	Zone diet modified for athletes, achieving predicted energy by maintaining carbohydrate and protein levels according to core Zone principles and increasing fat intake to meet remainder of energy needs
Female recreational runner and cyclist, 55 kg, 15% body fat, 1 hr moderate exercise each day. • Predicted energy requirements = 10,000 kJ/day • Zone protein allowance = 0.8 g/lb LBM (1.8 g/kg LBM)	Daily recommendations • Protein = 82 g (1.5 g/kg BM) • Carbohydrate = 110 g (2 g/kg BM) • Fat = 37 g • Energy = 4,600 kJ (1,100 kcal)	Daily recommendations • Protein = 178 g (3.2 g/kg BM) • Carbohydrate = 238 g (4.3 g/kg BM) • Fat = 80 g • Energy = 10,000 kJ (2,380 kcal)	Daily recommendations • Protein = 82 g (1.5 g/kg BM, 14% of energy) • Carbohydrate = 110 g (2 g/kg BM, 18% of energy) • Fat = 179 g (68% of energy) • Energy = 10,000 kJ (2,380 kcal)
Elite male rower, 90 kg, 10% body fat, 3-4 hr training per day • Predicted energy requirements = 19,000 kJ • Zone protein allowance = 1.0 g/lb LBM (2.2 g/kg LBM)	Daily recommendations • Protein = 178 g (2 g/kg BM) • Carbohydrate = 237 g (2.6 g/kg BM) • Fat = 80 g • Energy = 9,970 kJ (2,375 kcal)	Daily recommendations • Protein = 339 g (3.8 g/kg BM) • Carbohydrate = 452 g (5 g/kg BM) • Fat = 151 g • Energy = 19,000 kJ (4,525 kcal)	Daily recommendations • Protein = 178 g (2 g/kg BM, 16% of energy)) • Carbohydrate = 238 g (2.6 g/kg BM, 21% of energy) • Fat = 317 g (63% of energy) • Energy = 19,000 kJ (4,525 kcal)
Elite female swimmer, 65 kg, 15% body fat, ~3 hr training per day • Predicted energy requirements = 14,000 kJ • Zone protein allowance = 1.0 g/lb LBM (2.2 g/kg LBM)	Daily recommendations • Protein = 122 g (1.9 g/kg BM) • Carbohydrate = 163 g (2.5 g/kg BM) • Fat = 54 g • Energy = 6,830 kJ (1,625 kcal)	Daily recommendations • Protein = 250 g (3.0 g/kg BM) • Carbohydrate = 334 g (5.1 g/kg BM) • Fat = 111 g • Energy = 14,000 kJ (3,335 kcal)	Daily recommendations • Protein = 122 g (1.9 g/kg BM, 14% of energy) • Carbohydrate = 163 g (2.5 g/kg BM, 20% of energy) • Fat = 244 g (66% of energy) • Energy = 14,000 kJ (3,335 kcal)

BM = body mass, LBM = lean body mass.

Competition Eating

Although there are variations attributable to different competition scenarios, the typical race situation experienced by most rowers and swimmers involves one or more races in a session, repeated over a number of days of a carnival, meet, or regatta. Adequate carbohydrate and fluid levels are important for optimal performance but are not likely to be limiting for a single event if adequate prerace preparation and postrace recovery between races have taken place. This calls for a planned approach to race eating, especially when the athlete is competing in events away from her home base.

A key part of the competition eating plan is to understand the athlete's real energy needs over the racing period. The competition program will involve warm-up and cooldown activities in addition to the actual race program, as well as continued training on rest days. However, the energy cost of racing activities is usually substantially less than the usual training program. Therefore, strategic refueling and rehydration practices need to be organized within an eating program that achieves an adjusted energy intake. For some swimmers and rowers, racing is often a time of unnecessary gain of body fat, as the athlete overfuels himself in the belief that this will assist his race performance. Overeating can also occur during racing periods because the young athlete is away from his normal supervised nutrition plan or because the athlete is eating in response to the nervousness and anxiety generated by competition. Many swimmers and rowers also find themselves with spare time on their hands during the precompetition taper or race program, and they eat unnecessary amounts of food as part of entertainment activities or to fill time. By contrast, other rowers and swimmers with a busy race schedule and extensive travel commitments find that their access to food is limited. Poor food availability at the event location, a timetable that clashes with catering opportunities, and the distraction of racing activities can all interfere with the athlete's eating routine. In such cases the athlete will unnecessarily lose weight over the competition period and fail to achieve optimal recovery strategies between races.

The rower and swimmer can achieve adequate muscle glycogen stores for their events and preparation and recovery activities by ensuring at least 24 hr of tapered training and high carbohydrate intake (7-10 g/kg body mass per day). The daily racing routine should start with a high-carbohydrate prerace meal, which the athlete should choose from a range of familiar foods and following a plan that has been fine-tuned from previous racing experience. Typically, swimmers and rowers consume a prerace breakfast 1 to 3 hr before commencing prerace warm-ups. During and after warm-ups, and in recovery between events on the same program, carbohydrate-containing drinks (e.g., sport drinks) and light carbohydrate foods (sport bars, fruit, gels) are consumed to maintain body carbohydrate supplies and prevent hunger. After the competition session is completed, the athlete should consume a nutrient-rich meal to meet recovery goals of refueling, repairing muscle damage, and rehydrating. The traditional pattern of swimmers who compete in an evening session is to consume a carbohydrate-rich lunch after the morning heats, before resting or sleeping in the afternoon. A light snack is typically consumed before returning to the evening finals session, and the session is followed by dinner. The meal timetable should be arranged to allow the athlete quick access to food after sessions, both to provide rapid access to key recovery nutrients and to maximize the time available for rest and sleep.

Most swimmers and rowers, or the teams in which they compete, take a selection of portable snacks and drinks to the competition venue to allow refueling and rehydration after each event and during the competition program. Issues such as storage facilities, appetite appeal during a heavy racing program, and the need to comply with drug-testing protocols (i.e., only accepting food and drinks from sealed containers) often determine the suitable choices. Typical choices include specialized sport foods (sport drinks, bars and gels) as well as cereal and granola bars, fresh and dried fruit, jelly confectionery, and sandwiches. When swim meets or rowing regattas are held in hot locations, it is important to have ready access to a supply of fluids over the day and to monitor hydration levels in relation to general sweat losses into the environment as well as the specific losses during events and warm-ups. In summary, each athlete should develop a well-considered race-day eating schedule suited to his or her specific race program and should be proactive in ensuring that meals and snacks are accessible at key times.

Sport Foods and Supplements

With such a wide variety of nutritional interests and challenges (see the highlight box on page 147), it is understandable that rowers and swimmers would be interested in the range of sport foods and supplements that are manufactured or marketed for different purposes. Supplements and sport foods used by rowers and swimmers include products that address nutritional goals in a practical form as well as products providing ingredients claimed to directly enhance performance. The degree to which these products have become part of the daily programs of swimmers and rowers is demonstrated by the results of a survey of elite Australian swimmers (Baylis et al. 2001). Among the 77 national and international representatives who completed the survey, 99% reported the use of supplements and sport foods, naming 207 individual products.

The swimmers reported strong attitudes to issues related to sport safety and supplement use, which was defined in the survey as the absence of doping problems resulting from the use of these products. The majority of swimmers reported that it was very important (79%) or important (16%) to consider the risk of inadvertent doping from the use of a new supplement before deciding to take it. Only 5% of the swimmers expressed a neutral opinion on this issue. Professional advice from people such as dietitians, doctors, pharmacists, and sport scientists was the most popular source of information consulted in deciding to use a supplement; 53% of swimmers noted this as the most important type of advice and another 31% considered this the second most important information. The advice of a coach was considered highly as supporting information, ranking as the second most important (31%) or third-ranked (30%) source of information by swimmers. The list of ingredients stated on a supplement packet was highly ranked as primary information about a supplement, with 22% of swimmers reporting this as their most important knowledge source. Advice from alternative nutrition practitioners such as naturopaths, herbalists, or health food shop agents did not appear to rate highly in decision making; less than 10% of swimmers ranked such advice within their three most important information sources.

Eighty-seven percent of the swimmers reported the use of sport foods such as sport drinks, which can be valuable in helping such athletes to meet their special nutritional needs during training or competition (see table 6.3). On the other hand, 95% of athletes also reported using nutritional ergogenic aids including a range of vitamin and mineral preparations (95% of the group, with 71% reporting the use of more than one preparation), herbal products (61%), amino acid preparations (18%), and miscellaneous supplements such as inosine (16%) and coenzyme Q10 (7%).

Reviews of such supplements, both in chapter 3 and in the remainder of this chapter, suggest that only creatine (reported by 31% of the group), bicarbonate (3%), and caffeine (use undocumented) may provide definite benefits to sport performance for rowing and swimming when used in a specific manner. Therefore, in spite of or perhaps even because of professional advice, the majority of swimmers still appear to be following supplementation practices with little documented value.

This chapter finishes with a summary of supplements and sport foods that appear to be of some value in rowing and swimming (table 6.3) and a brief overview of research related to specific performance outcomes of the use of particular ergogenic aids in these sports (see tables 6.e and 6.f in appendix). Carefully examine these studies for an overview of the sport-specific literature on creatine, caffeine, bicarbonate and citrate, β-hydroxy β-methylbutyrate (HMB), colostrum, pyruvate, vitamin E, and several other products. The studies reviewed in these tables involve trained rowers and swimmers and an exercise protocol that has relevance to performance of real-life events. Of course, more research is needed using rigorous control and carefully chosen protocols to test the claims for most products. In the case of most of the supplements and proposed ergogenic compounds that are popular among swimmers and rowers, there are simply no studies that examine the claims made for training or performance benefits. The reader is therefore referred to the general conclusions reached in chapter 3 about such products.

Even in the case of products where supportive research exists, there is still a lack of well-controlled investigations on aspects of supplement use that are specific to the needs of rowing and swimming. For example, even though there is hypothetical support for the benefits of chronic creatine supplementation on interval and resistance training for swimming and perhaps rowing, there is a need for more studies that adequately track adaptation and changes performance over a sufficient period of training. This is also the case in chronic use of bicarbonate loading prior to interval training sessions to promote better training outcomes or greater training adaptations. Furthermore, these findings need to be tempered by the young age of swimmers and rowers, even at elite and subelite level—most experts believe that children and adolescents do not need such a supplement in light of the gains they are already making simply through maturation in age and training and in view of the lack of evidence that long-term creatine use is safe for such special populations. The results of supplementation studies undertaken with running and cycling protocols, even over similar durations and using energy systems similar to rowing and swimming races, need to be scrutinized for the special issues involved in technique-driven sports. Some supplements (e.g., caffeine) may have effects on fine motor control that are not necessarily important in activities involving only gross body movements and may translate into performance decrements rather than the anticipated performance enhancements.

Because rowers and swimmers compete in heats and finals to decide the final outcome of their events (often on the same day), there is a need to investigate the effects of supplementation protocols involving repeated use. For example, the lowest effective doses of bicarbonate and

Table 6.3   Sport Foods and Supplements That Are of Likely Benefit to Swimmers and Rowers

	Product	Comment
Use in achieving documented nutrition goals	Sport drinks	• Used to refuel and rehydrate during prolonged workouts and to rehydrate after the session. Contain some electrolytes to help replace sweat losses and increase voluntary intake of fluid.
	Sport gels	• Convenient and compact carbohydrate source that can be carried for use during prolonged dry land workouts (e.g., cycle sessions undertaken by swimmers and rowers) or on the water during rowing sessions.
	Sport bars	• Convenient, portable, and easy-to-consume source of carbohydrate, protein, and micronutrients for prerace meal or postexercise recovery. • Convenient and portable form of energy and nutrients that can help meet high energy needs, especially to support resistance training program or growth. • Convenient and compact source of energy and nutrients for the traveling athlete.
	Liquid meal supplements	• Convenient, portable, and easy-to-consume source of carbohydrate, protein, and micronutrients for postexercise recovery and "preexercise recovery" strategies. • Low-bulk and practical form of energy and nutrients that can help meet high energy needs, especially to support resistance training program or growth. • Well-tolerated preevent meal that can be consumed to provide a source of carbohydrate quite close to the start of a race or workout; liquid supplements seem to be better tolerated than solid food by some athletes with high risk of gastrointestinal problems. • Convenient and compact source of energy and nutrients for the traveling athlete.

	Product	Comment
	Multivitamin and mineral supplements	• Supplemental source of micronutrients for traveling when food supply is not reliable. • Supplemental source of micronutrients during prolonged periods of energy restriction (female athletes).
Strong potential for ergogenic benefit	Caffeine	• May enhance performance of rowing and swimming races when consumed prerace, but further sport-specific studies are needed to investigate the range of swimming events and the range of doses and consumption protocols (e.g., the timing of the prerace caffeine intake) that are effective for swimming and rowing events. There is some evidence from prolonged cycling and running protocols that small to moderate doses of caffeine (1-3 mg/kg) are as effective as larger doses (5-6 mg/kg) in achieving benefits and may reduce risk of side effects such as tremor and anxiety that can affect technique. Because rowing and swimming events are performed as a series of heats and finals, an additional benefit of finding the lowest caffeine dose at which performance enhancement occurs is to reduce the effect of preevent caffeine on postrace recovery and sleep patterns. Caffeine may be consumed in cola and energy drinks or as an ingredient in some sport products (e.g., some gels). There is conflicting evidence over the efficacy of coffee as a source of caffeine, because it contains other chemicals that might impair performance
	Bicarbonate or citrate loading	• There is reasonable evidence that the acute use of bicarbonate or citrate to increase blood buffering capacity (e.g., 300 mg/kg BM bicarbonate or 500 mg/kg BM citrate 1-2 hr prerace) might enhance the performance of events lasting 2-8 min (200-800 m swimming events and rowing events) via increased tolerance to production of H^+ ions via anaerobic glycolysis. Further field studies are needed with high-level athletes to confirm benefits. Risk of gastrointestinal problems should be noted but appear to be reduced by taking dose with large volumes of fluid (1-2 L). Swimmers and rowers who intend to load for a series of events over a day or consecutive days (e.g., heats and finals) should experiment with a lower dose for the second or subsequent races in view of residual increase in buffering capacity from earlier doses. Alternatively, a longer-term loading protocol can be used over a number of days leading up to the competition (e.g., 500 $mg \cdot kg^{-1} \cdot day^{-1}$ for 5 days spread into a series of doses over the day) to achieve a more sustained increase in blood-buffering capacity. There is new evidence that chronic loading of bicarbonate during training (loading immediately before interval training) may assist the swimmer or rower to train harder, as well as enhance the adaptations to the training that is undertaken. This needs to be confirmed in highly trained athletes.
	Creatine	• Creatine phosphate serves a number of important roles in exercise metabolism; the most well-known role is the rapid regeneration of ATP by the phosphagen power system. Studies show that creatine loading enhances the performance of exercise involving repeated high-intensity work bouts with short recovery intervals (<2 min recovery). Any performance benefits for a single sprint appear to be too small to detect, although there is limited evidence of enhancement of performance of high-intensity exercise lasting 6-8 min such as a rowing event. Although creatine loading may be useful for racing in a single rowing event, the most likely benefits for swimmers and rowers may come from using creatine in the training phase to enhance training adaptations to interval and resistance training. Performance benefits are seen only in those who experience significant increases in creatine stores following loading. Most studies have been undertaken in the laboratory, and relatively few have been undertaken with well-trained and elite athletes in sport-specific situations. Typical protocols for creatine use: loading dose: 20-30 g in multiple doses (e.g., 4 × 5 g) for 5 days followed by maintenance dose of 2-5 g/day. Uptake appears to be enhanced by consuming creatine with carbohydrate-rich meal or snack. Acute weight gain of about 1 kg occurs with creatine loading, presumably because of fluid retention. This is less likely to be of concern to weight-supported sports such as swimming and rowing.

ATP = adenosine triphosphate.

citrate and of caffeine should be determined to minimize side effects such as gastrointestinal discomfort or disturbances to postrace recovery and sleep. After all, although an acute supplementation protocol may enhance the performance of the immediate race, unwanted postrace side effects could jeopardize the outcomes of the following events. It is also important to investigate whether subsequent doses are still effective and without side effects at this level. It is possible that a lower dose may be effective in a repeated supplementation protocol, especially if the first dose has not been completely washed out. It is also possible that a subsequent dose may have a reduced or absent effect, leaving athletes to decide if the priority is to enhance performance to make a final or to wait until the final before using the supplementation protocol to achieve what they hope will be optimal performance. In the case of bicarbonate, a chronic or longer-term loading protocol involving 5 days of supplementation with 500 $mg \cdot kg^{-1} \cdot day^{-1}$ (spread into four doses over the day) has been investigated as an alternative to the acute loading dose (300 mg/kg, taken 1-2 hr preevent) (McNaughton, Backx, et al. 1999; McNaughton and Thompson 2001). This protocol was found to achieve an increase in plasma base excess that was sustained over the 5 days and enhanced the performance of a prolonged sprint undertaken on the day after the bicarbonate supplementation ceased. The persistence of the ergogenic outcome was suggested to be a desirable feature for sports involving a series of competition events.

Finally, because simultaneous supplementation practices are likely, the interaction between supplements such as caffeine and bicarbonate, or caffeine and creatine, need to be better investigated so that advice can be translated into guidelines for the real-life situations in which rowers and swimmers compete. The only available information on multiple supplement use by rowers or swimmers involves an investigation of acute creatine loading and bicarbonate supplementation. This study (Mero et al. 2004) examined the performance of two 100 m freestyle races held 10 min apart, when competitive swimmers undertook a 6-day creatine protocol (20 g/day) followed by bicarbonate loading (300 mg/kg) on the morning of the study. This combination was found to enhance the performance of the second swim compared with a placebo trial. However, mechanisms to explain the performance benefit and the individual contribution of each supplement were not provided in this study. Ideally, such studies should include designs that examine the single and combined effects of each intervention so that independent and interactive outcomes can be understood. At present, we are resigned to giving advice based on theory rather than real knowledge of all these factors.

RESEARCH TOPIC
Why Do Swimmers Carry Higher Body Fat Levels Than Other Endurance Athletes?

If you follow the world of swimming you will have heard not only of the world records and triumphs of swimmers but also of the battle that many female swimmers (and their coaches!) fight to control their levels of body fat. In the general literature on obesity and weight loss programs, several studies have found that swimming for exercise does not seem to provide an effective means of controlling body fat levels. Competitive swimmers typically complete 5,000 to 20,000 m per day in training, which obviously burns thousands of kilojoules. However, the typical body fat levels of these athletes, not withstanding the leanness of some individual swimmers, are generally higher than those of runners or cyclists who expend similar or even smaller amounts of energy in their training. Swimmers who struggle to control their weight and body fat levels are generally prescribed dry land training (running or cycling) in addition to their many laps of the pool in the belief that it is a necessary strategy to produce lower skinfold levels (body fat levels).

Research Priorities

Further research is needed to better understand the current practices of top athletes in these sports and to investigate various dietary strategies that can contribute to successful performance in various types of events. Areas that are of high priority for sport-specific research include the following

- Current nutrition practices of high-level swimmers and rowers
- The importance of weight and body fat levels in swimming performance, and strategies to assess and achieve ideal physique for swimming, especially for females and adolescents
- The importance of carbohydrate intake—within a session or in the overall training diet—for promoting optimal training adaptations and long-term performance
- The effect of the Zone diet on swimming performance (training and competition)
- Strategies for optimal recovery between workouts and between races within a competition program
- The current use of supplements and sport foods by swimmers and rowers and their specific benefit to performance in training and in competition in various events

There are several theories that could be put forward to explain these observations, even if they occur in isolated cases rather than being a universal truth. One, swimmers find it easier to achieve an energy imbalance through overeating; they have higher energy intakes than other athletes and eat more energy than they expend. It has been suggested that swimming doesn't cause the postexercise decrease in appetite that accompanies high-intensity running and cycling training. Many people observe that they feel like "eating a horse" after they have finished a swim workout and may overcompensate for their energy expenditure at the next meal. Some research suggests that this effect could be attributable to the cool environments (e.g., pool water) in which swimmers train and the attenuation of the increase in body temperature that usually accompanies prolonged or high-intensity exercise. By contrast, runners and cyclists usually experience an increase in body temperature during training, which may suppress appetite—at least in the short term.

Second, the overall daily energy expenditure of swimmers may be less than that of other athletes or less than their total energy intake because of a reduced contribution of incidental exercise. Swimmers may be less active outside their training sessions than other athletes—they may be so tired from the hours spent in the pool that they sleep, sit, or otherwise avoid any real energy expenditure outside their workouts. The culture of swimmers is to avoid walking, climbing stairs, or other exercise to save themselves for pool workouts. Even where additional dry land training is undertaken, sessions may not be of sufficient duration or intensity to create a substantial energy deficit.

Third, swimming is associated with different metabolic patterns during and after the exercise session, which are less reliant on fat metabolism and less able to contribute to loss of body fat.

Fourth, natural selection processes are at hand in determining who becomes a competitive runner or swimmer. Elite swimmers may be predisposed to have higher body fat levels because it is a help, or at least less of a disadvantage, to their swimming. Rounded shoulders and smooth curves may be more biomechanically sound than bony angles—at least up to the point where the extra weight of body fat creates a critical negative drag. Because higher body fat levels are of greater disadvantage to weight-bearing sports like running, those who are genetically gifted toward high-level aerobic capacities and power generation, but with a tendency toward higher body fat levels, may have headed for the water at an early age. Meanwhile, the very lean endurance athletes stayed on land!

Various studies have tried to pinpoint whether these discrepancies of energy or fat balance really exist in swimming.

Energy Balance in Competitive Swimmers and Runners

Jang et al. 1987

A crude measure of daily energy balance was undertaken on collegiate swimmers and distance runners. Ten athletes of each sex from each sport participated in the study by keeping detailed food records (3 days) and activity records (1 day). The activity records recorded the amount of time each individual spent sleeping, sitting, walking, standing, or training. The energy cost of these activities was estimated individually for each athlete by duplicating the activity in the laboratory and collecting data on oxygen consumption. The rate of energy expenditure in each activity was multiplied by the time spent, allowing an estimate of total daily energy expenditure. Body fat levels were lower in the runners by about 5%, whereas similar total daily energy intakes were reported by both swimmers and runners (see table 6.4).

Estimates of daily energy expenditure were in general agreement for swimmers and runners, with the values for the male athletes being roughly equal and similar to their reported intakes. The female swimmers were estimated to have higher energy expenditures than female runners and in fact appeared to be in slight negative energy balance. These results were not helpful in explaining an apparent greater tendency for female swimmers to gain body fat while training.

The major limitation of this study is that the methods of estimating each side of the energy balance equation are subject to considerable flaws (see chapter 2). It is well known that most people underreport their true energy

Table 6.4   Body Fat Levels and Energy Intakes of Swimmers and Runners

	Swimmers	Runners
BODY FAT LEVELS		
Male athletes	12%	7%
Female athletes	20%	15%
TOTAL DAILY ENERGY INTAKE		
Male athletes	3,380 kcal	3,460 kcal
Female athletes	2,490 kcal	2,040 kcal

intake when keeping food records, especially those who are dissatisfied with their body mass and body fat levels. It is also hard to accurately describe and complete normal daily activities while recording. Whether we would expect a correlation between mean energy intake from 3 days and expenditure from 1 day's activities is also questionable; generally, most people who are in energy balance achieve this over ~7 to 10 days.

Fat Storage in Athletes: Metabolic and Hormonal Responses to Swimming and Running

Flynn et al. 1990
Energy and fuel usage during training sessions and recovery in swimming and running were examined to see if differences in hormonal patterns and the oxidation of fat might explain differences in body fat levels. Swimmers and runners undertook their trained activity for 45 min at 75% to 80% $\dot{V}O_2$max and then recovered for 2 hr. Triathletes did one session of each mode of exercise so that results could be compared within the same individual. During exercise periods and recovery, blood samples were collected for measurement of hormones, glucose, and fatty acid levels. Respiratory gas exchange data were measured to monitor total energy expenditure and oxidation of various body fuels. Results showed that there were no differences in total energy expenditure during training or recovery between groups. There were some differences in substrate utilization and hormone levels. For example, swimming resulted in lower blood glucose levels than running, with some evidence of a greater reliance on carbohydrate as a fuel during swimming. This is likely to be further accentuated in the real-life training of swimmers, who undertake a high proportion of high-intensity interval work. During recovery, fat oxidation tended to be greater after swimming than running. The ratio of blood glucagon to insulin was greater in swimming trials than running during recovery. Overall, these differences were small and could not explain why swimmers have higher body fat levels.

Effects of Swimming and Running on Energy Intake During 2 Hr of Recovery

Lambert et al. 1999
Eight competitive triathletes undertook a 45 min session of either running or swimming at 70% $\dot{V}O_2$max and were then observed for 2 hr in a room with available foods and drinks. Ratings of hunger and thirst were obtained during recovery and did not differ between exercise trials. Blood glucose levels were higher after running than after the swim workout. There were no differences in voluntary energy intake during the 2 hr of recovery: (4,568 ± 611 kJ for running and 4,383 ± 484 kJ for swimming). This study failed to find evidence of differences in postexercise appetite and food intake based on mode of exercise. However, these results may not be representative of the effects of longer sessions undertaken at higher or intermittent intensities.

RESEARCH TOPIC

Protein and Carbohydrate— Does Co-Ingestion of These Nutrients Aid Recovery?

Recovery encompasses the following nutrition-related processes:

1. Restoration of muscle and liver glycogen stores
2. Synthesis of new protein following the catabolic state and damage induced by the exercise

It is clear that dietary carbohydrate intake is primarily involved with the first of these processes, whereas dietary protein is important for the second. There is also some evidence that speedy intake of these nutrients can enhance the rate of postexercise recovery, a strategy that is important for athletes who train or compete twice or more each day. It has been suggested that the combined intake of these nutrients in recovery meals and snacks is superior to consuming the primary nutrient alone—in other words, that the addition of protein to a carbohydrate-rich snack enhances glycogen storage and that the addition of carbohydrate to a protein-rich snack enhances net protein balance. What is the evidence for these theories, and how should athletes structure their recovery meals and snacks to promote optimal recovery outcomes?

Protein and Glycogen Storage

Typically, the most important dietary factor affecting muscle glycogen storage is the amount of carbohydrate consumed. Chapter 1 summarized the direct and positive relationship between the quantity of dietary carbohydrate and postexercise glycogen storage, suggesting that the daily muscle storage threshold is reached at around 7 to 12 g of carbohydrate per kilogram of body mass. Early intake of carbohydrate following prolonged exercise is valuable because it provides an immediate source of substrate to the muscle cell to start effective refueling, as well as taking advantage of a period of moderately enhanced glycogen synthesis (for review, see Burke, Kiens, et al. 2004).

However, it appears that total energy intake is also an important factor in the relationship between carbohydrate intake and glycogen storage (Tarnopolsky et al. 2001). The simplest way to consider this relationship is that dietary intake must provide for the body's immediate fuel requirements as well as storage opportunities. When energy intake is restricted, it is likely that greater proportions of available carbohydrate substrates (e.g., dietary carbohydrate) must be oxidized for immediate energy needs, whereas carbohydrate consumed during a period of energy balance or surplus may be available for storage within the muscle and liver. The addition of protein to recovery meals and snacks may enhance glycogen storage by increasing total energy intake—thus sparing dietary carbohydrate for muscle fuel stores. But it is also possible that the protein content of some carbohydrate-rich foods (e.g., flavored yogurt) or protein consumed at the same meal (e.g., milk on breakfast cereal) has independent effects on muscle glycogen storage, via its stimulatory effect on insulin secretion. An early study reported that the addition of protein (40 g) to carbohydrate feedings (112 g) consumed at 2 hr intervals after exercise caused a greater rate of muscle glycogen storage during 4 hr of recovery than either of these feedings alone. An enhanced insulin response was suggested to explain this response (Zawadzki et al. 1992). This study, despite methodological problems attributable to the failure to match the energy content of recovery meals, has been largely responsible for advice to consume protein with carbohydrate-rich meals to enhance refueling goals.

Over the last decade, a series of studies have continued to examine the effect of consuming protein (or amino acids), in addition to carbohydrate, on glycogen storage. A variety of outcomes have been reported: Some studies report an increase in glycogen storage when protein is added to a carbohydrate feeding (Ivy et al. 2002; Van Loon et al. 2000; Zawadzki et al. 1992), whereas others find no effect (Carrithers et al. 2000; Roy and Tarnopolsky 1998; Tarnopolsky et al. 1997; Van Hall, Shirreffs, et al. 2000; Van Loon et al. 2000).

Many of the conflicting results among studies, however, can probably be explained by differences in experimental design—including the frequency of supplementation and the amounts of carbohydrate and protein provided. For example, in studies demonstrating that the addition of protein to a carbohydrate supplement will enhance muscle glycogen storage, feeding intervals of 2 hr were used (Ivy et al. 2002; Zawadzki et al. 1992). Those studies that did not demonstrate a benefit of protein used 15 to 30 min feeding intervals (Carrithers et al. 2000; Jentjens et al. 2001; Tarnopolsky et al. 1997; Van Hall, Shirreffs, et al. 2000) and generally fed a high total amount of carbohydrate (Jentjens et al. 2001; Van Hall, Saris, et al. 2000) or a low amount of protein (Carrithers et al. 2000; Tarnopolsky et al. 1997). Regardless of the differences in experimental design, the majority of evidence suggests that consuming large amounts of carbohydrate at frequent intervals negates the benefits of added protein. However, the evidence is compelling that the co-ingestion of protein with carbohydrate will increase the efficiency of muscle glycogen storage when the amount of carbohydrate ingested is below the threshold for maximal glycogen synthesis or when feeding intervals are greater than 1 hr apart (Ivy et al. 2002; Van Loon et al. 2000; Zawadzki et al. 1992).

The effectiveness of protein to enhance muscle glycogen storage may also be limited to the first hour after supplementation. Ivy and colleagues (2002) reported that glycogen storage during the first 40 min of recovery after exercise was four times faster than with the carbohydrate from this snack alone and twice as fast as a larger carbohydrate feeding that was energy-matched to the carbohydrate–protein snack. This effect seemed to disappear in later recovery. These results may have important implications for recovery within a competition—for example, for sports such as soccer, which allow a very short recovery period (e.g., 20

min) between halves of a match. It is still uncertain whether the enhanced rates of glycogen storage resulting from the co-ingestion of protein and carbohydrate may be achieved via the increased insulin response from protein per se or as a result of the increase in energy intake.

It is prudent to conclude that the presence of other macronutrients with carbohydrate feedings does not substantially alter muscle glycogen synthesis when total carbohydrate intake is at the level for the glycogen storage threshold, at least in longer-term recovery. However, when the athlete's energy intake or food availability does not allow these amounts of carbohydrate to be consumed, the presence of protein in postexercise meals and snacks may enhance overall glycogen recovery.

Carbohydrate and Protein Synthesis

Net muscle protein balance is a result of relative changes in protein synthesis and protein degradation in the muscle cell, with an interchange between blood and intramuscular amino acid pools providing building blocks for protein synthesis. The goal of postexercise recovery is to achieve a relative increase in the ratio of protein breakdown and a decrease in protein breakdown in the muscle—which over time lead to a chronic improvement in net protein balance in the muscle and specific changes in the types of proteins within the muscle cell according to the exercise stimulus provided (for review, see Tipton and Wolfe 2001).

The consumption of a source of amino acids following resistance exercise causes net muscle protein synthesis, principally because of an increase in rates of muscle protein synthesis (Tipton et al. 1999). Postexercise carbohydrate intake stimulates insulin secretion and decreases the normal stimulation of muscle protein breakdown (Biolo et al. 1999). Theoretically, the combined intake of carbohydrate and amino acids should optimize net muscle protein synthesis, by changing both breakdown and synthesis in favorable directions. However, few studies have investigated this hypothesis. The available research suggests that added carbohydrate provides a small improvement in net protein balance compared with the intake of a source of amino acids alone (Miller et al. 2003). The response to carbohydrate intake also appears to be delayed, meaning that the best interaction might occur by staggering the intake of protein and amino acids until the peak of the carbohydrate-stimulated insulin action (Borsheim, Aarsland, et al. 2004). This hypothesis remains to be tested. Fewer studies have addressed nutritional interventions and postexercise protein balance following endurance exercise. However, there is some evidence that protein and carbohydrate intake enhances net protein balance following prolonged cycling and that early intake of recovery meals (1 hr) has greater benefits than delayed intake (3 hr) (Levenhagen et al. 2001).

There is some but not conclusive evidence that the co-ingestion of carbohydrate with protein can enhance the protein response to an exercise stimulus. Further work is needed to confirm these findings and to refine protocols including the timing and amount of carbohydrate that maximize this response. Importantly, end-point studies are needed in which greater outcomes of the training process—such as greater increases in muscle mass and strength or enhanced enzymatic adaptations—are demonstrated.

Other Effects on Recovery

Some studies have suggested that protein intake enhances functional aspects of postexercise recovery more than does carbohydrate alone. These end-points include indexes of muscle damage as well as the restoration of performance capacity itself. The consumption of a carbohydrate–protein drink immediately after a high-intensity workout by elite swimmers was reported to promote a more rapid recovery of plasma creatine kinase and lactate dehydrogenase concentrations during recovery than a glucose drink or water (Cade et al. 1991). Because the plasma levels of these enzymes were assumed to be markers of muscle damage, the protein–carbohydrate recovery drink was claimed to enhance the rate of postexercise muscle repair. Endurance-trained athletes who consumed two doses of a carbohydrate–protein drink (112 g carbohydrate and 41 g protein) after a glycogen-depleting treadmill run were reported to be able to run longer in a subsequent high-intensity run to exhaustion (541 vs. 446 s, $p < .05$) than when an energy-matched carbohydrate drink was consumed (153 g carbohydrate per serving). The recovery time between these bouts appeared to be 90 min, and the increased endurance was attributed to an enhancement of glycogen restoration with the protein–carbohydrate feeding, although this was not measured in any way (Niles et al. 2001).

A study involving team athletes investigated recovery in the 2.5 hr period separating a 70 min standardized session of intermittent exercise and a beep test of incremental intermittent exercise to fatigue (Maisey et al. 2003). Participants undertook the protocol on three occasions in a crossover designed study; between the two sessions of exercise they consumed either a placebo, a carbohydrate drink (1.5 g/kg BM), or an energy-matched carbohydrate (1.2 g/kg BM) and protein (0.3 g/kg BM) drink. Compared with the placebo trial, athletes ran longer on both the carbohydrate trial (11%) and carbohydrate–protein trial (14%). There was a wide coefficient of variation in the performance of the beep test (mean = 4%); the precision of estimates of mean finishing times was used rather than statistical significance to interpret the results of the study. Participants ran for 3.4% longer on the carbohydrate–protein trial than with carbohydrate only (95% confidence interval = 0.6-7.4%), giving a 37% chance of better performance in the carbohydrate–protein trial and a 63% chance that there would be no difference. Ratings of muscle soreness, perception of effort, and gastrointestinal comfort were collected for each trial; ratings of muscle soreness inversely tracked the differences in performance. Although it is difficult to interpret the results of this study in view of small participant numbers and low test reliability, these results at least encourage further research.

Postexercise recovery for many athletes and for many exercise situations involves a combination of goals such as

refueling and enhanced protein balance. Therefore, even if co-ingestion of nutrients does not enhance the outcome of a single process, it is likely that combining nutrients in postexercise meals and snacks is a clever strategy, because it allows each of the processes of recovery to proceed simultaneously.

PRACTICAL ISSUE

Strategies for High-Energy Eating in a Busy Day

Rowers and swimmers, particularly the adolescent males involved in these sports, have high energy requirements to support the fuel costs of a heavy training program, high levels of lean body mass, and the deposition of new body tissues associated with growth or specific resistance training programs. Although these requirements are fundamental to achieving training and competition goals, the eating practices of many athletes fall short of meeting energy and fuel needs. Factors that are implicated in the failure to achieve high energy needs include the following:

- A busy timetable or constant travel that limits access to food

- Inadequate time and opportunity to prepare or even to consume food

- Inability to eat before or during the hours of exercise because of the fear of gastrointestinal discomfort

- Depressed appetite following high-intensity training sessions or caused by the general fatigue accompanying a heavy exercise program

- The bulkiness and volume of carbohydrate-rich foods—particularly high-fiber choices—that limit total food intake

- Restrictions on variety of foods—for example, a fussy palate, food allergies or intolerances, overzealous interest in healthy eating

- Inadequate finances to purchase sufficient food or the specialized sport foods that can make high energy intakes more practical

Athletes with high energy requirements present an interesting challenge to the sports nutrition expert. Creativity is needed to find suitable foods and drinks to correspond with the athlete's busy timetable, food likes and dislikes, gastrointestinal comfort, appetite, and expense account. A comprehensive dietary history that explores the athlete's activities over a day and his or her usual food and fluid intake provides a basic assessment of the challenges impeding greater intake of energy or carbohydrate. A food diary is the next step and is often more revealing in identifying the real factors limiting present intake. Many athletes are unaware of their true eating practices and overestimate the number of times they eat each day or the size of food servings they consume. A food diary can allow both the athlete and the sports dietitian to identify long periods in the day without food intake, the occasions and activities that limit access to food, or the variations in appetite and gastrointestinal comfort over the day. Identifying the specific challenges allows the sports nutrition expert to develop a targeted plan of eating and drinking, along with behavioral changes that the athlete must make to guarantee that the plan can be implemented.

The typical issues that underpin the achievement of a high energy intake are summarized in table 6.5, together with guidelines that may assist an athlete to increase intake of total energy and important nutrients such as protein and carbohydrate. Many of these guidelines pertain to strategies that make food choices more compact and energy-dense or that increase the availability of food in the athlete's environment and lifestyle. One issue of particular interest is the timing and frequency of food intake, because there is some recognition that athletes with high energy intakes do not eat "three square meals a day." Rather, they adopt a pattern of constant meals and snacks, grazing over the day.

It appears that eating a series of small meals and snacks over the course of a day is a practical strategy that allows increased energy intake while also reducing the gastric discomfort of infrequent large meals. Strategic eating before, during, and after training sessions is a practice gaining much support from sports dietitians and nutritionists. Not only does this eating increase the total energy and nutrient intake for a day, but it may enhance training outcomes by matching the fuel needs of workouts or promoting more efficient recovery.

PRACTICAL ISSUE

Recovery Eating: Different Needs for Different Sports

Recovery has become a buzzword used ubiquitously throughout the sporting world, and principles of recovery nutrition have been prepared with an almost "one size fits all" approach. In fact, recovery can encompass a variety of different priorities or goals according to the individual athlete and his or her specific training or competition session. Our current approach to recovery nutrition could be enhanced, both in education programs or practical nutrition activities, by better recognizing the specificity of postexercise nutrition goals and teaching athletes to be more strategic about their postworkout eating practices.

The specificity of recovery nutrition goals is determined by a number of factors, including:

- The physiological or homeostatic challenges caused by the workout (e.g., fuel depletion, dehydration)
- Muscle damage or protein catabolism
- The goals associated with enhanced performance or adaptation to the exercise session
- The duration of the period between workouts
- Opportunities for energy and nutrient intake during the recovery period. Such opportunities can be lim-

ited both by food availability, as well as the athlete's total energy requirements and additional nutritional goals.

Table 6.g in the appendix summarizes a range of recovery scenarios that are commonly seen in sport, acknowledging the presence or absence of the need for a proactive approach to certain recovery goals and whether the athlete has a large or restricted energy budget with which to achieve nutrient needs. This approach does not completely account for the sophistication with which recovery situations can be individualized in theory, but it represents an improvement on the previous generic approach to recovery eating. It is of some concern to note that even by making this level of differentiation, we already challenge the boundaries of our current knowledge of sports nutrition to develop eating strategies that can be underpinned by rigorous science.

Many athletes face many practical challenges that restrict their ability to consume important recovery nutrients in the period after exercise. These challenges include the following:

- Fatigue—interfering with the athlete's ability or motivation to obtain or eat food
- Loss of appetite following high-intensity exercise
- Limited access to (suitable) foods at exercise venue
- The need to pay attention to other postexercise commitments (e.g., meetings with coaches, drug tests, equipment maintenance, warm-down activities)
- Cultural and social practices of postexercise nutrition (e.g., excessive alcohol intake)

It is difficult to provide exact guidelines for recovery eating, particularly because of the paucity of data regarding postexercise protein metabolism. We are unable to provide clear guidelines for the ideal type or amount of protein that should be consumed or for the timing of intake of various snacks or meals containing protein so that plasma amino acid concentrations peak at an appropriate time. Guidelines for carbohydrate intake can only be made on the basis of fuel requirements and may need to consider issues of pre-exercise carbohydrate intake if future research confirms that optimal recovery eating should start in the pre-exercise phase. It is presumed that these guidelines will also account for any benefits that carbohydrate intake may provide in enhancing net protein synthesis. However, timing or type of carbohydrate intake to optimize the insulin response in relation to protein recovery is not presently known.

The key exercise sessions for which optimal recovery is needed are as follows:

- Training or competition sessions that cause significant muscle glycogen depletion
- Exercise sessions undertaken to promote major functional adaptations in the muscle (e.g., quality training sessions, threshold training, interval sessions)

Table 6.5   Guidelines for Achieving High Energy Intakes

Issue	Strategies
Meal spacing	• A plan of frequent meals and snacks will maximize available eating time each day within gastric comfort. This should be programmed rather than haphazard. • A food diary may help to identify the athlete's actual intake rather than perceived intake and note the occasions or situations in which the athlete is unable to adhere to his or her plan of frequent meals and snacks. • Creative solutions should be found to allow food to be consumed in conjunction with other activities such as traveling, working, or studying; having medical or physiotherapy treatment; and attending team meetings or education sessions. • Carbohydrate should be consumed during prolonged exercises to provide additional fuel as well as contribute to total daily energy intake. • A postexercise snack providing carbohydrate and protein will enhance recovery as well as contribute to total daily energy intake.
Food availability	• The athlete is often faced with a chaotic and overcommitted lifestyle. Good skills in time management should see the athlete using quieter periods to undertake food shopping and meal preparation activities so that food is available during hectic periods. • The challenge of postexercise fatigue can also be overcome by preparing meals and snacks in advance. Such meals or snacks may just need to be reheated or served straight from the fridge as soon as the athlete returns from the session. • The traveling athlete should take a supply of portable and nonperishable snacks that can be easily prepared and eaten: e.g., breakfast cereal and powdered milk, cereal bars, sport bars, liquid meal supplements, dried fruit and nuts, and creamed rice. Some of these foods should be organized to suit the identified eating times for the day, whereas a nonperishable supply of "emergency foods" should be kept for times when the athlete is unavoidably detained from his or her normal eating routine. • Even at home, the athlete will need to be prepared to have snacks and light meals available during busy times of the day. Additional ideas, according to food storage and preparation resources, include fruit, yogurt, and sandwiches. • Specialized products such as sport drinks, sport gels, and sport bars provide a practical form of carbohydrate during exercise, whereas sport bars and liquid meal supplements provide an accessible form of carbohydrate and protein for postexercise recovery. Products may be available during competition events; however, in most training situations, athletes will need to provide their own supplies.
Appetite management and gastric comfort	• Gastric discomfort or limitations can be reduced by a pattern of small frequent meals rather than several large meals each day. • Energy-containing drinks such as liquid meal supplements, flavored milk, fruit smoothies, sport drinks, soft drinks, and juices provide a low-bulk way to consume energy and other important nutrients while meeting fluid needs. • Meals and snacks should be based on compact and energy-dense foods, including sugar-rich foods. • Although fiber intake is important in a healthy diet, excessive intake of high-fiber foods may limit total energy intake or lead to gastrointestinal discomfort. It may be necessary to moderate intake of whole-grain or fiber-enriched foods. • Appetite suppression may be overcome by presenting foods in small or easy-to-eat forms rather than forms requiring considerable cutting and chewing: e.g., fruit and sandwiches served as "finger-foods" or meats served in bite-size pieces in a stir-fry or kebabs rather than in large slabs. • The postexercise menu should consider environmental conditions and athlete's physical condition. For example, heat and dehydration may be matched by cool and liquid-based choices such as fruit smoothies, yogurt, or ice cream. By contrast, in cold conditions, warm soup, toasted sandwiches, or pizza may be a more appetizing choice.

- Resistance training sessions undertaken to promote gain in muscle size and strength
- Training or competition sessions that cause significant dehydration

It is assumed that athletes undertaking these sessions will be undertaking further sessions within 24 hr and need to recover to meet their subsequent goals. The simplest schema is to divide workouts into endurance and quality training and resistance training. Further subdivisions can be made on the basis of the athlete's energy requirements (high or restricted) and hydration status (mild or moderate to severe dehydration). The Australian Institute of Sport has attempted to provide athletes and coaches with education messages that integrate recovery guidelines (see table 6.h in the chapter appendix). We look forward to the results of future studies that will help to refine these guidelines further and allow more differentiation based on specific recovery needs.

chapter 7

Sprinting and Jumping

An athlete's ability to propel his body forward, upward, or sometimes in both directions at the same time has been of interest as far back as records of competitive sport exist. Sprinting was the original sport in the ancient Olympics and remained one of the key items of this competition as its program of events developed. In these ancient times, the title of fastest man on earth was bestowed on the winner of a race from one end of the Olympic stadium to the other, over a distance known as the stade or stadion (~190 m). The Olympiad—the period of the subsequent 4 years—was named after the winner of this sprint. In the present day, the 100 m race is the blue-ribbon event on the Olympic program and has evolved to include electronic timing and photo finishes that enable competitors to be separated to a thousandth of a second. Athletes who win this race receive the modern version of fame and fortune. The long jump was also part of sporting competitions in ancient times, being one of the events undertaken within the pentathlon. In ancient times, jumpers carried hand weights *(halteres)*

to increase their momentum and released these weights in the sand pit before landing.

This chapter covers the nutritional characteristics of sprint and jumping events of the track-and-field program that share the general feature of involving the development of speed over periods of up to 1 min. The track events are the 100, 200, and 400 m sprints and the hurdles (100 and 400 m for women, 110 and 400 m for men). Current world records for these events are summarized in table 7.1. The jumping events (long jump, triple jump, pole vault, and high jump) share some characteristics with sprints, because the development of kinetic energy via running speed in the approach to the jump is an important component of performance in the first three of these disciplines. Other events that are considered to fit within the scope of this chapter are the team relays (4 × 100 m and 4 × 400 m events) and the combined track-and-field events of heptathlon for women (7 individual events) and decathlon for men (10 individual events).

Table 7.1 World Records in Sprint Events

Event	World-record holder	World record (s)
100 m	M—Asafa Powell F—Florence Griffith-Joyner	9.77 10.49
200 m	M—Michael Johnson F—Florence Griffith-Joyner	19.32 21.23
400 m	M—Michael Johnson F—Marita Koch	43.18 47.60
110 m hurdles 100 m hurdles	M—Xiang Liu F—Yordanka Donkova	12.88 12.21
400 m hurdles	M—Kevin Young F—Yuliya Pechonkina	46.78 52.34

Unfortunately, because the major improvements in these sports over the past decades have occurred through developments in technique, training, and technology (competition surfaces, starting blocks, shoes), the nutritional issues of training and competition are less well developed than in other sports. As a result, this chapter is brief, and some of the recommendations or guidelines will need to be derived from sound theory or from studies of other sports, rather than specific research on track-and-field athletes. Some aspects of the preparation for track-and-field events, such as interval and resistance training, are further developed in the pursuant chapters on team and racket sports (chapters 8-10) and strength and power sports (chapter 11). The reader is directed to these chapters for insights on nutritional strategies to enhance the outcome of resistance and interval training programs, with the caveat that these athletes have somewhat different goals and competition outcomes.

Competition

Success in sprinting and jumping events involves various combinations of speed (a product of stride rate and stride length), fatigue resistance, and technique. A sprint is generally broken down into the phases of reaction at the start, acceleration phase, the phase of maximum speed, deceleration phase, and the finish (Williams and Gandy 1994). Fast reaction times, explosive power, and flexibility allow maximal velocities of up to 12 m/s and 11 m/s to be reached within 50 to 70 m by elite men and 40 to 60 m by elite women, respectively. In addition to an increase in speed endurance, the longer sprint events require the sprinter to master the technique of being able to run bends. The hurdling events call for special characteristics of strength and rhythm to allow the athlete to maintain his or her stride pattern between hurdles.

A shared characteristic of sprint events is that they are carried out at power outputs or exercise intensities that far exceed those needed to elicit maximal aerobic capacity. The power for these supramaximal events is derived mainly from the high-energy phosphates (adenosine triphosphate and creatine phosphate) and from anaerobic glycolysis derived from muscle glycogen stores. The metabolic requirements of such events have been best studied in relation to the 100 to 400 m sprints, but even then, the literature related to field studies of these events is limited.

In one study, seven male sprinters were monitored while sprinting over a variety of distances from 40 to 100 m on the track, with muscle biopsies being taken before and after the sprints (Hirvonen et al. 1987). Phosphocreatine content of the muscle decreased rapidly over the first couple of seconds, with stores being depleted within 5 to 6 s. It appeared from the constant rate of lactate accumulation that the contribution of glycogenolysis remained constant over the 100 m distance. In another study of eight elite male and female sprinters, it was estimated that anaerobic glycolysis contributed about 65% to 70% of total metabolic energy for a 100 m race (Locatelli and Arsac 1995). Race analysis

of the 100 m shows that maximal velocities, once attained, can typically only be held for 20 to 30 m by men and 15 to 20 m by women before deceleration occurs. There are several likely causes of the decline in speeds seen in most sprinters over the last 10 to 20 m of the race. Mechanical limitations include air resistance, failure of neuromuscular coordination, deceleration caused by the grounding foot, and the change in body position over the race (Nicholas 2000). Metabolically, the depletion of phosphocreatine stores appears to limit power output (Hirvonen et al. 1987). Despite a plentiful supply of glycogen and a subthreshold accumulation of lactate and H^+ ions, anaerobic glycolysis alone does not appear to be rapid enough to sustain the high rates of adenosine triphosphate utilization needed to achieve or maintain peak sprinting speeds. It is also possible that the accumulation of by-products of metabolism, such as inorganic phosphate, directly inhibits the cross-bridge recycling between actin and myosin filaments (Hultman et al. 1987).

The 400 m race has also been monitored in a sequential protocol (Hirvonen et al. 1992). National-caliber sprinters were asked to produce their best times for this distance on a track (~52 s), with splits being recorded for each 100 m. On subsequent occasions they were required to run 100, 200, and 300 m at the same speeds as these splits, with biopsies being taken before and after each run. Phosphocreatine content of the muscle was halved by the end of the first 100 m and depleted at the end of the 400 m. Muscle lactate concentrations rose over the 400 m, with maximal rates of accumulation in blood and muscle occurring between 100 and 300 m and a decline in the rate of glycolysis occurring over the last 100 m. Maximal concentrations of lactate in the muscle were reached after 35 s of sprinting, with maximal blood concentrations being achieved after about 27 s. Running speeds declined after 200 m, with a dramatic decrease over the last 100 m. This decline in running speed was associated with the low phosphocreatine concentrations, but particularly over the last portion of the race, with a reduced rate of glycogenolysis despite ample glycogen reserves (Hirvonen et al. 1992). It has been proposed that factors limiting the performance of the 400 m include the impairment of both glycolysis and the excitation–contraction process caused by the accumulation of H^+ ions (Hultman et al. 1987). Lacour and coworkers (1990) observed that postrace lactate concentrations following a 400 m race in top-level athletes were correlated with performance times, suggesting that good performers must be able to produce and tolerate high levels of lactate. In this study, mean values for postrace blood concentrations of lactate were ~20 mmol/L (Lacour et al. 1990). In addition, there is speculation that rising concentrations of ammonia in the muscle and blood might lead to central nervous system fatigue. Laboratory experiments on nonmotorized treadmills have confirmed the metabolic picture seen in these few field-based experiments (for further review of limitations to sprint performance, see Nicholas 2000 and Williams and Gandy 1994).

The International Association of Athletics Federations (IAAF), previously known as the International Amateur

Athletic Federation, is the international governing body for track-and-field events. The major competitions on the calendar for elite sprinters and jumpers are World Championships and Indoor World Championships, the Olympic Games, and meets on the professional circuit such as the Golden League and Grand Prix series. Some events involve a one-off race or straight final over a single day or night meet—for example, the Golden League and Grand Prix meets. By contrast, victory in the sprints and jump events at World Championships and Olympic Games is decided by a multiday program involving a series of heats, semifinals, and finals. The program of sprints, jumps, and combined events at the 2004 Athens Olympic Games is summarized in table 7.2 and illustrates that the winners of the sprint events must sustain their performance for three or four races over a 3- to 7-day period.

On some programs even within a multiday meet, the athlete must compete twice within the same session—for

Table 7.2 Timetable of Sprints, Jumps, and Combined Events on the 2004 Athens Olympic Games Track-and-Field Program

Day	AM session	PM session
2	100 m hurdles—W heptathlon Triple jump—1st round High jump—W heptathlon 100 m—W 1st round	Shot put—W heptathlon 100 m—W quarterfinal High jump—M 1st round 200 m—W heptathlon 400 m—M 1st round
3	400 m hurdles—W 1st round 400 m—W 1st round Long jump –W heptathlon 100 m—M 1st round	Javelin throw—W heptathlon Pole vault—W 1st round 100 m—M quarterfinal 100 m—W semifinal Triple jump—W 1st round 400 m—M semifinal 100 m—W final 800 m—W heptathlon
4		High jump—M final 100 m hurdles—W 1st round Triple jump—M final 100 m—M semifinal 400 m hurdles—W semifinal 400 m—W semifinal 100 m hurdles—W quarterfinal 100 m—M final
5	100 m—M decathlon Long jump—M decathlon 200 m—W 1st round Shot put—M decathlon	High jump—M decathlon Triple jump—W final 100 m hurdles—W semifinal 400 m hurdles—M 1st round 200 m—W quarterfinal 400 m—M final 400 m—M decathlon
6	110 m hurdles—M decathlon 100 m hurdles—M 1st round 200 m—M 1st round Discus throw—M decathlon Pole vault—M decathlon	Javelin throw—M decathlon Long jump—M 1st round 200 m—M quarterfinal Pole vault—W final 400 m hurdles—M semifinal 200 m—W semifinal 100 m hurdles—W final 400 m—W final 1,500 m—M decathlon

(continued)

Table 7.2   *(continued)*

Day	AM session	PM session
7		Pole vault—M 1st round Long jump—W 1st round 110 m hurdles—M quarterfinal 200 m—M semifinal 200 m—W final
8		High jump—W 1st round Long jump—M final 110 m hurdles—M semifinal 4 × 100 m relay—W 1st round 200 m—M final
9		Pole vault—M final Long jump—W final 4 × 100 m—M 1st round 4 × 400—W 1st round 4 × 400—M 1st round 110 m hurdles—M final 4 × 100 m—W final
10		High jump—W final 4 × 100 m—M final 4 × 400—W final 4 × 400—M final

M = men; W = women. Events are listed in program order.

example, semifinals and finals of the 100 m sprint (see table 7.2). This is a particular feature of the combined events in which the athlete undertakes three to five events on a single day (men's decathlon day 1: 100 m, long jump, shot put, high jump, and 400 m; day 2: 110 m hurdles, discus, pole vault, javelin, and 1,500 m; and women's heptathlon day 1: 100 m hurdles, high jump, shot put; day 2: 200 m, long jump, javelin, and 800 m). Jumping events may involve a qualifying round and final or a straight final program. However, within each session, each competitor must undertake a number of jumps, performing either a set number of jumps to determine the winner of the long jump and triple jump or following an elimination protocol to decide the winner of the high jump and pole vault. Some athletes may compete in more than one event across a track-and-field program—for example, the combinations of 100 and 200 m sprints, the 200 and 400 m double, or an individual sprint and relay. At the World Championship and Olympic level, exceptional athletes such as Americans Carl Lewis and Marion Jones have competed in five events on the same program (100 m, 200 m, long jump, 4 × 100 m relay, 4 × 400 m relay). Competing in a variety of events is more common at less elite levels of competition.

Even where athletes compete in single events, they may be part of a circuit or competition series in which a meet is scheduled every 3 to 14 days. Such is the nature of competition on the lucrative professional circuit in Europe or track meets within the National Collegiate Athletics Association (NCAA) season in the United States. Although athletes aim

to perform at their best on each occasion, this competition is generally used to help athletes peak for the major events of the season, such as regional and divisional championships in the NCAA or the World Cup Championship, World Championships, or Olympic Games.

Training

According to the characteristics of their events, sprinters and jumpers train for speed, speed endurance, power, technique, and flexibility. The training program is highly periodized to allow the athlete to peak for important competitions as well as to achieve benchmarks for each season toward long-term progress. The year may be arranged into a single-periodized or double-periodized program to suit the number of times that the athlete wishes to peak. Each competitive cycle is broken down into shorter phases and, finally, the weekly microcycle. At the elite level, sprinters and jumpers undertake one or two training sessions per day. Training activities include drills for starting action (e.g., squats, leg presses, reaction exercises), acceleration (e.g., power cleans, uphill acceleration, bounding for five strides, harness work, and tire towing), knee lift or pick-up phase (long bounding strides, rebound strides over hurdles, depth jumps), maximal velocity (towed running and down-slope sprinting, intervals such as 4-6 × 20-40 m with flying start), and holding form for the last 20 m (weight training with sets of 10-20 repetitions, fast endurance runs of 4 × 120 m with 8-10 min recovery). Williams and Gandy (1994) have provided examples of activities from each of these training techniques that could be undertaken by a 100 m sprinter to enhance various aspects of a race.

A variety of metabolic and functional adaptations are achieved by each of the training techniques undertaken by sprinters and jumpers. Resistance training is undertaken to increase the size and function of muscle mass; the principles and outcomes of this type of training are reviewed in chapter 11. The outcomes of speed or interval training are to enhance maximum power output during the initial part of a sprint, increase the total amount of work achieved in a sprint, and prolong the duration for which high-intensity work can be sustained. In one study involving 8 weeks of sprint training, peak power during a 30 s treadmill sprint on a nonmotorized treadmill was increased by 12%, with a 6% increase in overall work (Nevill et al. 1989). This laboratory protocol is considered to be similar to a 200 m sprint. The sprint enhancement was associated with a 20% increase in the contribution of anaerobic glycolysis to adenosine triphosphate regeneration and a concomitant increase in muscle lactate concentration. No changes were observed in phosphocreatine or aerobic metabolism (Nevill et al. 1989). According to the review by Nicholas (2000), the increased capacity for anaerobic glycolysis achieved by sprint training may be explained by a variety

of adaptations; these include an increase in proportion of type IIa muscle fibers, an increase in the activity of the rate limiting enzyme phosphofructokinase (PFK), an increased efflux of H^+ from the cell, and enhanced muscle buffering capacity. Changes in the sodium–potassium pump, improved potassium regulation, and other factors that influence muscle contraction and development of tension are also involved.

Plyometric training, which involves drills of bounding, jumping, and hopping, is undertaken to achieve a number of goals related to the elastic properties of the muscle. These goals include increasing explosive power, learning to better attenuate ground forces, and increasing the stiffness of the muscle so that it tolerates greater stretch loads. Muscle stiffness enhances explosiveness and the body's ability to store and reuse the elastic energy from running and jumping. Various combinations of jumping (two-leg landings), hopping (one-foot landings), and bounding (alternate-leg takeoffs) are classified according to the number of ground contacts and the horizontal or vertical displacement of the body's center of gravity. Specific sessions of plyometric training are typically undertaken two to three times per weekly microcycle, depending on the sport and the phase of training. Low-amplitude drills may also be built into the warm-ups for other sessions. Because of the high neural demand of such training, it is generally not undertaken

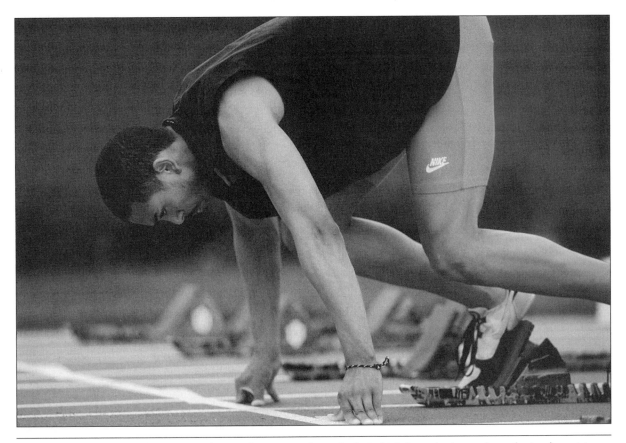

According to the phase of training and type of event, workouts include high-intensity intervals on the track, resistance training, flexibility work, technical drills, and plyometrics.

when the athlete is fatigued, except for events such as the longer sprints (e.g., 400 m and 400 m hurdles) where speed and power endurance are required. Plyometric training is often undertaken within a resistance or speed training session but is undertaken early in the session or carefully integrated into the session according to the athlete's age and training status.

Physique and Physiology

Joe Douglas has been on to me about my weight. He thinks I'm too big and that the excess baggage is slowing me down. . . . I stepped on the scale and I registered two hundred pounds. . . . So as of this morning, the fight is on. Me against the pounds. I need to be at one-eighty-five or below. . . . I even wrote a memo on my computer, printed it out, and taped it to the door of the refrigerator, as a constant reminder. There is nothing else there, just that memo to Ruth, who has been with me for years, cooking and cleaning, and to myself, so we can't possibly miss it.

TO: Ruth and Carl

FR: Carl

Re: revised new diet

Breakfast: Grapefruit juice

              20 almonds

              Vitamins

Lunch: Vegetable juice

              Sandwich

Snack   Fresh fruit/vegetable juice

Dinner   Fresh vegetable juice

              Dinner salad

              Main course

              Vitamins

Knowing me, I won't be able to stay away from the scale. I'll probably be on it two or three times a day, keeping an eye on the progress until I'm back where I need to be. I don't think it will take more than two or three weeks.

Carl Lewis from One More Victory Lap
(Lewis and Marx 1996, pp. 92-93)

Gone are the long locks now, joining the teeth braces, belly button ring, earrings, watch, bracelet—anything that might add a tiny bit of weight and slow down Jana Pittman a fraction of a millisecond. . . . "I'm running with nothing but a light pair of socks, a light pair of shoes, a tiny body suit. I made the ultimate sacrifice yesterday and went and cut all my hair off, which was shattering." Pittman kept the chopped-off hair, which reached halfway down her back, took it with her and weighed it—another 400 g in weight gone.

"Pittman shaves for gold," The Melbourne Age *newspaper, Australia, August 5, 2004, p. 12. World 400 m hurdles champion Jana Pittman prepares for the Athens Olympic Games.*

Power-to-weight ratio is an important characteristic in sports where athletes are required to move their own body mass. For sprints, the emphasis is on increasing the power side of this ratio. Typically, sprinters carry a large lean body mass, with high levels of muscularity in both their upper and lower bodies that is capable of producing explosive power over short distances. Resistance training programs are undertaken to increase this muscularity and enhance speed and strength. There is also some consideration of the weight side of the balance, with sprinters achieving a leanness and muscular definition that they often like to showcase during the warm-up or postrace "parade." Low levels of body fat and concern for total body mass become more important in longer sprints or where the athlete must achieve vertical movement against gravity (e.g., high jumps, hurdles, and pole vault). Although many sprinters and jumpers achieve their leanness and preferred racing weight as a natural consequence of genetics and training, others undertake deliberate weight loss programs or at least make this a focus of their eating plans.

Body height, or more particularly leg length, plays a role in sprint performance by influencing stride length. Hurdlers need to be tall, or at least have proportionally long legs, to aid hurdle clearance. Height provides an important advantage in high jump because it means that the jumper's center of gravity, which must be raised above the bar to successfully complete a jump, is already high. Elite female jumpers can typically clear their body height by a maximum of 25 cm, whereas men can jump 50 cm above their body height. Athletes who compete in the combined events of heptathlon and decathlon must achieve a physique that allows them to be competitive over a range of sports with different biomechanical and physiological characteristics. A study of elite female heptathletes by Houtkooper and colleagues (2001) found these athletes to have low levels of body fat and high levels of muscularity.

Lifestyle and Culture

Sprinters tend to be outgoing and flamboyant. This is shown by the rituals seen at high-level meets where the men strut around the track—often with bared torsos—during the warm-up or postrace laps and where the women adorn themselves with jewelry and painted nails. Sprinters' emphasis on muscularity aligns them with the nutritional culture of the strength and power athletes described in chapter 11. As a consequence, most are focused on protein intake and the use of nutritional supplements, and they are prey to information (and advertising hype) from the body-building industry. Such issues are discussed in greater detail in chapter 11. Unfortunately, because specific research on nutritional interventions for sprinters and jumpers is lacking, it is difficult to provide strong recommendations to guide the dietary practices of these athletes. When such information is available, however, it will need to be communicated with marketing and presentation styles that can compete against existing messages and successfully capture the athletes' attention.

Dietary Surveys

Historical accounts document some unusual dietary beliefs by sprinters throughout the ages. According to books on the ancient Olympics, the evolution of special eating practices by athletes can be traced back to these times (Perrottet 2004; Zissomou 2004). During the first century of Olympic competition, athletes apparently ate the typical Greek diet of the time, consisting of bread, cheese, olives, olive oil, vegetables, fruits, honeyed cakes (Perrottet 2004), and small quantities of fish and meat (Zissomou 2004). Information from the 5th and 6th centuries BC describes the development of special eating patterns by individual athletes designed to achieve better results. Charmis, a sprinter from Sparta, espoused eating nothing but figs, whereas Dromeus of Stymphalos won two footraces in 480 BC following an all-meat diet (Perrottet 2004). A high-protein diet became all the rage among many athletes after this time and, in combination with harder training, caused a massive change in body mass and strength and an increased need for sleep and rest. The hours associated with training, eating, and sleep became so great that these athletes were not able to undertake other activities—thus becoming the first professional athletes. The specialization of medical gymnastics—the development of specialists in medicine and nutrition related to sport performance—also began in these times (Zissomou 2004).

There has been little formal investigation of the current dietary practices of sprinters and jumpers. The few available dietary surveys of sprinters, jumpers, and multievent athletes are summarized in the appendix to this chapter (table 7.a). The most comprehensive of these studies provides an overview of the dietary practices of an elite group of female heptathletes and tracks their interest in eating for performance, hydration status, competition planning, and supplement use (Mullins et al. 2001). It is impossible to draw any major conclusions from these studies about widespread nutrition beliefs and practices of sprinters and jumpers. There is anecdotal evidence that many sprinters are focused on muscular power and strength rather than fuel needs and share the nutritional interests of weight-training athletes. These interests include high-protein diets and supplements that are promoted to enhance muscular development. Such concerns are addressed in more detail in chapter 11. There is an urgent need for comprehensive dietary surveys of track athletes.

Nutritional Issues and Challenges

The nutritional issues faced by sprinters and jumpers have not been as well developed for research or education activities as the characteristics of other sports. Nevertheless, it is possible to identify a number of challenges that arise in training and competition; these issues are summarized in the highlight box on page 176. Because there is a lack of specialized or sport-specific information related to many aspects of nutrition for sprinters or jumpers, this chapter tackles only a small number of issues in some detail. The reader is directed to chapter 1 for an overview of the principles of the general nutritional strategies that could be applied to track-and-field athletes. Some of the topics or themes that are regarded as important by sprinters and jumpers are addressed in greater detail in other chapters, as follows:

- Eating to reduce weight and body fat: chapter 4, including tables 4.3 through 4.5
- Eating to gain muscle mass and strength: chapter 11, the first practical issue
- Protein needs for strength and power athletes: chapter 11, including the first research topic on timing and type of protein intake
- Nutrition for the traveling athlete: chapter 10, the first practical issue

The information provided in this book on the first three of these topics may contradict the current beliefs and practices of sprinters and jumpers. For example, low-carbohydrate diets and fat loss supplements are likely to be popular strategies used for weight loss by some contemporary athletes, and there is a large range of supplements promoted to enhance the gain of muscle mass. Neither of these approaches is considered optimal or necessary to reduce body weight or fat. It appears that many sprint athletes also believe in the need for high-protein diets and specialized protein supplements. The evolution of the science and practice regarding protein needs of athletes is discussed in more detail in chapter 11. This summary will show that current opinion does not support the need for high intakes of protein (>2 $g \cdot kg^{-1} \cdot day^{-1}$) by strength and power athletes (Tipton and Wolfe 2004). Because dietary surveys of other strength and power athletes show that varied eating patterns based on moderate to high energy intakes can provide protein amounts of up to 2.0 $g \cdot kg^{-1} \cdot day^{-1}$, sprinters do not need protein-only supplements or protein-focused diets that exclude other foods or energy sources. However, there is new information suggesting that the strategic timing of protein intake in relation to training may provide an effective strategy to promote gains in muscle mass and strength. The current knowledge is discussed in greater detail in chapter 11 but needs to be studied in relation to performance outcomes in sprint-based sports.

Common Nutritional Issues Arising in Sprint and Jump Events

Physique Issues

- Increasing and maintaining high levels of lean mass for power within ideal body mass
- Maintaining low body fats levels to optimize power-to-weight ratio

Training Issues

- Consuming adequate energy intake to maintain high level of body mass and lean body mass and to optimize gains in lean body mass achieved through resistance training
- Consuming adequate energy intake to maintain ideal body mass and lean body mass; optimizing gains in lean body mass achieved through resistance training
- Consuming adequate carbohydrate to provide fuel for resistance and sprint (interval) training sessions and to optimize net protein synthesis response to training; consuming carbohydrate at strategic times to optimize these goals
- Considering creatine supplementation to optimize the response to resistance and sprint (interval) training
- Judiciously using supplements and sport foods with focus on those with proven benefits or an ability to assist the athlete to meet nutritional goals
- In sports with antidoping code, avoiding supplements with high risk of contamination with banned substances

Competition Issues

- Preevent meal
- Between-event intake for sports with multiple rounds or races: developing strategies to keep the athlete well hydrated, well fueled, and comfortable
- Eating while traveling to major competitions and on race circuit

Carbohydrate Needs

Interval training, either on the track or with resistance exercises, can draw heavily on muscle glycogen reserves. High-intensity sprints involve high rates of utilization of muscle glycogen for anaerobic glycolysis. Muscle glycogen has been found to decline by 20% to 25% from resting levels during an all-out 30 s sprint undertaken on a nonmotorized treadmill, with type II fibers having a greater presprint concentration and a greater decline in glycogen content than type I fibers (Greenhaff et al. 1994). A single 6 s cycle sprint can deplete glycogen content by 14% of resting levels (Gaitanos et al. 1993). Sprint performance is generally not considered to be limited by muscle glycogen availability (Vandenberghe et al. 1995) unless glycogen concentration falls below a critical threshold of around 25 mmol/kg wet weight muscle (Nicholas 2000). However, Jacobs and coworkers reported a 10% to 15% reduction in the performance of maximal exercise associated with such levels of glycogen depletion (Jacobs, Kaiser, et al. 1982). The recovery of muscle glycogen stores between training sessions may be compounded in the case of resistance and plyometric training, because the eccentric component causes muscle damage and delayed glycogen resynthesis.

Research on the effect of dietary intake on the performance of a single sprint is conflicting. According to a review by Maughan and others, dietary strategies that enhance muscle carbohydrate availability sometimes, but not consistently, enhance the performance of maximal exercise, although low-carbohydrate diets have a more consistent effect in reducing capacity for such high-intensity work (Maughan et al. 1997). For example, in one investigation, participants increased power output by 9% during a 30 s Wingate cycling test when they consumed a diet providing 50% of energy as carbohydrate compared with a low intake (5% of dietary energy) of carbohydrate (Langfort et al. 1997). By contrast, other studies have failed to find differences in performance of a single high-intensity exercise bout when carbohydrate intake was altered to manipulate muscle glycogen content (Hargreaves et al. 1997, 1998). Wooten and Williams (1984) reported that carbohydrate failed to enhance power output either during a 30 s cycling test or a second Wingate test performed 15 min later.

In studies where the manipulation of carbohydrate intake enhances the outcome of high-intensity performance, benefits may be more related to changes in blood acid–base balance than to muscle glycogen availability (Maughan et al. 1997). In particular, a low-carbohydrate diet that is high in protein results in metabolic acidosis that may limit maximal exercise by reducing the rate of efflux of lactate and H+ ions from the exercising muscle. This effect has been seen in protocols of high-intensity exercise lasting 1 to 6 min rather than supramaximal exercise of 60 s or less; nevertheless, it may have some relevance to 400 m events in which the impairment of anaerobic glycolysis is associated with a performance decline. Overall, there is no strong evidence for direct benefits of a high carbohydrate intake on the performance of a single sprint race compared with a mixed diet. However, the athlete is advised against a low-carbohydrate diet that may cause prerace glycogen content to be depleted below critical levels.

Investigations of the metabolic profile of repeated sprints show that muscle glycogen content can be substantially depleted by such a work bout, although there is a decline in anaerobic glycolysis and increased reliance on aerobic metabolism as the sprints progress. For example, in a cycling protocol of 10 × 6 s cycling sprints with 30 s recovery, muscle glycogen was reduced by 14% after the first bout and 36% after the 10 sprints (Gaitanos et al. 1993). The effects of dietary carbohydrate stores on prolonged bouts of repeated sprints have been investigated in several studies. Balsom and coworkers exposed participants to 48 hr of a high- or low-carbohydrate diet before an intermittent protocol involving 6 s cycling bouts at 30 s intervals (Balsom, Gaitanos, et al. 1999). The low-carbohydrate preparation reduced glycogen concentrations in the vastus lateralis by at least 50% of the values achieved in the high-carbohydrate treatment and was associated with a dramatic reduction in the work performed in both a ~10 min protocol and a ~30 min protocol of these intervals.

In another study, highly trained cyclists undertook a glycogen depletion ride and 36 hr of either a high (80-85% of energy) or low (5-10% of energy) carbohydrate diet before performing a protocol involving repeated 60 s cycling sprints with 3 min active recovery (Rockwell et al. 2003). There was a superior performance in the high-carbohydrate trial, with participants completing a mean of 14.3 versus 10.4 sprints and increasing exercise time by 37% (57.5 vs. 42 min). Although there was no difference in the peak power output in the first sprint or the time taken before sprints reached a 15% fatigue index (reduction of sprint pedaling revolutions by 15%), there was an 87% enhancement of the time from 15% fatigue to the cessation of the protocol at 30% fatigue. The high-carbohydrate diet was associated with higher preexercise glycogen content than the restricted carbohydrate intake but a similar rate of glycogen utilization during exercise and overall glycogen decline (~40% of resting levels), leaving

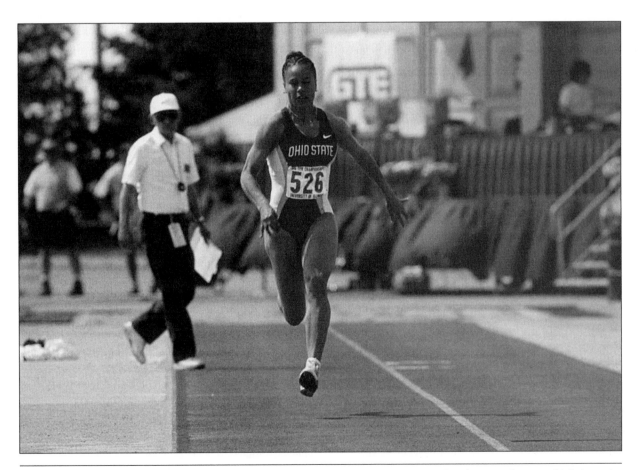

Because many situations, particularly in training, require the sprinter or jumper to undertake more than one high-intensity effort within the session, the carbohydrate requirements for repeated sprint performance must be considered.

muscle glycogen higher at fatigue in the high-carbohydrate trial. Baseline muscle content of creatine phosphate and adenosine triphosphate was similar between trials and declined to a similar extent in both trials at the point of fatigue. There was a trend for a smaller decline over time in the calcium release from sarcoplasmic reticulum (SR) with the high-carbohydrate trial. Limitations to the performance of repeated sprints in this study could not be explained by either depletion of creatine phosphate and limitations of the phosphagen system or the achievement of critically low glycogen content. However, because measurements were made only of the total muscle content of glycogen, it is possible that depletion occurred selectively in type II fibers or specific cellular compartments such as the SR (Rockwell et al. 2003).

Studies of intermittent sprint protocols involving team sports have also reported benefits to exercise capacity or performance following strategies to enhance carbohydrate availability, even when compared with a moderate-carbohydrate diet (Akermark et al. 1996; Balsom, Wood, et al. 1999). These studies are reviewed in the next chapter on field-based team sports. The carbohydrate needs for resistance training should also be considered, because resistance training plays a key role in the conditioning programs undertaken by sprinters and jumper and provides another example of repeated high-intensity or interval exercise. Carbohydrate intake could play a role in optimizing the gains achieved by a resistance program in two separate ways: as a fuel for the exercise session or as a promoter of the anabolic hormonal environment needed to optimize protein synthesis following the session. Although the results are not always consistent, a number of studies have shown that strategies that enhance carbohydrate availability during a resistance workout can allow the athlete to train harder (Haff et al. 1999; Lambert et al. 1991). In addition, carbohydrate consumed in conjunction with protein, immediately before or after resistance training, may enhance net protein balance in response to the session (Borsheim, Cree, et al. 2004; Tipton et al. 2001). The literature on carbohydrate intake and resistance training is reviewed in chapter 11.

There is evidence that a high intake of carbohydrate is important in enhancing recovery between bouts of intermittent sprint training, such as back-to-back sessions of interval-based track work. In one study, participants undertook an interval exercise protocol on two occasions separated by a 2-day recovery period. Each protocol consisted of five sets of five all-out sprints with 30 s recovery between sprints and 5 min active recovery between sets, followed by a final set of 10 × 6 s sprints with 30 s recovery (Fulcher and Williams 1992). During the recovery period between protocols, participants consumed either their normal (moderate) intake of carbohydrate (~450 g/day) or a low-carbohydrate diet (<100 g/day). In the moderate-carbohydrate trial, participants showed a significant increase in peak power output during the five sets of sprints in the second exercise protocol. This improvement in performance in the second trial was not seen with the low-carbohydrate trial (Fulcher and Williams 1992).

Another investigation monitored performance of 5 × 60 s maximal cycling sprints separated by 5 min recovery (Jenkins et al. 1993). This intermittent sprint protocol was undertaken twice, separated by a 3-day recovery period involving high (83% of energy), moderate (58% of energy), or low (12% of energy) intakes of carbohydrate. The low-carbohydrate trial was associated with a decline in performance on the second occasion; this was not seen with the moderate- and high-carbohydrate intakes. Nevill and coworkers (1993) tested a similar range of carbohydrate intakes on 24 hr recovery between two hour-long treadmill tests involving 30 × 6 s sprints. Power outputs during the sprints declined over the duration of the test on day 1 and were even lower on day 2. There was no difference between trials when the total 60 min of the trial on day 2 was examined; performance declined by 5%, 0.5%, and 0.2% compared with day 1, for low-, normal-, and high-carbohydrate trials, respectively (not significant). However, over the first 20 min of the test on day 2, there was evidence of better performance in the high-carbohydrate trial compared with the low-carbohydrate diet (Nevill et al. 1993). This study shows the difficulty of repeating performance of intermittent high-intensity sprints on successive days but suggests that better restoration of muscle carbohydrate stores can enhance recovery.

In summary, sport scientists have failed to address the specific carbohydrate needs for training and competition performance in sprinters and jumpers. There are no studies that directly investigate the effects of everyday intakes of carbohydrate on daily training outcomes or one-off performance in these events. The effects of acute strategies to enhance carbohydrate availability in training—that is, intake before, during, or after a session—have not been studied in relation to sprinters and jumpers or their specific workouts. Ideally, these studies need to be conducted over long periods to see if benefits to single sessions translate into superior training outcomes and adaptation. The evidence supporting the benefits of a high-carbohydrate diet for competition performance is not strong and cannot justify the development of rigid recommendations for the carbohydrate intakes of sprinters and jumpers in training or competition. However, the results of laboratory studies of supramaximal exercise and resistance training, and investigations of interval-type performance in team sports, provide circumstantial evidence to support general nutrition guidelines for these athletes. It appears prudent to advise sprinters and jumpers to consume at least a moderate intake of carbohydrate in daily eating patterns and to avoid carbohydrate-restricted diets. This is particularly important for training situations involving repeated high-intensity sprints within a single session or for recovery between multiple sessions of interval and resistance training. Indeed, the translation of results of studies from resistance training athletes and team sports suggests that strategic intake of carbohydrate before, during, and after prolonged sessions of training might lead to better training and enhance the stimulus for gains in muscle size and strength. These outcomes need to be investigated using protocols of relevance to sprinters and jumpers.

Eating for Multiple Races and Events

The nutritional issues underpinning the performance of a single sprint event are not as physiologically challenging as those of endurance sports. Carbohydrate and fluid status are unlikely to be limiting factors in one-off performance, especially if the sprinter or jumper has followed a well-chosen meal pattern over the 24 hr period before the event. The general principles of the preevent period, including the preevent meal, are outlined in chapter 1, goals 12 and 13, and in table 4.5 in chapter 4. However, as shown in the following list, there are often significant practical challenges to eating well in the competition situation:

- Finding suitable foods for pre- and postevent eating when traveling and away from usual food supply or reliable access to food.

- Integrating competition eating (preevent and postevent meals) into a daily meal plan, especially when the event is scheduled at an inconvenient time—for example, late at night. If the athlete is competing on a circuit so that competition days make up a substantial part of the weekly schedule, this can become a chronic issue over the competitive season, even effecting overall nutrition status.

- Managing fluid and food intake over a prolonged session or day of competition, when the athlete's events or rounds are spread over a number of hours. This is especially challenging for the athlete who is competing in more than one event or the combined events (heptathlon and decathlon). Even if the athlete's actual event involves only a brief period of high-intensity energy expenditure, he or she may be involved in activities or environments that incur sweat losses and increased energy expenditure for prolonged periods. Being involved in an event, or simply being at the competition venue, can distract the athlete from attending to her dietary needs. In some cases, foods and fluids are not readily available.

The keys to meeting these challenges are good preparation and tracking. Athletes should work with their coach and sports dietitian or nutritionist to consider the nutritional needs of the competition program. Fluid, energy, and carbohydrate intake must be matched with the general considerations for hydration status, gastrointestinal comfort, and fuel requirements over the hours of a competition session as well as the specific needs incurred by warm-up, events, and cool-down activities. Special nutritional needs related to a new environment should also be considered. The athlete should then examine the competition timetable to pencil in his or her likely schedule of activities for the day—this should include logistical tasks such as travel to the track and event registration as well as exercise tasks such as warm-ups and events. In some competitions and events, it may be hard to predict a definite timetable. Nevertheless, the process will allow the sprinter or jumper to develop a rough outline of when fluid and food breaks will be needed—including the last substantial (preevent) meal, fluid top-ups after a warm-up or between rounds, and snacks to promote more substantial recovery between events that are more widely spaced. In a multiday meet, the athlete will need to plan for recovery meals at the end of each session or the end of the day.

Once a blueprint for the day's meals, snacks, and fluid breaks has been prepared, the athlete should turn attention to the availability of foods and drinks within the competition environment. The wider issues of eating away from home are discussed in chapter 10 (practical issue). This discussion encourages the athlete to investigate information about the general food supply at the competition destination and any specific catering plans that may be in place. Such information may indicate that the athlete needs to bring a special food supply, including specific foods and fluids that can be consumed before the event, between rounds of an event, or for postevent recovery. These items may include specialized sport products such as sport drinks, gels, bars, and liquid meal supplements (see table 7.3). In addition to bringing a specific supply of foods, drinks, and sport products to the competition site, many athletes find it useful to prepare a recording sheet that keeps track of their actual intake over a day. It is easy in the heat of the moment to lose sight of what has been

Table 7.3 Sport Foods and Supplements That Are of Likely Benefit to Sprint and Jump Performance

	Product	Comment
Use in achieving documented nutrition goals	Sport drinks	• Use to refuel and rehydrate during prolonged workouts in the heat and to rehydrate after the session. Contain some electrolytes to help replace sweat losses and increase voluntary intake of fluid. • In sports that extend over prolonged periods in the heat with the athlete remaining on the field (e.g., jumps, heptathlons, decathlons), a sport drink may help to keep the athlete refueled and hydrated between rounds or events.
	Sport bars	• Convenient, portable, and easy-to-consume source of carbohydrate, protein, and micronutrients for prerace meal or postevent recovery. • Convenient and compact source of energy and nutrients for the traveling athlete or for competition schedules that conflict with athlete's usual meal pattern.

(continued)

Table 7.3 *(continued)*

	Product	Comment
	Liquid meal supplements	• Convenient, portable, and easy-to-consume source of carbohydrate, protein, and micro-nutrients for "recovery eating strategies" before and after the workout. • Low-bulk and practical form of energy and nutrients that can contribute to high energy needs, especially to support resistance training program or growth. • Well-tolerated preevent meal that can be consumed to provide a source of carbohydrate and energy quite close to the start of the event or during gaps of 1-2 hr between events, heats, or finals when solid food may not be well-tolerated by some athletes. • Convenient and compact source of energy and nutrients for the traveling athlete or for competition schedules that conflict with athlete's usual meal pattern.
	Sport gels	• Convenient and compact carbohydrate source that can be carried for use during prolonged workouts and between efforts in multievent sports (e.g., between events in decathlon and heptathlon or between rounds in jumps).
	Multivitamin and mineral supplement	• Supplemental source of micronutrients for traveling when food supply is not reliable. • Supplemental source of micronutrients during prolonged periods of energy restriction (female athletes).
Documented ergogenic benefit	Creatine	• Serves a number of important roles in exercise metabolism; the most well-known role is the rapid regeneration of adenosine triphosphate by the phosphagen power system. Studies show that creatine loading enhances the performance of exercise involving repeated high-intensity work bouts with short recovery intervals (<2 min recovery). Performance benefits for a single sprint appear to be too small to detect. The most likely benefits for jump and sprint athletes may come from using creatine in the training phase to enhance training adaptations to interval and resistance training. Performance benefits are seen only in athletes who experience significant increases in creatine stores following loading. Most studies have been undertaken in the laboratory and are yet to be confirmed with well-trained and elite athletes in sport-specific situations. Typical protocols for creatine use: Loading dose of 20-30 g in multiple doses (e.g., 4×5 g) for 5 days followed by maintenance dose of 2-5 g/day. Uptake appears to be enhanced by consuming creatine with carbohydrate-rich meal or snack. Acute weight gain of about 1 kg occurs with creatine loading, presumably attributable to fluid retention. This is less likely to be of concern to sprint events (or to weight-supported sprint sports such as track cycling) but may be of concern to weight-sensitive sports such as jumping events.
Potential for ergogenic benefit	Caffeine	• Has the potential to increase performance in events lasting as little as 60 s (Graham 2001a, 2001b). It is unlikely to increase strength or maximal capacity but can increase endurance and resistance to fatigue during prolonged or repeated efforts. Therefore, although there may be application to the competition situation, the main benefits may be found as a training aid that allows the athlete to work at a higher output for longer. It is less well studied in brief, anaerobic-based events, particularly in sport-specific situations. Unresolved issues include the optimal dose and timing of intake of caffeine and the potential for large doses to have negative effects on technique or to interfere with recovery and sleep between multiple events. Caffeine may be consumed in cola and energy drinks or as an addition to some sport products (e.g., some gels). Conflicting evidence over the efficacy of coffee as a source of caffeine, because it contains other chemicals that might impair performance.
	Bicarbonate or citrate loading	• There is some evidence that accumulation of H^+ ions limits the performance of sprint events lasting ~60 s (e.g., 400 m sprint and hurdles). The use of bicarbonate or citrate to increase blood-buffering capacity (e.g., 300 mg/kg body mass bicarbonate or 500 mg/kg body mass citrate 1-2 hr prerace) might enhance the performance of such events. Field studies are needed with high-level athletes to confirm benefits. Risk of gastrointestinal problems should be noted but appear to be reduced by taking dose with large volumes of fluid (1-2 L). Athletes who intend to load for a series of events over consecutive days (e.g., heats and finals) should experiment with a lower dose for the second or subsequent races in view of residual increase in buffering capacity from earlier doses. Alternatively, a longer-term loading protocol can be used over a number of days leading up to the competition (e.g., 500 $mg \cdot kg^{-1} \cdot day^{-1}$ for 5 days spread into a series of doses over the day) to achieve a more sustained increase in blood-buffering capacity. There is recent evidence that chronic bicarbonate loading (loading immediately before interval training) may enhance training adaptations. This may also allow the athlete to train harder.

consumed, especially if weather and competitor delays significantly alter the predicted timetable. An objective account of fluid and food intake may help the athlete stay focused on his or her nutrition goals, particularly during multiday and multievent competition. It may also assist the athlete to undertake a thorough debriefing after the session to consider which aspects of the preparation and competition performance were successful and which may need fine-tuning.

Sport Foods and Supplements

Sprinters share with strength and power athletes an intense fascination with dietary supplements. The types of supplements promoted in the muscle-building industry are reviewed in the chapter on strength and power sports (chapter 11). The discussion in that chapter reveals that most of the popular supplements used by resistance-trained athletes either are unstudied or have failed to achieve claims made by word of mouth and advertisements. A summary of the available literature on supplements purported to increase gains in muscle mass and strength is presented in tables 11.c and 11.d. In the present chapter, the results of studies related to sprint or jumping performance, or the types of training sessions undertaken by these athletes, are discussed. Again, there is a scarcity of investigations of many of the popular supplements, particularly studies involving top-level sprinters and jumpers as participants or performance protocols with direct relevance to the competitive outcomes in these events.

Table 7.3 summarizes the range of sport foods and supplements that are likely to contribute to the nutrition goals or performance of sprinters and jumpers. Products such as sport drinks, sport bars, gels, and liquid meal supplements may be used by sprinters and jumpers before, during, or after a track workout to meet needs for carbohydrate, protein, or fluid and thus enhance performance and recovery in such a session. Some products may also be of value in promoting a desired increase in muscle mass and strength, increasing energy intake, or providing a source of nutrients after sessions of resistance training. It is logical that maximizing the outcomes of a training program will better prepare the athlete for competition. There may also be occasions for the athlete to use sport foods to remain hydrated or well fueled in the competition scenario—particularly in multievent sports or events involving multiple rounds spread over a session. Because the logistics of many track-and-field competitions interfere with access to everyday foods, specialized sport foods may be useful for meal replacements or recovery snacks. Although there are no scientific studies to show direct benefits to performance from these suggested uses of these sport foods, these uses may be recommended on the basis of sound nutrition practice.

Among ergogenic aids, creatine, caffeine, and bicarbonate are identified as the only products with a reasonable level of scientific support for benefits to sprint performance or training outcomes (table 7.b in the chapter appendix). In the case of creatine, there is strong evidence that supplementation may be of benefit to the training process, as discussed in greater detail subsequently. Studies that have investigated the effects of creatine supplementation on the performance of single or repeated sprints are summarized in table 7.b. Studies that support beneficial uses of caffeine and bicarbonate or citrate loading for sprint events are fewer in volume and suffer from a lack of sport-specific protocols and well-trained athletes. In the case of bicarbonate and citrate, there is some preliminary evidence that the chronic practice of loading with a buffer prior to interval training sessions may provide a greater training response, but this requires further investigation in well-trained runners. In terms of acute supplementation for race performance, beneficial uses appear to be limited to the longer sprints (400 m sprints and hurdles), where there is evidence that speed is reduced at the end of a race because of a decline in anaerobic glycolysis, potentially caused by the build-up of metabolic acidosis. The available studies on protocols lasting a minute, including a field study of a 400 m race (Goldfinch et al. 1988), support possible benefits to competition performance. However, these effects need to be studied with highly trained sprinters and in the context of a competition program that may require the athlete to undertake a series of heats, semis, and finals. How to manage a repeated pattern of bicarbonate loading, or take into account the effects of supplementation on performance of a subsequent bout, deserves particular investigation. The longer-term loading protocol for bicarbonate supplementation, involving loading with split doses over 5 days, may be useful in this situation (see chapter 3). The use of caffeine in sprint events, single and repeated, also merits study because there is some evidence that this supplement might enhance speed endurance in trained participants (Doherty 1998; Doherty et al. 2002). Whether this translates into enhanced sprinting performance, and whether caffeine supplementation provides other benefits such as faster reaction times, are of interest.

A range of other supplements are taken by sprint-focused athletes in the belief that these products will enhance reaction, speed, recovery, or body fat levels. Unfortunately, the specific claims for many of these products have been not been investigated, but supplements that have received attention with a sprint-related protocol such as bovine colostrum, inosine, and ribose have failed to show evidence of detectable benefits (see table 7.c). In fact, in the case of inosine, there is evidence that this supplement might actually impair the performance of high-intensity exercise. Two studies involving running (table 5.e) and cycling (table 4.f) protocols have found that participants showed better performance of high-intensity tasks while on the placebo treatment than on the inosine trial (Starling et al. 1996; Williams et al. 1990). Potential mechanisms for exercise impairment include an increased formation of inosine monophosphate (IMP) in the muscle, either at rest or during exercise. High IMP concentrations have been found at the point of fatigue in many exercise studies;

furthermore, IMP has been shown to inhibit adenosine triphosphatase activity (Sahlin 1992). It is possible that increased resting concentrations of muscle IMP reduced the duration of high-intensity exercise before critically high levels were reached, causing premature fatigue. Such a theory can only be investigated by direct measurements of muscle nucleosides. Another possible mechanism of performance impairment is an increase in levels of uric acid, a product of inosine degradation. In studies of inosine supplementation in athletes, 5 days and 10 days of intake doubled blood concentrations to levels above the normal range (McNaughton, Dalton, and Tarr 1999; Starling et al. 1996; Williams et al. 1990). Thus, chronic inosine supplementation may pose a health risk because high uric acid levels are implicated as a cause of gout. In summary, because there is a lack of evidence of performance benefits, and the possibility of performance decrements and side effects, there is little to recommend the use of inosine supplements by sprint athletes.

It is unfortunate that the literature on dietary supplements and sprint or jump performance is so scarce. Both the scientific community and the supplement industry are encouraged to address the paucity of information on the effects of such products on these basic and popular sports. In the absence of sport-specific information about a purported ergogenic aid, the reader must settle for a general understanding of the literature provided in the appendix to chapter 3. This chapter will finish with a brief discussion of two supplements targeted at the power systems underpinning sprint performance; one that has achieved success by commercial and scientific benchmarks and one that has so far failed to reach either of these standards.

Creatine

Muscle creatine, or more specifically phosphocreatine, is the critical power source for sprint and jump events, in both training and competition. Muscle phosphocreatine concentrations are depleted within 5 to 6 s of all-out sprinting, and the depletion of this high-energy fuel is responsible for the decline in speed seen at the end of the 100 m sprint (Hirvonen et al. 1987). A laboratory study of 30 s maximal treadmill sprinting showed that peak power declined by a mean of 65% during this exercise and that participants who started the trial with highest phosphocreatine content in type II fibers showed a smaller decline in power output (Greenhaff et al. 1994). Although sprint training does not appear to cause an adaptive increase in muscle creatine stores, there is evidence of a response to oral intake of creatine. A typical meat-containing diet provides approximately 2 g of creatine per day, roughly equivalent to daily turnover. However, vegetarians have reduced body creatine stores, suggesting that endogenous production cannot totally compensate for the lack of dietary intake (Green et al. 1997).

For more than 50 years it has been known that oral intake of creatine is largely maintained in the body (Chanutin 1926). However, it is only recently that changes in muscle creatine and phosphocreatine following supple-

mentary creatine intake have been documented using skeletal muscle biopsy procedures and imaging techniques. In a watershed study, Harris and colleagues (1992) showed that muscle creatine content was increased following repeated doses of oral creatine large enough to sustain plasma creatine levels above the threshold for maximal transport into the muscle cell. Their rapid loading protocol—four to six doses of 5 g of creatine monohydrate for 5 days—increased total muscle creatine concentrations by an average of 20% to reach a muscle threshold of 150 to 160 mmol/kg dry weight. About 20% of the increased muscle creatine content was stored as phosphocreatine, and saturation occurred after 2 to 3 days. Increases in muscle creatine stores were greatest in those individuals who had the lowest presupplementation concentrations and when coupled with intensive daily exercise (Harris et al. 1992). Similar increases in muscle creatine levels can be achieved by a slow loading protocol, with supplemental doses of 3 g/day for a month (Hultman et al. 1996). Creatine supplementation protocols are summarized in the appendix to chapter 3.

The widespread use of creatine supplementation by sprint athletes is well recognized. In fact, the initial popularity of creatine owes much to the publicity surrounding its use by British track-and-field athletes in their preparation for the 1992 Barcelona Olympic Games. Linford Christie, the unexpected winner of the 100 m sprint, was rumored to be one of the first satisfied customers of a creatine supplementation program. Today, creatine is the subject of a textbook (Williams et al. 1998) and more than 200 peer-reviewed studies, review papers (Branch 2003; Greenhaff 2000; Hespel et al. 2001; Juhn and Tarnopolsky 1998a, 1998b; Kreider 1998), and position statements (American College of Sports Medicine 2000). By 2000, creatine had amassed annual sales of more than 5 million kilograms (Hespel et al. 2001).

Theoretically, increased muscle phosphocreatine levels could enhance the performance of a single supramaximal bout of exercise or the ability to repeat high-intensity work bouts with a short recovery interval as a result of the increased rate of phosphocreatine resynthesis during this recovery. This provides a hypothetical benefit to the performance of a single sprint (competition performance) or the ability to undertake conditioning techniques such as interval and resistance training. The magnitude of the number of studies of creatine supplementation provides several luxuries—meta-analyses and reviews to look at overall trends rather than the results of a single investigation as well as a reasonable body of literature involving specifically trained participants. Studies that have investigated the effects of creatine supplementation on performance of single or repeated bouts of high-intensity exercise in sprint-trained athletes are summarized in table 7.b. The reader is also directed to reviews of other creatine studies with application to the preparation of sprint-based athletes in this book. These include the effect of creatine supplementation on resistance training in strength and power athletes in chapter 11 (see text and appendix in chapter 11) and on repeated sprints in team and racket sport players (tables in appendixes to chapters 8-10 and chapter 10, research topic).

Those who have reviewed the creatine literature have generally concluded that the major benefit of creatine supplementation is to enhance the performance of repeated 6 to 30 s bouts of maximal exercise, interspersed with short recovery intervals (20 s to 5 min), where it can attenuate the normal decrease in force or power production that occurs over the course of the session (Branch 2003; Juhn and Tarnopolsky 1998a; Kreider 1998). According to table 7.b, most (Bosco et al. 1997; Harris et al. 1993; Havenitidis et al. 2003; Schedel, Terrier, et al. 2000; Skare et al. 2001; Ziegenfuss et al. 2002) but not all (Delecluse et al. 2003; Finn et al. 2001; Redondo et al. 1996) studies of acute supplementation in sprint-trained athletes show that it is of benefit to a protocol involving repeated sprints. Thus, the major benefit of creatine supplements for sprinters and jumpers would appear to be as a training aid, allowing the athlete to train harder and gain greater adaptations to interval and resistance training. More studies are needed to investigate whether training enhancements actually translate into a better competition performance. Only two studies have examined the effect of chronic protocols of creatine supplementation on sprint and jump performance, and the results are unclear (Kirksey et al. 1999; Lehmkuhl et al. 2003).

By contrast, although two studies report favorable results in sprint-trained athletes (Bosco et al. 1997; Skare et al. 2001), creatine supplementation is not generally considered ergogenic for a single bout of supramaximal exercise, either because the contribution of phosphocreatine is not the limiting factor to performance or because any benefit is too small to be consistently detected (Kreider 1998). One reason for the lack of consistency in the literature regarding acute creatine supplementation and exercise function is the failure of most studies to accept changes in performance that are considered nonsignificant by a statistician but worthwhile in the world of competitive sport (Tarnopolsky and MacLennan 2000). The issue of detecting important changes in research on sports supplements is discussed in chapter 3 (research topic).

There are valid reasons for sprinters and jumpers to consider creatine supplementation at an established phase of their career, during appropriate times of the training and competition calendar. The decision to use creatine should be made with consideration of appropriate protocols of use and the possibility of side effects. The purported increase in the prevalence of muscle cramps, strains, and injury associated with creatine supplementation is discussed in more detail in chapter 10, in the third research topic. Anecdotal reports of these problems are often raised by sprint athletes, but there is currently no documented support for a true increase in these problems.

Ribose

Ribose is a pentose sugar that provides part of the structure of a variety of important chemicals in the body, including the adenine nucleotides adenosine triphosphate, adenosine

monophosphate, and adenosine diphosphate. It is found in the diet, but purified forms have also recently been released onto the market, finding their way into sport supplements. Oral ribose is quickly absorbed and tolerated even at intakes of 100 g; however, at US$400 per kilogram, ribose powders are an expensive form of carbohydrate.

In the body, the pentose phosphate pathway is a rate-limiting pathway for the interconversion of ribose-5-phosphate and glucose. Ribose-5-phosphate can be converted to phosphoribosyl pyrophosphate (PRPP), which is then involved in the synthesis or salvaging of the adenine nucleotide pool. It has been suggested that suboptimal amounts of PRPP may limit these processes. Indeed, ribose infusion is known to enhance adenosine triphosphate recovery and exercise function in animal models of myocardial ischemia where baseline levels of PRPP levels were low (see Op 't Eijnde et al. 2001). In humans, repeated bouts of high-intensity exercise (e.g., training) may reduce muscle adenosine triphosphate content and total adenine nucleotide pool, possibly because the rate of nucleotide salvaging and synthesis falls behind the massive rates of nucleotide degradation (Hellsten et al. 1993; Stathis et al. 1994). It has been suggested that oral intake of ribose might increase the rate of nucleotide salvaging and synthesis and achieve quicker recovery of the reductions in muscle total adenine nucleotides after exercise. Sport supplements have been produced, typically delivering 3 to 5 g doses of ribose, with claims that they will dramatically reduce recovery from 72 hr to 12 hr. Ribose in combination with creatine is claimed to provide the most sophisticated energy support system.

Several studies have examined ribose supplementation in athletes undertaking repeated bouts of high-intensity exercise, with reports of performance enhancements. However, the consensus from studies that have been published in full in the peer-reviewed literature does not support the value of ribose supplementation. Eight studies involving oral ribose intake and performance of repeated high-intensity sprints in active or sprint-trained participants are available. In comparison to the manufacturers' recommended dose of 3 to 5 g/day, most studies provided participants with daily amounts of 10 to 20 g of ribose (Berardi and Ziegenfuss 2003; Dunne et al. 2006; Kreider, Melton, Rasmussen, et al. 2003; Op 't Eijnde et al. 2001; Van Gammeren et al. 2002), whereas a higher intake of ~45 g/day was consumed in one investigation (Hellsten et al. 2004). The results of each study failed to provide evidence of a worthwhile benefit to the sprint performance of participants on the ribose trial (see tables 6.f, 7.c, and 11.d). Although there were individual cases or indexes that were apparently enhanced in the ribose trial compared with placebo (Berardi and Ziegenfuss 2003; Kreider, Melton, Rasmussen, et al. 2003), these results were not consistently seen within or across studies.

Two of the studies involved a sophisticated protocol that monitored changes in the muscle adenine pool as well as performance changes. One study investigated these characteristics during two intermittent training sessions undertaken 24 hr apart (Op 't Eijnde et al. 2001). The protocol was undertaken on two occasions: as a baseline measure on active participants, and following a 7-day training program involving two bouts of intermittent exercise each day while participants were taking ribose (four doses of 4 g/day) or placebo. The first exercise bout in each testing occasion decreased muscle total adenine nucleotide, with muscle adenosine triphosphate content being reduced by 20% at the time of the second bout. However, ribose supplementation did not alter the loss or recovery of adenosine triphosphate resulting from this exercise protocol, nor did it change muscle force or power characteristics during maximal testing (Op 't Eijnde et al. 2001). The authors acknowledged that plasma ribose concentrations achieved by the supplementation were too low to achieve a significant change in nucleotide synthesis and salvage. However, the doses used in the study were already higher than the dose recommended by most supplement manufacturers. The other study tracked 72 hr recovery between a 7-day protocol that reduced muscle adenosine triphosphate content by about 25% and a bout of intermittent high-intensity exercise (Hellsten et al. 2004). Although muscle adenosine triphosphate was still reduced at 24 hr into recovery, regardless of treatment, and at 72 hr in the placebo trial, ribose supplementation was associated with a return to pretraining levels by 72 hr. Despite differences in the restoration of adenosine triphosphate content between trials, there was no difference in muscle power characteristics in the subsequent performance protocol between the trials. This study noted that ribose supplementation at high levels (45 g/day) and for prolonged periods (>24 hr) can enhance the rate of resynthesis of muscle adenosine triphosphate following an exercise-related decline in this nucleotide. The authors concluded that although ribose may be a limiting factor for the rate of resynthesis of adenosine triphosphate, the reduction in muscle adenosine triphosphate observed after intense training does not appear to be limiting for the performance of high-intensity exercise (Hellsten et al. 2004).

There is currently no evidence to promote the benefits of ribose supplementation on the performance of sprint training or competition. If benefits do apply, they are likely to require doses of ribose that could not be supported by a cost–benefit analysis. Further work is needed to explore this area, but the ultimate outcome might be challenged by the practicality and expense of consuming larger doses of oral ribose.

Research Priorities

Areas of interest for immediate research include these:

- Nutrition beliefs and practices of high-level jumpers and sprinters during training
- Carbohydrate needs of interval and resistance training sessions, and effects of varying intake on training adaptations and event-specific performance outcomes
- Effects of variation in amount and timing of protein intake on the adaptations achieved by resistance training and on event-specific performance outcomes
- Race-day eating practices of high-level jumpers and sprinters, especially those undertaking multiple rounds or multievent competition
- Use of supplements and sport foods by sprinters and jumpers, and their specific benefit to performance in various events in these sports

chapter 8

Field-Based Team Sports

The next three chapters of this book deal with sports based on intermittent high-intensity exercise. There will not be sufficient space to consider all the characteristics of individual sports that fall into these categories; rather we take a broader view of common characteristics of such sports. Although many of the features will be shared across sports, we divide intermittent high-intensity sports into three more manageable sections: field-based team sports, court sports, and racket sports.

Most team sports can be considered as prolonged events or even endurance sports, because they typically involve playing time of 60 to 120 min. Because previous chapters of this book focused on prolonged, *continuous* exercise activities, it is worth considering some of the different and defining characteristics of field and court sports. The following features of these sports are in contrast to the nutritional issues discussed in the previous chapters covering prolonged continuous exercise:

- Team and racket sports are characterized by high-intensity passages of play interspersed with low-intensity activities such as standing, walking, and jogging. This is likely to present a different challenge for the body in terms of fuel utilization and thermoregulation.

- These sports incorporate breaks in play: formal breaks between sets, quarters, or halves of a game and informal breaks such as substitutions and stoppages for injury and rule infringements. These breaks allow further recovery between high-intensity passages and provide opportunities for intake of fluid and carbohydrate.

- The game characteristics of different positions or playing styles within a team can vary markedly. Therefore, even within a sport, players may have different physique characteristics and face different nutritional issues and challenges.

- There is no predictable work requirement during competition in team or racket sports. Each match

in a sport is literally a new ball game. It can be difficult to make precise judgments of the nutritional challenges faced in a match.

- Although match or game analysis of various team and racket sports can estimate typical activity patterns in a sport (e.g., the total distance covered, time or distance spent at different running speeds), these calculations underestimate the energy expenditure in a game. Studies show that many of the activities undertaken while moving (e.g., handling the ball, tackling, defending) add considerably to the energy cost. The energy cost of constantly accelerating, decelerating, and changing direction must also be taken into account.

- Performance in team and racket sports is determined by a complex and changing mixture of physical and skill-based talents. Players not only must be able to run to the ball or scene of play but must be able to execute skills involving cognitive function (e.g., reading the play, making tactical decisions) and motor control. In contact sports, players must possess the strength and speed to apply or withstand tackles. There is a considerable amount of jostling even in noncontact team sports. Nutrition plays a complex role in promoting optimal performance during competition by ensuring that the muscles and central nervous system are adequately fueled. It is likely that inadequate nutritional strategies during competition have a greater negative impact on performance than in most prolonged continuous sports, because these shortcomings will also affect the skill and cognitive function that overlay the player's performance.

- In team and racket sports, competitions are undertaken under two different protocols: a seasonal fixture or a tournament. Both call for clever recovery tactics between matches, because players may be required to play full-length games with a recovery period of 1 to 2 days, or in some case hours.

However, another feature of the match schedule is that it can blur the traditional differentiation between training and competition. At higher levels, players usually undertake a pronounced preseason campaign to prepare for the competition season, or they undergo specific training between tournaments. However, even at this level it can be difficult to integrate training and everyday nutritional goals within a weekly or twice weekly competition schedule.

The integration of training and competition nutrition strategies into the athlete's eating program may provide a challenge to many team and racket sport players and is explored over the next three chapters of this book.

Competition

The term *field-based team games* includes the various codes of football (soccer, Australian football, rugby and rugby league, American gridiron football), field hockey, and other sports such as lacrosse. The sports of baseball, softball, and cricket also fall within the scope of this chapter, although because competitive matches involve less movement overall, with the majority of play generally being focused on a couple of players at any one time, these sports receive less attention in the chapter. Because the size of the playing arena in field sports is larger than a court, and the game duration is typically 60 to 120 min, team players in these sports may cover a considerable distance during a game. Time–motion studies on team games show that this movement is achieved in a highly intermittent nature, with the player's position or playing style and the flow of each game dictating the time spent sprinting, accelerating, decelerating, changing direction, jumping, jogging, walking, or standing. Depending on the game, additional activities superimposed on these movement patterns include tackling or withstanding contact, lifting or pushing other players, and handling the ball. In some codes, there are specialist teams of offensive and defensive players who alternate on the ground according to the characteristics of play or the unlimited rotation of a smaller number of players from a substitution bench. Other games provide limited opportunities for substitutions and most players are on the ground for the whole duration of the game. Although it is not possible to provide a comprehensive discussion of the specific characteristics of each team sport, a brief review of the activity patterns of several well-studied field games is presented to highlight the range of the physiological and nutritional challenges involved in these sports. The reader is also directed to table 8.1, which summarizes the characteristics of a larger range of common field games, and table 8.2, which outlines factors that help to shape the overall nutritional issues faced by team sport players.

According to time–motion analyses conducted in the 1970s on players from the English First Division league (Reilly and Thomas 1976), each game of 90 min duration involves about 1,000 discrete bouts of action, with players typically changing activity every 5 to 6 s. The typical movement pattern requires the player to run every 30 s, including a ~15 m sprint every 90 s, with a rest period of about 3 s every 2 min. The total distance covered during a game in the 1970s was seen to vary not only from game to game but also according to playing position, at least for teams playing in a conventional team formation. Midfielders were found to cover 9 to 11 km per match, compared with 8 to 9 km for the outfielders. Goalkeepers typically covered about 4 km, mostly undertaking activities needed to maintain arousal. The distances covered in a game were shared between walking (~25%), jogging (~37%), cruising (~20%), sprinting (~11%), and running backward (~7%). Less than 1% and up to 4% of these activities were undertaken while the player was in possession of the ball. Both the total distance covered and the time spent in high-intensity activities were seen to decrease in the second half of matches, suggesting fatigue (Reilly and Thomas 1976).

According to the excellent review by Reilly (1990a), various studies have found that the average intensity of a soccer match is around 75% of the player's aerobic capacity. However, the regular bursts of anaerobic activity add considerably to the metabolic load incurred during a game. A simple time–motion analysis of the running distances and speeds incurred during a match can be misleading in determining the total energy requirements of a player. After all, the energy costs of running activities are increased when the player is required to accelerate, decelerate, change direction, run at an angle, or handle the ball. Energy for brief periods of high-intensity soccer play can be supplied by the alactic phosphagen system and anaerobic glycolysis; blood lactate levels collected at halftime and the end of the match are 4 to 6 mmol/L, and evidence indicates that peak lactates of 7 to 8+ mmol/L can occur regularly throughout play (for review, see Reilly 1990a).

A more recent study reexamined the activity patterns of high-level professional soccer players, playing in both elite and lower-level European leagues (Mohr et al. 2003). Analysis of 129 matches showed that the top-class players performed 28% more high-intensity running and 58% more sprinting than moderate-level professional players. In the laboratory, these top-class players scored higher on a soccer-specific test combining anaerobic and aerobic fitness. Comparison of games at different times of the season revealed that top-class players covered greater distances at high intensity during the later matches, suggesting that fitness and performance increased over the season. This outcome might be explained by a reduction in the playing schedule from two matches to one match a week in the second half of the season, allowing more time for specific training between games. Examination by position found that midfielders, fullbacks, and attackers completed greater distances during a game (~10.5-11 km) than the defenders (~9.5 km) and a greater distance at high intensity (2.2-2.5 km vs. 1.7 km).

Regardless of playing position and the competitive standard of the game, the amount of high-intensity running in the last 15 min of a match was 35% to 45% less than

Table 8.1 Characteristics of Commonly Played Field Games

Sport	Game time	Dimensions of field	Number of players	Other game characteristics
Association football (soccer)	2 × 45 min halves	Rectangle: Length: 100-130 m (110-120 m for international matches) Width: 50-100 m (70-80 m for international matches)	11 players from each team on field at one time; substitution bench of 3 players allows replacements but benched player cannot return to field	• Noncontact game • Major differences in game characteristics of players with extremes ranging from "midfield" players to goalkeeper • Jumping to head ball
American football	4 × 15 min quarters plus substantial time on (clock stopped for time-outs and interval between plays)	Rectangle: Length: 100 yd + 2 × 10 yd end zones Width: 53.5 yd	11 players from each team on field at one time Separate offensive and defensive teams alternate according to play	• Contact (blocking and tackling) a feature of the game • Uniforms feature heavy protective wear • 45 s between plays allows more recovery than Canadian football • Smaller field means players are less mobile and larger than Canadian football players
Canadian football	4 × 15 min quarters plus substantial time on (clock stopped for time-outs and interval between plays)	Rectangle: Length: 110 yd + 2 × 20 yd end zones Width: 60 yd	12 players from each team on field at one time Separate offensive and defensive teams alternate according to play	• Contact (blocking and tackling) a feature of the game • Uniforms feature heavy protective wear • 20 s between plays requires greater endurance than American football
Australian football	4 × 20 min quarters plus substantial time on—total game time is typically 120 min	Oval: Length: 135-155 m Width: 110-155 m	18 players from each team on field at one time; unlimited substitutions from 4 players on interchange bench	• Major differences in game characteristics of "on ball" and "key position" players • Tackling and contact allowed; minimal protective wear • Frequent jumping to "mark" (catch) or punch ball
Gaelic football	70 min for championship or county games (2 × 35 min) 60 min for league games (2 × 30 min)	Rectangle: Length: 137 m Width: 82 m	15 players from each team on field at one time; substitution bench of 3 players allows replacements but benched player cannot return to field	• Running game with limited tackling • Major differences in game characteristics of players with extremes ranging from "midfield" players to goalkeeper
Rugby union	2 × 40 min halves	Rectangle: Length: 100 m Width: 60 m	15 players from each team on field at one time; substitution bench of 7 players with maximum of 6 substitutions in game. Replaced player cannot return to field except for time spent in "sin bin" or "blood bin"	• Contact, tackling, scrums a feature of the game • Jumping in line-outs and to "mark" (catch) ball • Game style differs between positions on field—generally divided into backs (mobile) and forwards (big and powerful)

(continued)

Table 8.1 (continued)

Sport	Game time	Dimensions of field	Number of players	Other game characteristics
Rugby league	2 × 40 min halves	Rectangle: Lengthp: 100 m Width: 60 m	13 players from each team on field at one time; substitution bench of 4 players with unlimited number of substitutions during game	• Contact, tackling, scrums a feature of the game • Game style differs between positions on field—generally divided into backs (mobile) and forwards (big and powerful)
Field hockey	2 × 35 min halves	Rectangle: Length: 91 m Width: 55 m	11 players from each team on field at one time; substitution bench of 5 players with unlimited number of substitutions during game	• Noncontact game • Major differences in game characteristics of players with extremes ranging from "midfield" players to goalkeeper
Lacrosse	4 × 15 min quarters	Rectangle: Length: 110 yd Width: 60 yd	10 players from each team on field at one time; unlimited substitutions permitted from up to 10 players	• Contact game • Protective gear worn as part of uniform • Major difference in game characteristics of players with a goalie, 3 defense players, 3 midfielders, and 3 attack players

Table 8.2 Characteristics of Team Sports That May Have Relevance to the Athlete's Nutrition Goals or Challenges

Game characteristic	Nutritional implication
• Elapsed time of game • Duration of playing periods within game time	• Duration of time that players are exposed to environment • Duration of time that players may have limited access to nutritional support (e.g., opportunities for intake of fluid and carbohydrate)
• Actual playing time • Distance covered in game	• Heat production (sweat losses, fluid needs) • Carbohydrate utilization, risk of carbohydrate depletion (muscle glycogen, blood glucose) • Importance of low body fat content for endurance
• Number, duration, and frequency of high-intensity work bouts during game • Work–recovery ratio between high-intensity work bouts and low-intensity activities	• Heat production (sweat losses, fluid needs) • Carbohydrate utilization, risk of carbohydrate depletion (muscle glycogen, blood glucose) • Opportunity for creatine phosphate resynthesis during recovery between high-intensity work bouts (potential for benefits from creatine loading) • Limitations on performance derived from acid-base disturbances (potential for benefit from bicarbonate loading)
• Number of formal breaks during match (quarters, halves) • Availability of rotational or unlimited player substitutions during game	• Opportunities to periodically reduce workload (and rate of heat production and substrate utilization) in individual players • Opportunity for intake of fluid and carbohydrate within game
• Rules regarding carriage of fluids onto field of play • Rules regarding access of trainers to field of play during playing time or informal breaks in play	• Opportunity for intake of fluid and carbohydrate within game
• Season of play • Typical playing environment (heat, humidity, altitude)	• Heat production (sweat losses, fluid needs) • Carbohydrate utilization
• Jumping, changing movement patterns and direction within game play	• Importance of low body fat content for speed and agility
• Scrums, tackling, pushing within game play	• Importance of high body mass and lean body mass for strength and momentum • Tolerance of higher body fat content • Potential for direct muscle damage and contact injuries that may interfere with muscle repair and refueling between matches
• Uniform characteristics: use of heavy protective gear (helmets, padding)	• Heat load, impairment of evaporation of sweat losses • Impairment of ability to drink during game
• Seasonal fixture or tournament draw • Number of games, and period between matches • Length of season or tournament	• Opportunities for recovery (refueling, rehydration, repair) between matches • Relative importance and integration of training (and training nutrition goals) within competition program • Opportunity for changes in physique (both positive during preseason and negative during off-season)

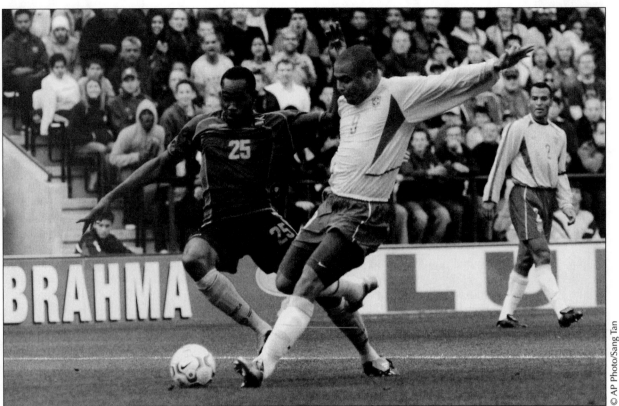

© AP Photo/Sang Tan

Soccer, also known as association football, is the most widely played team game in the world.

that undertaken in the first 15 min of a match (Mohr et al. 2003). Furthermore, the 5 min period immediately following the period in which most high-intensity work was undertaken was associated with a temporary decrease in the amount of high-intensity play. Although it could be argued that the reduction in high-intensity play during the last segment of the game resulted from change in game tactics once the match outcome had been decided, time–motion analysis found that substitute players who came onto the ground during this period carried out more high-intensity work than the players who had been on the ground for the full 90 min. Therefore, it appears that players experience fatigue during a match—both in temporary patches throughout the game and as a long-lasting outcome during the final and often deciding period of the game.

Australian football is another free-flowing game played on a large field, which allows players to cover considerable distances over the match duration of ~100 to 120 min. Eighteen players take the field for each team at any time, with an interchange bench of another five players who are continually rotated on and off the field. The modern game has evolved to a faster style of play, and the specialization of the traditional field positions has been blurred. Nevertheless, players can be divided into on-ball players, who typically follow the play, interspersing low-intensity jogging with high-intensity sprints (up to 60 m), and key position players, such as fullbacks and full forwards, who perform a high number of short sprints over a smaller

territory. There are few published studies of time–motion analyses of Australian football; one study from the 1970s reported that a "follower" covered 14.94 km over a game, whereas a fullback covered only 4.58 km (Jacques and Pavia 1974). It is likely that the modern style of game requires a match distance of 12 to 20 km for the most mobile players, although unpublished observations of some extraordinary players in the national competition have claimed distances of 20 to 25 km in matches. Such reports need to be confirmed. Activity patterns also involve tackling and evading tackles, bumping opponents, leaping to mark (catch) or punch the ball, bouncing or carrying the ball, and kicking and hand-passing the ball. The game places high physical demands on its players: In addition to requiring specific game skills, Australian football can be seen as a hybrid of the speed and endurance of soccer and the heavy physical contact of rugby codes and American football.

Although rugby union only became a professional sport in 1995, it has a long history of play, and its World Cup held every 4 years is considered the fourth largest sporting event in the world. According to game analyses discussed in the excellent reviews by Reilly (1990a) and Duthrie and colleagues (2003), the ball is typically only in play for about 30 min of the 80 min game, with the remaining time being taken up by injury stoppages, periods when the ball is out of play, the setting up of scrums and line-outs, and kicking for penalty goals and try conversions. Each 15-member team is made up of eight forwards and seven backs, although there are specialist positions within these groupings. The large and powerful forwards are considered the ball winners, who compete in brief, high-intensity activities in contact with or close proximity to the opposition team to gain possession of the ball. Meanwhile, the backs (known as the ball carriers), stand and walk until required to sprint—either to move the ball forward, provide decoy running lines, or run back in support and to cover defense. Although rule changes have apparently allowed the game to adopt a faster and more free-flowing style in recent years, it appears that the breakdown of game time into 85% lower-intensity activities and 15% high-intensity work (9% running and 6% tackling, pushing, and competing against the opposition) has held constant.

There are few, particularly recently conducted, time–motion studies of high level games, but existing analyses suggest that the typical distance covered during the game is 5.8 km, with 2.2 km at walking pace, 1.6 km jogging, and 2.0 km sprinting. The typical sprint distance is ~20 m, with the backs covering greater distances, both over the total game and at sprinting speeds. Most high-intensity activities of the forwards involve body contact rather than running; in fact, these activities mean that the forwards have a higher total workload for the game than the backs. Ninety-five percent of all activities are carried out over periods of less than 20 to 30 s, with the recovery period exceeding the duration of the preceding work. Anaerobic glycolysis and phosphagen systems provide power for the high-intensity passages of play. Blood lactate concentrations, admittedly collected at times of convenience rather than in specific relationship to high-intensity activities, generally range from 3 to 6 mmol/L and are higher in forwards than backs. The generous work-to-recovery ratios in the game are generally believed to prevent the accumulation of high blood lactate levels.

The common element of competition in field-based team sports is the heavy reliance on anaerobic power systems to fuel periods of high-intensity play, supported by a pronounced contribution of aerobic power systems in the recovery periods between activities. Depending on the code, the particular game, and the playing style of the individual player, performance in a game may be limited by total substrate availability or the recovery of the substrate pool within the game as well as by hydration and thermoregulation. Nutritional strategies during competition must not only target the muscle's ability to produce work but also support the optimal function of the central nervous system for the skills, concentration, and decision marking that ultimately determine performance outcomes. Developing nutritional strategies to support competition performance requires specific knowledge of the game and of the requirements for individual players as well as flexibility to address changing needs between games and between players. An additional and substantial consideration is that competition within team sports is organized within a seasonal fixture or tournament so that the final outcome of competition involves recovery between a series of games.

The competition structure of field-based team sports can be divided into tournaments or seasonal fixtures. Tourna-ments are typically held over periods ranging from a week (lower-level competitions) to 6 weeks (World Cups and championships), with matches being played every 1 to 3 days. Some tournaments involve pools in which groups of teams are selected to play each other in a series of games, with the top teams advancing to a knock-out final series. Draws for other tournaments are organized with a knock-out approach to all matches. A seasonal fixture typically lasts 4 to 6 months and can also be decided according to different rules. In some cases, teams in the league or conference are simply each drawn to play a designated number of times in a home and away fixture, with the winning side being the one that has accumulated most points at the end of this draw. In other competitions, the home and away fixture is used to rank teams, with the top group going on to play in a finals or championship series or in a separate competition such as a bowl, which can include teams from another regional fixture. The team competition structure can involve local, national, and international associations and leagues, which can mean substantial travel to attend games.

Many field-based team sports started as winter-based competitions, with all games between teams in the competition being played simultaneously in a weekly fixture. However, at the top level of professional sports, factors such as the pressure for media coverage, the desire to maximize crowd attendances at games, and the increased number of teams in the competition have led to an irregular draw, with teams being scheduled to play every 5 to 9 days. In some professional sports, teams are entered into more than one league or cup—for example, English soccer teams may play in the English Premier League, European Champions League, and FA cup—meaning that players can be scheduled to play every 3 to 4 days over a significant part of the competition season. Although the fixtures for such competitions usually take major international tournaments into account, the playing year is often extended by additional competitions such as Olympic Games and World Championships or World Cups. Players in professional competitions must add the requirements of their national team preparation to their already crowded team-based playing season. Even at lower or junior levels of competition, talented team athletes may choose to play for a number of teams (age-group and open competitions, or the school or college league and the local competition), which also increases the number of matches undertaken by an individual player in a season. Clearly, the nutritional principles of recovery are of high priority for team sport players, especially for players in mobile positions in lengthy duration sports and those in contact sports where injuries and muscle damage impair the rate of postgame recovery.

Training

Careful periodization is a hallmark of preparation for team sports. The year can generally be broken down into three periods: the preseason, the competition season, and the off-season. The duration and priority of each of these phases depend on the level of competition, with lower-level competitions and younger players generally enjoying a longer off-season. At high school and sometimes at the collegiate level, it is not unusual for team sport players to adopt another code or sport in the off-season of their winter-based team game; for example, football players often play cricket in the Australian summer or play lacrosse or run track in the American summer. However, for many recreational or low-level competitors, the off-season can also be a time of deconditioning, where inactivity and poor eating patterns replace the training and dietary commitment shown during the season. The off-season in most professional or elite team sports is now very short—as little as 4 weeks for some players—and even during that time there may be a club requirement or personal commitment to undertake an individual training program. For other players, the off-season may be a time for having corrective surgery or rehabilitation of a chronic injury.

The preseason may last 4 to 16 weeks depending on the level of competition. Typically, it involves a series of individual and team-based training programs, with players often being sorted into groups with different training goals depending on their style or position or play, their perceived weaknesses and goals for the upcoming season, or their need for injury rehabilitation. Different philosophies exist between and within team sports about the proportion of time spent on general and specific conditioning activities (endurance, speed, strength) and the introduction or positioning of game-based skills. At the elite or professional levels of some codes such as American football or soccer, an intensive two-a-day practice routine may be implemented for special camps or times of the preseason. The final phase of the preseason phase usually involves actual match play, in the form of friendly matches between clubs or a brief preseason tournament competition. Although many field-based team games are considered winter sports, the extended duration of the competition season and the early start of preseason conditioning often mean that players undertake preseason training in hot conditions. This presents a particular challenge for players undertaking an intensive training program.

During the season, players must continue to train between games to maintain or even enhance their conditioning and skill levels. It is challenging to organize a training program that achieves these goals yet allows recovery and repair between games played 3 to 9 days apart. The training week is organized into a series of team-based and individual sessions, with the proportion of each activity depending on the level of competition and the philosophy of the team coach and fitness and conditioning experts. Sessions can be dedicated to specific fitness and conditioning issues (e.g., endurance, strength, power, speed, agility, flexibility) or to improving skills and practicing team play. In the case of professional team sport players, training sessions can be scheduled throughout the day. However, at junior or lower levels of competition, training must be organized around the player's school or work commitments, and most team-based training sessions are undertaken in the afternoon and early evening.

The periodization of micro- and macrocycles of training within the competitive season is as much an art as a science, and it varies according to the coach's philosophy, the actual match draw (frequency of games, positioning of games designated as more important), and the method of deciding the competition outcome. For example, in leagues where the championship is awarded to the team who wins most games or points over the duration of the season, there is greater emphasis on maintaining consistency over the whole period and perhaps peaking for matches against key opponents. However, in tournaments and competitions that involve a playoff, players must play well enough throughout the season and for key games so that their team is included among the teams in the playoff yet save their peak until the finals, particularly the championship match. The typical philosophy is to divide the season into training blocks that are focused around a key goal or event—such as the build-up to matches against key opponents or to a series of matches with short recovery periods. During phases where there are longer recovery periods between matches, or where matches or opponents require less focus, there may be an opportunity to focus training volume and intensity on fitness and conditioning goals. Between matches there is normally a short period to allow promote recovery, a more intensive period of training, and then a taper and focus on team play.

Physique and Physiology

The physique requirements of team sport players vary across and within sports, and it is beyond the cope of this chapter to provide more than a brief summary of common issues. In most codes, the physique characteristics of players vary across playing positions or playing styles. Some team sport players play a fast and agile game, covering significant distances during a match; these characteristics are generally aided by a lean physique. Generally, body fat levels of team sport players do not reach the low levels typical of endurance athletes such as runners and triathletes, although in recent years there have been trends for a gradual reduction in body fat levels of professional team sport players (Duthrie et al. 2003). Indeed, some professional team sport players in mobile positions (e.g., midfielders in soccer and Australian football) have set new standards of leanness for their codes. In many situations, however, a common issue faced by many team sport players is the need to reduce high levels of body fat. Periods of inactivity, such as the off-season or an injury break, are often a time of significant gain of body fat. Team sports are filled with case histories illustrating that reduced exercise levels, coupled with inappropriate eating (and drinking) patterns, quickly lead to energy imbalance and weight increase.

At lower or recreational levels of competition, many team sport players begin a new season out of shape and gradually lose body fat over the competition schedule. At elite levels, most coaches expect players to retain a reasonable level of fitness and physique all year round and to fine-tune this during the preseason. Indeed, a study of Australian football teams found a clear delineation between standards of competition and changes in body composition of players over the competitive season: Professional players were leaner at the beginning of a season and showed minor changes in physique over the year, whereas semiprofessional players and amateur players showed a graded response, starting the season with higher levels of body fat and gradually reducing body fat and increasing lean body mass over the season (Burke et al. 1986). Nevertheless, even at top levels of competition there are many well-publicized cases in which team sport players have struggled to reduce their body fat levels to meet a team standard.

Strength, speed, and power are game characteristics favoring the development of lean body mass; these features are particularly important for sports or positions involving physical contact. Many team sport players undertake resistance training to increase their muscle size and strength. In addition to desiring high levels of muscle mass, many players in contact sports strive simply to be big; for example, rugby union forwards and American football players often weigh in excess of 120 kg. Higher levels of body fat are sometimes common in these players, and in some players and codes like American football, this appears to be tolerated. In certain games and playing positions, bulk is a desirable characteristic and the player must balance the advantages of increased momentum against a possible loss of speed and agility. Many players follow the nutritional strategies of strength-training athletes (discussed in chapter 11), emphasizing protein intake and using purported muscle-gain supplements. However, the optimum nutritional strategy for gain of muscle mass and strength involves a positive energy balance (often requiring high total energy intakes), adequate carbohydrate intake to fuel training and recovery, and strategically timed intake of protein in relation to training sessions.

Lifestyle and Culture

When entering competitive team sports, the young player can expect to face a busy lifestyle, juggling practice and games around the commitments of high school and college. For players who participate in amateur and semiprofessional team sports throughout their adulthood, the pressures of work or family make take precedence over training. When team training sessions are scheduled for afternoon and late evening, with some individual sessions being undertaken in the early morning, the players (and their families) may need to reorganize their meal schedule to accommodate a breakfast on the run and a late dinner in the evening. Other meals and snacks eaten during the day must be fit around work and study commitments. Such a chaotic or displaced eating pattern may challenge the player's ability to meet the high energy requirements associated with growth and training. It may be particularly difficult to fuel the prolonged sessions of high-intensity work or resistance training programs designed to increase muscle

size and strength. One study of collegiate football players undertaking an intensive 10-week off-season conditioning program found that the control group (no intervention) failed to make any progress in terms of gains in body mass, strength, or power over this period (Pearson et al. 1999). The authors suggested that the lifestyle changes associated with an intensive training program reduced opportunities for these players to eat, thus reducing their energy intake.

Some team players involved in collegiate or other institutionalized programs have the luxury of residential scholarships, including access to special training tables, or athlete dining halls. Of course, these facilities provide their own challenges to meeting nutritional goals, which are discussed in more detail in chapter 9. Meanwhile, most young team players are expected to be more self-sufficient or self-funded in looking after their nutritional needs. The expense of a large food bill or the cost of specialized sport products can be a drain for those starting out. In addition, many young team sport players leave home to pursue a career in the junior ranks of a team or club before they have had a chance to learn domestic skills. Many struggle with lack of skills in shopping and meal preparation or even just the time management skills needed to look after themselves. In the absence of good domestic or organizational skills, many players resort to takeaway, or fast, foods and haphazard eating patterns (Burke and Read 1988b; Jonnalagadda et al. 2001). This time can make or break a promising career, and many teams and clubs recognize the problem by organizing homestay or foster family programs for young recruits as well as nutrition activities and personal development schemes designed to teach athletes the necessary skills to survive. Supermarket tours and cooking classes are popular components of these activities and demonstrate the club's commitment to the importance of eating well in addition to providing an informal opportunity to create rapport between the player and sports nutrition experts.

Professional team sport players have the luxury of spreading their training schedule, and other commitments such as medical and testing appointments or team activities, over the day. Sometimes, particularly during periods of two-a-day practice or competition travel, the player is faced with a busy timetable that interferes with a normal eating schedule. At other periods, professional (or otherwise full-time) players are left with a considerable amount of time on their hands during the day. In some situations, eating becomes an entertainment, with the intake of unnecessary amounts or inappropriate choices of food leading to nutritional problems. In both situations, players need to understand their nutritional goals and to formulate an eating routing that can achieve such goals, whatever the requirements of the day.

Finally, travel plays a large role in the lives of many team sport players. They may be required to travel regionally, interstate, or even to other countries to fulfill the requirements of the primary leagues or competitions in which they play. Depending on the distance, the draw, and the importance given to preparation for the upcoming match, the travel commitment may span one to several days and involve transport by plane, bus, train, or car. The mode of

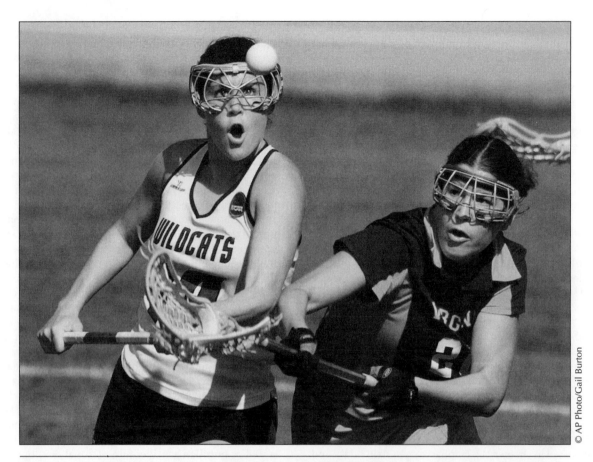

AP Photo/Gail Burton

Team sport players need to master the challenges of eating on the road or away from home, using their own food plan, as well as the opportunities organized for eating with the team, to ensure that they meet their nutrition goals.

transport can create special nutritional needs (e.g., the need to increase fluid losses in pressurized or air-conditioned environments) as well as determine the opportunities for food intake. Meanwhile, the duration of the trip will determine the player's exposure to the immediate challenges of travel nutrition as well as determine the priority of travel nutrition in the player's total diet. In the case of tournaments or specialized training camps, players may be required to leave their home base for substantial periods.

Dietary Surveys

The available literature on the reported dietary intakes of athletes in field-based team sports is summarized in tables provided in the appendix to this chapter (table 8.a for males and table 8.b for females). These include studies of soccer, American football, and Australian football players, at levels of play ranging from high school to elite professional. There are fewer data available on female players because most of these sports are male-dominated. The range of types of sports and the spread of time periods of the data collection make it difficult to make firm conclusions about the dietary practices of contemporary

team sport athletes. However, the results of several studies generally show that absolute energy intakes are highest in male team players with large physiques (e.g., American football players), especially during phases of growth or resistance training to gain muscle mass (Short and Short 1983). Intakes relative to body mass are highest in players in sports requiring high levels of activity during game play and in players who must undertake conditioning to maintain or enhance fitness (e.g., professional soccer players) (Bangsbo et al. 1992; Jacobs, Westlin, et al. 1982; Rico-Sanz et al. 1998). Some sports or athletes within these sports share a mixture of these characteristics—for example, some players in Australian football desire to have both a high degree of muscularity and the endurance to run large distances during a game. The only studies of energy balance in team sport players have been undertaken in soccer players. One study, undertaken in Japanese professional soccer players, found that mean reported energy intake accounted for only 88% of energy expenditure, estimated from doubly-labeled water techniques (Ebine et al. 2002); the authors concluded that this discrepancy was the result of underreporting. The other study, which used daily activity records to assess energy expenditure, found closer agreement with estimates of energy intake and expenditure of a group of soccer players from the Olympic team from Puerto Rico (Rico-Sanz et al. 1998).

For many team sport players, daily carbohydrate intakes within the range of 5 to 7 g/kg body mass would seem adequate for the moderate fuel cost of training and match play. This target appears to be met by some (Bangsbo et al. 1992; Caldarone et al. 1990; Hickson, Johnson, et al. 1987; Lundy et al. 2006; Schena et al. 1995; Short and Short 1983; Van Erp-Baart et al. 1989a) but not all (Hickson, Johnson, et al. 1987; Hickson, Wolinsky, et al. 1987) groups of athletes in field-based team sports. Higher intakes, within the range of 7 to 10 g/kg body mass, might be considered more suitable for professional athletes in soccer and Australian football, especially for the midfield players in teams fueling for more than one game each week or during phases of intensive training. Such intakes have been reported in a few studies of professional male soccer players (Jacobs, Westlin, et al. 1982; Rico-Sanz 1998; Zuliani et al. 1996) but are generally the result of high energy intakes rather than focused carbohydrate-rich eating, because the carbohydrate content of the diets of male team sport players in most of the available studies appears to be in the range of 40% to 50% of total dietary energy intake. Male team sport players typically report protein intakes within the range of 13% to 20% of dietary intake energy; this appears to provide daily protein intakes that meet or exceed 1.5 g/kg body mass. Studies in which reported micronutrient intakes have been estimated typically find that male team sport players are also able to meet the relevant recommended daily allowances for vitamins and minerals, at least as assessed by mean intakes of the group (Burke et al. 1991; Hickson, Wolinsky, et al. 1987; Lundy et al. 2006; Millard-Stafford et al. 1989; Rico-Sanz et al. 1998; Van Erp-Baart et al. 1989b). Further research on the dietary practices of high-level players in team sports is welcomed, especially to see the influence of the sports dietitians who have become part of the sports medicine support teams for most professional sports teams over the last decade. There is at least some preliminary evidence, from comparing the results of dietary surveys of Australian football players from professional teams in the national league, of a trend to greater intakes of carbohydrate and lower intakes of fat and alcohol, both in absolute terms and as a proportion of total dietary intake of energy (Burke et al. 1991; Graham and Jackson 1998; Shokman et al. 1999; Wray et al. 1994). The alcohol intake of team sport players deserves special mention and is discussed in a later section of this chapter. In general, alcohol is either excluded or left unreported in dietary surveys of athletes, leaving incomplete data on the alcohol intake practices of athletes. However, there is at least some evidence, including anecdotal reports, of poor alcohol practices occurring in sport, particularly among team sports.

The literature on dietary practices of female team sports players paints a less favorable picture of the typical intakes of these athletes (table 8.b in appendix). In general, the energy intakes reported by these athletes are less than those of male athletes (relative to body mass) and are often not substantially different than the intakes expected of sedentary females. Whether this reflects inadequate dietary survey methodology, a light training load attributable to the low caliber of play, or a deliberate energy deficit to achieve loss of body fat is uncertain. Several of these studies have compared dietary intakes during the season with postseason dietary practices and report lower energy intakes in the off-season as a result of reduced activity levels (Clark et al. 2003; Nutter 1991). Low energy intakes limit the opportunity for intake of macronutrients; typical daily carbohydrate intakes reported by female team sport players appear to be within the range of 3 to 5 g/kg body mass. Although reported protein intakes generally exceed the recommendations of 0.8 to 1.0 g/kg body mass set by nutrition experts in most countries, in many groups or individuals, protein intakes appear to fall short of the guidelines (1.0-1.5 g/kg body mass per day) set by some sports nutrition experts (see chapter 1).

Several studies of female team sport players have reported intakes of micronutrients—particularly minerals—that are below the relevant dietary reference values. For example, diets reported by field hockey players were found to provide micronutrient intakes below daily allowances for iron, magnesium, zinc, and calcium in one study (Tilgner and Schiller 1989) and for iron and calcium in another (Nutter 1991). Clark and colleagues (2003) observed, during the season, that mean reported intakes of a group of collegiate soccer players for some vitamins (e.g., folate, vitamin E) and minerals (e.g., magnesium) were less than 75% of daily allowances, indicating a risk of suboptimal intakes in some individuals. Iron was the micronutrient at most risk of inadequate intake in a study of international-level soccer players (Martin et al. 2006). Intakes of micronutrients were even lower during postseason because of lower energy intakes, with intakes of calcium and iron falling below 75% of daily allowances. Vitamin and mineral supplements were not routinely taken by this group. Further work is needed to explore the suitability of dietary survey methodology in female team sport players and to validate the reports of apparently low energy intakes. Whether apparently suboptimal intakes of carbohydrate and micronutrients occur frequently and affect nutritional status and performance also needs further examination. There are conflicting reports on iron status in female players of field-based team sports. Whereas one study reported a progressive decline in serum ferritin concentrations over three seasons in a group of female field hockey players (Diehl et al. 1986), another study did not find evidence of changes in hematological status of female soccer and hockey players over 14 weeks of training and competition (Douglas 1989).

Nutritional Issues and Challenges

The nutritional needs and challenges of field-based team sports are complex, and they change over the week and over the season according to the phase of training or competition. There are differences in the nutritional needs of players across sports but also within the same team, creating a challenge to those who educate the players or organize nutritional support for a team. The highlight box on this page summarizes some common issues faced by team players in field-based sports, including issues related to achieving optimal physique, optimizing training, and preparing for and recovering from games. Unusual features of many team sports, which create special nutritional requirements or practices, include the need to integrate training nutrition goals and competition goals in different ways at different times, the traveling lifestyle, and the opportunity to consider strategies that affect mental function as well as muscle function. Sports dietitians who work closely with successful teams in two different professional sports share some of the strategies they use to tackle these special nutritional needs in the second and third practical

issues. Discussion of the scientific background and guidelines for many of these issues is provided here and in the following two chapters.

Achieving Ideal Body Fat Levels

There is anecdotal evidence that over the last decade, team players in many field games have become interested in the better management of body fat levels. This may be because of the increased involvement of specialists in nutrition and conditioning as team staff, less deconditioning during breaks and injuries, and the belief that a lower body fat level might enhance performance on the field. As with all sports, it is hard to distinguish between the pure effects of a loss of body fat on performance and the effects of the strategies that were used to achieve it—for example, better attention to eating and an increased volume and intensity

Summary of Common Nutritional Issues Arising in Field-Based Team Sports

Physique Issues

- For some sports and positions: increasing and maintaining high levels of lean body mass for strength
- For some sports and positions: maintaining moderately low body fat levels to aid speed and agility
- Reducing or maintaining ideal body fat levels after period of inactivity because of off-season or injury

Training Issues

- Achieving high energy intake to maintain high body mass and size, especially during period of growth such as adolescence or aggressive resistance training
- Achieving high carbohydrate intake during interval between matches and training to promote optimal refueling.
- Consuming adequate protein to meet increased requirements attributable to heavy training and to promote recovery from matches and adaptation to training
- Considering creatine supplementation for training adaptations (match simulation, interval training, resistance training)
- Monitoring risk of reduced iron status, especially in female athletes and athletes undergoing growth spurts
- Addressing fluid and carbohydrate intake during prolonged training sessions
- Enhancing nutrition knowledge and domestic skills in young players
- Integrating training and match goals in a weekly fixture

Competition Issues

- Fueling up before events
- Consuming the prematch meal
- Managing fluid and carbohydrate intake during matches
- Refueling and rehydration between matches, especially in a tournament
- Determining optimal nutrition for the traveling athlete
- Using alcohol in a healthy manner, especially after a match
- Considering creatine and caffeine supplementation for competition performance

of training. It is likely that, compared with their predecessors, modern team sport players are better able to reduce their risk of gaining large amounts of body fat as well as to undertake more effective fat loss programs when these are desired. General dietary strategies for achieving loss of body fat were discussed in chapter 4 and summarized in tables 4.2-4.4. Some of the specific risk factors for unwanted gain of body fat among team sport players are summarized in table 8.3, together with strategies to prevent or reduce high body fat levels.

Table 8.3   Risk Factors and Strategies to Combat Unwanted Gain of Body Fat Among Team Sport Players

Risk factor	Strategies to address risk factor
Drastic reduction in activity levels during the off-season	• Recognition of energy cost of normal training and competition, to allow an appropriate reduction in energy intake • Encouragement of self-monitored off-season activity program, especially involving novel and enjoyable modes of exercise and cross-training
Poor eating and drinking practices during the off-season, ranging from relaxation of during-season "discipline" through to food and alcohol binges	• Development of individualized off-season dietary plan, allowing greater food flexibility and enjoyment than during the season, but with appropriate energy intake to match reduced energy expenditure • Counseling regarding food and alcohol binges to allow a more moderate approach to social eating occasions
Energy imbalance during injury because of a reduction or cessation of activity levels, compounded by boredom- or stress-related eating	• Development of individualized eating plan, integrated with injury rehabilitation program, so that nutrients needed for repair are provided within an appropriately reduced energy budget • Counseling and behavior modification education to identify inappropriate eating and replace with alternative activities or more constructive responses to eating cues
Poor nutrition knowledge and practical skills leading to poor food choices and reliance on takeaway foods	• Nutrition education activities to improve nutrition awareness and identify nutrient-dense, less energy-dense foods • Individual counseling and development of dietary plan with appropriate energy balance or deficit to allow weight maintenance or loss • Practical nutrition activities (e.g., supermarket tours, cooking classes) to teach domestic skills and self-reliance with preparation of appropriate meals • Specific activities related to making sound choices in restaurants and takeaway outlets
Chaotic meal patterns and displaced meals leading to poor awareness of actual food intake in a day	• Counseling in time management and domestic skills to develop a sound eating routine • Development of an eating plan with routine of appropriate meals and snacks • Where this problem commonly occurs among players and is exacerbated by team commitments, provision of meals and snacks within team environment or facilities for players to store or prepare their own supplies
Residential situation (e.g., college, foster family) exposing athlete to inappropriate food choices	• Development of nutrition education resources or activities for caterers (large and small quantity), promoting messages about the special nutritional needs of athletes • Education of players to make sound choices from available options or take proactive role in requesting modifications to menu • Identification of food items that can be added to, or substituted in, present meals to improve overall menu
Constant travel leading to disturbance of home routine; game schedule of frequent matches where emphasis is on proactive fueling and recovery	• Development of an individualized eating plan that provides adequate opportunities to meet player's fuel needs for match preparation and recovery, without exceeding appropriate energy budget

(continued)

Table 8.3 *(continued)*

Risk factor	Strategies to address risk factor
Poor nutrition knowledge, leading to reliance on short-term fad diets and unsafe or ineffective weight loss practices rather than long-term energy restriction	• Development of nutrition education resources providing objective and non-judgmental information about the ineffectiveness of fad diets or short-term measures • Individual counseling of overfat players to include discussion of realistic short-term and long-term fat loss goals and structured monitoring program to provide feedback and support
Regular excessive intake of alcohol, often in conjunction with inappropriate eating	• Development of nutrition education resources providing objective and non-judgmental information about the role of excessive intake of alcohol in gain of body fat; for example, energy content of alcohol per se, risk of poor eating practices during alcohol binge and "hangover" phase • Individual counseling to negotiate contract regarding appropriate alcohol intake practices

Of course, as in all sports, team sport players may need guidance to choose a playing weight and body fat level that are suited to their game and to their individual characteristics. Valid and reliable methods of assessment of body composition, which can be applied in the field, are an important tool for the coach, fitness advisor, and player. Such measurements should be taken at various times of the season to develop an individual history for each player and to select the range of physique characteristics at which the player appears to be performing at her or his best. This will be expected to vary over the season, according to the phase of training or competition, as well as over the player's career as he or she matures in age and training. Some players in strength- and power-based team sports may desire a high body mass, without considering the disadvantages of being overfat, such as reduced speed and agility or impaired thermoregulation in hot weather. For example, many defensive linemen and linebackers in American football carry high body fat levels. This phenomenon appears less prominent than in past times. On the other hand, there is some anecdotal evidence that many team sport players may be overfocused on achieving very low body fat levels without direct evidence that this enhances their on-field performance. It is harder to measure the impact of body composition on the performance of complex sports in which skill and tactics play such an important role. Nevertheless, it is apparent from observation of the best players in any team sport that a wider range of body types is tolerated than in many other simpler sports. This argues strongly against the imposition of team standards in which each player is expected to achieve a rigid standard of body fat or body mass. Instead, individual goals should be set for each player.

The achievement of ideal body fat level and playing weight should occur before the competitive season—from the combined efforts of staying in better shape during the off-season and undergoing conditioning during the preseason program. The player should allow sufficient time for any loss of body mass or fat to be achieved without compromising the preseason or within-season training

program. This doesn't always happen in practice, even in the more enlightened times or professionalized codes of team sports. There are still examples in most field-based team sports of weight loss practices involving fad diets, extreme energy restriction, abuse of fat-loss supplements containing stimulants such as ephedrine or ephedra, and dehydration techniques (e.g., training in sweatsuits, use of saunas, and restriction of fluid during training). At best, these techniques can lead to the frustration of failing to achieve fat loss goals or to fatigue and impaired performance. Tragically, the extreme use of these practices can lead to serious outcomes including death. There has been much speculation that the recent heatstroke deaths of some college or professional footballers and a baseball player in the United States were associated with their extreme weight loss practices. In particular, players need to know that techniques based on dehydration may temporarily reduce body mass but do not address the real goal of loss of body fat. Instead, dehydration simply adds another risk factor to the development of heat stress, as discussed in the later section on fluid needs during training and matches. Players who need to lose weight and body fat must be provided with access to nutrition education and counseling services.

Eating to Gain Muscle Bulk and Strength

Many field-based team sports (e.g., American football and rugby codes) require speed, strength, and power. Consequently, high levels of muscle mass and strength are requirements for high-level performance, and there is evidence over recent times of a general increase in lean muscle mass of elite players in these codes (see reviews by Reilly 1990 and Duthrie et al. 2003). However, strength or bulk is also required in other team sports, at least for some players or positions on the team. Consequently, resistance training is a feature of most field-based team games, ranging from playing an assistive to a primary role in training programs according to the player or code.

Preseason preparation provides the major opportunity for programs to increase muscle bulk and size, although in power-based codes, players still undertake substantial resistance training loads during the competitive season to maintain the fruits of their preseason labors. Resistance training includes specific programs undertaken in a gym as well as game-specific drills such as practicing scrums or using tackle dummies. Although in some codes, the player is aspiring to a long-term and substantial increase in muscle mass and strength over the years of a playing career, in other codes, the young player is simply aiming to accelerate his maturation into an adult physique and to consolidate his playing style and skills.

The key components for success in gaining muscle size and strength are a well-designed resistance training program, genetic potential, and well-timed nutritional support. Curiously, the exact components of the optimal diet for gain of muscle size and strength are still unknown, despite centuries of debate among athletes and coaches and, more recently, sport scientists. Clearly, adequate energy is important, as are adequate amounts of protein and micronutrients involved in the development of new tissues. The most recent scientific studies suggest that the timing of nutrient intake, particularly in relation to training sessions, may be as important as meeting total nutritional needs. The current understanding of nutrition to support resistance training goals is discussed in greater detail in chapter 11. The reader is also directed to chapter 6, in which the strategies for achieving a high energy intake in a busy day (the first practical issue) and for postexercise recovery (the second practical issue) are covered in the context of rowing and swimming. Many field-based team sport players, particularly in the more mobile sports such as Australian football, soccer, or hockey, may share the issues faced by rowers and swimmers in needing to combine the goals of training for endurance as well as strength. In such cases, the gain of muscle bulk and strength is a function not only of the outcomes of a specific resistance training program but also of minimizing the catabolic outcomes that may occur as a result of prolonged sustained or intermittent high-intensity exercise. Thus, the team player needs to take special care in the nutritional support of all training sessions, supplying adequate fuel both for the session and for high energy needs over the day, as well as providing a timely supply of the nutrients needed during recovery to optimize the adaptations achieved by the session. Tables 6.5 (high-energy eating) and 6.h (nutritional guidelines for recovery) contain information that will be useful for the team sport player in addressing goals for muscle bulk and strength. Sport foods and supplements may also play an important role in meeting such goals (discussed subsequently).

Team sport players need expert guidance regarding realistic expectations for gains of muscle mass and strength. Their goals should be considered as a long-term project requiring long-term commitment. There is evidence that team sport athletes are also susceptible to the claims for many so-called muscle gain practices that should be considered ineffective (or at least lacking scientific support),

ad hoc, and often risky. These practices include restrictive high-protein diets and the use of supplements, including prohormones that are considered banned substances in some but not all team sports. These practices are discussed in greater detail in chapter 11.

Ironically, many of the factors summarized in table 8.3 that place the team sport player at risk of unwanted gain of body fat can also interfere with the achievement of optimal gains of muscle bulk and strength. A chaotic and overcommitted lifestyle, in which the player fails to establish a suitable routine of meals and snacks or to develop an awareness of her total food intake, is a major impediment to achieving optimal returns from a resistance training program. As outlined in table 6.5, a high-energy, high-nutrient intake is best achieved by a pattern of small, frequent meals and snacks, spread over the day and in conjunction with the training program. Good organization is needed to ensure access to suitable foods and drinks, whatever the day's activities. In some situations this may be the sole responsibility of the player, but in other cases, a team may decide to offer some form of nutritional support within the club environment, especially in conjunction with the training program. The provision of sport foods, drinks, and snacks in the training environment is valuable because it ensures that players can meet their immediate nutrition goals after a workout, under supervision. It also provides an education opportunity, illustrating practical ways of meeting sports nutrition goals and demonstrating that the team or club places importance on the achievement of nutrition goals.

Specialized sport foods such as sport bars, liquid meal supplements, and sport drinks provide a practical and portable source of the energy, protein, carbohydrate, and micronutrients needed to support a program for gaining muscle bulk and strength. However, the cost of such products often is a burden for a young player or for a team that needs to cater for a large number of players. In such cases, these products should be used only in situations in which everyday foods are impractical to eat. Features such as low perishability, simple preparation characteristics, delivery of a desired amount of key nutrients, and general ease of consumption make these sport foods useful for an outdoor training situation, for the player on the move between a series of commitments, or for an athlete with a suppressed appetite. However, lower-cost alternatives are available for other situations or for the motivated player—for example, cartons of flavored yogurt, flavored milks, fruit smoothies, cereal bars, and dried fruit and nut mixes. Chapter 11 provides greater discussion of alternatives to sport foods.

Teaching Nutrition Awareness and Domestic Skills to Young Players

The talent identification and draft programs that exist in many team sports have seen an increase in the number of young players apprenticed to clubs and teams. This often means that players leave home to relocate to the club or training program before learning the life skills and domestic skills necessary to support an independent existence. Player welfare programs and career and education services will be important in helping young athletes make the huge adjustments to their lifestyle. Programs that increase nutrition awareness and practical nutrition skills will also assist young players to become self-reliant and able to meet important nutritional goals during a crucial time of their career development. Many professional teams or collegiate programs hire sports dietitians to provide an integrated nutrition education program for players, with special activities targeted to young players and those living away from home for the first time. Such programs can include the following:

- Group education sessions and workshops, targeting special challenges (e.g., travel, weight gain, hydration, and fueling issues)

- Supermarket tours with education on time management skills, reading food labels, and low-budget food purchasing

- Cooking classes in specialized kitchens or in the players' own homes

- Visits to restaurant and takeaway outlets to develop skills in menu selection

The experience of the Department of Sports Nutrition at the Australian Institute of Sport, and others who have developed integrated nutrition programs for professional teams (Burns and Dugan 1994) and collegiate programs (Vinci 1998), is that interactive and practical activities that address athletes' lifestyle issues are highly successful in improving nutrition knowledge and eating behavior. There are many benefits in undertaking education activities such as a cooking class or supermarket tour:

- Opportunity to create rapport between the player and the sports nutrition expert, outside the artificial or formal atmosphere of an individual counseling session. Such rapport can enhance the educative potential of the immediate session as well as create interest by the player for future education opportunities.

- Opportunity, when sessions are undertaken in the players' homes, to observe signs of lifestyle, self-sufficiency, and domestic skill rather than rely on self-reports from athletes.

- Opportunity to teach and supervise the development of practical skills, rather than rely on the player to convert theoretical information into behavior changes.

- Demonstration of commitment by the club or team to achievement of good nutrition practice by players.

The principles and skills involved in preparing meals suited to a busy lifestyle and the nutritional goals of sport are discussed in more detail in the first practical issue in this chapter.

Recovering During the Training Week and Fueling Up for Matches

There are few studies of the fuel demands of team sport players during training or competition, with the available evidence being focused on the match play of soccer players. The scarcity of data makes it difficult to develop rigorous guidelines for the carbohydrate intake of team sport players. However, it is intuitive that athletes involved in mobile codes (e.g., soccer, Australian football, field hockey, lacrosse) or with mobile playing styles should be proactive in ensuring adequate carbohydrate stores for the aerobic and anaerobic production of fuel, during both training and matches. This may require special attention to match preparation, refueling during games, postevent recovery, and fueling during the training week.

Several older studies used biopsy techniques to monitor muscle glycogen concentrations in soccer players as a result of actual match play. These studies reported considerable depletion of muscle glycogen content after a game, with some players showing a low glycogen content at halftime (Saltin 1973). Players with depleted muscle glycogen stores have been reported to cover less distance at a lower average speed during the second half of the match (Ekblom 1986). In one study, players with the lowest glycogen levels were found to cover 25% less distance in the second half than players with highest muscle glycogen content. Walking and sprinting contributed 50% and 15% of the distance covered by the former group and 27% and 24% for the latter group, respectively (Saltin 1973). Magnetic resonance spectroscopy was used to provide a noninvasive estimation of glycogen degradation during a laboratory-based shuttle test simulating soccer play. A correlation between glycogen utilization and time to exhaustion was found, indicating a role for muscle glycogenolytic capacity in the onset of fatigue in soccer (Rico-Sanz et al. 1999). Another outcome of this study was the confirmation that fatigue may occur well before the end of the game; mean time to fatigue by the well-trained soccer players who undertook the protocol was around 42 min.

The value of fueling up in preparation for a match has been demonstrated in both field and laboratory studies. Participants followed 48 hr of either a high- or low-carbohydrate diet before short-term (<10 min) and prolonged (>30 min) protocols of intermittent exercise (6 s bouts at 30 s intervals). The low-carbohydrate preparation, which reduced glycogen concentrations in the vastus lateralis by at least 50% of values achieved in the high-carbohydrate treatment, was associated with a dramatic reduction in the work performed in both protocols (Balsom, Gaitanos, et al. 1999). In another investigation, professional soccer players completed an intermittent high-intensity protocol of field and treadmill running lasting ~90 min, after 48 hr of high-carbohydrate (~8 g·kg^{-1}·day^{-1}) and control (~4.5 g·kg^{-1}·day^{-1}) diets (Bangsbo et al. 1992). The high-carbohydrate diet increased intermittent running to fatigue at the end of the protocol by ~1 km ($p < .05$), although the performance enhancement was more marked in some participants than others (Bangsbo et al. 1992). These studies show that higher preexercise glycogen stores enhance capacity to undertake repeated bouts of exercise, even as short as 6 s in duration.

Other studies using applied or real-life protocols have confirmed these findings. Movement analysis of a four-a-side indoor soccer game lasting 90 min was undertaken following 48 hr of high (~8 g · kg⁻¹ · day⁻¹) or moderate (~3 g · kg⁻¹ · day⁻¹) carbohydrate intake (Balsom, Wood, et al. 1999). Compared with the moderate carbohydrate intake, the high-carbohydrate diet increased muscle glycogen content by 38% and allowed soccer players to complete ~33% more high-intensity work during the game. Another investigation found that elite-level ice hockey players who carbohydrate-loaded before a game were able to skate for longer distances and at higher intensities that when their normal dietary preparation was undertaken (Akermark et al. 1996). Players from two elite Swedish ice hockey teams were randomly allocated to either a carbohydrate-enriched (8.4 g · kg⁻¹ · day⁻¹) or mixed (6.2 g · kg⁻¹ · day⁻¹) diet in the recovery period between games held 3 days apart. Muscle glycogen concentrations were reduced after the first game for all players (43 mmol/kg wet weight [ww]), but restoration levels were 45% higher in the carbohydrate-loaded players before the next game (99 vs. 81 mmol/kg ww, $p < .05$). Distance skated, number of shifts skated, amount of time skated within shifts, and skating speed were all increased in the carbohydrate-loaded players compared with the mixed diet group, with the differences being most marked in the third period. Individual differences in performance were said to be related to muscle glycogen metabolism (Akermark et al. 1996).

Twenty-four-hour recovery was studied in team sport players who undertook a 60 min treadmill test involving multiple sprints and were then randomized into groups of low (12% of energy), normal (47% of energy), and high (79% of energy) carbohydrate intake. Power outputs during 6 s sprints interspersed over the 60 min declined over the duration of the test on day 1 and were even lower when repeated on day 2. Day 2 performance was not different between dietary groups for the total 60 min; performance declined by 5%, 0.5%, and 0.2% compared with day 1 for low-, normal-, and high-carbohydrate trials (not significant). However, over the first 20 min of the test on day 2, the high-carbohydrate group performed better than the low-carbohydrate group (Nevill et al. 1993). This study shows the difficulty of repeating performance of high-intensity exercise on successive days but suggests that better restoration of muscle carbohydrate stores can enhance recovery.

An even shorter recovery period of 2.5 hr was provided to team sport athletes who undertook a 70 min intermittent exercise protocol before consuming a placebo, carbohydrate (1.5 g/kg), or iso-energetic drink providing carbohydrate (1.2 g/kg) and protein (0.3 g/kg) (Niles et al. 2001). The outcomes of the subsequent intermittent shuttle run to fatigue lasting 7 to 8 min were interpreted using mean

results and confidence intervals rather than the traditional view of statistical significance. Participants ran 10% to 14% longer with carbohydrate-containing drinks compared with placebo, with confidence intervals suggesting that the range of the true likely effect of the improvement would be 2% to 20%. There was a trend to further improvement with the carbohydrate–protein beverage; however the mean enhancement of ~3% was likely to be within the range of a 1% deterioration to a 7% improvement. Although there was no explanation of these findings apart from a lower self-reported level of muscle soreness, the authors suggested that enhanced muscle glycogen restoration might account for differences in the second exercise bout. Further research is needed to investigate the timing and amount of nutrients needed to promote recovery after team sport activities. Superior recovery might not only directly promote better match performance when games are close together but also allow better training during the week, ultimately promoting better adaptations and outcomes. This theory has not been directly tested in team sports.

Whether muscle fuel status is involved in the apparent deterioration of skills toward the end of the game in many team sports is hard to determine. Different dietary preparations (carbohydrate intakes of 8 vs. 4 g · kg⁻¹ · day⁻¹) were consumed by recreational soccer players over the 48 hr period before a simulated soccer match (Abt et al. 1998). Shooting and dribbling tasks were undertaken before and after a 60 min intermittent treadmill run. The performance of these drills did not deteriorate over time in the control trial; therefore, it is not surprising that the high-carbohydrate treatment did not change the outcome. The authors concluded that either their treadmill protocol failed to achieve sufficient glycogen degradation to impair the execution of skills as seen during real match play or factors other than fuel depletion are responsible for this decline (Abt et al. 1998). However, the ability of the test protocol to provide a reliable and valid measure of match skills in these participants must also be questioned.

Overall, the literature supports the value of restoring glycogen between matches and of providing adequate fuel for training sessions requiring high-intensity intermittent exercise. However, there has been little systematic study of the amounts of dietary carbohydrate needed to achieve optimal refueling by real-life players. Older studies of professional soccer players found an inability to replete muscle glycogen during the 48 hr after a match, despite minimal training and a mean daily carbohydrate intake of 8 g/kg (Jacobs, Westlin, et al. 1982). Muscle glycogen concentrations determined from biopsy samples increased from ~46 to ~69 mmol/kg ww during the first 24 hr of sedentary recovery, with restoration correlated to the degree of post-match depletion. However, no further refueling appeared to take place during the second 24 hr recovery period, which included light training; muscle glycogen concentrations were 73 mmol/kg ww at the end of this period. The reported values for glycogen content in this study are low compared with other literature values for well-trained and rested athletes and are in contrast to more recent studies suggesting that the well-trained muscle can normalize or even supercompensate glycogen stores within 24 to 36 hr of the last exercise bout (Bussau et al. 2002). This may reflect an artifact of the study or a specific impairment of glycogen resynthesis in team sport players—for example, as a result of muscle damage from high-intensity running or contact injuries.

In contrast, a study using magnetic resonance spectroscopy monitored muscle glycogen utilization during a simulated soccer match and its repletion over 24 hr of recovery while players consumed their habitual diets (Zehnder et al. 2001). Mean muscle glycogen content decreased from 134 to 80 mmol/kg ww over the exercise protocol but was almost restored to prematch levels (122 mmol/kg ww) after 24 hr. Players consumed 327 g of carbohydrate (4.8 g/kg body mass) during this period. Whether this is a suitable simulation of the real fuel demands of actual matches, and whether players would benefit from a higher carbohydrate to ensure full glycogen repletion, could not be addressed by this study.

Further study is needed before clear guidelines for daily carbohydrate intake can be provided to team sport players (Burke, Loucks, et al. 2006). However, it is reasonable to set goals of 5 to 7 g·kg⁻¹·day⁻¹ for high-level players in less mobile sports, situations with a less demanding training and competition schedule, or players with lower energy requirements. For mobile players who want to maximize muscle glycogen refueling between matches and training, targets of 7 to 10 g·kg⁻¹·day⁻¹ may be required. Historically, many team sport athletes have considered carbohydrate intake a priority only for the night before the game or for the pregame meal. It may take a change in culture for some modern players to eat adequate carbohydrate to keep pace with the daily fuel demands of training and match play.

Pregame Meal

The pregame meal has held a special place in the nutrition of team sport players. In the early days of sports nutrition, the preevent meal was considered to have an almost magical role in the athlete's preparation—as if the right combination of foods, eaten at the right time and in the right amounts, could transform a player or team into championship form. Superstition was involved with the belief that one meal could overcome a week of inattention to eating as well as the choice of foods. A high-protein meal such as steak or bacon and eggs was often promoted, perhaps a legacy of the old beliefs that protein fueled the muscles or, from even earlier times, that some attribute of the animal that was consumed could be conferred on the athlete's own performance.

The modern approach is that the preevent meal provides a chance to fine-tune nutritional preparation for the upcoming match, especially with regard to fuel and fluid status. This is especially important in tournament situations or where games are otherwise scheduled close together, leaving insufficient time for recovery from the previous match or training session. Gastrointestinal comfort also needs to be considered, ensuring that the player neither becomes hungry over the hours of the prematch warm-up and competition itself nor suffers from gut discomfort from excessive intake. In the team environment, there is a motivational aspect of having players eat together. Many teams organize a communal meal to address preevent nutritional needs, both for bonding opportunities and to address the logistics of interstate or even international travel. Because games can be played at various times of the day or evening according to the code and level of competition, the preevent meal may take the form of breakfast, lunch, dinner, or even a substantial snack. In most cases, the preevent meal is consumed within the 2 to 4 hr period before the game, and the menu for the rest of the day is adjusted accordingly.

Chapter 1 (table 1.3) provided suggestions for menu plans based on carbohydrate-rich foods, with some players needing to modify intakes of protein, fat, or fiber to ensure a low risk of gastrointestinal problems during the game. In most team situations, the communal preevent meal adheres to a tried-and-true formula—the second and third practical issues in this chapter outline the approach taken by two different and very successful professional football teams. Many team sport players are happy with a narrow range of menu selections, liking the confidence that familiarity or routine provides. However, the menu needs to provide sufficient choice to cater to the various preferences of each team member. Buffet-style eating is generally used to achieve maximal flexibility with menu choices (see section of catering for athletes in chapter 9).

Whether in the team setting or as a result of their own organization, some players select unusual menus and foods in the preevent meal, sometimes falling outside the sports nutrition guidelines. Because the psychological value of the preevent meal is considered important, many sports dietitians and nutritionists who work with these players choose not to intervene unless the player experiences problems or requests advice. In many cases, the athlete's general nutritional preparation or her firm belief in her preevent meal choices can overcome any theoretical disadvantages of apparently inappropriate eating patterns. Nutritionists should respect the athlete's own belief system, especially at crucial times such as competition day.

Fluid and Fuel Needs During the Match and Training

Match play and training for team sports can lead to significant muscle glycogen utilization and loss of fluid. The replacement of fluid and carbohydrate during the exercise session provides an opportunity to address the fluid deficit incurred through sweating as well as provide additional carbohydrate for the muscle and central nervous system. The needs and opportunities for intake of fluid and carbohydrate during various team and racket sports are underpinned by issues that are distinctly different than those in continuous sports. These issues are discussed in greater detail in separate sections of chapter 9 (the first and second research topics, and the first practical issue). The remainder of this section focuses on refueling and hydration practices of field-based team sport players.

The available information on fluid losses and voluntary intakes in field-based team sports during training and competition sessions is summarized in table 8.c in the appendix to this chapter. Unfortunately, there are few published data on real-life practices of modern players across the full range of team sports, particularly at high levels of competition and during match play. However, the available observations suggest at least the potential in field-based team sports for a significant mismatch between sweat losses and fluid intakes to occur during training and games. Across most field-based team sports, mean sweat rates of 800 to 1,000 ml/hr are common, but losses may occur at 150% to 200% of these rates in hot and humid conditions or in individual players (see table 8.c). Success with fluid replacement appears to vary markedly between, but even within, team sports. Reported fluid intakes range from 200 to 1,400 ml/hr, replacing less than 10% of sweat losses in some players (Mustafa and Mahmoud 1979) to nearly 90% in others (Kirkendall 1993). Typically, studies report mean fluid deficits of 1.5% to 2% body mass accruing across team games; of course, some players exceed these levels (e.g., 4-5%), whereas other players are able to maintain better hydration status. Even when the mean level of fluid deficit accruing across a session appears moderate (<2% of body mass), it is possible that team players were already dehydrated at the start of the session (Godek, Godek, et al. 2005; Godek, Bartolozzi, et al. 2005; Maughan et al. 2004). Under these circumstances, even a small to moderate fluid deficit incurred during the game is likely to cause greater physiological detriment.

Even when opportunities to drink are not limited, it appears that many team sport players fail to consume fluids at rates that keep pace with sweat losses (Broad et al. 1996; Maughan et al. 2004; Shirreffs et al. 2005; Stofan et al. 2003, 2005). The choice and availability of fluid appear to play a role. In one study, football players were found to consume less fluid during a session when the drink supply was warm (from on-field water fountains) than when cold water was available (Godek, Godek, et al. 2005). The environmental temperature appears to play a role in determining fluid intake, independent of actual fluid needs. For example, one study that compared fluid balance during training in the same group of soccer players under winter and summer conditions found little difference in overall fluid deficits; although sweat rates were reduced in cold conditions, players also reduced their fluid intakes compared with drinking practices during summer (Broad et al. 1996). Another investigation of fluid balance during a winter training session undertaken by professional soccer players also reported very low rates of fluid intake, leading to a significant level of hypohydration (Maughan et al. 2005). Thus, even in cold weather, team sport players may need encouragement to hydrate adequately.

The effects of hypohydration on the performance of team sports are discussed in greater detail in chapter 9 but may be expected to impair both movement patterns and skill levels. It is possible that overall effects of hypohydration are greater in team sports than in other exercise activities, because the negative effect of fluid deficits on mental skills and concentration is an important factor in determining match outcomes beyond any simple effect on muscular work output. Although the etiology of heat cramps is not fully understood, there are anecdotal observations that susceptible team sport players experience unusually high rates of fluid and electrolyte loss during exercise and should pay attention to replacing these losses to prevent heat cramps (Stofan et al. 2005). This issue is covered in greater detail in chapter 10 (research topic 2).

In some team sports, poor drinking practices may cause a health risk to players as well as performance deficits, because dehydration may contribute to the development of heat illnesses. Many modern team sports may be played in conditions, or with rules and customs, that do not allow temperature regulation. Many field-based team games, which evolved as winter sports or originated in countries with cool climates, are now played in hot environments. For example, cricket has spread from temperate English summers to tropical and hot climates such as those found in the Indian subcontinent, the Caribbean, Australia, and South Africa; similarly, soccer is now played in many countries with hot climates. The evolution of national and international competitions, and the repositioning or lengthening of playing seasons, have forced traditional winter sports to be undertaken in hot locations or summer or transitional months. Rules governing the time of play, the length of play without rest, and the uniforms worn by players may be suitable for cool environments; however, they may not have been adapted in recognition of the marked increases in heat loads in hot environments. Team players may not be prepared for increased heat accumulation in terms of sound acclimatization practices before playing in a hot location or the sensible choice of exercise patterns during training. Inappropriate practices in the summer training for American football include wearing full protective gear or undertaking excessive training loads, sometimes in the belief that players can be toughened through training under thermal stress in a dehydrated condition (Knochel 1975).

It has been claimed that at least 50 American football players died from heat stroke in the 10 years from 1965 to 1975 (Knochel 1975). Although education appeared to eradicate some dangerous beliefs and practices, reducing the rate of deaths from heat illnesses in American football players over the next two decades, since 1994 there has been an apparent increase in deaths (Bailes et al. 2002). Some experts have speculated that this reversal has been caused by the use of ephedrine-containing fat loss supplements that increase metabolic heat production and by extreme weight loss practices that cause dehydration (Bailes et al. 2002). It is hard to prove these theories because these practices generally coincide with other risk factors such as hot weather, impairment of thermoregulation by high levels of body fat and heavy protective uniforms, and the imposition of twice-a-day training in underconditioned players. Nevertheless, dehydration may add another component to this dangerous mixture and should be minimized.

Team sport players face different challenges to understanding or anticipating their sweat losses than other athletes, because each match and even training session have an unpredictable workload. Because each match in team sports is unique and differs between players in the same team, the individual athlete must be aware of his likely sweat losses across a range of scenarios. Regular monitoring of changes in body mass over a training session or match is a practical way to gauge sweat losses and replace these over the session. Despite the lack of data in the published literature, this appears to be a common activity undertaken by the sport scientists and sports dietitians and nutritionists advising professional team sports (see the second and third practical issues in this chapter). Players need to consider the specific opportunities provided by their sports to drink during the match and training sessions. This includes a range in the occasions available for fluid intake (from between the formal periods of a game to opportunities on the ground during play) and the availability of fluids (from sports in which official rules limit fluid intake on the field to codes in which trainers can take fluids to players during play). These issues and strategies to achieve good hydration practices in team sports are covered in detail in the first practical issue in chapter 9.

Given the restrictions on fluid intake during some team sports, or the brief duration of the recovery period between some training sessions and matches, there has been some interest in the benefits of preexercise hyperhydration strategies for team sports or at least the practical strategies that can ensure better hydration over the whole day between exercise sessions. This would appear important in light of evidence that some players commence a training session with a significant fluid deficit, presumably as a result of failing to fully restore sweat losses from the previous session (Godek, Godek, et al. 2005; Maughan et al. 2004). Dabinett and coworkers (2001) undertook an intervention strategy in female field hockey players in which they monitored weight changes during exercise sessions and urine characteristics and prescribed fluid intakes to ensure adequate hydration during a period of acclimation training in the heat. This strategy allowed players to achieve the behavioral changes needed to increase their fluid intakes to meet fluid requirements under conditions of thermal stress. There has been some interest in the potential benefits of hyperhydration to prepare for competitions in hot weather. One intervention study involved a small group of players from the Puerto Rico national soccer team who increased fluid intake to achieve overhydration before a match played in hot conditions (Rico-Sanz et al. 1996). Players were randomly allocated to a week of voluntary hydration (fluid intake ~2.7 L/day) and a week of hyperhydration (fluid intake ~4.6 L/day) before the match. Total body water increased with hyperhydration, despite a significant increase in urine output. Analysis of testing before, during, and after the match found that additional water intake in these heat-acclimated players improved temperature regulation during the soccer match but had no significant effect on the performance decrement of some soccer-specific tasks observed at the end of a soccer match. In light of the new recognition of the dangers of excessive fluid intake by individuals, such strategies cannot be universally recom-

mended, and education programs regarding hydration need to stress the potential dangers of overdrinking.

Nutritional practices during training and competition must consider the need for carbohydrate replacement as well as fluid intake. In fact, team sports have played an interesting role in the development of refueling practices for athletes. In 1967, the Miami Orange Bowl playoff in American college football saw the Florida Gators in competition against Georgia Tech. The Gators were being badly beaten and at halftime used a new drink designed for them by Dr. Robert Cade of the University of Florida. The drink, containing electrolytes and carbohydrate, was designed "to replace what the game was taking out of them." The Florida Gators played well enough in the second half to overcome their opponents and win their first Bowl. Their drink, called Gatorade, was released commercially. It took another 20 years for sport scientists to embrace the performance benefits of consuming carbohydrate–electrolyte drinks during a wide range of sports. Today, sport drinks are the most widely accepted form of specialized sports foods and are a lucrative niche in both the beverage and supplement industries.

The benefits of consuming carbohydrate during a training session or match in team sports will depend on the type, duration, and intensity of the activity. Research Topics 1 and 2 in chapter 9 consider the effects of refueling on both the muscle and the central nervous system—looking at both the movement patterns of team sport players and the maintenance of important cognitive aspects of a game such as execution of skill, concentration, and decision making. Some (Kirkendall et al. 1988; Muckle 1973; Ostojic and Mazic 2002; Welsh et al. 2002) but not all (Criswell et al. 1991; Nassis et al. 1998; Zeederberg et al. 1996) studies show that carbohydrate intake during a session can enhance various aspects of team sport performance. Of course, the available studies barely scratch the surface of the complexity or range of team sports; therefore, we lack definite proof of the specific performance advantages of refueling during the full range of training or competition settings in team sports. However, it is intuitive that such a strategy would be of greatest importance to the more prolonged field-based sports (e.g., soccer and Australian football) and to players with a mobile playing style. Refueling strategies should also be considered in tournament situations or in a busy competition or training schedule that leaves insufficient time for complete recovery of muscle fuel stores between each session. The use of commercial sport drinks or other carbohydrate-containing fluids can address fluid needs as well as fuel requirements; in fact, the provision of a flavored drink is likely to enhance overall intake of fluid compared with plain water and may be one tactic to improve fluid intake practices of team sport players. It is unlikely that the intake of such a drink will provide any disadvantages in a team sport, although for some players, the cost and energy content of the drink may need to be taken into account. However, for some players with high fuel and energy needs, carbohydrate replacement during training and matches will provide the additional benefit of contributing to overall daily needs.

Alternative products and strategies are used by team sport players to address fuel needs during training and competition sessions. Sport bars and gels provide a compact form of fuel that can be consumed in the break between the warm-up and the game or at longer formal breaks (e.g., halftime). Gels have become a popular source of carbohydrate replacement in many team sports, with some players preferring to take a more concentrated form of carbohydrate at certain times (e.g., just before the start of the game or at halftime) and consume plain water during play. This choice is often made when the code requires mouth guards or other equipment that might otherwise become sticky when sport drinks are the sole source of fluid. Other carbohydrate choices of team sport players include fruit, such as oranges and bananas, and confectionery items. The player should experiment with the amount and timing of intake during training sessions and practice matches before implementing a strategy during important competitions.

Alcohol

David Boon [Australian cricketer] may still hold the record for the number of cans of beer consumed on a flight between Australia and England—believed to be 54—but there certainly isn't a shortage of sports types trying to snatch it from him. Hot on the heels of English Rugby [Union] star Mike Tindall sinking "just under 50" on his return from the team's World Cup triumph last week, news now is that Australian Legends rugby league second-rower Gavin Miller also went very close to knocking off the record on his recent return flight to Sydney. According to reports at the weekend, Miller reached the magical 50 mark before calling it a day. But what made his performance all the more remarkable was that friends reckon he had 10 beers before he boarded the plane at Heathrow, and also drank three scotches and three small bottles of wine on the trip just to break the monotony.

The Age newspaper, Melbourne, Australia, December 2, 2003, p. 12

Westham [English soccer team] defender Hayden Foxe has reportedly been fined two weeks' wages [$A40,000] by the club for urinating on a bar in a drunken night out with teammates in London this week. Fox . . . had earlier dismissed reports that the players had behaved like "animals" and "appallingly" before they were thrown out of the bar after racking up a $5200 drinks bill.

The Age newspaper, Melbourne, Australia, December 22, 2001, p. 13

On this spot on September 17, 1984, Val Perovic of Carlton Football Club drank 37 × 375 ml cans of (beer) in two hours. Witnessed by hotel patrons, teammates and a very nervous doctor.

From a plaque on the wall of the Duke of Wellington Hotel, Melbourne, Australia

Melbourne Storm players Ben Roarty and Danny Williams have been involved in an end-of-season trip brawl that left Roarty in need of medical care and Williams' future at the club in doubt . . . . Storm's CEO Chris Johns said . . . "we are not dealing with choir boys here. We are dealing with footballers. . . . .while I am not condoning what they did, these things do happen. . . .This can happen when the boys have had a few drinks under their belts."

The Sunday Age newspaper, Melbourne, Australia, October 21, 2001, p. 15

Collingwood [Australian Football League] Football Club was in mourning today for its star, Darren Millane, killed in an early morning car crash. Its 1990 premiership flag hung at half mast as tearful staff answered scores of calls from its fans. . . . Millane, 26, died instantly when his car hit the back of a slow-moving truck . . . just before 3 am this morning.

D. Ballantine, Herald Sun newspaper, Melbourne, Australia, October 7, 1991, p. 1

Darren Millane was six times the legal alcohol limit for driving when he died. . . . Police sources confirmed yesterday that Millane's blood-alcohol level was 0.322.

L. Talbot, Herald Sun newspaper, Melbourne, Australia, October 28, 1991, p. 7

At the height of his boozing, just before he [English soccer player, Paul Gascoigne] checked in for rehab . . . London's The Sun newspaper ran a front page story headed "what Gazza drank in just one night". The accompanying picture showed 20 bottles of Hooch alcoholic lemonade, a bottle of Archers peach schnapps (20 double shots) and two tumblers filled with a rainbow concoction that was apparently made of Pernod, Baileys, Tequila, Galliano and Sambuca. A couple of days later the newspaper offered a carton of Newcastle Brown Ale to the first person to see him in a pub. He has beaten his wife, been in countless drunken fights, and only last year had a drinking binge in his hotel room that left a friend dead. In between times he has played some scintillating football for Newcastle, Tottenham, Lazio, Rangers, Middlesborough and England.

Jim White, The Sunday Age newspaper, Melbourne, Australia, January 30, 2000, p. 20

There are few reliable data on the alcohol intakes and drinking practices of athletes. First, because alcohol provides a minor component of dietary energy intake, it is often excluded from the results of dietary surveys. More important, even when the general limitations of dietary survey methodology are taken into account, it is likely that self-reported data on alcohol intake are particularly flawed. Because alcohol is regarded so emotively, people are unlikely to report their intake accurately. Athletes can both underreport and overreport their true intake of alcohol, depending on whether they believe their audience is likely to disapprove of, or promote, heavy alcohol use.

The dietary surveys of athletes that include estimates of alcohol intake suggest that it contributes 0% to 5% of total energy intake in the everyday diet. However, these figures can provide a misleading view of the alcohol intakes of athletes. For example, professional football players from the leading team in the national Australian Rules Football League reported a mean daily alcohol intake of 20 g, accounting for 3.5% of total energy intake (Burke and Read 1988b). However, these players rarely drank alcohol during the training week, in accordance with the club policy, and instead confined their intake to weekends, particularly after the weekly football match. The mean reported postmatch intake of alcohol was ~120 g (range = 27-368 g), providing 19% of total energy intake on match day (range = 3-43% of total energy intake). Such binge drinking practices were confirmed in a separate study in these same athletes. Blood samples were taken from 41 players who attended a 9:00 a.m. training session on the morning following a weekend match. Fourteen of these players still registered a positive blood alcohol level (BAL) from their previous evening's intake, with levels ranging from 0.001 to 0.113 g/100 ml. Blood alcohol level in four players exceeded the legal limit for driving a motor vehicle in Australia (0.05 g/100 ml).

As illustrated in the introduction to this section, the lay press provides ample anecdotal evidence of binge drinking patterns of some athletes, particularly in the immediate celebration or commiseration of their competition performances or in the off-season. In some cases, these episodes are romanticized, and the drinking prowess of the athletes is admired. Whether total alcohol intake, or the prevalence of episodes of heavy alcohol intake by athletes, is different from that of the general population remains unclear. Surveys that have examined this issue report conflicting results. Various hypotheses have been proposed to explain likely associations between sport and alcohol use. It has been suggested that athletes might have a lower intake of alcohol because of increased self-esteem, a more rigid lifestyle, and greater interest in their health and performance. Equally, alcohol has been associated with the rituals of relaxation and celebration in sport, and it has been suggested that athletes might be socialized into certain behaviors and attitudes to drinking as a result of their sport participation. Alcohol has a strong relationship to sport through the sponsorship of events and teams by companies that produce beer and other alcoholic drinks and through the licensed clubs or fund-raising strategies that often provide the financial underpinning of sports clubs.

Several dietary surveys comparing different groups of athletes have reported that the mean daily alcohol intakes of team sport athletes are significantly greater than those of athletes involved in endurance, strength, or weight-conscious sports (Burke et al. 1991; Van Erp-Baart et al. 1989a). Although these studies were not specifically designed to collect data on alcohol intake, the findings are supported by data collected in some population surveys on alcohol

use. Watten (1995), in a national survey of Norwegian adults, reported that men and women involved in team sports reported a higher intake of alcohol, particularly beer and liquor, than those involved in individual sports or those with no sports involvement. However, some of these differences can be explained by the age and educational backgrounds of participants.

Clearly, although anecdotal evidence suggests that some team sport players consume alcohol in excessive amounts, on at least some occasions, further studies are needed to fully determine athletes' alcohol intake and patterns of use. Information on athletes' attitudes and beliefs about alcohol is also desirable, because it would allow education about current drinking practices that are detrimental to the athlete's performance or health. Although alcohol is not a necessary component of a diet, it is intricately involved in the social aspects and enjoyment of eating—factors that are also important to the athlete. Athletes must find a balance between these lifestyle aspects of nutrition and the dietary practices needed to optimize their performance. The excessive intake of alcohol, particularly at important times such as postexercise recovery, is clearly at odds with optimal dietary practice. Many of the quotes in the introduction of this section provide evidence of the serious negative consequences that can arise from the unsafe drinking practices that have been allowed to continue, or even flourish, in team sports. A more complete picture of the issues involved in alcohol and sports performance is provided in research topic 1 in this chapter—covering the acute effects on alcohol on exercise and sport performance, the effects of alcohol on processes of postexercise recovery, exercise performance following excessive alcohol intake (the hangover effect), and the chronic effects of heavy alcohol use on performance. This section concludes with some guidelines for sensible approaches to alcohol intake by athletes.

Frequently throughout this chapter, attention has been drawn to the culture of team sports. Alcohol intake practices appear to one of the most obvious examples of the strong traditions and shared beliefs supported by the culture of team sport. These traditions are handed down as players become coaches or by the group of trainers or other support staff who work with clubs and teams over many years. These traditions are also reinforced by the financial and social infrastructure of the team or club and by the wider environment provided by the media. It is difficult to compete against such a culture—to expose coaches and players to new ideas and research, to replace long-held beliefs and attitudes, or to change the team structure, customs, and activities. Alcohol intake practices are one of the areas of sports nutrition that seem most resistant to change or reason, and it may take many generations in sport before attitudes and behavior can be shifted.

Nevertheless, there are signs that at least some sporting organizations are taking proactive steps to address problem drinking within team sports. Many teams, leagues, and organizations have begun to develop and implement specific alcohol and drug education programs within their environments. Education messages that focus on long-term health issues do not appear to have great currency for young athletes. Messages that have greater success are those related to sports performance and to professionalism, particularly in addressing the public image that is most likely to attract sponsorship and financial reward to players. Many teams have introduced other strategies to support these education messages with infrastructure changes or with player-involved codes of conduct that promote professional behavior and punish episodes of alcohol-related misconduct. We await the outcome of these programs.

Sport Foods and Supplements

Given the large number of people involved in team sports around the world, and the range of nutritional issues and challenges involved in these activities, it is not surprising that team sport players provide a lucrative market for the supplement and sport food industry. Many companies vie for the sponsorship of professional sporting teams, or they seek endorsement of their products from sports teams. The close-knit culture of team sports provides a fertile environment for spreading ideas and testimonials about the use of various products.

Sport foods and supplements that are likely to contribute to the nutritional goals and optimal performance of team sport players are summarized in table 8.4. Few studies have directly tested the specific benefits of various supplements to the performance of team sports. The classification of these products is mostly based on the nutritional profile of these products in comparison with the common sports nutrition issues seen in team sports or from the results of research undertaken on protocols of intermittent high-intensity exercise. There are clear cases for using various sport foods to achieve nutritional goals of training and competition for many team sport players. These situations include using a product to provide nutritional support before, during, and after a match or key training sessions or to provide a compact and portable supply of energy and nutrients when everyday food is unavailable or difficult to consume. It is often hard to consume everyday foods during a busy day, while traveling, or when energy and fuel needs are greater than gastrointestinal comfort. In some teams, sport foods are made available in a group environment, which presupposes that either all players have the same nutritional needs or that each player has sufficient nutritional knowledge to choose a supplementation protocol suited to her specific needs. Because it is most likely that players vary in their nutritional needs, even within the same team, each player must be taught to recognize when and how sport foods can be made part of her own nutrition program.

There is a clear need for more applied and sport-specific studies on the effects of various supplements on the wide range of popular team sports. Within many team-based

sports, creatine is the supplement of greatest current interest, and there is a sound basis to this interest. A large body of evidence supports the beneficial effects of creatine loading on the performance of repeated high-intensity bouts of exercise with a short recovery interval, an exercise protocol reliant on the recovery of the phosphocreatine power system. This description broadly describes the movement patterns of match play in team and racket sports. It also underpins many of the training protocols undertaken in these sports—resistance training to gain muscle size and strength, interval training to increase speed and anaerobic fitness, or specific match practice. As such, creatine supplementation could be of theoretical benefit as a training aid (chronic supplementation) or to optimize competition performance (acute preparation for a single match or chronic supplementation protocols for a tournament or seasonal fixture). The general picture of creatine supplementation for team and racket sports is discussed in greater detail in chapter 10 (research topic 3). Meanwhile, table 8.d in the appendix to this chapter summarizes the results of published studies examining the results of acute creatine supplementation on field-based team sports players or protocols of relevance to match play in such sports. As noted in chapter 10, the literature is insufficient in both quantity and design to provide clear proof of performance benefits. In particular, no studies have examined the effect of creatine supplementation on the outcome of an actual game—for example, an increase in the goals scored or defended. There is a leap of faith that the enhancement of movement patterns in a sport or an increase in the strength of players will change the score at the final siren. However, this issue is not unique to the creatine literature. Some of the challenges and techniques involved in studying performance enhancement in unpredictable games such as team and racket sports are discussed in chapter 10 (research topic 1)

Table 8.e summarizes the results of other studies that have been undertaken on supplements involving field-based team sport players or exercise protocols of direct relevance to team sports. Because of the challenges in undertaking such research, it is not surprising that so few studies exist. In general, the studies conclude that there is no evidence to support the use of other supplements that are commonly used in team sports, including supplements claimed to directly increase muscle size and strength (e.g., β-hydroxy β-methylbutyrate or HMB) or decrease body fat (e.g., chromium picolinate). This comment should not be confused with the supported use of sport foods within a dietary program that has been specifically developed to target a nutritional goal—for example, the use of a liquid meal supplement providing energy, carbohydrate, and protein to meet high energy needs or specific recovery needs following a resistance training session. These conclusions about the lack of efficacy of other dietary supplements are based on the general literature regarding these compounds or products (see chapter 3) rather than the specific research available in team sport players. In some cases, table 8.e provides examples of studies that have found an apparent benefit arising from the use of a supplement in field-based

Table 8.4   Sports Foods and Supplements That Are of Likely Benefit to Field-Team Sport Players

	Product	Comment
Use in achieving documented nutrition goals	Sport drinks	• Use to refuel and rehydrate during prolonged training sessions and matches and to rehydrate after the session. Contain some electrolytes to help replace sweat losses and increase voluntary intake of fluid.
	Sport gels	• Convenient and compact carbohydrate source that can be used for additional refueling during matches and prolonged training sessions, especially if water is used for hydration goals.
	Sport bars	• Convenient, portable, and easy-to-consume source of carbohydrate, protein, and micronutrients for prematch meal or postexercise recovery. • Low-bulk and portable form of energy and nutrients that can contribute to high energy needs, especially to support resistance training program or growth. • Convenient and compact source of energy and nutrients for the traveling athlete.
	Liquid meal supplements	• Convenient, portable, and easy-to-consume source of carbohydrate, protein, and micronutrients for postexercise recovery, including "recovery" intake before resistance exercise • Low-bulk and practical form of energy and nutrients that can contribute to high energy needs, especially to support resistance training program or growth. • Well-tolerated preevent meal that can be consumed to provide a source of carbohydrate quite close to the start of a match or workout; seems to be better tolerated than solid food by some athletes with high risk of gastrointestinal problems. • Convenient and compact source of energy and nutrients for the traveling athlete.
	Multivitamin and mineral supplement	• Supplemental source of micronutrients for traveling when food supply is not reliable. • Supplemental source of micronutrients during prolonged periods of energy restriction (female athletes).
	Electrolyte supplements	• May provide additional source of sodium for replacement during exercise by cramp-prone players with heavy sweat and electrolyte losses.
Strong potential for ergogenic benefit	Creatine	• Creatine phosphate serves a number of important roles in exercise metabolism; the most well-known role is the rapid regeneration of adenosine triphosphate by the phosphagen power system. Studies show that creatine loading enhances the performance of exercise involving repeated high-intensity work bouts with short recovery intervals (<2 min recovery). Chronic creatine supplementation may enhance the responses of many field-based team sport players to various training protocols—resistance training undertaken by team sport players to enhance muscle mass and strength, interval training undertaken to enhance anaerobic fitness, and match-specific play. Some studies in the field have shown that acute supplementation enhances the performance of match-simulation protocols, or movement patterns within actual field play, and may therefore be seen as a competition aid. More studies of this type are needed across a wider range of field-based team sports. Typical protocols for creatine use: loading dose of 20-30 g in multiple doses (e.g., 4 × 5 g) for 5 days followed by maintenance dose of 2-5 g/day. Uptake appears to be enhanced by consuming creatine with carbohydrate-rich meal or snack. Acute weight gain of about 1 kg occurs with creatine loading, presumably because of fluid retention.
	Caffeine	• May enhance performance of prolonged exercise (e.g., matches) by reducing perception of fatigue. More studies need to be undertaken in team sports to confirm either enhancement of movement patterns or attenuation of decline in skills and concentration over the prolonged period of a match. New studies show that intakes of small to moderate amounts of caffeine (~2 mg/kg) may be as effective as the traditional larger doses (6 mg/kg), especially when taken just prior to the onset of fatigue.
Possible potential for ergogenic benefit	Bicarbonate or citrate	• The use of bicarbonate or citrate to increase the blood-buffering capacity (e.g., 300 mg/kg body mass bicarbonate or 500 mg/kg body mass citrate 1-2 hr pregame) might enhance the performance of team sports involving repeated sprints. Field studies are needed with high-level team sports to confirm benefits. Risk of gastrointestinal problems should be noted but appear to be reduced by taking doses with large volumes of fluid (1-2 L). There is also recent evidence that chronic bicarbonate loading (loading immediately before interval training) may enhance training adaptations. It may also allow the athlete to train harder.

Research Priorities

The results of sports nutrition research undertaken on endurance athletes may not apply to intermittent high-intensity sports; to address the overlay of skill and cognitive performance, specific research on team sports is required. Such research should investigate the following issues:

- The development of protocols that are sufficiently reliable and valid to detect changes in performance that would enhance the outcome of team sports. This includes protocols addressing activity patterns during the game as well as the key mental and motor skills involved.

- The range of physiques in each sport, including specific positions, that are consistent with optimal performance.

- The current dietary practices of team sport players across all levels of play, with specific interest in the possible energy restrictions practiced by female players.

- Carbohydrate requirements for specific sports, including refueling between matches played in tournaments, road trips, and other situations of limited recovery.

- Current hydration and fuel intake practices of team sport players and whether these contribute to optimal performance.

- Use of supplements and sport foods by team players, and their specific benefit to performance in various codes and situations.

team sports. However, in the absence of confirmation from other studies, a plausible hypothesis to explain the specific results of the study, or a theory to explain why unique benefits would be expected in a team-based sport, we have deferred to the consensus of the general literature. Sport scientists, especially those who work with elite team athletes, are encouraged to investigate supplement use in team sport.

RESEARCH TOPIC

Alcohol and the Athlete

Alcohol is strongly linked with modern sport. The alcohol intakes and drinking patterns of athletes are not well studied; however, it appears that some athletes undertake binge drinking practices, often associated with postcompetition socializing and with team sports. The issues involving alcohol and the athlete include the acute effects on alcohol on exercise and sport performance, the effects of alcohol on postexercise recovery, exercise performance following excessive alcohol intake (the hangover effect), and the chronic effects of heavy alcohol use on performance. The variety of effects of alcohol on different body tissues and the variability of participant responses to alcohol make it difficult to study the direct effects on sport performance. The scarcity of studies of alcohol and performance can also be explained by other practical challenges: the reluctance of ethics committees to allow study participants to drink alcohol in amounts that are in well in excess of healthy drinking guidelines and the difficulty of finding a way to control the placebo effect—it is hard to provide an alternative treatment to an athlete to mimic the effects of a large intake of alcohol!

Alcohol (ethanol) can be consumed in a variety of drinks, and table 8.5 shows the amount of a beverage needed to provide a standard 10 g serving of alcohol. Following absorption from the stomach, alcohol is metabolized primarily by the liver at rates that vary widely between individuals. It is unclear whether exercise affects the rate of metabolism of alcohol. Reviews of the acute effects of alcohol ingestion on exercise metabolism (American College of Sports Medicine 1982; Williams 1991) conclude that alcohol does not contribute significantly to energy stores used for exercise, but in situations of prolonged exercise it may increase the risk of hypoglycemia resulting from the a suppression of hepatic gluconeogenesis. Increased heat loss may be associated with this hypoglycemia as well as the skin vasodilation caused by exercise, impairing temperature regulation in cold environments. Studies of the effects of alcohol on cardiovascular, respiratory, and muscular function have provided conflicting results, but ingestion of small amounts of alcohol does not appear to significantly alter the cardiorespiratory and metabolic responses to submaximal exercise (for reviews, see American College of Sports Medicine 1982; Williams 1991).

Effects of Acute Alcohol Ingestion on Exercise Performance

In previous times, athletes consumed alcohol before or during exercise in the belief that it would enhance performance. The major benefits from such alcohol intake are likely to be psychologically driven—alcohol has been used to decrease sensitivity to pain, improve confidence, and remove other psychological barriers to performance. However, alcohol may also be used in the belief that it stimulates the cardiovascular system or lessens the tremor

Table 8.5   Alcoholic Drinks: A Standard Serving Contains Approximately 10 g of Alcohol

Drink	Amount (ml)
Standard beer (4% alcohol)	250
Low-alcohol beer (2% alcohol)	500
Cider, wine coolers, alcoholic soft drinks	250
Wine	100
Champagne	100
Fortified wines, sherry, port	60
Spirits	30

and stress-induced emotional arousal in fine motor control sports. Although it is no longer on the general banned list of the World Anti-Doping Agency, alcohol is still considered a banned substance in some sports such as shooting and fencing. In some sports such as darts and billiards, alcohol is still popularly consumed during exercise, but this may reflect the culture of sports that are widely played in a bar environment as well as the belief that is a performance aid (for review, see Williams 1985).

The few studies of acute alcohol ingestion and actual sport performance show variability in results and responses. The ingestion of small amounts of alcohol (keeping BAL below 0.05 g/100 ml) did not have a significant effect on the performance of a 5-mile treadmill time trial, although there was a trend toward performance deterioration at higher blood alcohol levels (Houmard et al. 1987). Meanwhile, McNaughton and Preece (1986) tested the performance of runners over various distances ranging from 100 to 1,500 m, at four different levels of alcohol consumption (BAL estimated at 0-0.1 g/100 ml). Alcohol intake did not affect performance of 100 m times in sprinters, but it reduced performance over 200 m and 400 m as alcohol intake increased. Middle-distance runners showed impaired performance in 800 and 1,500 m run times, with these effects also being dose-related (McNaughton and Preece 1986). An earlier study showed no effect of alcohol (0.6 ml of 94% ethanol/kg body mass) on isometric strength but a 6% reduction in vertical jump height and a 10% decrease in performance in an 80 m sprint (Hebbelinck 1963).

There is a limited amount of information on the effects of acute ingestion of alcohol on motor control and the performance of skilled tasks. However, it is clear from the controlled studies that have been conducted that alcohol has an adverse effect on tasks in which concentration, visual perception, reaction time, and coordination are involved (Williams, 1995). In 1982, the American College of Sports Medicine published a position statement concluding that small to moderate amounts of alcohol had a detrimental effect on reaction time, hand–eye coordination, accuracy, balance, and complex skilled tasks, with no evidence cited to support the purported beneficial effects of reduced tremor (American College of Sports Medicine 1982). The final advice of this expert group was to avoid ingestion of alcohol before or during exercise.

Effects of Acute Alcohol Ingestion on Postexercise Recovery

The postcompetition situation is often associated with alcohol intake and binge drinking, and it is likely that social rituals after training in some sports may also involve moderate to heavy intake of alcohol. Given that athletes may be dehydrated and have eaten little on the day of competition, it is likely that alcohol consumed after exercise is more quickly absorbed and has increased effects. Therefore, we need to examine the effects of alcohol on processes that are important in the recovery from prolonged exercise and on the performance of subsequent exercise bouts.

Restoring the body fluid deficit incurred during exercise is a balance between the amount of fluid that the athlete can drink after exercise and his ongoing fluid losses. The palatability of postexercise fluids is an important factor in determining total fluid intake, whereas replacement of sodium losses is a major determinant of the success in retaining this fluid (see chapter 1). It has been suggested that beer is a valuable postexercise beverage because at least some athletes are able to consume it voluntarily in large volumes. However, the diuretic action of alcohol and the absence of a worthwhile sodium content (unless accompanied by the intake of salty foods) are likely to increase urine losses. Indeed, Shirreffs and Maughan (1997) examined the effect of alcohol on postexercise rehydration from an exercise task that dehydrated participants by 2% of body mass. Participants replaced 150% of the volume of their fluid deficits with drinks containing 0%, 1%, 2%, or 4% alcohol within 90 min of finishing the exercise. The total volume of urine produced during the 6 hr of recovery was positively related to the alcohol content of the fluid. However, only in the 4% alcohol drink trial did the difference in total urine approach significance, with a net retention of 40% of ingested fluid compared with 59% in the no-alcohol trial, equating to a difference of about 500 ml in urine losses. Participants were still dehydrated at the end of the recovery period with the 4% alcohol drink, despite having consumed 1.5 times the volume of their fluid deficit. Although individual variability must be taken into account, this study suggests that the intake of significant amounts of alcohol will impede rehydration (Shirreffs and Maughan 1997).

Low-alcohol beers (<2% alcohol) or beer shandies (beer mixed in equal proportions with lemonade, thus diluting the alcohol content and providing some carbohydrate) may not be detrimental to rehydration. Furthermore, notwithstanding other effects of small to moderate amounts of alcohol, these drinks might be useful in encouraging large fluid intakes in dehydrated athletes, especially when consumed in combination with sodium-containing foods. However, drinks with a more concentrated alcohol content are not advised, because the combination of a smaller fluid volume and a greater alcohol intake will reduce the rate of effective fluid replacement.

Because alcohol has a number of effects on the intermediary metabolism of carbohydrate, it is possible that postexercise intake might impair the restoration of depleted glycogen stores. In the absence of carbohydrate intake, alcohol intake is known to impair the carbohydrate status of the liver by inhibiting hepatic gluconeogenesis and increasing liver glycogenolysis. Alcohol intake has been reported to impair muscle glycogen storage in rats following depletion by fasting or exercise (for review, see Palmer et al. 1991). We have undertaken studies on well-trained human participants, with separate studies being undertaken to investigate muscle glycogen storage after 8 and 24 hr of recovery in exercise-depleted muscles. These time periods, apart from representing common time intervals between training sessions, also represented periods during which blood alcohol levels were first substantial and then largely metabolized. Our studies were designed to test the direct effect of alcohol (equivalent to 10 standard drinks) added to a high-carbohydrate recovery diet, as well as its indirect effect in displacing carbohydrate from the postexercise diet. Muscle glycogen storage was significantly reduced on the alcohol displacement diets in both the 8 and 24 hr studies compared with the high-carbohydrate diets. There was a trend toward a reduction in glycogen storage over 8 hr of recovery with the alcohol + carbohydrate diet; however, glycogen storage on the alcohol + carbohydrate diet during the 24 hr study was identical to the control diet. Therefore, there was no clear evidence of a direct impairment of muscle glycogen storage by alcohol when adequate substrate was provided to the muscle; however, this may have been masked by intersubject variability. The results of these studies suggest that the major effect of alcohol intake on postexercise refueling is indirect; high intakes of alcohol are likely to prevent the athlete from consuming adequate carbohydrate to optimize muscle glycogen storage. In general, athletes who participate in alcoholic binges are unlikely to eat adequate food or make suitable high-carbohydrate food choices. Furthermore, food intake over the next day may also be affected as the athlete sleeps off a hangover. Further studies are needed to determine the direct effect on alcohol on muscle glycogen storage.

Alcohol is known to exert other effects that may impede postexercise recovery. Many sporting activities are associated with muscle damage and soft tissue injuries, either as a direct consequence of the exercise, as a result of accidents, or as a result of the tackling and collisions involved in contact sports. Standard medical practice is to treat soft tissue injuries with vasoconstrictive techniques (e.g., rest, ice, compression, elevation). Because alcohol is a potent vasodilator of skin vessels, it has been suggested that the intake of large amounts of alcohol might cause or increase undesirable swelling around damaged sites and might impede repair processes. Although this effect has not been systematically studied, case histories report these findings. Until such studies are undertaken, it seems prudent that players who have suffered considerable muscle damage and soft tissue injuries should avoid alcohol in the immediate recovery phase (e.g., for 24 hr after the event).

Another likely effect of skin vasodilation following alcohol intake is an increase in heat loss from the skin. This may be exacerbated by hypoglycemia, which results from the combined effects of carbohydrate depletion and impaired liver gluconeogenesis. Therefore, athletes who consume large quantities of alcohol in cold environments may incur problems with thermoregulation. An increased risk of hypothermia may be found in sports or recreational activities undertaken in cold weather, particularly hiking or skiing, where alcohol intake is an integral part of "after-ski" activities. As in the case of postexercise refueling, it is likely that the major effect of excessive alcohol intake comes from the athlete's failure to follow guidelines for optimal recovery. The intoxicated athlete may fail to undertake sensible injury management practices or to report for treatment; he may fail to seek suitable clothing or shelter in cold conditions or to notice early signs of hypothermia. Although studies that measure the direct effect of alcohol on thermoregulation and soft tissue damage are encouraged, these effects are likely to be minor or at least additive to the failure to undertake recommended recovery practices.

Finally, the effect of alcohol intake on judgment and high-risk behavior during the postgame wind-down must be considered. Alcohol consumption is highly correlated with drowning, spinal injury, and other problems in recreational water activities (O'Brien 1993) and is a major factor in road accidents. A number of elite athletes have died in motor car or other accidents following excess alcohol intake. The lay press frequently contains reports of well-known athletes being involved in brawls or other situations of domestic or public violence while intoxicated. Clearly, athletes are not immune to the social and behavioral problems following excess alcohol intake; there is some discussion that certain athletes may be more predisposed to these outcomes (see O'Brien 1993). Further studies are required before it can be determined whether athletes, or some groups of athletes, are more likely to drink excessively or suffer a greater risk of alcohol-related problems. However, it appears that athletes should at least be included in population education programs related to drunk driving and other high-risk behavior.

Effect of Previous Day's Intake on Performance

Some athletes are required to train (or even compete again) on the day after a competition and its postevent drinking binge. In other situations, athletes may choose to drink heavily the night before a competition, as a general part of their social activities, or in the belief that this will help to relax them before the event. The effect of an alcohol hangover on performance is widely discussed by athletes but has not been well studied. Next-day performance after the consumption of large amounts of alcohol (about eight standard drinks) was found to be constant for power or strength but impaired in terms of high-intensity cycling (Karvinen et al. 1962). Another study involved aerobic and anaerobic testing of rugby union players on a Friday night and the following Saturday after consuming their typical Friday night's alcohol intake—subsequently reported at ~130 g (range 1-38 standard drinks). A standardized sleep time and breakfast were followed. Although $\dot{V}O_2$max was significantly reduced by any level of alcohol intake (O'Brien 1993), without the presence of a control trial, it is hard to dissociate the effects of alcohol from the variability of repeated testing. Research in other areas of industrial work (e.g., machine handling and flying aircraft) suggests that impairment of psychomotor skills may continue during the hangover phase. Clearly this will be of detriment in team sports and court sports, which demand tactical play and a high skill level.

Effects of Chronic Alcohol Intake on Sport Performance

Athletes who chronically consume large amounts of alcohol are liable to the large number of health and social problems associated with problem drinking. Early problems to affect sport performance include inadequate nutrition and generally poor lifestyle. Weekend binge drinkers tend to maintain their food consumption, because alcohol does not seem to regulate total energy intake in the short term. Alcohol is an energy-dense nutrient (providing 27 kJ or 7 kcal per gram), and frequent episodes of heavy alcohol intake can be expected to increase total energy intake. However, erratic eating patterns and choice of high-fat foods in conjunction with alcoholic binges can also lead to excess energy consumption and contribute to weight gain. A common issue, particularly in team sports, is the significant gain in body fat during the off-season resulting from increased alcohol intake coupled with reduced exercise expenditure. Many players need to devote a significant part of their preseason (and even early season) conditioning to reversing the effects of their off-season activities. Clearly this is a disadvantage to performance and to the longevity of a sports career.

The following guidelines have been proposed to represent a sensible approach to alcohol intake by athletes (Burke and Maughan 2000):

- Alcohol is not an essential component of a diet. It is a personal choice of the athlete whether to consume alcohol at all. However, there is no evidence of impairments to health and performance when alcohol is used sensibly.
- The athlete should be guided by community guidelines that suggest general intakes of alcohol that are safe and healthy. This varies from country to

country, but in general, it is suggested that mean daily alcohol intake should be less than 40 to 50 g (perhaps 20-30 g per day for females) and that binge drinking is discouraged. Because individual tolerance to alcohol is variable, it is difficult to set a precise definition of heavy intake or an alcohol binge. However, intakes of about 80 to 100 g at a single sitting are likely to constitute a heavy intake for most people.

- Alcohol is a high-energy (and nutrient-poor) food and should be restricted when the athlete is attempting to reduce body fat.
- The athlete should avoid heavy intake of alcohol on the night before competition. It appears unlikely that the intake of one to two standard drinks will have negative effects in most people.
- The intake of alcohol immediately before or during exercise does not enhance performance and in fact may impair performance in many people. Psychomotor performance and judgment are most affected. Therefore, the athlete should not consume alcohol deliberately to aid performance and should be wary of exercise that is conducted in conjunction with the social intake of alcohol.
- Heavy alcohol intake is likely to have a major impact on postexercise recovery. It may have direct physiological effects on rehydration, glycogen recovery, and repair of soft tissue damage. More important, athletes are unlikely to remember or undertake strategies for optimal recovery when they are intoxicated. Therefore, the athlete should attend to these strategies first before any alcohol is consumed. An athlete who has suffered a major soft-tissue injury should consume no alcohol for 24 hr.
- The athlete should rehydrate with appropriate fluids in volumes that are greater than her existing fluid deficit. Suitable fluid choices include sport drinks, fruit juices, soft drinks (all containing carbohydrate), and water (when refueling is not a major issue). However, sodium replacement via sport drinks, oral rehydration solutions, or salt-containing foods is also important to encourage the retention of these rehydration fluids. Low-alcohol beers and beer–soft drink mixes may be suitable and seem to encourage large volume intakes. However, drinks containing greater than 2% alcohol are not recommended for rehydration.
- Before consuming any alcohol after exercise, the athlete should consume a high-carbohydrate meal or snack to aid muscle glycogen recovery. Food intake will also help to reduce the rate of alcohol absorption and thus reduce the rate of intoxication.
- Once postexercise recovery priorities have been addressed, the athlete who chooses to drink is encouraged to do so in moderation. Drunk-driving education messages in various countries may provide a guide to sensible and well-paced drinking.

- Athletes who drink heavily after competition or at other times should avoid driving and other hazardous activities.
- It appears likely that it will be difficult to change the attitudes and behaviors of athletes with regard to alcohol. However, coaches, managers, and sports medicine staff can encourage guidelines such as these and specifically target the myths and rationalizations that support binge drinking practices. Sport staff should reinforce these guidelines with an infrastructure that promotes sensible drinking practices. For example, alcohol might be banned from locker rooms and replaced with fluids and foods appropriate to postexercise recovery. In many cases, athletes drink in a peer-group situation and it may be easier to change the environment in which this occurs than the immediate attitudes of the athletes.

PRACTICAL ISSUE
Cooking Skills for the Busy Athlete

Athletes face many challenges in achieving self-sufficiency in food purchasing and preparation. Some of these are common to all young people living in a modern, busy world, where it is no longer usual for a family to eat together or for parents to provide training in domestic skills to prepare their children to leave home. However, other issues are peculiar to the world of sport. Common challenges include the following:

- The talented athlete suffers from a lack of time or opportunity to develop cooking skills while growing up, because the family's activities were organized to allow him to concentrate on training or competing. Moving into a college or institute with a training table or athlete dining hall meets the athlete's immediate food needs without opportunity to contribute to their preparation. The athlete then leaves these sheltered environments and is suddenly required to become self-sufficient.

- The athlete is sharing accommodation with other athletes who have the same problems—inadequate time and knowledge.
- The day is overcommitted with training, work or school, medical and conditioning appointments, and media requests. There is little time to fit in shopping and cooking as well.
- The first training session is undertaken early in the morning, and most of the day's food is eaten on the run.
- Training sessions or competition sessions finish late at night. The athlete returns home too hungry or too tired to take the time to cook.
- Sports nutrition tactics for enhanced refueling and repair recommend a recovery meal within 30 to 60 min of finishing the workout or event. How do you get a nutritious meal on the table so quickly?
- It is impossible to coordinate timetables within the athlete's household. No one eats at the same time, and the athlete ends up cooking for one. It is hard to be motivated to prepare a real meal for one or to adjust recipes.
- The athlete often has to apply his or her existing cooking skills to the travel situation, where the environment is a bare apartment with even more limited cooking resources and a limited number of ingredients. How do you manage to make a flavorsome meal without leaving lots of leftovers or wasted ingredients?

Table 8.6 provides a number of tips and skills that can help the athlete develop adequate, if not accomplished, skills in food preparation and cooking. Where possible, it is valuable for athletes to undertake cooking classes—especially classes focused on the lifestyle and nutritional needs of the particular sport—to allow them to learn skills in a hands-on manner and enjoyable atmosphere. Small group classes, involving other athletes and possibly undertaken in the athletes' homes, offer many learning advantages, and are a popular activity.

Table 8.6   Principles and Skills of Food Preparation and Cooking for the Busy Athlete

Principles	Strategies
Using teamwork in a group household	• When time or money is scarce, it helps to pool resources. A household meeting should be called to discuss a central plan and coordinate a roster of shopping and cooking. • Communication can be managed via a central notice board or lists. • Conflicting timetables mean that athletes have different periods of "free time." Each athlete should be encouraged to contribute some of her "free time" to the roster, knowing that her housemates will do the same for her on their busy days.
Acquiring new skills	• Cooking classes, especially those organized for athletes in small groups, are a valuable tool in teaching skills, fostering an enjoyment of cooking, and creating rapport between the athlete and nutrition educator. It is often quicker for the novice cook to learn by example and when supervised than by trying to read recipe books.

(continued)

Table 8.6 *(continued)*

Principles	Strategies
Acquiring new skills *(cont'd)*	• A number of recipe books have been especially written for athletes and are suited not only to nutritional needs of sport but also to lifestyle issues such as lack of time and need for quick preparation. • The athlete should be reminded that many recipes are simply variations on a certain style of cooking. Once one style has been mastered (e.g., a stir-fry or a risotto) it is easy to experiment with a few new ingredients to increase the overall repertoire of menu items. • It helps to collect tips from other athletes or good cooks. Many ideas or recipes can be adapted to meet the needs of athletes: for example, to lower the fat content, increase the carbohydrate content, or shorten the cooking or preparation time. Keeping a resource file on such tips is often even more valuable than having a large collection of individual recipes.
Planning ahead and using time management skills	• Counseling in time management often prepares the busy athlete to have the time and skills to take on a new challenge. It is difficult to implement order and organization from a baseline of total chaos and lack of awareness of basic planning. The house and kitchen should be kept clean and tidy, so that cooking time is productive. • Supermarket shopping is more efficient when undertaken outside peak hours. Times when the athlete is tired or hungry should also be avoided. If finances permit, online supermarket shopping can also save time. • A shopping list should always be prepared to streamline the time spent in the supermarket and reduce unnecessary or impulse purchases. It helps to have a checklist of useful items for the pantry and freezer (long shelf-life) and refrigerator (short shelf-life). The shopping list should be prepared by listing perishable and unusual items from the week's menu roster, as well as adding "depleted" items from the general checklist. • Taking advantage to stock up on "supermarket specials" can help with the food budget; however, the athlete should only buy products that can be properly stored and consumed within their "use-by" date. • Even when an athlete is only cooking for one, he or she should cook the whole recipe, or even double the recipe, to create leftovers. Freezing leftovers in single-serve portions is a valuable idea because they thaw and reheat more quickly and provide a rapidly prepared meal on a late night or a meal to take to work or school. • Recipes that are most valuable for batch cooking are those that are "complete meals" (carbohydrate base, a protein source, and vegetables in one dish). It is helpful when relying on leftovers or a late evening "freezer to microwave" meal to have all ingredients intact in one container. • In a very busy lifestyle, it often suits to use the "rest day" to cook meals for the week (for refrigeration or freezing) and to make up a loaf of filled sandwiches or rolls for the freezer. Planning ahead also means that the week's meals can be balanced for nutritional needs and enjoyment, rather than ending up unbalanced and monotonous. • A good supply of portable snacks and quick meals should always be on hand, such as single-serve breakfast cereals, cartons of yogurt, cereal bars, and fruit. Cool-packs and insulated containers and bottles can all help to increase the range of food and drink items that can be taken "on the run" in a busy day. • The preparation or cooking for some meals can be done in stages, leaving the last part for a quick finish when the athlete arrives home from training or competition. In some cases, the meal can be left in the oven on automatic timing, to cook while the athlete is at training. Such strategies mean that the meal can be on the table within 30 min of arrival home—promoting rapid refueling or maximizing the time for recovery and sleep.
Using creative shortcuts	• It is good to invest in a few cooking tools or household items that save time and produce quality outcomes. These items include a good wok or large nonstick frying pan, microwave oven, sharp knives, well-sized oven dishes, and a rice cooker. • Where expenses permit, it is useful to buy meats that are already trimmed and diced for the recipe, or fresh or frozen vegetable stir-fry mixes. In a busy lifestyle, it is often worth paying for the convenience of having most of the preparation done for you. • There are many nutritious, time-saving food products than can be used as the basis of a meal or as a long-life ingredient to replace the lack of a fresh one. Examples include low-fat pasta sauces and stir-fry mixes, fresh pasta, frozen vegetable medleys, canned vegetables and legumes, canned salmon and tuna, long-life milk, fresh or frozen pizza bases, fresh soups, prepared custards and rice puddings, minced herbs, pancake, bread, and muffin mixes, spray-on oils, and fresh pasta and noodles. Fresh ingredients can be added to these items to add additional flavor and nutrients and create a wholesome meal.

PRACTICAL ISSUE

Catering for a Team Sport on Match Day

An interview with Trevor Lea, sports dietitian to Manchester United Football Club.

Trev, how long have you been working with Manchester United, and how did you become involved with the team?

I have been working with Manchester United for the last 16 seasons. I had been working in the area of sport nutrition with various athletes and various sports for some time, when Manchester United asked if I could advise their players.

Can you explain the competition program undertaken by the team? How many competitions or leagues do they play in? How many games are played over the season in total? What is the average length of time between games?

The team plays in a number of leagues and cups involving up to 60 games a season. This means two games a week for most of the season, usually with 3 days between games.

How many home games does the team play in a season? What do the away games entail? How far might the team have to travel and do the players travel as a team? When and how is the travel undertaken?

Approximately 25 matches are played at home. The players travel as a team to the various away matches, which are mainly played in England, the furthest being 250 miles away from Manchester. For matches in England, the players travel on the team coach. The remaining matches are played in mainland Europe and the team travels by plane to these games.

What time of day are matches commonly played? What would a player's typical routine be on a match day prior to the game, both in terms of activities and eating patterns?

Matches are usually played at 15:00. A typical day would involve the player getting up, having a breakfast at home, and then resting until lunch. The players then go to the ground 3 hr before the match for the prematch meal. After lunch, the player then prepares for the match.

Do you organize a team sitting for the prematch meal for all or any of the matches? What sort of menu do you organize? What sort of menu do you advise when players are organizing their own prematch meals?

All prematch meals involve a team sitting with the food being prepared by our own chef. I work with the chef to plan the menu and recipes. The meal is a light meal with soup and bread, rice or pasta, chicken or fish with a low-fat sauce, vegetables, or salad. It's a little bit boring but the players have the same meal for away matches in their hotel before traveling to the ground.

What is the team nutrition plan for refueling and rehydration during a match? Who are the people involved in implementing this plan? Do you have a program for monitoring how well individual players achieve the plan?

It is quite rare that the players have an opportunity to drink once the match has started. At halftime they are provided with isotonic sport drinks and snacks in the form of biscuits and fruit, to help go some way to help with replacing lost fluids and carbohydrates. The players are truly professional in their attitude and with support from the staff they take responsibility for their own fluid and food intakes. To give the players a guide as to how much to drink, weighing of the player before and after training along with monitoring fluid intakes is useful.

Is there a team plan for postmatch nutrition—in the locker rooms? In the club rooms? On team travel home from the match? How is this organized?

The team plan is to refuel and rehydrate in the hours following a match. There is always food and drink available for players after the match or on the way home. The players choose from a selection of sport drinks, soup, bread, sandwiches, biscuits, fruit, and scones.

Is there a team policy regarding alcohol intake in the match period—for example, the night before a match, or in the postmatch period? What sort of education do you provide about this issue?

We educate the players with regard to the effect of alcohol on performance and recovery. The players choose not to drink alcohol in the 24 hr before a match. A few may have a social drink after matches; however, with having a training session the next morning the emphasis is on sleep and recovery.

Like most Premier League teams, Manchester United has a large number of players from other countries and cultures. Its players are among the highest-paid athletes in the world, and many would regard themselves as being the ultimate professional athlete. How do you approach the situation of trying to meet different food likes, different nutritional needs, and different ideas about nutrition within the same team plan? How do you approach the situation where players want a menu choice or want to follow an eating plan that you feel isn't suitable?

I spend a lot of my time talking with individual players about their nutritional needs and their ideas. I make sure they understand their requirements with explanations of the exercise physiology involved. I then show them how they can meet their food and fluid needs with the foods we have available in England.

PRACTICAL ISSUE

Providing Nutrition Services for a Team Sport

Following is an interview with Michelle Cort, sports dietitian for the Brisbane Lions, during their winning spree of Australian Football League premierships in 2001, 2002, and 2003, and current dietitian to the Sydney Swans, winner of the Australian Football League premiership in 2005.

Michelle, what is the pathway to becoming involved as a sports dietitian with a professional football team? For example, how did you become involved with the Brisbane Lions?

I first started with the Lions at the end of 1998, when a new coach (Leigh Matthews) and his new assistant coaching staff also came on board. I was working in a sports medicine center with sports physiotherapists, massage therapists, and other sports medicine practitioners. Together we put in a proposal to provide sport science and sports medicine services to the Lions and we were accepted. This ensured a team approach to the provision of these services was possible from the outset.

Can you explain the competition program undertaken by an AFL team? How many games does the team play in a season? What is the average length of time between games?

There are 22 games played in the regular home and away season from March to September. Teams play 11 games and then have a bye weekend, followed by the remaining 11 games. Eight teams then qualify for the finals series (played in September), which can be one to four games. A preseason competition also exists during February and March. Up to four games can be played in this knockout, or tournament style, competition. Games are usually separated by 6 to 8 days.

How many home games do the team play in a season? What do the away games entail? How far might the team have to travel and do the players travel as a team? When and how is the travel undertaken?

Brisbane and Sydney typically play 11 games in their home cities during the regular season. The remaining games are played in Melbourne, Perth, and Adelaide and occasionally in Hobart. Ideally the team would prefer not to play two away games in a row because of the effect of travel on recovery and performance. However, because of the nature of the draw this is unavoidable.

Because of the frequency of travel by the team, numerous strategies have been tested and put into place to minimize the risk of negative effects to recovery and performance. Travel to an away game is always by plane and undertaken the day before the game. Flight times vary from 90 min to 6 hr depending on the destination. Return after the game is dependent on the time the game is played. The team will travel back hours after the game if a day game has been played or the following morning if a night game has been played.

Several nutritional issues arise as a result of flying to and from games. Avoiding dehydration on the flight is critical. Players are supplied with additional fluid for the flight based on the amount of time spent in the pressurized cabins. Additional food items are also taken to supplement the meals provided on the plane and help with providing fuel for upcoming training sessions (at destination) or for refueling after games.

What time of day are matches commonly played? What would a player's typical routine be on a match day prior to the game, both in terms of activities and eating patterns?

Day games are usually played between 1 and 4 p.m. and night games start around 7 p.m. and finish at approximately 10 p.m. Emphasis is placed on the player adhering to his usual routine as much as possible with respect to activity or eating regardless of whether playing at home or away. A player's activity patterns on game day are individualized with some players choosing to do light activity while others prefer to relax.

Before day games the players will consume a breakfast that is similar to their training day breakfast. A pregame meal is then consumed 2 to 3 hr before the game. For night games, a player's eating plan is reasonably similar to his training diet with the emphasis on carbohydrate food choices. Breakfast, a mid-morning snack, lunch, and then a pregame meal will be consumed. Fluids are encouraged at all meals, with particular attention being paid to fluid intake in the couple of hours prior to a game.

Do you organize a team sitting for the prematch meal for all or any of the matches? What sort of menu do you organize? What sort of menu do you advise when players are organizing their own meals?

When traveling away for games, the players usually eat meals as a group at the hotel where they stay. I send the required menu for each meal to the hotel catering staff about 1 week prior to arrival. The specified menu is always buffet style. This allows for the players to choose foods that they prefer in the quantities they desire. The menu is constructed so that the players have access to foods that they are comfortable and familiar with at each mealtime. The meals are high in carbohydrate and contain good-quality protein sources. Extra fruit, vegetables, and salad are also always available at meals. Two to three meal options are available at each mealtime. Snacks such as fruit, low-fat yogurt, and cereal bars are also available in the dining rooms at meals. This allows the players to take the snacks away for use at other times. Plenty of fluid choices are also available for the players at meals. These include jugs of fluid at the tables and serving areas as well as bottled fluid that the players are able to take away from the meal area for use during the day or night.

During the preseason and season I like to see players individually on a regular basis and am able to develop individualized meal plans that ensure they are able to meet their training and competition goals. If players are eating outside the hotel environment while traveling away, they possess the skills and knowledge necessary to choose correct meal choices. Maintaining usual eating habits and routine before games is always stressed to the player. Never trying new food experiences and practicing pregame eating before training sessions is important. Based on this, the player knows what works for him and what he feels comfortable with.

Let's use the Brisbane Lions experience as an example, because it has some special challenges. What is the team nutrition plan for refueling and rehydration during a match? Who are the people involved in implementing this plan? Do you have a program for monitoring how well individual players achieve the plan?

The Brisbane Lions place a major focus on refueling and rehydration during games to ensure they are able to perform at a high intensity throughout the entire period. This is more important for the Lions than many other teams, because although football is a winter sport, Brisbane is located in the northern part of Australia and enjoys warm weather conditions throughout the year. This focus is valuable, however, because the finals are played in early spring and can often be played in atypically hot conditions. This could give an advantage in being better acclimatized and better practiced at warm weather play.

Team plans that I have constructed for rehydration and refueling are practiced during training sessions so that the players adapt to consuming specific items regularly throughout exercise. I regularly used group education sessions attended by the players, coaching staff, medical and sport science staff, and trainers to communicate the rehydration and refueling strategies throughout the season and preseason. This helps to ensure a common message is delivered to the players by all of the support staff with regard to these strategies. Fluid balance studies (weighing players before and after a workout) are also regularly conducted at training in an effort to encourage good hydration strategies and fluid choices. Sport drinks are stressed as the fluid of choice to the players, both as a means of rehydration and in providing additional fuel. Different types of sport drinks and sport food (e.g., carbohydrate gels) choices are all trialed during training sessions.

My teams have considered it advantageous for the dietitian to attend both home and away games to ensure that nutritional strategies and plans are followed by the players at all times. My role during games is very hands-on. Players would be weighed before, at halftime, and at the end of the game as a system of monitoring their fluid deficit. This provides instant feedback to the player regarding the amount of fluid he needs to consume to rehydrate. Several players who have a history of cramping have mentioned that this strategy has improved their confidence in return-

ing to the game in the second half knowing that they have consumed appropriate amounts of fluid.

There are good opportunities for players to obtain regular drinks during games as trainers run onto the field with a bottle of water and a bottle of sport drink at breaks in play or when the ball is at the opposite end of the ground. I can obtain feedback from the trainers during training and games as to which players aren't drinking regularly and which fluid they are choosing. This allows me to speak with specific players and encourage them to improve strategies at these times. It also provides useful feedback for targeting certain topics the following week at group education sessions.

At quarter-time, halftime, and three-quarter-time breaks I can provide players with their specific drinks and check that each has consumed his required amount. At times, certain players may prefer a carbohydrate gel and water at breaks instead of a sport drink, and it is my role to ensure these are consumed appropriately. It's very encouraging to hear the head coach and assistant coaches reminding the boys to "grab a drink" before they will talk to them at quarter-time, halftime, and three-quarter time.

Is there a team plan for postmatch nutrition? How is this organized?

My role as team dietitian includes organizing the postmatch recovery foods and fluids. Once again, the players have a good understanding of the importance of recovery nutrition because of the ongoing education they receive from me throughout the preseason and season, reinforced by input from the conditioning and medical and sport science staff.

Postmatch foods and fluids are provided to the players in their dressing rooms at home and away matches. A range of fluids for rehydration and carbohydrate- and protein-containing snacks for refueling and muscle repair are provided. Certain players will not feel like eating solid foods after games; therefore, liquid meal supplement drinks are provided as an alternative to solid foods. The players have been educated to then eat a carbohydrate- and protein-containing meal within 2 hr after leaving the ground. This is provided at the hotel when playing away games.

Is there a team policy regarding alcohol intake in the match period—for example, the night before a match or in the postmatch period?

No policy exists regarding alcohol intake the night before the match, and no official policy exists in the postmatch period. Prematch, the players are extremely focused and alcohol intake is not an issue. I educate players regarding the possible negative effects of alcohol consumption postmatch. Over the past few years, the senior players have taken an extremely professional approach to recovery after matches, and the majority will always avoid alcohol consumption the night after the game (especially when traveling). This attitude from the senior players has influenced the younger team members who have learned from them and also follow similar practices.

How do you approach the situation of trying to meet different food likes, different nutritional needs, and different ideas about nutrition within the same team plan? How do you approach the situation where players want a menu choice or want to follow an eating plan that you believe isn't suitable?

When you are dealing with the players on an almost a daily basis, their food likes and dislikes and meal plans become very familiar. You can provide for the different tastes and needs of the players when we travel by offering buffet-style meals (which allows for players to make choices based on their likes and dislikes and preferred quantities). I would ensure that all of the players have their preferences catered for within the two to three meal options available.

Although AFL is a team game, individual players can have different nutritional goals and strategies depending on the position played, how much game time they receive, and whether they are injured. Different body composition goals also result in the players often having different nutrition strategies. Therefore, ongoing individual advice is provided to the players to ensure these goals are met and the appropriate nutritional strategy is implemented. Supplement and sport food programs were developed for the team; however, an individualized approach is taken with the provision of these to the players.

Several nutrition issues are common to the whole team, however (e.g., importance of recovery), and are discussed with the group as a whole as well as individually. I have found that using group (team) sessions is a useful way of reinforcing nutrition messages that have been discussed in individual sessions. Occasions have arisen where a player wishes to try an eating plan that nutritionally doesn't appear to be advantageous. On these occasions I discuss individually with the player the reasons as to why the current meal plan will not be ideal for performance and the possible negative effects that can occur. I then ask them to watch out for signs that indicate the nutritional strategy may not be ideal (e.g., reduced energy levels, decreased intensity at training, reduced strength in the gym). This often helps to back up or reinforce the importance of adhering to the strategy recommended by the dietitian.

Like a lot of elite athletes, in an effort to gain a performance edge over competitors, the players will come to me seeking advice and information regarding a new or special supplement or idea that they have come across. I will provide the player with my advice based on current scientific knowledge of the supplement and whether it would be of specific benefit to them. I think that it is important to never discount and ignore the player's opinion regarding a certain strategy he feels works best for him, regardless of whether I agree with the principles. Being willing to discuss different ideas without judgment, while also giving an opinion based on scientific evidence, helps to ensure that the player feels comfortable discussing future nutrition ideas.

Fortunately, the medical and sport science and conditioning team and coaching staff meet each week to discuss player issues. This allows the team to ensure that a common message and strategy regarding preparation and recovery strategies are presented to the players. The team approach and unified message help to ensure that the players have confidence that they are receiving the correct nutrition messages and strategies.

What innovative strategies have you tried in terms of nutrition at your teams? How do you sell these ideas to the rest of the medical and sport science team? How do you handle the situation when other people on this panel want to take on nutrition strategies for which you believe there is little scientific evidence?

Over the past few years I have been able to set up systems and strategies that allow the players to receive what they require to ensure that their nutritional strategies and goals can be achieved. Spending such a large amount of time with the players over many years has enabled me to continually fine-tune and improve on these strategies. The continual idea of seeking for improvement and more effective ways of providing and implementing all of the sport science and sports medicine services including nutrition is a philosophy that the players are well aware of. This has given them confidence that they receive up-to-date, cutting-edge advice and practical strategies from the sports medicine and sport science staff. This consequently allows them to be confident in a game situation that they have been able to do everything possible to prepare for competition and optimal performance.

Nutrition strategies that I have implemented include these:

- Monitoring of hydration status using specific gravity measures and weighing of players before and the day after a game. Feedback to the players regarding hydration status and strategies from this has been extremely useful.
- Manipulation of the sodium content of rehydration fluids to aid in improved rehydration.
- Recovery food and fluid program for after games and training.
- Development of a sport food and sports supplement program within the club. This helps to ensure the players receive appropriate supplements and sport foods and that they receive them at the correct times with respect to training and games.

Other strategies have ensured players receive up-to-date, practical, relevant nutrition messages. These include the following:

- Football nutrition courses that all new drafted players to the club complete with me during the preseason. Sessions are held weekly and include group discussions and workshops on football-specific topics such as hydration, recovery, pretraining eating, cooking classes, shopping tours, and food court tours.
- Themed nutrition displays in players' dressing rooms targeting issues discussed in the previous week with the players.

- Nutrition diary and record sections in the players' weights program folders.
- Trials of new products at training sessions.
- Nutrition travel packs for players for flights to and from games.

It works well when medical and conditioning team meetings are held regularly to discuss new and better ways of implementing strategies in all areas of sport science and sports medicine, including nutrition. This approach helps to ensure that the sports medicine and sport science team provides a unified message to the players and coaching staff. Each professional is regarded as the expert in his or her field. Ideas are discussed (often for lengthy periods!), and ultimately the expert in the field will decide whether it would be of benefit to the team or player if the strategy was implemented.

chapter 9

Court and Indoor Team Sports

This section continues our exploration of sports based on intermittent high-intensity exercise, moving the emphasis to court sports such as basketball, netball, and volleyball as well as other games on a smaller playing arena such as ice hockey, water polo, and beach volleyball. These games can be played on outdoor courts, but at the elite level they are often played inside stadiums with an environment controlled by air-conditioning. The game characteristics again feature high-intensity efforts of running and jumping, interspersed with low-intensity movements. A smaller playing area will generally lead to a faster game (e.g., shorter duration movements with more frequent changes in activity) and lower total distance covered during the game.

Many of the nutritional issues of court and indoor sports are shared with field-based team sports, and once such issues are identified, the reader will be directed to the relevant sections of chapter 8 and other chapters of this book to explore the information that is presented elsewhere. The focus of this chapter is limited to the unique issues of court and indoor sports and to a summary of the scientific underpinning and guidelines regarding fluid and carbohydrate needs of intermittent high-intensity sports.

Competition

Court and indoor sports share and differ in a number of characteristics. For example, there is a range in the ratio of activity and inactivity between various sports, because of breaks between playing periods and time-outs. There are also differences in the substitution of players on and off the court. Some court sports are won by the team that scores the most points within a set period of play (e.g., basketball, netball, ice hockey, and water polo). By contrast, the duration of some games (e.g., volleyball) is open-ended, with victory being awarded to the team that first achieves a certain number of points. Many of these sports date back over a century, with some codes being

invented or adapted from existing sports to provide an activity that could be played indoors—and thus protected from inclement weather. Other court sports are deliberately played in an outside environment, even at the elite level (e.g., beach volleyball).

Because there are too many sports to discuss in individual detail, this section discusses and compares the competition features of two popular court sports—basketball and volleyball. These sports enjoy worldwide popularity for male and female players over a range of ages and skill levels. They are represented on the Olympic Games program and hold world championships at both junior and elite levels. Both sports are represented in the National Collegiate Athletics Association (NCAA) program, with college basketball being a particularly important and highly watched sport within this system.

A regulation game of basketball is played over two 20 min halves or four 12 min quarters. These figures denote the live time (actual playing time), and at high levels of play, the frequent stopping of the time clock when the ball is out of play substantially increases the total duration of the game. The game is played with five players from each team on the court at any one time, and additional players may be rotated into play from the bench throughout the match. Physical characteristics—particularly height—play an important role in performance, perhaps at a greater level than in most other sports (see "Physique and Physiology"). Success as a basketball player is also determined by speed, agility, skill, and tactical sense.

Typical activity patterns of a basketball game were described in a time–motion study on matches played from the National Basketball League in Australia (McInnes et al. 1995). According to this study, basketball players make a large number of discrete movements each game (~1,000), changing their activities every 2 s. This is similar to other court sports but is greater than that seen in field sports. About 100 high-intensity activities are undertaken by each player per game, occurring approximately every 20 s of actual playing time. Because of the small size of the court and the duration of activity, players rarely achieve maximum running speed during a game. Instead, considerable energy is expended overcoming movement momentum to change direction or to accelerate and decelerate. Jumping, passing, shooting, and blocking shots are other common activities, and although basketball is technically a noncontact sport, there is generally a high level of physical interaction between players on opposing teams.

Basketball is an intense activity with a heavy aerobic component and moderate to high rates of energy expenditure while the player is on the court (MacLaren 1990). There has been little direct study of fuel utilization patterns during basketball games. Although there is no information on glycogen utilization over a match in basketball players, the detection of high concentrations of blood lactate throughout the game indicates that glycolysis of carbohydrate provides an important fuel source for basketball competition. High heart rates are seen during live time in basketball; in some players and during some passages of play, heart rates approach maximal values (McInnes et al. 1995). Across the game, mean heart rates of 170 beats/min and a mean aerobic consumption equivalent to 70% $\dot{V}O_2$max are typical, which are in contrast to values of 110 to 125 beats/min and 55% $\dot{V}O_2$max during a typical volleyball match (MacLaren 1990). However, mean heart rates during play remain high despite only 15% of live time being devoted to high-intensity activities. The contribution of psychological arousal and anxiety toward heart rate values has not been identified. Studies based on heart rate values suggest that the physiological demands of men's basketball and elite-level competition are greater than that of women's competition or subelite and recreational games. Nevertheless, there is considerable individual variability in game heart rate responses depending on fitness levels, positions played, and the amount of time spent on the court.

Studies of football codes have reported a reduction of distance covered and running speed in the latter part of a game, but basketball players in the games studied by McInnes and coworkers (1995) showed no changes in movement patterns between quarters of the game. Thus, there was little evidence that physiological fatigue factors affected the intensity and pattern of play, at least for the single games studied. This may not be the case for all situations of play, particularly during tournaments or road trips where players may carry some level of fatigue, fuel depletion, or hypohydration from one game to the next. However, within any individual game there are opportunities for substantial recovery between high-intensity activities. The majority of low-intensity activities such as standing and walking occur during stoppages in play—for example, breaks between quarters or halves, time-outs, substitutions, and free throws. Coaches can use time-outs and substitutions not only to impart tactical advice but to provide valuable rest periods following prolonged periods of uninterrupted intense play. The opportunities also allow nutritional strategies such as intake of fluid and carbohydrate to be achieved.

Volleyball matches have an open-ended duration until one team wins three sets, each consisting of 15 points. A review of studies of elite-level tournaments from the 1970s reported that the mean duration of a set in volleyball was 20 to 23 min for women and 22 to 26 min for men, with a mean total game time of 72 to 84 min and 84 to 95 min, respectively (MacLaren 1990). Of course, the time for individual games within these tournaments covered a wide range—from 28 to 149 min (women) and 36 to 178 min (men). This uncertainty in competition demands is compounded in the case of tournaments, where a team may progress through to the finals with a series of brief matches or, at the other extreme, a number of prolonged games. The overall winner may be either the team with the greatest endurance or the team that has faced the fewest or shortest sets (i.e., expended the least energy) in the lead-up to the final game.

In addition to requiring skill and tactical sense, success in volleyball is determined by jumping ability, speed, agility, and specific strength. Like basketball, volleyball is a game of high-intensity activities interspersed with rest intervals. Various time–motion analyses on elite-level volleyball matches have found that the typical duration of a rally is 6 to 10 s, with the typical duration of the rest period being 12 to 14 s and a rally-to-rest ratio ranging from 1:1.2 to 1:2.2 (MacLaren 1990). Although games at subelite and recreational level have longer rallies, volleyball players typically spend greater amounts of time at rest than in active play during a game. High-intensity activities during a game include serving, retrieving, setting, and the jumping activities of spiking and blocking. Such activities occur each 20 to 40 s during a game, being more frequent when the player is rotated to the front court. Technical and tactical aspects of the game mean that players have various roles and different activity patterns during a game. In a typical 85 min match, setters spend less total time in jumping activities (3.5-8.5 min) and greater proportions of their activity on setting, whereas blockers or spikers typically spend 7.5 to 15 min in jumping activities and only a small amount of time on setting (MacLaren 1990). The main energy system for the explosive nature of jumping activities in volleyball is the phosphagen system, and rest periods allow regeneration of adenosine triphosphate and creatine phosphate. Lactate levels are low to moderate over the game, suggesting that anaerobic glycolysis does not make a significant contribution to the fuel used over the game. Studies of glycogen utilization patterns over a volleyball match show substantial depletion in slow-twitch fibers but also that some players may start a match with low glycogen stores from previous games or training sessions (for review, see MacLaren 1990).

Like field-based team sports, court and indoor sports can be played both in a seasonal fixture and in a tournament format. As such, competition outcomes are decided by a series of matches with recovery intervals ranging from 1 to 7 days. In some lower-level competitions, players may be scheduled to play in a weekly match. However, in other situations players undertake games more frequently and attend practice between matches. This can occur when a player is registered in more than one team or competition, during tournaments, and in professional leagues where the popularity of the game and the number of teams in the draw have led to a heavy competition schedule. For example, in the American National Basketball Association, a team can expect to play more than 80 games in the main draw of the season and, if they are successful in the final series, a playoff between the two top teams involving the best of seven matches. In some national or continental leagues or associations, a team may travel to a particular city or region and play two to three games over successive or alternating days against local teams in the same league. Issues arising from the breakdown of the year into off-season, preseason, and competition seasons, and the various competition scenarios, are covered in greater detail in the section on competition characteristics in chapter 8: Field-Based Team Sports.

Training

A variety of skills and physical attributes are needed in court and indoor sports, with a range of characteristics occurring between sports but also between players within the same sport according to position or style of play. Trainable characteristics are aerobic and anaerobic endurance, body fat levels, speed and agility, strength, jumping ability, and specific game skills. The principles of periodization of training were discussed in greater detail in chapter 8; refer to this chapter for a better understanding of the general issues of training for team sports. Overall, the training undertaken by players in court-based and indoor team sports will involve sessions specifically aimed at enhancing fitness and conditioning or the individual physical attributes desired for the sport, as well as sessions based on skill and tactics, including game simulations and match play. Depending on the sport and the level of play, these sessions may be self-initiated or prescribed or conducted by the club. They may also be undertaken as team practices or as individual or one-on-one sessions to work on specific aspects of conditioning or skill. One type of training undertaken by athletes in many court sports, but less commonly in other team sports, is plyometrics. This form of training, undertaken to enhance jumping ability, is discussed in more detail in chapter 7 within the training characteristics of sprint athletes.

Physique and Physiology

Athletes involved in court and indoor team sports need to have good levels of aerobic and anaerobic fitness. Generally, elite players in sports such as basketball and volleyball have above-average values for maximal aerobic capacity (MacLaren 1990). However, these values fall short of the very high scores recorded by elite endurance athletes, particularly when they are expressed per kilogram of body mass. Within sports, athletes have different aerobic capacities depending on their positions of play. Typically, the playmakers in each code (e.g., guards in basketball and

centers in netball) have a higher maximal aerobic capacity than other teammates. Because court sports require speed, agility, and specific strength, players are expected to have above-average levels of muscularity and lower levels of body fat. Again, these characteristics vary between sports and positions of play and are not as prominently expressed as in other sports, for example, the low body fat levels of endurance athletes or the high levels of lean body mass in rugby and American football players. A recent development in many court sports has been the pursuit of low body fat levels, at least among female players, largely driven by aesthetic reasons rather than performance advantages. This phenomenon is discussed in greater detail in the section titled "Bodysuits and Body Fat Levels."

Two distinguishing and interrelated characteristics seen in court-based team sports such as basketball, volleyball, and netball are height and jumping ability. In the case of basketball, goals are scored (or blocked) through a ring that is positioned 305 cm (10 ft) above the ground, whereas analysis of the volleyball matches in elite players has shown that the main action in the game takes place at a height above ground of 330 cm for males and 300 cm

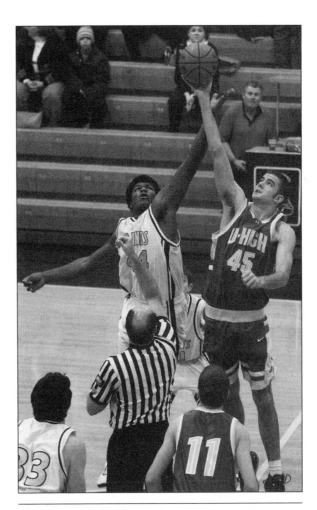

Almost all of the professional players in major leagues in center position are in excess of 200 cm in height.

for females, some 70 to 85 cm above the height of the net (MacLaren 1990). Clearly, players need both height and jumping capacity to be able to reach the aerial playing zone. Studies of national volleyball teams have reported mean heights ranging from 185 to 195 cm for males and 178 to 180 cm for females (for review, see MacLaren 1990). Basketball players are typically taller; studies report mean heights across a range of top-class players of 195 to 200 cm for males (for review, see MacLaren 1990). Within a basketball team there is a general graduation in heights among players from the small but skillful play-making guards to the forwards and the centers. For the center, height is an absolute requirement, and there is less need for speed and agility. Volleyball players have been recorded as having the greatest vertical jumping ability of all groups of athletes, with mean values for vertical jump of 50 to 75 cm across a range of studies of top-class players (for review, see MacLaren 1990). Basketball players also possess good vertical jump ability but to a lesser extent than volleyball players, perhaps as a result of being taller and heavier. Again, there seems to be some degree of variability within the team according to the requirements of the position.

Lifestyle and Culture

Most of the lifestyle and cultural issues that concern court and indoor team sport players were presented in chapter 8: Field-Based Team Sports. These include meeting nutrient needs in a busy day, the challenges of starting out as an aspiring young player (e.g., moving away from home with limited domestic skills and a tight budget), frequent travel, and the collegiate or sports institute scene. See chapter 8 for a discussion of these issues. One personal observation of relevance to height-focused sports such as basketball and volleyball is that aggressive talent identification programs often identify potentially very tall athletes at an early age and feed them into specialist developmental programs with either camp-based or semipermanent residential structures. It can be difficult for caretakers, coaches, sport scientists, and other personnel who work with these athletes to remember their true age. When one is dealing with a 15- or 16-year-old who is 195 cm, it is easy to assume that he has the intellect and maturity of an adult. Education activities, levels of responsibility, and other program attributes need to be clearly targeted to the real needs and capabilities of a young adolescent rather than an older person, despite the physical appearance of these athletes.

Dietary Surveys

High energy demands are expected to occur in conjunction with the unusually large and rapid growth spurts experienced by some adolescent players. Even after many athletes achieve their height potential, they need to continue high energy intakes while they fill out, or undertake special training programs aimed at increasing lean body mass. The energy requirements of the fully mature player are also expected to be reasonably high to support both the training and match program and the player's large body mass. Of course, when energy intakes or requirements of such players are expressed relative to body mass, these values become more modest in comparison with those of other athletic populations. Unfortunately, it is difficult to see these principles demonstrated by the few available dietary surveys of court sport athletes, which are heavily focused on collegiate basketball players in the case of males (table 9.a in the appendix to this chapter) and collegiate volleyball players in the case of females (table 9.b). Consistent with the dietary survey literature from other sports, females report relatively lower energy intakes than their male counterparts, and there is no information to distinguish whether this is an artifact of dietary survey methodology, whether it can be explained by restricted dietary practices related to weight loss goals, or whether it reflects lower energy expenditure in training.

It is unwise to draw too many conclusions about the adequacy of macronutrient and micronutrient intake of court sport players from such limited data, but it appears that male players typically report daily protein intakes equivalent to ~1.5 to 2.0 g/kg BM and carbohydrate intakes of ~5 to 6 g/kg BM (Nowak et al. 1988; Schena et al. 1995; Van Erp-Baart et al. 1989a). These protein intakes easily meet the increase in protein requirements for heavily training athletes recommended by some sports nutrition experts (see table 1.1). Guidelines for carbohydrate fuel needs of training and competition will depend on the frequency and duration of play, but at least two studies of court sport players suggest that they do not always eat sufficient carbohydrate to fully recover fuel stores daily. In these studies, researchers found that the pregame glycogen stores of a group of volleyball players were already partially depleted (Conlee et al. 1982; Viitasalo et al. 1982). This is likely to be even a greater risk in female court sport players, because their reported daily intake of carbohydrate is lower at ~3 to 4 g/kg BM (Ersoy 1995; Nowak et al. 1988; Papadopoulou et al. 2002; Risser et al. 1990; Van Erp-Baart et al. 1989a). Reported protein intakes of female players of ~1 to 1.2 $g \cdot kg^{-1} \cdot day^{-1}$ meet guidelines for sedentary populations but may not meet the increased requirements for either growth or heavy exercise suggested by some authorities (see table 1.1). Intakes of micronutrients are likely to be adequate in the case of male players but appear to be inadequate for female court sport players. For example, in one survey of female collegiate basketball players, mean intakes of some vitamins and minerals (riboflavin, niacin, vitamin C, and calcium) met 100% of the country-specific recommended daily allowances, but substantial numbers of individual participants recorded intakes below 70% of these levels (Hickson et al. 1986). Furthermore, mean intakes of the group were less than 70% of the guidelines for iron, vitamin B_6, magnesium, and zinc. Similarly, Papadopolou and colleagues (2002) reported mean daily intakes of vitamin B_6, iron, and zinc that were below 70% of the recommended intakes in a group of junior basketball players.

There is a clear need for more dietary surveys of contemporary court and indoor team sport players, including professional and elite players as well as collegiate and junior teams. Given the nutrient needs for growth, it would be of interest to study the iron status of court sport players in more detail. One Australian study reported a decline in serum ferritin concentrations in a group of junior elite female netball and basketball players across a season; however, there were no other changes in indexes of iron status, leaving the meaning of this decline unclear (Ashenden et al. 1998). Meanwhile, another study that undertook hematological screening of a number of adolescent and adult players from national basketball competition in Israel reported a high prevalence of iron depletion (22% of players) and iron-deficiency anemia (7% of players). The prevalence of these conditions was substantially higher in female players than in male players.

Nutritional Issues and Challenges

A summary of commonly seen challenges is presented in the highlight box on this page and includes issues related to achieving optimal physique, optimizing training, and preparing for and recovering from games. Chapter 8 discusses the scientific and practical aspects of most of these issues. This chapter focuses on a few unique requirements or characteristics of court and indoor sports before undertaking an overview of the benefits of hydrating and fueling during games based on intermittent high-intensity exercise.

Common Nutritional Issues Arising in Team Court Sports

Physique Issues

- For some sports and positions: increasing and maintaining high levels of lean body mass for strength
- For some sports and positions: maintaining moderately low body fat levels to aid speed and agility
- Reducing or maintaining body fat levels after period of inactivity such as the off-season or during injury
- Bodysuits: adding additional stress to achieve lean physique and low body fat levels

Training Issues

- Achieving high energy intake to maintain high body mass and size, especially during periods of growth such as adolescence or aggressive resistance training
- Consuming adequate carbohydrate during the interval between matches and training to promote optimal recovery
- Consuming adequate protein to meet increased requirements resulting from heavy training and to promote recovery from games and adaptation to training
- Considering creatine supplementation for training adaptations (match simulation, interval training, resistance training)
- Monitoring reduced iron status, especially in female athletes and athletes undergoing growth spurts
- Monitoring fluid and carbohydrate intake during prolonged training sessions
- Enhancing nutrition knowledge and domestic skills in young players
- Integrating training and match goals in a weekly fixture

Competition Issues

- Fueling up before events
- Planning the pregame meal
- Monitoring fluid and carbohydrate intake during games
- Refueling and rehydrating between games, especially in a tournament
- Evaluating nutrition for the traveling athlete
- Using alcohol wisely, especially in postmatch situation
- Considering creatine and caffeine supplementation for competition performance

Bodysuits and Body Fat Levels

Sepp Blatter, Swiss president of [soccer] world governing body FIFA said women should show off their bottoms to increase the game's popularity. "Let the women play in more feminine clothes like they do in volleyball," he said. "They could, for example, have tighter shorts. Female players are pretty, if you excuse me for saying so, and they already have some different rules to men—such as playing with a lighter ball . . . so why not do it in fashion?"

Rachel Wells, The Melbourne Age *newspaper, Melbourne, Australia, accessed August 25, 2006, from http://www.theage.com.au/articles/2004/01/16/1073878029209.html*

I am so excited that I am finishing my Olympic career so that I won't have to worry about what I eat or drink so that I can fit into that darn body suit. I have to keep in some sort of shape for the WNBA but at least there you get to wear baggy clothes.

Michele Timms, captain of the silver medal winning basketball team at the 2000 Olympic Games, explaining her decision to retire from the Australian national team but to continue playing one or two more seasons in the U.S. Women's National Basketball Association. From The Bulletin *magazine, Sydney, Australia, October 17, 2000, p. 109*

In the section on physique characteristics of court and indoor team sport players earlier in this chapter, it was noted that low to moderate body fat levels may assist the performance of some players in mobile sports or positions. Nevertheless, a range of body fat levels is tolerated in court sports, and values are generally above those typically found in endurance athletes. Interestingly, in recent years there has been a renewed interest by female team athletes in achieving low body fat levels—not with the primary goal of improving performance on the court but to enhance their appearance. The catalyst for this interest appears to have been the introduction of form-fitting bodysuit uniforms by many women's teams as competition attire. These uniforms have been chosen by various netball, basketball, and volleyball teams in the belief that they make female sport look more appealing to spectators, television, and sponsors because they are more revealing of body contours and size than the traditional uniforms of shorts or skirts and singlets. A similar situation is seen in beach volleyball, where skimpy swimwear is the regulation uniform. These prescribed uniform changes have added an unnecessary level of pressure to females regarding their physique, even to already successful athletes, as demonstrated by the quote at the opening of this section.

Many sports dietitians and nutritionists who work with women's teams have noted an increase in interest in weight loss strategies among the athletes who now wear bodysuits during competition. In some cases, use of these uniforms is even believed to have increased the prevalence of disor-dered eating within a sport (personal communication, Jill McIntosh, former National Head Coach of the Australian Netball team). Although there are no data to support this hypothesis, it is a believable outcome considering that the necessity to wear revealing or figure-hugging uniforms is a key risk factor for the development of disordered eating among athletes (Otis et al. 1997). The issues of disordered eating are discussed in greater detail in chapter 5 related to distance running, and chapter 13 related to gymnastics. Further discussion on dietary strategies to assist with loss of weight and body fat can be found in the section titled "Achieving Low Body Mass and Body Fat Levels" in chapter 4. Individualized and specific advice from a sports dietitian or nutritionist is valuable in helping help team sport athletes who want to get in shape to set realistic goals for body mass and body fat levels and a suitable time frame in which to achieve these goals. As is the case for all athletes, female team sport players should be prepared to set their ideal physique based on trial-and-error observations over an adequate period of time. These athletes need to consider measures of long-term health and performance, rather than aesthetics alone. In addition, the player should be able to achieve her targets while eating a diet that is adequate in energy and nutrients and free of unreasonable levels of food-related stress.

In the meantime, it appears that female team sport athletes, especially those who wear competition bodysuits, may constitute a previously unidentified group at high risk of fad diets, problem weight loss behaviors, and disordered eating. Research is needed to confirm the extent and the severity of these problems, to develop effective education strategies to reduce athletes' risks, and to alert those who work with these team sports to make an early diagnosis of problems. This likely will represent a cultural change in some sports, which athletes, coaches, trainers, and sport science and sports medicine teams may be ill-equipped to handle without specialized assistance. If a link to impaired health of the athlete can be proven, perhaps the whole concept of the bodysuit should be reexamined by sports administrators, because it constitutes such a peripheral issue to performance in these sports.

Fluid and Fuel Needs

There has been little research on the specific fluid and fuel requirements of court and indoor sports, but it is likely that training and competition can lead to reasonable levels of muscle glycogen utilization and loss of fluid, particularly for the playmakers on a team. The different needs and opportunities for intake of fluid and carbohydrate during various team and racket sports are discussed in greater detail in separate sections of this chapter (research topics and the first practical issue). Characteristics of court-based sports that may predict lower requirements for carbohydrate and fluid than in field-based games include the possibility of a cooler or controlled environment in air-conditioned stadiums and the shorter duration of movements and smaller distances covered in a match attributable to the smaller size of the playing arena.

Analysis of the movement patterns in elite-level basketball does not always show evidence of fatigue during the last phases of the game (McInnes et al. 1995), suggesting either that physiological factors do not limit performance in this game or that the nutritional practices undertaken by the players in these studies have already addressed their fuel and fluid needs. However, the literature does suggest that in some situations, substantial fluid deficits are likely to occur despite the drinking practices of players (Broad et al. 1996; Minehan et al. 2002). Even when the fluid deficit incurred across a single game or training session appears small (< 2% body mass), players may have started the session already dehydrated (Burke 2006b, 2006c; Godek, Godek, et al. 2005; Maughan et al. 2004), compounding the effects of this fluid loss. Further investigation of hydration issues in court sports should be undertaken since there is some evidence that moderate levels of dehydration (~2%) can impair skills and movement patterns seen in basketball (Dougherty et al. 2006). Furthermore, significant depletion of glycogen stores has been found during volleyball matches (Conlee et al. 1982; Viitasalo et al. 1982), and there is support for the enhancement of performance in both an intermittent high-intensity exercise protocol undertaken by basketball players (Dougherty et al 2006; Welsh et al. 2002) and a real-life ice hockey game (Simard et al. 1988) when players consume carbohydrate during the session. Therefore, although no clear guidelines can be provided regarding fluid and carbohydrate needs during court and indoor team sports, it seems prudent for each player to experiment with strategies to supply these nutrients before and during matches and prolonged practices.

The sections at the end of this chapter provide greater discussion of the scientific support and the practical issues involved in fueling and rehydration strategies during court sports. There are surprisingly few data on the current practices of court sport players, particularly at the elite and professional level. The available literature is summarized in table 9.c (appendix) and includes information on the practices of junior elite basketball and netball players (Broad et al. 1996) and elite water polo players (Cox et al. 2002). These data, collected during both training and competition, probably represent proactive drinking practices in real-life situations, because the players involved were scholarship holders in a sports institute where education regarding fluid intake was frequently provided and where fluids were made available during games and workouts. This may not be the case in all teams. It is also interesting to note that although the stadium environment reduced the difference in temperature between summer and winter conditions, players appeared to be influenced by the season in terms of their hydration practices. For basketball players, there was a trend in both training and game situations for smaller fluid intakes during winter conditions. This often meant that the total fluid deficit by the end of the session was similar to or even greater than that seen in summer conditions (Broad et al. 1996). In most other sports, summer conditions pose the greater threat to hydration status. Fluid losses in the aquatic environment of water polo were significantly

smaller than in the land-based sports; this finding is supported by data from swimmers (see chapter 6).

A separate study was subsequently undertaken on these same athletic populations to see whether the choice of drink influenced fluid intake practices during training sessions (Minehan et al. 2002). This study was initiated in response to a comment by the coaches of the female basketball and netball teams that players had ceased to consume the sport drink provided during practice, preferring to drink water. We believed that this aversion to consuming an energy-containing fluid during practice may have been driven by body weight issues related to the wearing of bodysuits (see preceding section). Therefore, we decided to investigate the effect of flavor and awareness of the kilojoule content of drinks on fluid balance in training sessions undertaken by these female court sport players. Male basketball players who undertook a similar court practice session and who had received similar education about sport drinks were used as a comparison group. At nine separate practices, players were provided with a clearly labeled bottle providing either water, a carbohydrate–electrolyte solution (sport drink), and an identically flavored but artificially sweetened version of this drink (diet sport drink). Questionnaires completed at the end of each practice found that water was rated significantly higher than either flavored drink for mouth-feel, gastrointestinal comfort, and desire to use the fluid again. However, measurements of the voluntary fluid intakes over the sessions found that both the regular and diet versions of the sport drink were associated with better fluid balance than water. Contrary to our initial hypothesis, in the case of flavored drinks, the kilojoule content of the beverage did not significantly influence voluntary intake in athletes. This finding supports the results of other studies that have reported greater voluntary intakes of flavored drinks compared with water during exercise (Passe et al. 2000; Szlyk et al. 1989; Wilk and Bar-Or 1996) but is unique in finding that this situation continues to occur even when the participants claim to prefer water.

A separate finding of this study was that the netball players had a lower rate of fluid intake than basketball players (Minehan et al. 2002). This may reflect innate differences such as thirst arising from a specific exercise activity as well as extrinsic differences such as education and encouragement to drink. In fact, we observed apparent differences in the latter. The basketball coaches appeared to place greater emphasis on the importance of regular fluid intake and encouraged frequent (four or five per hour), short (1-2 min) breaks during the session for the primary purpose of consuming drinks. Netball players appeared to have fewer (one or two per hour) but longer (5-10 min) breaks per session, with breaks serving the primary purpose of providing coach feedback. It appeared that the opportunity to drink was a secondary outcome of the breaks. Because training sessions are not controlled by competition rules and should therefore be less restrictive in determining opportunities for fluid intake, it is interesting that the structure of the session still appears to have some influence on fluid balance and that encouragement to drink by the coach or trainer is an important factor in determining intake.

In summary, players of court and indoor team sports should develop an appropriate plan for hydration and refueling during games and training sessions. Further details on practical ways to approach this and evidence to support the benefits are provided in the research and practical sections of this chapter. Although the fuel costs of training and competition sessions may be less than those of field-based team sports, there may be situations or individual players who will benefit from refueling during a session. In any case, the use of a sport drink can be valuable in encouraging fluid intake, even when there is little need for carbohydrate intake per se during the session.

The Road Trip

Travel is a standard part of the competition structure of teams that play in national or regional associations and leagues. One specific aspect is the road trip, where a team will travel to a city or area for 3 to 5 days, playing two to three games during this period. Privately owned and professional teams in elite competitions sometimes have the luxury of traveling in a private or chartered jet, or a specially fitted team coach, which is organized to meet the needs and timetable of the team. Most teams, particularly at less elite or lucrative levels of play, are reliant on public transportation. The general challenges of travel are discussed in greater detail in chapter 10.

The double- or triple-game road trip provides a number of nutritional challenges. There may be a 48 hr period of recovery between games on some occasions, but in some circumstances games are played less than 24 hr apart (e.g., a Saturday night game followed by Sunday afternoon competition). Sometimes the team will change locations between games. In some court or indoor team sports, or at least for some players within a team, each game leads to fatigue and substantial depletion of fuel and fluid levels, which must be replenished before the next game. In general, most of these sports do not involve the heavy physical contact of field-based team sports; however, high-intensity play can lead to some level of muscle damage or perhaps an injury (e.g., an acute incident or exacerbation of a chronic condition) that also requires recovery and repair. Speedy replacement of key nutrients will play a role in enhancing these recovery processes. In addition, a more aggressive approach to hydration and fueling during the next game can help to compensate for less than optimal rehydration and glycogen resynthesis.

Teams approach the nutritional needs of the road trip in a variety of different ways. At one end of the spectrum, the team may enjoy the services of a sports dietitian or nutritionist, who will organize a catering plan and develop special menus for postgame recovery snacks, the postgame meal, and the preevent meal for the following game. This approach, followed by a number of successful clubs in professional field-based team sports, was illustrated in interviews presented in the practical issues sessions of chapter 8. In this system, nutritional plans are organized in advance and undertaken at a team level, although they are usually developed with the flexibility to meet specific needs of individual players. However, the team is expected to eat together and will travel with a supply of additional snacks and sport foods to complement catered meals or to provide access to nutritional support at key times—for example, in the locker room immediately after the game, or in the team bus on the way to a game. Sometimes the team dietitian will travel with the team to ensure that the plan is properly implemented and to provide on-the-spot education or feedback to the players. This is particularly useful in terms of organizing and monitoring nutritional practices during a game—for example, ensuring that each player has access to her own drink bottle and that appropriate fluids and sport products are supplied to meet carbohydrate and fluid needs. In extreme environments, it may also be valuable to provide feedback about the rate of fluid loss and each player's success in replacing this during and after the game. Depending on the team, a manager, team trainer, or even sports medicine professional (e.g., sports doctor or physical therapist) may undertake this role on the road.

In some competitions, it is traditional for the host team to organize some of the catering arrangements for both teams—particularly the preevent and postevent meals. The postevent meal may serve a dual function of supplying recovery nutrition for the players and providing a social opportunity for players from both teams to mingle with each other and perhaps with the media, team sponsors, or key people from the competition organization. Unfortunately, in some circumstances the social and business aspects of this function are given priority over the player's recovery needs, and challenges arise in the form of unsuitable choices of food and drinks, inconvenient timing of the function, and the interruption to sleep, injury treatment, and other recovery modalities. The team may need to find creative ways of adding to a menu or consuming recovery snacks before attending the official function.

Finally, some teams require their players to assume responsibility for their own game preparation and recovery on the road trip. Players are often simply supplied with a per diem or daily allowance and are expected to organize their own meals. The disadvantages of this approach are that it assumes that the players are suitably motivated and educated to address their nutritional goals and that there are adequate opportunities and facilities for them to purchase suitable meals and snacks. These factors cannot always be assumed—especially when players and young and have poor practical nutrition knowledge. Most clubs abound with stories of the purchases made with per diems, to the exclusion of food needs! In addition, where games are played late at night or travel schedules demand early morning departures, the player may find themselves having to balance the need for sleep against the need for food or may find that they have missed the hours of normal hotel and restaurant catering. When a club chooses to discharge the responsibility for feeding its players on road trips, the players need to be educated on the best strategies for meeting their nutritional needs on the road.

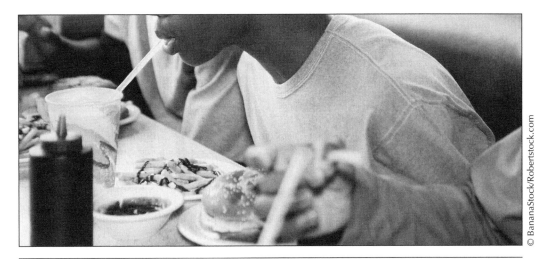

When players purchase meals, they often succumb to the lure or convenience of fast foods and takeaway restaurants, where their food choices do not adequately address the needs of postexercise recovery.

Sport Foods and Supplements

Sport foods and supplements that are likely to meet nutritional goals and ensure optimal performance of court and indoor team sport players are summarized in table 9.1. As is the case with most sports, this list is a small subgroup of the products actually used by players, even at a junior level. There are very few direct studies of supplements and performance in court and indoor sports; the literature from peer-reviewed publications is limited to studies of carbohydrate and fluid intake (see research topics 1 and 2) and creatine (see table 9.d in the appendix). Again, these products are classified based on their application to the common sports nutrition issues seen in court and indoor team sports or based on research undertaken in laboratories or general protocols of prolonged or intermittent high-intensity exercise.

There are clear cases for the use of various sport foods to achieve nutritional goals of training and competition for many players. These situations include provision of nutritional support before, during, and after a match or key training sessions or the provision of a compact and portable supply of energy and nutrients when everyday food is unavailable or difficult to consume. Sport drinks and foods can often help to address the challenges of the road trip or tournament or the high energy needs of the adolescent player undergoing a growth spurt. As is the case for field-based sports, in some teams, supplies of sport foods or supplements are often made available to players in a group environment. Players need to be educated about using such supplements to enhance their effectiveness.

There is a clear need for applied and sport-specific studies on the effects of various supplements on the wide range of popular court and indoor team sports. The conclusions about the lack of efficacy of other dietary supplements are based, in the absence of evidence from studies in other team or intermittent high-energy sports, on the consensus from the general sports nutrition literature. Although one group reported that supplementation with antioxidant vitamins over several weeks during the competition season reduced markers of oxidative stress in a group of professional basketball players, the significance of this finding on the health and performance of the players was not measured and remains uncertain (Schroder et al. 2000, 2001). Sport scientists, especially those who work with elite teams, are encouraged to research the effects of supplements in court and indoor team sports.

RESEARCH TOPIC
Effect of Carbohydrate Replacement and Hydration Strategies on Prolonged Intermittent Exercise

There is general agreement that exercise capacity and performance of prolonged submaximal activities are impaired by hypohydration, especially when the exercise is undertaken in the heat (Sawka and Pandolf 1990). The exact mechanisms underpinning the decrements in endurance or performance are debated, but there is evidence of impairments of cardiovascular and thermoregulatory function as well as an increased perception of effort. The decline in these parameters occurs in proportion to the degree of fluid deficit (Montain and Coyle 1992). At high levels of hypohydration (e.g., >4% loss of body mass as fluid), there is an increased risk of gastrointestinal dysfunction and upset (Rehrer et al. 1990), which can impair performance in its

Table 9.1 Sport Foods and Supplements That Are of Likely Benefit to Court and Indoor Team Sport Players

	Product	Comment
Use in achieving documented nutrition goals	Sport drinks	• Used to refuel and rehydrate during prolonged training sessions and games and to rehydrate after the session. Contain some electrolytes to help replace sweat losses and increase voluntary intake of fluid. May be useful, even when carbohydrate replacement is not beneficial, for encouraging better hydration. May be more important for use in tournament situation where there is inadequate opportunity for refueling between games.
	Sport gels	• Convenient and compact carbohydrate source that can be used for additional refueling during matches and prolonged training sessions. Particularly useful as a compact carbohydrate supply when water is used for hydration goals.
	Sport bars	• Convenient, portable, and easy-to-consume source of carbohydrate, protein, and micronutrients for prematch meal or postexercise recovery. • Low-bulk and portable form of energy and nutrients that can contribute to high energy needs, especially to support resistance training program or growth. • Convenient and compact source of energy and nutrients for road trips and other travel.
	Liquid meal supplements	• Convenient, portable, and easy-to-consume source of carbohydrate, protein, and micronutrients for postexercise recovery and "preexercise recovery" strategies. • Low bulk and practical form of energy and nutrients that can contribute to high energy needs, especially to support resistance training program or growth. • Well-tolerated preevent meal that can be consumed to provide a source of carbohydrate quite close to the start of a match or workout; seem to be better tolerated than solid food by some athletes with high risk of gastrointestinal problems. • Convenient and compact source of energy and nutrients for road trips and other travel.
	Multivitamin and mineral supplement	• Supplemental source of micronutrients for traveling when food supply is not reliable. • Supplemental source of micronutrients during prolonged periods of energy restriction (female athletes)
Strong potential for ergogenic benefit	Creatine	• Creatine phosphate serves a number of important roles in exercise metabolism; the most well-known role is the rapid regeneration of adenosine triphosphate by the phosphagen power system. Studies show that creatine loading enhances the performance of exercise involving repeated high-intensity work bouts with short recovery intervals (<2 min recovery). Chronic creatine supplementation may be valuable in enhancing the response of court and indoor team sport players to various training protocols—resistance training undertaken to enhance muscle mass and strength, interval training undertaken to enhance anaerobic fitness, and match-specific play. Studies in field-based team sports have shown that acute supplementation enhances the performance of match-simulation protocols, or movement patterns within actual field play, and may therefore be seen as a competition aid. More studies of this type are needed across a wider range of court and indoor team sports. Typical protocols for creatine use: loading dose 20-30 g in multiple doses (e.g., 4 × 5 g) for 5 days followed by maintenance dose of 2-5 g/day. Uptake appears to be enhanced by consuming creatine with carbohydrate-rich meal or snack. Acute weight gain of about 1 kg occurs with creatine loading, presumably attributable to fluid retention.
	Caffeine	• May enhance performance of prolonged exercise (e.g., matches) by reducing perception of fatigue, but studies are yet to be undertaken in court-based and indoor team sports to show either enhancement of movement patterns or attenuation of decline in skills and concentration over match. Caffeine may be consumed in cola and energy drinks or as an ingredient in some sport products (e.g., some gels). There is conflicting evidence over the efficacy of coffee as a source of caffeine, because it contains other chemicals that might impair performance.

own right as well as exacerbate poor hydration status. Many studies show that fluid replacement during continuous submaximal exercise enhances endurance or performance. Replacement of carbohydrate during such exercise is also beneficial, with some evidence that the effects are independent and additive to those achieved by fluid intake (Below et al. 1995). Mechanisms for the benefits of carbohydrate intake during prolonged continuous exercise include prevention or reversal of hypoglycemia and, at least in cycling, the provision of an alternative fuel source to sustain high rates of carbohydrate oxidation once muscle glycogen stores become depleted (Coyle et al. 1986). There is some controversy regarding the effect of carbohydrate intake on constant pace running, with some (Tsintzas, Williams, et al. 1993) but not all (Arkinstall et al. 2001) studies reporting glycogen sparing, perhaps confined to certain muscle fibers (Tsintzas, Williams, Boobis, et al. 1996). Carbohydrate intake may also provide some benefits by reducing central fatigue or enhancing the function of brain and central nervous system to improve pacing strategies.

Because the physiological and biochemical characteristics of prolonged intermittent high-intensity exercise differ from those of continuous exercise, we need to examine the effects of nutritional strategies on the capacity to perform such activities. Unfortunately, few studies of such protocols are available, particularly with direct relevance to the movement patterns of team and racket sports. The characteristics and results of the relevant literature are summarized in table 9.e and include studies that use athletes or protocols suited to the sports of soccer (McGregor et al. 1999), cricket (Devlin et al. 2001), tennis (Magal et al. 2003), and basketball (Dougherty et al. 2006; Hoffman et al. 1995). Despite the scarcity of studies, it seems reasonable to conclude that hypohydration impairs the capacity for intermittent high-intensity exercise. Two studies undertaken in a mild environment (13-16°C) found clear evidence of a reduction in speed or capacity for sprinting after 60 to 75 min of an intermittent running protocol when participants incurred fluid deficits of 2% to 3% of BM (Devlin et al. 2001; McGregor et al. 1999). This reduction in sprint capacity was attenuated or absent in the trial in which fluid was provided to better match sweat losses. Data from the other three studies indicated performance impairments with hypohydration, in both a hot (Magal et al. 2003) and a moderate (Dougherty et al. 2006; Hoffman et al. 1995) environment, although issues regarding the study design or low statistical power make such an interpretation less clear. It is difficult to provide a placebo condition in hypohydration studies, although researchers who investigated shuttle running by cricket players tried to address this by having participants suck on artificially flavored ice cubes during the "no-fluid" trial with the explanation that these were a new performance-enhancing sport product (Devlin et al. 2001).

The present literature cannot provide a complete explanation for the mechanisms underpinning the performance impairment with hypohydration. McGregor and coworkers noted a higher mean heart rate during intermittent exercise in a no-fluid trial compared with a trial in which fluid was consumed (McGregor et al. 1999). They also noted higher blood cortisol concentrations and an increased perception of effort over the last 15 min block of the intermittent shuttle test, corresponding with the performance decrement. Although body temperatures were not measured in this study, it was suggested that an increased thermal load might occur in the no-fluid trial. An earlier achievement of a critical core temperature has been hypothesized to explain reduced endurance or premature fatigue during prolonged submaximal exercise in the heat. In these conditions, fluid replacement has been shown to better maintain skin blood flow and attenuate the increase in core temperature, possibly by preventing an increase in serum osmolality (Montain and Coyle 1992). The increase in core temperature also seems to play an important role in explaining the reduction in exercise capacity when intermittent running is undertaken in the heat (Maxwell et al. 1996; Morris and Maxwell 1998). Maxwell and coworkers (1996) investigated high-speed treadmill sprinting followed by intermittent sprinting and found that the number of sprints achieved in the heat (~30°C) was significantly less than when the protocol was undertaken in a cooler environment (~20°C). Morris and Maxwell (1998) used a protocol involving 75 min of the Loughborough Intermittent Shuttle Test followed by intermittent sprints to exhaustion and showed that participants fatigued sooner in the heat (~30°C; mean distance 8,842 m) than in a cooler environment (~20°C; mean distance 11,280). This difference occurred despite a lack of differences in the level of hypohydration, ratings of perceived exertion, and blood metabolites. Differences in sprint capacity were attributed to differences in rectal temperatures (39.4 vs. 38.0°C). Another advantage of fluid replacement in the heat, at least during submaximal exercise, is that it attenuates the increase in muscle glycogen utilization that would otherwise occur (Hargreaves et al. 1996). This probably results from an attenuation of the effect of heat or dehydration on both circulating epinephrine concentrations and muscle temperature.

The effect of carbohydrate intake during prolonged intermittent exercise has been examined in a number of studies, which are summarized in the appendix table 9.e. The studies include investigations in both hot (Criswell et al. 1991; Morris et al. 2003) and moderate environments (Dougherty et al. 2006; Ferrauti et al. 1997; Kipp et al. 2003; Kirkendall et al. 1988; Muckle 1973; Nicholas et al. 1995; Vergauwen et al. 1998; Welsh et al. 2002) and with specific relevance to the sports of soccer (Kipp et al.

Research Priorities

It is important that specific research is undertaken on the nutrition issues involved in team sports. The range of issues described in Chapter 8 is also pertinent to court sports.

2003; Kirkendall et al. 1988; Muckle 1973), tennis (Burke and Ekblom 1982; Ferrauti et al. 1997; Mitchell et al. 1992; Vergauwen et al. 1998), ice hockey (Simard et al. 1988), basketball (Dougherty et al. 2006; Winnick et al. 2005), and American football (Criswell et al. 1991). The general consensus from these studies is that carbohydrate intake enhances the ability to undertake prolonged intermittent high-intensity exercise (see table 9.e). However, this effect may not always be seen under hot environmental conditions (Criswell et al. 1991; Morris et al. 2003), presumably because in such situations the major limiting factors relate to thermoregulation rather than fuel status. In fact, data from some studies have suggested that the consumption of a carbohydrate–electrolyte drink caused a more rapid increase in rectal temperature compared with the intake of a flavored water placebo, perhaps because of a decrease in rates of gastric emptying and overall fluid delivery (Morris et al. 2003). Performance improvements in sport-simulated protocols have been seen in terms of enhanced endurance in a high-intensity run to fatigue at the end of the intermittent exercise protocol (Nicholas et al. 1995; Welsh et al. 2002) or better sprint times or speed in tests undertaken at the end of the protocol (Ferrauti et al. 1997; Kipp et al. 2003; Vergauwen et al. 1998). Under field conditions, carbohydrate intake has been associated with greater distances undertaken at high speed or more contact with the play of the game in the second half of a match (Kirkendall et al. 1988; Muckle 1973; Simard et al. 1988).

Mechanisms to explain the beneficial effects of carbohydrate intake on exercise capacity or performance of prolonged intermittent activities include the maintenance of higher blood glucose concentrations throughout the exercise or late in exercise (Ferrauti et al. 1997; Nicholas et al. 1995; Welsh et al. 2002). There is also evidence of glycogen sparing over the exercise protocol compared with the placebo condition (Leatt and Jacobs 1989; Nicholas et al. 1999), with this effect resulting either from a reduced utilization of muscle glycogen during the exercise or from resynthesis of glycogen during the activity. In a cycling protocol involving variable intensity of exercise of longer intervals (8 min at 45% $\dot{V}O_2$max interchanged with 8 min at 75% $\dot{V}O_2$max), a lower decline in muscle glycogen concentration with carbohydrate intake was hypothesized to be attributable to a slower rate of muscle glycogen utilization because this effect was seen only in the type I muscle fibers (Yaspelkis et al. 1993). Although glycogen synthesis is known to occur during low-intensity exercise in the presence of adequate substrate, it is generally limited to the nonactive or type II fibers (Kuipers et al. 1987). This issue needs further investigation in intermittent exercise protocols simulating team sports. Overall, despite the lack of a large body of literature, there is reasonable evidence to support the intake of fluid and carbohydrate during prolonged intermittent high-intensity sports such as team and racket sports. Such strategies appear to benefit the movement patterns involved in competitive play in such sports. Further research is needed to elucidate the mechanisms underpin-

ning these benefits, and sport-specific investigations provide opportunities to define the exact range of sports and playing conditions under which these benefits are most clearly seen. Whether the benefits of carbohydrate intake during prolonged intermittent exercise are also preserved during hot conditions needs further investigation.

RESEARCH TOPIC

Effect of Carbohydrate Replacement and Hydration Strategies on Skill and Decision Making

Athletes in team and racket sports undertake a complex array of skills and cognitive tasks involving fine motor control, concentration, and decision making. There is some evidence of mental and central nervous system fatigue toward the end of the match in at least some of these sports, as shown by a reduction in skills and concentration and an increase in errors. The final outcome of a match is decided by a complex interplay between the movement patterns of players, which allow them to reach strategic positions in relation to the ball or other players, and the execution of specific skills and cognitive tasks. In prolonged submaximal exercise, there has been an increasing interest in the role of fatigue or functioning of the brain and central nervous system on performance and on the effects of carbohydrate and fluid replacement strategies on issues such as perception of effort and pacing strategies. Because team and racket sports offer an even greater role for cognitive performance in the outcome of a sports event, it is important for such effects to be investigated in this environment. Table 9.f summarizes the available literature in which cognitive performance has been monitored under conditions of prolonged intermittent high-intensity exercise, with and without fluid replacement and with or without carbohydrate intake.

Under resting conditions in the heat, hypohydration has been shown to impair the performance of various measures of cognitive performance. A series of psychomotor tests in heat-acclimatized participants who were hypohydrated by 1%, 2%, 3%, and 4% of BM revealed that body fluid deficits of >2% were associated with significant and progressive reductions in the performance compared with a well-hydrated state (Gopinathan et al. 1988). Compared with trials involving fluid replacement, hypohydration during intermittent high-intensity exercise has been shown to increase blood cortisol concentrations and perception of effort, indicating a greater degree of mental as well as physical stress faced by the participants. The challenge of undertaking studies of nutritional strategies and cognitive performance in sport is in finding a test protocol that is both reliable and valid for the specific code. This issue is discussed in more detail in chapter 10 (research topic 1). In the literature regarding fluid and skill or cognitive performance, researchers have taken a variety of approaches, including the comparison of baseline and postexercise performance of well-known psychomotor tests or drills and skills that are important in a sport. The total number of studies that have investigated this issue is small but includes investigations of specific relevance to soccer (McGregor et al. 1999), basketball (Dougherty et al. 2006; Hoffman et al. 1995), cricket (Devlin et al. 2001), and tennis (Magal et al. 2003), with studies undertaken in hot (Magal et al. 2003) or moderate (Devlin et al. 2001; Dougherty et al. 2006; Hoffman et al. 1995; McGregor et al. 1999) conditions. These studies generally provide support for the benefits of hydrating during team and racket sports to maintain skill and cognitive performance. Some studies have reported a significantly better performance in the fluid versus no-fluid condition (Devlin et al. 2001; McGregor et al. 1999); others found no clear-cut performance differences but acknowledged problems with study methodology, including an underpowering in statistics (Hoffman et al. 1995; Magal et al. 2003).

The effects of carbohydrate replacement during intermittent exercise protocols on skills and cognitive performance have been investigated in a number of studies with specific relevance to soccer (Kipp et al. 2003; Muckle 1973; Ostojic and Mazic 2002; Welsh et al. 2002; Zeederberg et al. 1996), tennis (Ferrauti et al. 1997; Vergauwen et al. 1998), basketball (Dougherty et al. 2006; Welsh et al. 2002), and squash (Bottoms et al. 2006; Wallis and Galloway 2003). Conditions have included both hot (Ferrauti et al. 1997) and moderate (Burke and Ekblom 1982; Dougherty et al. 2006; Ostojic and Mazic 2002; Zeederberg et al. 1996) temperatures. Again, skill and cognitive performance have been measured in a number of ways: using well-known psychomotor tests (Welsh et al. 2002), studying drills and skills that are important in a sport (Bottoms et al. 2006; Ferrauti et al. 1997; Ostojic and Mazic 2002; Wallis and Galloway 2003; Welsh et al. 2002), monitoring skills throughout a sport-specific simulation test (Dougherty et al. 2006;Vergauwen et al. 1998), and monitoring skills of players during actual games (Muckle 1973; Zeederberg et al. 1996). The consensus is that carbohydrate intake during prolonged intermittent exercise helps the player to maintain skill and cognitive performance for the duration of the protocol (see table 9.f). Such effects seem most apparent when the protocol is prolonged and the no-carbohydrate trial leads to a reduction ;. in blood glucose concentrations during the latter phases of exercise and an increase in the perceived rates of exertion. There are insufficient studies to determine whether these effects are greater under hot conditions, although it is known that central nervous system fatigue is aggravated by hyperthermia (Nybo and Nielsen 2001). Mechanisms underpinning reduced function of the central nervous system include alterations to neurotransmitters, inadequate supply of blood glucose for uptake into the brain, and depletion of brain glycogen stores. Further research is needed to explore these mechanisms and to identify the specific range of team and racket sports in which carbohydrate supplementation is of benefit.

PRACTICAL ISSUE

Strategies for Staying Hydrated in Team, Court, and Racket Sports

A range of factors govern fluid intake during exercise, including access to fluid, opportunities to drink, cultural beliefs about the importance of hydration, palatability of the fluid, gastrointestinal comfort, and external cues. Most of the guidelines for fluid intake during exercise have focused on prolonged continuous events, but the needs and opportunities for fluid replacement during team and racket sports differ from those in endurance sports. These differences include, possibly, the greater rewards of fluid replacement strategies—because the effect of dehydration on mental skills and concentration provides an additional factor in determining performance outcomes. Exercise characteristics and workloads in team and racket sports vary between players, positions, and playing styles. Furthermore, each match is a unique game. As a result, it is difficult to predict the fluid needs of a team athlete, and each athlete needs to be treated individually.

The opportunity to ingest fluids during team and racket sports is governed by different factors than are found in prolonged continuous activities. Fluids may be consumed while the athlete is sedentary—for example, during formal breaks in activity (quarter-time or halftime breaks, change of ends in tennis), during player substitutions, and during informal stoppages of play (e.g., after a rule infringement or break for injury). These opportunities vary between sports according to the style of play and the rules of the game. An increased frequency of formal breaks and a shorter playing time between breaks increase the potential to maintain fluid balance during team competition, both by reducing the duration of sustained activity (i.e., reducing sweat rate) and increasing opportunities to drink. Games permitting unlimited player substitutions (e.g., hockey, basketball, Australian football) or rotations (e.g., American football) increase the potential to match fluid loss and consumption. Similarly, games that allow liberal fluid intake during official playing time by allowing trainers to provide drink bottles to players on the field when they are not involved in play (e.g., Australian football, rugby codes) also increase the opportunity for hydration. In contrast, rules that place *any* restriction on fluid replacement during playing time or the carriage of fluid onto the field of play (e.g., soccer) increase the likelihood of a fluid mismatch. The various rules and opportunities for fluid intake in various team and racket sports are summarized in table 9.2.

The opportunity to drink is limited by an available fluid supply, and if optimal fluid intake is to be achieved, access to fluids should be maximized. Individual drink bottles are good for hygiene practices and ensure an available supply of fluid while also providing constant feedback to a player regarding the volume she has consumed. Where team officials are not permitted to take drinks to players

Table 9.2 Opportunities to Drink Fluids During Various Team Games and Racket Sports

Sport	Game characteristics	Opportunities to drink	Special comments
American football	• 4 × 12 min or 4 × 15 min + substantial "time on"[a] • Unlimited substitutions[b] • Time-outs	• Breaks after each quarter • Time-outs • Substitutions • Pauses in play	Trainers may run onto field with drink bottles during breaks or pauses in play.
Australian rules football	• 4 × 20 min + substantial "time on" • Unlimited substitutions	• Breaks after each quarter • Substitutions • Pauses in play	Trainers may run onto field with drink bottles during breaks or pauses in play.
Basketball	• 4 × 12 or 2 × 20 min + substantial "time on" • Unlimited substitutions • Time-outs	• Breaks after each quarter or half • Substitutions • Time-outs	Fluids must be consumed on the court sidelines.
Badminton	• Best of 3 sets • Set won by first to reach 15 points (11 points women), with only the server scoring a point	• Breaks after sets	
Cricket	• Test matches: 3 × 2 hr sessions over 5 days • Limited over matches: 2 × 50 over innings in single day • Fielding team and two players from batting team on field on each occasion	• Breaks between sessions • Some competitions: one official drink break within each session of a test match (after 60 min) and two drink breaks during each session of a limited over match (after 70 min) • Other competitions: Drinks may be taken during pauses in play from drink bottles kept on the field	Traditional rules (Marylebone Cricket Club 1992) provide one official drink break per hour of play. Updated rules of International Cricket Council give discretion to the umpire under conditions of extreme heat to take extra drink breaks or to allow an individual player to take a drink from a bottle kept on the field provided that no playing time is wasted (International Cricket Council 2004).
Field hockey	• 2 × 35 min • Unlimited substitutions	• Break between halves • Substitutions • Pauses in play	Drinks must be consumed at sidelines. Drinks cannot be carried or thrown onto the field. Players must not leave the field unless substituted.
Ice hockey	• 3 × 20 min + substantial "time on" • Unlimited substitutions • Time-outs	• Breaks between periods • Substitutions • Time-outs	Players must drink at bench.
Lacrosse	• 4 × 15 min • Time-outs • Unlimited substitutions	• Breaks after each quarter • Time-outs • Substitutions	

234

Sport			
Netball	• 4 × 15 min or 2 × 20 min • Time-outs • Limited substitutions	• Breaks after each quarter or half • Time-outs • Substitutions	Fluids must be consumed on court sidelines.
Rugby league	• 2 × 40 min plus small amount "time on" • Unlimited substitutions	• Break after each half • Substitutions • Pauses in play	Trainers may run onto field with drink bottles during pauses in play.
Rugby union	• 2 × 40 min plus small amount "time on" • Limited substitutions—players can be replaced but cannot return to play	• Break after each half • Pauses in play	Trainers may run onto field with drink bottles during pauses in play.
Soccer	• 2 × 45 min plus small amount "time on" • Limited substitutions—players can be replaced, but cannot return to play	• Break after each half • Pauses in play (drink must be taken at sideline)	Official rules amended in 1994 to allow drinks during play stoppages. "Players are entitled to take liquid refreshments during a stoppage in the match but only on the touch line. It is not permitted to throw plastic water bags or any other water containers onto the field" (Federation International de Football Association 2003, p. 68).
Squash	• Best of five games • Game won by first to reach 9 points, with only the server scoring a point	• Breaks between games (90 s interval)	
Tennis	• Singles or pairs • Best of 3 or 5 sets depending on gender and tournament • Each set first to 6 games • Each game first to 4 points	• Short break at change of ends after each 2 games • Break between sets	Players keep their own drink supplies (and extra equipment) at their courtside chair and return to these during breaks.
Volleyball	• First to 3 sets • Limited substitutions • Time-outs	• Time-outs • Substitutions • Breaks between sets	Official rules prohibit fluid on court—drinks must be taken on sideline.
Water polo	• 4 × 7 min + substantial "time on" • Unlimited substitutions • Time-outs	• Breaks after each quarter • Substitutions • Time-outs	

aTime on refers to additional time played in each period to compensate for "stopping of clock" when ball is considered out of play; it adds considerably to the duration of the total session time; bSubstitutions refer to players who are able to return to the game after substitution. "Unlimited" means that players may be rotated any number of times during the game; "limited" means that the rules restrict substitutions to a finite number per game or that a player cannot return to the field after being substituted.

on the court or field, drinks should be kept close to the site of play. Access to drink supplies may be a limiting factor where fluids can only be consumed on the sidelines of large fields or pitches (e.g., soccer and hockey). Restrictions may also be encountered in indoor arenas; in addition to official rules dictating that fluid must be consumed on the court sidelines, some stadiums prohibit the carrying of fluids near any playing surfaces because of concerns that spillage may create slippery conditions and increase the risk of accidents and injury.

The impact of gastrointestinal (GI) discomfort following fluid intake in team sports has not been systematically studied. GI problems may also be increased because of the high-intensity workloads associated with team sports as well as the opportunity for high rates of fluid intake: Both factors have been implicated in the development of GI disturbances during exercise (Brouns et al. 1987; Robinson et al. 1995). There is some evidence of reduced rates of gastric emptying of fluids during intermittent team games (Leiper, Broad, et al. 2001; Leiper, Prentice, et al. 2001). On the other hand, the large body sizes of many team sport athletes will mean that greater absolute losses of fluid and tolerance of fluid intake are likely, compared with smaller endurance athletes (Broad et al. 1996). This makes it even more important to avoid generic recommendations across sports concerning optimal fluid intakes.

The coach appears to play an important role in influencing hydration practices during training, by structuring the session and providing opportunities and encouragement to drink (Minehan et al. 2002). Other external cues such as environmental temperature (Broad et al. 1996) or players' cultural beliefs are also important determinants of fluid intake but are often dissociated from real fluid needs.

Although fluid balance in team sports has not been extensively studied, there is a potential for significant hypohydration to occur, especially when games or training sessions are undertaken in hot environments. This hypohydration may be superimposed on a pre-existing fluid deficit, for several studies have found that team and racket sport players may already be dehydrated when they arrive at an exercise session (Bergeron, Waller, and Marinik 2006; Burke 2006b, 2006c; Godek, Godek, et al. 2005; Maughan et al. 2004). Therefore, some effort needs to be made to hydrate well from day to day, and to fully rehydrate after workouts or matches. During sessions, at least in moderate conditions, it appears that most sports provide the opportunity for adequate fluid intake to keep fluid deficits below 1% to 1.5% of body mass; in extremely hot conditions, a goal of maintaining fluid deficits below 2% may be more practical. Strategies are required to educate team sport players about the importance of hydration and about ways to use or create opportunities within their sport to optimize their fluid intake. Specific guidelines are impractical because they do not take into account the differences between sports with respect to opportunities for ingesting fluids; nor do they account for the considerable inter- and intra-individual differences in fluid needs in players of team sports, even among those involved in the same sport. The following general guidelines are suggested and should be adapted to each individual and each sporting situation.

- In hot environments (i.e., >25°C, 60% humidity), an excessive heat load can accumulate during training or competition. Issues such as the time of day of play, the length of play without a formal break, conditions in indoor venues, and the suitability of playing uniforms, strapping, and protective gear should be examined. It may be possible to modify some of these factors to reduce heat overload. Appropriate acclimatization should be undertaken in preparation for competition in a hot environment.

- Players can become aware of their typical sweat losses by weighing themselves before and after training or games in different environmental conditions. This should be undertaken at regular intervals to develop and evaluate the success of individual fluid intake strategies. In extreme weather conditions or during tournament competitions, it may be useful to monitor body mass changes as a team activity. In this way individuals most at risk of hypohydration can be identified (those with highest sweat losses or reluctant drinkers), and a team fluid intake plan can be implemented.

- The player should begin each match or game well hydrated, particularly when competition is to be undertaken in hot conditions. This may involve strategies to restore fluid losses from previous competition or training sessions and to hydrate in the 1 to 4 hr before competition and between warm-up and the game.

- Opportunities to consume fluids during each team sport should be assessed and optimized, to best match but not exceed the rate of fluid loss. Opportunities include

  - *official break periods between quarters and halves of matches,*

  - *stoppages in play (e.g., breaks attributable to injury or rule infringement, and*

  - *times when players are substituted or rotated off the field of play.*

Individual opportunity and gastric tolerance may dictate how much fluid can be consumed at each drink break; some players may be able to drink regularly throughout a match whereas others may only manage small amounts during informal breaks, topped up with another fluid bolus at the halftime break. Ideally a fluid intake plan should be able to replace about 80% of sweat losses; this may not be practical or possible when sweat rates are in excess of 1 to 1.5 L/hr. It seems that team sport players can learn to tolerate an hourly fluid intake of up to 10 ml/kg (600-1,000 ml/hr).

- The governing bodies or officials of some sports may need to assess and revise current rules limiting fluid intake to formal breaks that are greater than 30 min apart. In situations of extreme heat, it may be possible to instigate new rules that reduce the duration of uninterrupted playing time (e.g., introduce quarters rather than halves in a game) or insert a formal drink break during the playing time. Alternatively, players may find strategies that can work within existing regulations to arrange access to fluids within playing time. For example, to cope with the present rules of soccer, which prevent drink bottles being carried onto the pitch, bottles should be placed around the periphery of the ground, or behind the goals, to allow players to leave the field quickly and take a drink during informal stoppages in the game.

- Access to fluid during games should be organized rather than ad hoc. Issues and strategies include the following:

  - *Ensuring suitable clean fluids when traveling to countries with an unsafe water supply.*

  - *Providing an adequate supply of fluid at the site of the match to allow players to meet their fluid needs before, during, and after the match. Fluids, even water, may not be readily available when games are played in remote outdoor locations, and teams are advised to purchase large drink containers that can provide the 30 to 60 L of fluid that may be needed by a team playing in hot conditions.*

  - *Providing individual drink bottles to players so that they have separate and continuous access to fluid and continuous feedback about the volume of fluid they have consumed.*

  - *Organizing trainers to carry drinks to players on the field as allowed by the games rules and flow of play, so that fluid is available when there is even the briefest opportunity to consume it.*

  - *Providing encouragement and reminders to players to drink during games, particularly during breaks when game strategies are evaluated and discussed.*

- The palatability of fluids is important in determining voluntary intake. Cool, pleasant-tasting drinks should be made available; there is evidence that sport drinks and other sweetened beverages may be consumed in larger amounts than plain water.

- Sport drinks and other carbohydrate-containing drinks offer the additional advantage of supplying fuel in situations where muscle and liver glycogen stores have become depleted during the match. Supplying additional fuel may improve performance in terms of both work output and maintenance of skill and motor performance. Carbohydrate intake during matches may be of most benefit in team and racket sports of longer than 60 to 90 min duration (e.g., soccer, Australian football, tennis), especially for running players with the largest workloads. Carbohydrate intake may become more critical during tournament play when a busy match schedule does not provide adequate opportunity for full recovery of body carbohydrate stores between matches.

- Postmatch rehydration is an important part of recovery and requires an aggressive strategy when moderate to severe levels of hypohydration have been incurred or when another match or training session is scheduled within 24 hr (e.g., in a tournament). Drinks containing carbohydrate and electrolytes should be chosen to promote recovery of fuel stores and to enhance the retention of ingested fluid. Excessive intake of alcohol after competition is frequently observed in team sports and should be discouraged.

- All competition strategies should be well practiced in the training situation. This will allow players to develop their individual fluid intake plan and learn to tolerate fluid intake during exercise. Training performances may also benefit from better hydration (or supplementary carbohydrate intake).

PRACTICAL ISSUE

The Athlete Communal Dining Facility—Perspectives for the Athlete and the Caterer

When athletes live in communal facilities such as a college, sports institute, or training camp, they may rely on the catering facilities to supply the majority of their food intake over long periods. The athlete villages organized for major sporting competitions can also provide the majority of dietary intake of athletes during these key times, via special athlete dining halls. Several studies have noted that residential dining facilities influence dietary intake of athletic groups both to enhance (Hickson, Johnson, et al. 1987) or to decrease (Ellsworth et al. 1985) the athletes' ability to meet their nutrition goals compared with their usual home practices. This highlights the responsibility of such catering services to organize a suitable menu and optimize food availability during the times that it is important for the athlete to eat. However, the athlete must also recognize the special challenges of eating in such an environment.

Athlete's Perspective

Imagine a situation where there is free food—maybe even served 24 hr a day—with numerous choices on offer, plenty of company to enjoy it with, and no sight of Mum to make sure that vegetables are eaten. This is the scenario provided by the dining halls of the athlete villages organized for many of the world's major sporting competitions. Many of the same characteristics are found in the communal dining facilities organized at residential sports institutes or the special training tables provided to collegiate athletes within the campus catering. As perfect as this situation sounds, it presents a number of challenges for the athlete. Some of the same challenges are faced when eating in "all you can eat" restaurants and even the buffet-style catering that is recommended because of the flexibility it offers for athletic groups (see chapter 10). For young and inexperienced athletes, the temptations and challenges often interfere with achieving nutritional goals. Athletes need to understand the special challenges of communal eating and to adopt special eating strategies.

Challenges for the Athlete (Burke, Bell, et al. 2004)

• Great quantities of food. Athletes can serve themselves as much as they want from an almost inexhaustible supply. It is easy to eat more than usual and more than is needed.

• Many choices of food all at once, which also leads to overconsumption.

• Different and unusual foods. Some people find it difficult to adjust to food that is different than the way they eat at home or to food that has been batch-cooked rather than individually prepared.

• Lack of supervision. Many young athletes are unused to the responsibility for their food intake.

• Distraction. Surrounded by a large group of people with different eating habits, many athletes find it difficult to concentrate on their own nutritional goals. And, given the competitive nature of athletes in general, it isn't surprising that official and unofficial eating competitions can take place.

• Anxiety about food availability. Eating with a large number of people or needing to line up for food can make the athlete anxious about food availability. It is tempting to grab extra food or favorite foods when they are available, in the belief that this may be the last opportunity to obtain such items.

• Eating for entertainment. Food provides an emotional and social role for athletes and, perhaps, some stress release during the nail-biting weeks of competition. If the dining room becomes a hangout, extra food can be consumed in the name of unwinding and relaxing together.

• Food monotony. Although there may be plenty of variety within and between meals, after a while the experience of eating in the dining hall becomes monotonous.

Tips for Eating Well

• The athlete should clearly know her nutritional goals and how to choose food to achieve these. If athletes are unsure of what to choose or are used to having other people organize their meals, it is valuable to consult a sports dietitian for some specific advice.

• Buffet-style eating tends to promote "a bit of this, a bit of that" approach to meals. The athlete should consider the total menu available—making use of menu boards or surveying the food choices—and then plan the meal while waiting in line.

• Piling a bit of everything on the plate is haphazard and leads to a meal that is unbalanced and usually more than needed—quickly leading to unwanted weight gain. It also promotes boredom with the catering, because there is no sense of difference between meals. Athletes can increase the longevity of their interest in the menu by having a different theme or food choice each night. This is especially important when the athlete will be eating from this same

menu for long periods (e.g., more than 2 weeks), or where the menu cycle is short (less than 7 days).

• The athlete should learn to take a relaxed attitude to eating among a large group—feeling confident that there is plenty of food for everyone and menu items will often be repeated.

• The athlete should use available information, such as nutrition cards or education sheets, to learn more about the food that is being served. When unsure about food items, the athlete should ask the dining hall supervisor or chef. In some situations, a dietitian or nutritionist may also be at hand to answer questions.

• Athletes should not concern themselves with the amount and type of food that other athletes are consuming. Instead they should recognize that the nutritional needs of other athletes, even from the same sport, may vary quite markedly from their own. Each athlete needs to have confidence in his or her personal nutrition plan.

• Athletes should remove themselves from the food environment once they have finished eating, to avoid exposure to the potential for boredom eating.

Caterer's Perspective

It is hard to think of a greater challenge in catering than to organize the dining hall at a major sporting event such as the Olympic Games. In this specific event, the dining hall is open 24 hr a day, serving meals to the 15,000 athletes and coaches who reside in the Olympic village over 4 weeks. In some cases, this facility operates from temporary accommodation that has been assembled and dismantled within a matter of days. The menu must cater for

• cultural, religious, and social preferences of athletes and coaches from more than 190 different countries;

• wide variation in the nutritional needs of a variety of sports;

• variation in nutritional needs of athletes as they transition between training, tapering, competing, and then celebrating;

• opportunities to showcase the local cuisine of the host city or country; and

• special needs for athlete with food allergies and intolerances or other special nutritional requirements.

Of course, important issues related to hygiene and food presentation must also be taken into account. Although the dining halls and training tables that operate within sports institutes or college dining facilities deal with a smaller-scale version of these issues, they are often faced with an additional overlay of

• budgetary constraints,

• timetabling constraints (providing food service around the athletes' training and competition schedules within the minimum number of service hours), and

- conflict with mainstream nutritional needs if non-athletes share the food service facility.

Tips for Catering for Athletes
Strategies that have proved useful in running the Australian Institute of Sport (AIS) dining hall (Cummings et al. 2006) and in developing catering plans for AIS athletes when they travel to other residences are summarized next:

- A buffet-style or self-service food service is most suitable for feeding athletes because it offers the advantages of

  ○ *fast service for athletes who are hungry and challenged for time,*

  ○ *maximum flexibility in allowing athletes to choose the quantity and type of food they need from the menu selection, and*

  ○ *cost-savings because of bulk cooking, reduced staffing requirements, and low food wastage.*

- The number and variety of menu items need to be balanced within a meal and across the menu cycle. Generally, the larger the group size, the greater the number of selections that may be needed or justified within the meal. Too many choices within the menu for a single meal can lead to overeating—which is expensive for the caterer and creates nutritional problems for the athlete. However, too little choice can make it difficult for the individual athlete to compile a meal to suit his or her specific needs and food preferences. With experience, the caterer will learn the right balance for their specific athletic group.

- When catering for a large number of athletes, caterers usually can provide for the special dietary needs of some individuals (e.g., vegetarian, lactose-free choices) within the basic menu for each meal. However, when menus are developed for a small group, it is usually easier for such special needs to be handled as an individual request.

- The specific menu items for each meal should be dictated by the nutritional needs and preferences of the athletic populations eating in the hall. In general, meals should offer a range of carbohydrate-rich, moderate-fat food items, including foods that are valuable sources of protein and micronutrients. Depending on the specific training and competition requirements of the athletic groups, there may be a need for additional focus on fuel needs, energy concerns (e.g., care with fat content of meals, and portion control), or the provision of at-risk nutrients (e.g., calcium, iron). Specialized groups will require specialized menus. Traditional cooking styles may need to be modified to achieve these goals; there are now a number of recipe books targeted at the special needs of athletes.

- The menu should also consider the cultural and social aspects of the food preferences of athletic groups. Depending on the age and background of these athletes, there may be a need to keep to plain and simple food items or to offer more adventurous and cosmopolitan choices.

- The day-to-day variety of meals should be dictated by the duration of the stay of the athletic group. Food monotony is a common complaint from athletes who are long-term residents of colleges and institutes. Strategies to deal with this challenge include having a long menu cycle (e.g., 2-4 weeks) in which favorite items can appear more frequently, including "wild card" or seasonal items within the basic menu, or off-setting the menu to 10 days or 20 days so that meals are not repeated according to days of the week. Short menu cycles (<7 days) should only be used when the duration of stay of the athlete is also brief.

- The buffet menu is generally based on foods that are presented in large quantity serving dishes, allowing the athlete to determine his or her own serving size. However, foods that are expensive or considered treats in terms of their nutritional profile should be provided as portion-controlled or individual servings, to encourage appropriate eating restraint.

- The dining hall menu should cater for the between-meal snacks and postexercise eating needs that play an important role in the diets of most athletes. If the dining facility is not open for extended hours, particularly during the day, the menu should include portable food items that can be taken away for such snacks.

- Athletes welcome information about the nutritional characteristics of the food items in the dining hall. It is useful to provide nutrition cards detailing the energy and nutrient profile of standard serving sizes of food items—these should be available at the point of service to assist the athlete in making food choices. Other education resources such as posters or printed table mats can provide general information about appropriate sports nutrition strategies. The motto of the AIS dining hall food service is "Feeding athletes for today, educating them for tomorrow."

- It is valuable to run education programs regarding the special nutritional needs of athletes for the chefs and staff of the dining hall. Many of these concerns are unknown within the general catering industry. Such education programs allow the catering staff to appreciate the needs of the athletes and to feel involved in helping the athletes to meet their nutritional goals. This appreciation is crucial if staff are to follow modified recipes, meet individual requests for special food needs, or devise creative ways to meet the food challenges faced by athletes.

chapter 10

Racket Sports

Racket sports are played around the world, at extremes ranging from a social hit to the lucrative but demanding professional tennis circuit. Competition is undertaken between two, and sometimes four, players on a variety of playing areas. The formats involve either hitting over a net onto a divided court (e.g., tennis, badminton, table tennis) or hitting against a wall in a shared court (e.g., squash and racquetball). Other variations between racket sports include the size and type of racket, the type of missile, the game duration, and the rules of competitive play. Games can be played indoors and outdoors; playing surfaces vary between and even within sports and include grass, clay, wood, concrete, and synthetic materials. Common elements to all racket sports are the intermittent nature of the activity, the involvement of both upper and lower body in play, and the importance of fast reaction, agility, speed, and often power.

The major racket sports at an international level are tennis, squash, badminton, racquetball, and table tennis. However, there are many less popular or more localized racket games, including variants played with the hand instead of a paddle or racket. This chapter focuses on tennis, because the potential for prolonged matches and the demands of the tournament circuit arguably create the greatest nutritional challenges seen in racket sports. In addition, the majority of the available literature concerns tennis; there are few observational or intervention studies involving other racket sports. Nevertheless, the characteristics of other racket sports will be compared with tennis when of interest, and any available studies of nutritional issues in racket sport players will be sought.

Competition

Essentially, competition in racket sports involves a series of rallies where the players hit the ball to each other until it is no longer in play. The physiological characteristics of each sport vary according to the typical duration of each rally, the ratio of rest to activity during the game, and the number of rallies or points that a player must win to ultimately decide the match. These factors vary markedly between racket sports but also within each sport according to the skill level of the players, the surface of the court, and the rules of the particular competition. The environment can also add an overlay to the physiological demands of a racket sport, with many matches being played in hot and humid conditions. Although some sports are usually played indoors (e.g., squash and badminton), air-conditioning of the playing arena is usually only guaranteed at the top level of competition. Many of the elite tennis tournaments are held in extremely hot weather with little acknowledgement of these conditions.

Tennis is played on a relatively large playing arena. Rallies are generally brief—range 2 to 10 s, mode 2 to 4 s—and involve short maximal sprints of 8 to 12 m per point (Op 't Eijnde et al. 2001; Reilly 1990). The length of rallies varies according to the surface and the players' style, with longer rallies being associated with slower surfaces and a baseline playing style. The rally-to-game ratio in tennis is generally low (20-30% of game time), with relative inactivity during standard rest periods between games when players change ends, as well as the time between points when the ball is being retrieved and the player then prepares to serve (for review, see Lees 2003; Reilly 1990b). Mean heart rates are elevated to around 70% to 85% of maximal rates for the duration of the match (Lees 2003). For further information, the reader is directed to the excellent review of the applied physiology of tennis performance by Kovacs (2006).

Badminton, which is also played on a court divided by a net, has a typical rally length similar to tennis interspersed with shorter recovery intervals. Despite a more challenging work-to-rest ratio, it is generally considered to place similar or marginally lower metabolic demands on players compared with tennis, because the smaller playing arena reduces the movement patterns of players. Tennis also requires greater force production and the involvement of a larger muscle mass in stroke play. Squash games involve longer rallies (4-8 s) than both tennis and badminton, with the duration of points being greater with more experienced players compared with novice or recreational players. The work-to-rest ratio in squash is greater than in other racket sports, often accounting for more than 50% of game time. The longer playing times and shorter respites increase the metabolic demands of this sport compared with other racket games. Although rallies in racquetball are of similar duration to those of squash, mean recovery times in this game tend to be longer than in squash. Overall, the rate of energy expenditure associated with tennis is considered to be slightly greater than badminton but less than squash and racquetball. The metabolic cost of doubles play (e.g., tennis, badminton) is less than for a singles match. For a more detailed description of the metabolic and game characteristics of various racket sports, see the reviews of Reilly (1990b) and Lees (2003).

The duration of matches in racket sports is open-ended and variable. The outcome is decided when one player wins a requisite number of points; depending on the relative skill levels of opponents, the code, and even the rules of the particular competition within a sport, a match can

vary from less than 10 min (e.g., squash) to more than 5 hr (e.g., tennis). In tennis, men play the best of three or five sets, whereas women play the best of three sets. At the time of writing this book, the record for the longest match in a high-level racket sport was 6 hr 33 min, set at the 2004 French Open between Arnaud Clement and Fabrice Santoro. However, typical match play in most racket sports is 30 to 90 min. The variability of nutritional requirements of competition from game to game creates a challenge for players in planning both their preevent and during-event eating strategies.

Racket sports involve a complex mixture of physical and mental skills. The characteristics of play include anticipation, fast reaction time, quick limb movements, and footwork. Players must demonstrate speed and agility not only in movement patterns but also in the mental processes of anticipating, tracking, decision making, and executing an accurate shot. In tennis particularly, high levels of muscular force are required to successfully execute the initial serve as well as strokes such as the forehands and backhands. As is the case for other intermittent high-intensity activities, fuel requirements during racket sports are provided by both aerobic and anaerobic pathways. Depending on

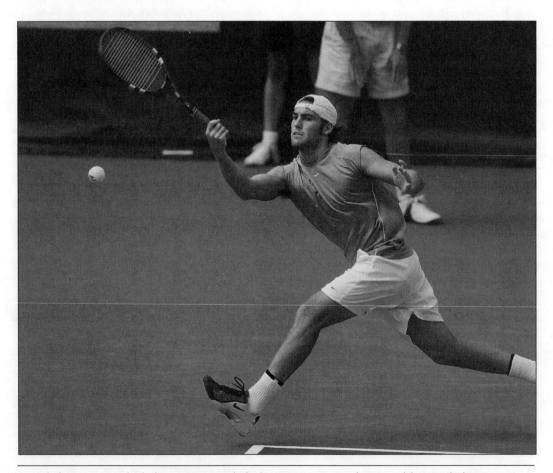

Actual playing time, which determines muscle fuel requirements, is a fraction of the match duration. However, elapsed playing time is also important because it determines the players' exposure to environmental challenges as well as the interval from the pregame meal.

the length of the rally, the phosphocreatine system and anaerobic glycolysis provide substantial contributions to fuel needs. There are conflicting data over the relative importance of each of these power systems to overall play and to the accumulation of lactate during matches. In sports or situations where rallies are consistently short (<5 s), blood lactate concentrations will probably remain low (<3-4 mmol/L). However, elevated lactate concentrations, up to or even exceeding 10 mmol/L, have been reported in tennis (Bergeron et al. 1991; Ferrauti et al. 2003) and squash (Sharp 1998), and can cause fatigue during play.

Other causes of fatigue and performance decrements during match play in racket sports include carbohydrate depletion and losses of fluid and electrolytes. Although there are no published studies of glycogen utilization in racket sports, it is likely that prolonged matches draw heavily on muscle glycogen stores. Blood glucose concentrations generally increase during a match as hepatic glucose output is stimulated to match or exceed muscle glucose uptake. However, studies of prolonged match play in tennis have shown a decline in blood glucose levels after several hours (Ferrauti et al. 1997; Mitchell et al. 1992). Carbohydrate intake during such play is associated with better maintenance of glycemia (Ferrauti et al. 1997) and enhanced performance (Ferrauti et al. 1997; Vergauwen et al. 1998). In one study, many elite tennis players reported at least occasional episodes of symptomatic hypoglycemia, occurring more frequently during tournaments than in training, and particularly during warm-ups to matches as a transient response to the combination of activity and preexercise carbohydrate intake (Ferrauti et al. 2003). Such rebound hypoglycemia has also been reported at the onset of squash matches, but its significance is uncertain (Noakes et al. 1982). Strategies to maintain glycemia during tennis play are discussed subsequently.

Millions of people around the world play racket sports on a social or recreational level, and at subelite level many play as individuals or within a team or club in competitions with a weekly fixture. The issues involved in weekly competition, including the periodization of the training program, were discussed in greater detail in chapter 8. In this chapter, the focus is on tournament play, because this is the major format by which elite or professional competition in racket sports is conducted. Typically, tournaments are organized with a knockout format: A pool of players are seeded to play each other, and winners progress to the next round until the last two players meet in the final. In major competitions such as the Grand Slam events in tennis (Wimbledon, Australian Open, French Open, and the U.S. Open), the competition draw involves 128 players (or 64 pairs in the doubles competition), with the title being won over seven matches spread over a fortnight of competition. At this level, players undertake matches every second day, and sometimes every day in the case of rain delays, to progress to the final. Other competitions are conducted with a smaller draw of players and a shorter time frame (7-10 days) and generally require daily match play. Of course, many players may enter more than one competition within a tournament (singles, doubles, and,

in the case of Grand Slams, mixed doubles), meaning that they often play more than once each day. A variation on the tournament is the team competition—for example, the century-old Davis cup, which is the International Tennis Federation (ITF) team championship for men. In this competition between nations, two teams of three to four players compete over 3 days with two singles matches on the first day, a doubles match on the following day, and the reverse singles matches on the final day.

The tournament protocol compounds the nutritional challenges of competition at a number of levels. First, the successful player must compete in a series of matches, and recovery between matches requires the replacement of fluid levels and carbohydrate stores that are often substantially depleted. Because the time between matches may be insufficient for complete recovery, the player may start the next match with suboptimal hydration and fuel status. The variable nature of matches and the competition timetable mean that it is difficult for players to anticipate their true needs for the next event or, sometimes, even the time of the start of play. As a result, depending on the player's decision to enter more than one event in the competition or even the outcome of matches in the single draw, players may have a widely different experience in the same tournament. For example, in the pathway to the 2003 Wimbledon men's singles title, eventual winner Roger Federer lost one set and accumulated 10 hr and 28 min of playing time, compared with Mark Philippoussis, who played 15 hr and 46 min and dropped six sets during his progress to the final.

Professional tennis involves an international circuit in which players travel from tournament to tournament, not only to compete in each competition but to accrue points toward an overall player ranking. The international nature of the sport is reflected not only by the diversity of locations of the top tournaments but also by the spread of nationalities of the world's best players. The advent of all-weather courts and indoor stadiums has extended the duration of the competitive season, even at subelite levels. However, at the professional level it has become an almost year-long tour, with the calendars of the ITF, ATP, and Women's Tennis Association (WTA) featuring events from the first week of January to the end of November. The major tournaments for the year are interspersed throughout the calendar. To aim to win the four Grand Slam tournaments or to enhance their rankings, players must maintain high levels of fitness and match preparation over a long duration, strategically peaking for key events.

Competition has been identified as an important factor in player development in racket sports (Crespo et al. 2003), and a busy competition schedule can start at an early age. A thriving junior tennis circuit operates at regional, national, and international level. Furthermore, it is not unusual in tennis for very gifted players to emerge into, and even dominate, the professional ranks while in their teenage years. This is particularly common in the women's competition—for example, the 2004 Wimbledon Championship was won by the 17-year-old Maria Sharapova. Many tennis players enjoy a lengthy career or maintain their competitiveness until an age that would be considered very old in other sports. In 2004, Martina Navratilova was still competing successfully in the singles and doubles competitions of Grand Slam tournaments at the age of 47. Generally, however, players peak in their 20s; according to the ATP Web site, the mean age of a player ranked in the top 200 of the ATP is around 25 years (www.atptennis.com).

Training

Training for racket sports is generally divided into three areas:

- Off-court conditioning such as fitness work or resistance training that is undertaken to achieve the desired physiological or physical characteristics for successful play
- On-court physical and technical practice
- Game situations

Many top racket sport players spend 4 to 6 hr per day undertaking such activities, with the focus varying according to the athlete's perceived weaknesses and goals, the time of the year and competition program, and prevailing theories about training. These vary between players and their fitness advisors and coaches and change over time. The emergence of a new and dominating champion in any sport often changes training practices. For example, in earlier times, the emphasis of training was to undertake match play. However, the athleticism of champion players such as Martina Navratilova and Ivan Lendl in the 1980s, achieved by specialized conditioning programs and attention to diet, revolutionized training ideas. The concept of training periodization over a year and between competitions was discussed in chapter 8: Field-Based Team Sports, and the reader is directed to this chapter for an understanding of this theory. Although periodization can be practiced in racket sports, it is often more difficult to achieve because of the long duration and uncertainty of the tournament circuit. In fact, because tennis is an almost year-round sport, there is typically only a brief off-season.

Physique and Physiology

The most important characteristic of racket sport athletes is sport-specific skill. Overall, successful racket sport players do not appear to possess unique physiological or physical characteristics. Aerobic capacity is typically above average but not extraordinary, and there are a mixed range of physiques among successful players in most racket sports (Reilly 1990b). Many of the world's best players of badminton and squash come from Asian countries, where the typical physique is small and lightly muscled. Therefore, height and lean body mass do not appear to be important determinants of performance in these racket sports.

Examination of the physiques of elite tennis players suggests that height can provide some benefits to performance in this racket sport, although there are clear exceptions to this rule among the world's best players, such as Lleyton Hewitt and Roger Federer. Height provides an advantage in the execution of several shots (e.g., service, volleys) and in general reach around the court. According to several studies reviewed by Reilly (1990b), tennis players from many countries tend to be taller than the average populations that they represent. The typical player in the top 200 of the ATP rankings is tall and lean with a mean height of 183 cm and body mass of 78 kg (www.atptennis.com). Female players are even more likely to be taller than the average population.

High levels of muscle mass and low levels of body fat can also provide an advantage in terms of the power behind shots as well as speed and agility on the court. Thus, we would expect elite tennis players to have higher levels of muscle mass and lower body fat levels than the general population. From time to time, tennis players with striking physiques arising from their genetics or intensive conditioning programs have emerged to dominate play. It is unclear how much the muscular development or leanness displayed by these athletes contributes to their on-court performance per se. It is difficult to isolate the specific characteristics that make a champion in such complex sports or to separate the effects of the outcome of a training program from other benefits of the drive and work ethic that are involved in achieving it. Although the physiques of these champions are used to set a new benchmark for the tennis world, the sport allows players with very different body sizes to be successful. The issue of body fat levels of female players is discussed later in this chapter.

Lifestyle and Culture

Racket sports are played in a variety of cultural environments, including junior competition, collegiate sport, and the professional circuit. Lifestyle and cultural issues for the first two levels of play were discussed in chapter 8. The tennis circuit provides a unique environment with features including almost constant travel and a competition calendar of lengthy duration with almost no off-season. At the junior level and for players down the rankings, traveling is usually undertaken on a shoestring budget and without a support crew. The issues and challenges of travel are discussed in detail in the first practical issue in this chapter.

Most high-level professional players surround themselves with a group of specialists with expertise in various aspects of the game or performance—for example, a conditioning specialist, coach, psychologist, and medical or physical therapy practitioners. The positive outcomes of this practice include an organized and self-sufficient approach to match preparation. This approach assists the player to cope with an isolating lifestyle. One down side of the self-sufficiency, however, is that it may support an insular approach to sport science and sports medicine. It is challenging under tour conditions to find opportunities for cross-fertilization of ideas and interests with professionals in other sports or even within the sport. The culture of the close-knit entourage may exacerbate the principle of keeping secrets or strategies within the group rather than sharing and developing information throughout the sport. There is a lack of studies—both observational and interventionist—involving racket sport players of subelite and elite levels.

Dietary Surveys

At various times, tennis has been responsible for generating interest in sports nutrition, with high-profile players experimenting with different nutritional strategies or adopting special diets as part of their training and competition preparation. Martina Navratilova provided publicity for the high-carbohydrate eating plan espoused by nutritionist Robert Haas in the best-selling book *Eat to Win* (1983). Other players who apparently worked with Haas and followed this dietary plan were Ivan Lendl and Jimmy Connors. This book was one of the first popular publications both to publicize the special nutritional needs of athletes and to promote the role of carbohydrate-rich foods in providing fuel for exercise. However, long before that, players from Harvard University in the era of the 1890s apparently experimented with different dietary strategies for competition, following dietary advice from Dr. James Dwight, a medical doctor and doubles tennis champion. This group, which included Dwight Davis, after whom the Davis Cup competition is named, was reported to try nutrition strategies including the consumption of cold oatmeal between sets (www.daviscup.com).

Unfortunately, there are no published data on the dietary practices of contemporary tennis champions or indeed other racket sport players. The results of the sparse literature concerning dietary surveys of racket sport athletes are summarized in table 10.a (appendix to this chapter) and are isolated to two studies of female collegiate tennis players (Gropper et al. 2003; Nutter 1991) and one report from female tennis players who represented the United States at the Olympic Games (Grandjean and Ruud 1994b). Consequently, there is insufficient information to draw any conclusions about typical eating patterns of racket sport players. The only comment that is warranted from the available literature is that female collegiate tennis players appear to continue the pattern that has been seen in other studies, in which female athletes report energy intakes that are below their expected energy requirements (Gropper et al. 2003; Nutter 1991). As such, reported intakes of carbohydrate by these players appear to be well below the guidelines for athletes undertaking prolonged training and competition play. Intakes of at-risk micronutrients such as iron and calcium are also below relevant daily recommendations (Nutter 1991). The validity of these data and effect of such dietary intakes need to be investigated.

There is a clear need for dietary surveys to be undertaken on racket sport players, particularly to investigate how professional and elite players address the challenges of constant travel and tournament play.

Nutritional Issues and Challenges

The nutritional requirements and challenges in racket sports (see highlight box on page 246) share similarities with those seen in field- and court-based team sports. Strategies for achieving optimal physique and fueling for training and weekly competition fixtures are discussed in chapters 8 and 9, and the reader is directed to these chapters for nutrition strategies for players undertaking games based on intermittent high-intensity activity. At the serious level of play, whether elite or junior, racket players face unique nutrition issues related to a constant travel schedule, unpredictable competition scenarios, and the recovery challenges of tournament play. This chapter deals specifically with these unique issues and several nutritional concerns that are topical in tennis. In completing this series of chapters on intermittent high-intensity activities, we review the research and practical issues related to creatine supplementation for team and racket sports players.

Weight Concerns in Female Tennis Players

Former Wimbledon champion Pat Cash has accused modern women tennis players of being out of shape and overweight. . . . "These days, girls can take it easy and still earn millions. Look at Lindsay Davenport. She's a big girl. When you look at her, you think whoah, there is no way she is going to be a tennis player—put her in the shot put instead.". . . Former Wimbledon champion Richard Krajicek, was forced to make a groveling apology three years ago after he branded the stars of the women's game "fat lazy pigs."

From "Our women stars are overweight: Pat Cash's amazing outburst." The Sunday Telegraph newspaper, Sydney, Australia, January 14, 2001, p. 48

Professional tennis players are in the public eye and often gain publicity or media comment for issues other than their on-court performance. A recurring story that has no doubt created stress and misery for a number of prominent female players is the assertion that many of the top women are out of shape or overfat. Such comments are often accompanied by an unflattering photo of nominated players. There have been suggestions that such pressures do not only exist at the top level of play; rather, there is pressure even at junior levels of competition for female players to achieve an ideal physique. Harris (2000) cited a string of lay articles in magazines, books, and newspapers discussing issues of weight control in tennis players over a range of levels, including allegations that tennis players who were judged overweight by their coaches received punishments, including threats of loss of scholarship funding.

Common Nutritional Issues Arising in Racket Sports

Physique Issues

- For some individual players: achieving and maintaining moderately low body fat levels to aid speed and agility and enhance heat tolerance
- For some individual players, particularly in tennis: increasing and maintaining high levels of lean body mass for strength and power
- For some female players: achieving ideal physique and dealing with risk of inappropriate or disordered eating when subjected to pressure regarding body fat levels

Training Issues

- Integrating training and competition goals when playing in a weekly fixture
- Establishing sound eating patterns and meeting training nutrition goals within the short periods between tournaments during prolonged competitive season
- Achieving high energy intake to support heavy training or match program and perhaps growth (e.g., for adolescents or players undertaking aggressive resistance training)
- Consuming high carbohydrate intake during interval between matches and training to promote optimal refueling
- Achieving adequate protein intake to meet increased requirements resulting from heavy training and to promote recovery from matches and adaptation to training
- Considering creatine supplementation for training adaptations (match simulation, interval training, resistance training)
- Reducing risk of reduced iron status, especially in female athletes, and athletes undergoing growth spurts
- Maintaining fluid and carbohydrate intake during prolonged training sessions
- Enhancing nutrition knowledge and domestic skills in junior players, especially when involved on the circuit

Competition Issues

- Tournament eating: achieving the cycle of fueling up before events and recovering between matches
- The prematch meal: achieving nutritional needs and gastric comfort, especially when the exact time of the match may be uncertain in a tournament timetable
- Monitoring fluid and carbohydrate intake during matches
- Achieving adequate nutrition for the traveling athlete
- Achieving total or long-term nutritional goals in addition to immediate needs for refueling and rehydration, especially when the duration of the competition season is prolonged
- Considering creatine and caffeine supplementation for competition performance

In response to this concern, 107 female tennis players and 26 coaches from a range of colleges in the United States were surveyed on issues related to weight concern, body image, and disordered eating (Harris 2000). Although these players were involved in tennis teams within division I collegiate competition, they were not considering a professional or elite career in tennis. Their attitudes to their own weight (generally within the normal range) were typically positive, and their answers suggested normal eating behaviors and self-concept. However, weight was seen as being important and they agreed that they played

better when they weighed less. Furthermore, they agreed that most female tennis players think that they need to lose weight. A small number of respondents exhibited more extreme attitudes and problematic ideas. The coaches who responded to the survey reflected a similar approach to their players' careers, caring about the outcome of their tennis performances but being more concerned about their success in gaining college degrees. They were happy with their players' body weight. Furthermore, coaches' attitudes to weight and performance could also be considered healthy, because they professed that decisions about the need to lose weight were driven by issues of speed, stamina, and conditioning rather than measurements of body fat and weight per se. Thus, the results of this study suggest, at least at the collegiate level, that tennis players are not at greater risk of weight concerns and problems than other females. Further investigations need to be undertaken to confirm these findings and extend the study to more elite groups.

There is no scientific support that low body fat levels are necessary for successful player in general or for improved performance in individual players. However, the periodic emergence of dominant female players with a strikingly lean and muscular physique, such as Martina Navratilova or Venus and Serena Williams, provides circumstantial evidence of the benefits of low body fat levels. Whereas leanness is likely to assist with some aspects of the game, such as agility and heat tolerance, it is uncertain how much it contributes directly to game performance. Furthermore, in the case of successful players, it is impossible to isolate the effects of leanness from other genetically determined characteristics of the individual or to separate the effect of a loss of body fat from other effects of the training and dietary practices undertaken to achieve it.

Of course, there are some individuals in racket sports who may benefit from a reduction in weight and body fat, especially where a chronic energy surplus has caused the player to stray from his ideal playing weight. This can happen during a break from play or training or while injured. It may also occur because the player is unable to keep track of his or her energy intake because of constant travel or play. Although the challenge for many players in a tournament play is to consume *enough* carbohydrate fuel and total energy, it is possible for other players to overcompensate when fueling. A series of brief matches or an early exit from the tournament may mean that a player does not use expected energy requirements and may have overeaten during preparation. Young players on tour may not always make good nutrition choices because of a lack of supervision or inadequate finances and may become reliant on fat-rich, energy-dense takeaway foods. Guidelines for loss of weight and body fat can be found in the section titled "Achieving Low Body Mass and Body Fat Levels" in chapter 4. Individualized and specific advice from a sports dietitian is valuable in helping racket sport athletes set realistic goals for body mass and body fat levels and a suitable time frame in which to achieve them. The sports dietitian can also advise on sound eating practices that contribute to the player's overall nutritional goals. The player should be able to achieve his or her weight loss goals while eating a diet that is adequate in energy and nutrients and free of unreasonable levels of food-related stress. The ideal physique to which the player aspires should be based on observations of health and performance over an adequate period of time. The issues of disordered eating and the female athlete triad are discussed in greater detail in chapter 5, related to distance running, and chapter 13, related to gymnastics. Where such problems arise in racket sports, the player should be referred at an early stage for expert assistance.

Fuel, Fluid, and Electrolyte Needs During Matches

The metabolic demands of racket sports generally predict moderate rates of sweat loss during play. However, the hot environmental conditions in which training or competition is undertaken in many racket sports often add a significant overlay of heat stress. Many racket sports are played indoors, where there is a restriction of the airflow that could otherwise offer convective and evaporative cooling. Even when courts or stadiums are air-conditioned, the ventilation characteristics and the heat generated by lighting in these venues add a substantial thermal stress. Tennis is technically a summer sport, and many of the major tournaments are played in countries where summer temperatures regularly exceed 30°C. The Australian Open Tennis Championship is well known for exposing players to ambient temperatures of 35°C to 40°C, with court temperatures being even higher because of the enclosure of the space, reflection of radiant energy, and retention of heat in the playing surface. Such extreme conditions, especially when combined with high humidity, provide a high risk of heat stress illness.

Issues related to dehydration in team and racket sports were examined in chapter 9. The reader is directed to this chapter for reviews of the effect of dehydration on movement patterns and skill aspects of these sports (see research topics), as well as a discussion of the practical challenges of matching fluid intake to sweat losses in such sports (see the first practical issue). Despite the apparent likelihood of high rates of sweat loss and the publicity given to dramatic situations in major tennis tournaments where players have cramped on court or required intravenous rehydration after games, there are few scientific studies of actual sweat rates and fluid intakes in racket sports. The available literature on fluid balance during training and competition in racket sports is summarized in table 10.b (appendix) and is limited to tennis and squash. This information suggests that sweat rates ranging from 1 to 2.5 L/hr can be expected across these sports, although the extreme rates at the top of this range may be limited to individual players and extreme environments (Bergeron 2003). Among a group of 17 male tennis players with a history of cramping during matches who were studied by Bergeron (2003), four players were estimated to incur sweat rates of greater than 3 L/hr during singles match play.

Factors predicting high rates of sweat loss in a racket sport include play involving prolonged rallies, high ambient and court temperatures, and restricted airflow in the playing venue. On the other hand, a player's ability to consume fluid during a match to counter such sweat losses includes individual issues such as innate drinking behavior and gastrointestinal comfort as well as sport-related factors such as the rules governing availability of fluids and opportunities to drink. In sports such as badminton and squash, fluid intake is limited to the periods between games and sets. One study of squash players reported a mean fluid intake of only 67 ml over an observed 16 matches (Hansen and Brotherhood 1988). However, tennis rules permit players to have a more regular drinking schedule with a standardized rest period of 90 s as the players change ends every two games within a set and between sets themselves. Observation of matches and the limited literature suggests that most top tennis players are aware of the need to hydrate during events and organize a supply of drinks courtside for these occasions. However, there is a range in the drinking behavior of players in most racket sports; for example, in one study of tennis players, fluid intake ranged from 328 to 1,750 ml over a match (McCarthy et al. 1988).

Some players appear to manage a substantial rate of fluid intake during competitive play—for example, mean fluid intake during singles match play in one study was 1,600 ml/hr (Bergeron 2003). Furthermore, 3 of the 17 players included in this cohort reported an intake of more than 2 L/hr—an intake likely to approach the limits posed by gastrointestinal comfort during high-intensity exercise and by the opportunities to drink during rest periods. Despite such high rates of drinking, these players accrued a mean fluid shortfall of 1,000 ml or more than 1% BM per hour. These data show that with matches lasting up to 5 hr, a substantial fluid deficit can accrue in "heavy sweaters" despite the best hydration strategies. It is unlikely that all racket sport players experience sweat losses of this volume, at least during many of their matches. But it is also uncertain that most players are as motivated or organized to drink such large amounts of fluid on all occasions. Therefore, it is likely that a physiologically significant level of hypohydration occurs during match play and high-level practice for many racket sports players. The literature review in chapter 9 (see the first research topic) provides evidence that fluid replacement during prolonged intermittent activities can enhance exercise capacity (Devlin et al. 2001; McGregor et al. 1999). The sport-specific studies on racket sports support the theory that hypohydration will impair the movement patterns and endurance of players. For example, exercise-induced dehydration of ~3% caused a reduction in 5 and 10 m sprint times in tennis players (Magal et al. 2003). In this study there were no detectable changes in the performance of an agility test or tennis-specific skill tests. However, other studies of intermittent high-intensity exercise protocols have reported that fluid deficits are associated with a reduction in motor skills and mental functioning (Devlin et al. 2001; McGregor et al. 1999).

Racket sport players should monitor their actual fluid losses during match play and practice and should follow an appropriate fluid intake plan. General guidelines regarding fluid intake for team and racket sports are provided in chapter 9, the first practical issue. The choice of fluid seems to be important, at least in matches of a prolonged nature or within a tournament setting. The addition of carbohydrate to a fluid (e.g., a sport drink), or other strategies for carbohydrate intake during play such as the use of carbohydrate gels, can provide an additional fuel source for the muscle and central nervous system and reduce the risk of hypoglycemia. The literature review provided in chapter 9 (see the first and second research topics) includes stud-

ies in which carbohydrate intake was shown to enhance movement patterns in prolonged intermittent activities (Kirkendall et al. 1988; Nicholas et al. 1995; Simard et al. 1988; Welsh et al. 2002; Winnick et al. 2005), as well as sport-specific skills (Dougherty et al. 2006; Kipp et al. 2003; Muckle 1973; Ostojic and Mazic 2002; Wallis and Galloway 2003). In these studies, the control treatment or trial was associated with a decline in performance over the duration of the protocol that was prevented or attenuated with carbohydrate intake.

Studies that are specific to racket sports also support the benefits of carbohydrate supplementation on performance (see tables 9.e and 9.f in appendix for specific details of studies). Ferrauti and coworkers (1997) investigated the effect of carbohydrate intake in male and female tennis players on the performance of a battery of tests undertaken after 4 hr of tennis practice. Carbohydrate intake prevented the decline in blood glucose concentrations over the latter stages of this play seen in the placebo trial and was associated with superior performance of a sprint running test. However, there was no enhancement of hitting accuracy or overall success (games won) during the tennis play. The authors suggested that in the lower-intensity situation of tennis practice, factors such as motivation and concentration were able to compensate for the reduced fuel status in the placebo trial; this may not be the case during a competitive event (Ferrauti et al. 1997). However, it is also possible that benefits to individual components of performance do not translate into a detectable improvement in overall match play (see the first research topic).

Whether carbohydrate intake enhances racket sport performances may be determined by whether the match would otherwise expose the player to fatigue secondary to low blood glucose levels. Consumption of a carbohydrate-containing drink was associated with better jumping ability and ball accuracy at the end of 2 hr of tennis play compared with trials undertaken with water intake or no fluid (Burke and Ekblom 1982). By contrast, others failed to find any benefits of carbohydrate supplementation to a protocol monitoring serve velocity and accuracy and error rates during 3 hr of tennis (Mitchell et al. 1992). In the former study, the control condition was associated with a decline in blood glucose concentrations and a deterioration in performance (Burke and Ekblom 1982). However, in the latter investigation, blood glucose concentrations and performance were maintained in the control condition, making it unlikely for performance enhancement to be found with carbohydrate intake (Mitchell et al. 1992).

Finally, benefits to both sprint ability and stroke performance were found when a tennis-specific protocol devised to evaluate stroke quality and a 70 m shuttle run were undertaken before and after 2 hr of tennis practice (Vergauwen et al. 1998). Performance in the shuttle run was maintained in the carbohydrate trial, in contrast to the 2.5% reduction in placebo trial. In the placebo trial, postpractice testing revealed a reduction in stroke quality for first service and for defensive rallies. However, carbohydrate intake attenuated the reduction in stroke precision with a smaller decrease in error rate and nonreached balls;

players were able to produce more powerful and precise shots compared with the control condition. The authors noted that a change in sprint ability might have some effect on stroke quality; a decrease in speed would increase the time taken to achieve body stability and control during stroke execution, thus reducing the power and precision of shots and increasing errors. However, the maintenance of running speed over 2 hr of tennis practice could not fully explain the ergogenic action of carbohydrate on stroke quality in this study. Other mechanisms, perhaps related to better concentration and coordination, may also be implicated.

The prevalence of hypoglycemia during tennis has been investigated both by questioning players about their experiences and by observing changes in blood glucose concentrations during practice and actual tournament play (Ferrauti et al. 1997, 2003). It appears there is some risk of a decline in glycemia toward the end of a prolonged passage of play (Ferrauti et al. 1997). However, hypoglycemia occurs most frequently at the onset of exercise following a rest period, with this phenomenon appearing to be self-correcting despite carbohydrate intake (Ferrauti et al. 1997, 2003). The prevalence was greater during tournaments than training and at the commencement of a second bout of activity (e.g., the second match in a day) compared with the first workout. The authors explained this outcome as a rebound hypoglycemia, occurring when liver glucose output falls behind muscle glucose uptake. Action to address such alterations in glycemia includes ensuring an appropriate warm-up before the commencement of play to stimulate sympathetic activity and mobilization of substrates (Ferrauti et al. 2003). However, carbohydrate consumed during a first match and in the break between matches might help to overcome the depletion of liver glycogen stores and better allow the defense of glucose homeostasis.

Information on the effects of carbohydrate ingestion on the performance of other racket sports is limited to two studies involving squash. In one investigation, squash players experienced a 19% decrease in performance accuracy after playing three simulated games when consuming a placebo drink (Graydon et al. 1998). However, carbohydrate supplementation during the games allowed performance to be maintained. In the other study, players undertook skill tests before and after 20 min of moderate-intensity treadmill running and 9 min of on-court, high-intensity "ghosting" (Wallis and Galloway 2003). Scores on the postexercise skill test were higher in the carbohydrate trial than placebo trial, and the performance difference was attributed to better positioning of the player on court relative to the ball.

Finally, there is increasing interest in proactive replacement of electrolytes during prolonged matches and tournaments, especially in individuals or situations where sweat losses are high and lead to large electrolyte losses. This is believed to be a risk factor for the development of heat-related muscle cramps in susceptible players (see the second research topic). There are also single case histories of hyponatremia occurring in players as a result of large sweat and electrolyte losses treated by intake of large amounts of

low-sodium fluids (Bergeron 2003); however, most serious cases of hyponatremia in athletes occur through excessive intake of fluid (Almond et al. 2005). Some experts call for players at risk of high sodium losses to increase their dietary salt intake and possibly add salt to their on-court drinks. Old practices such as the consumption of pickle juice, salt tablets, or bananas (for potassium replacement) during matches are less likely to be effective because they may not assist the player to address fluid and sodium needs simultaneously. For more discussion of this topic, the reader is directed to the second research topic.

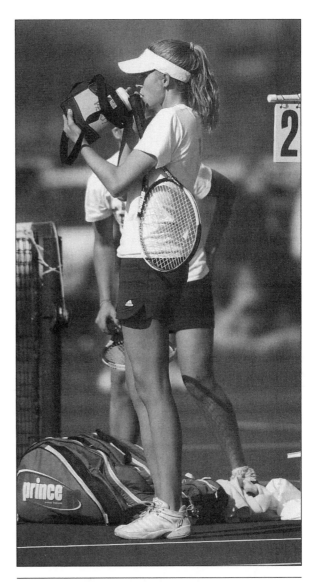

There is sound reason for racket sport players to consider consuming carbohydrate during competition and practice sessions, especially where there is evidence of a performance decline over the duration of play. Each player should experiment with the use of sport drinks during play, particularly in games or situations involving prolonged sessions of activity or for multiple bouts such as in the tournament setting.

Tournament Play

The program of multiple matches during tournament play creates a major challenge for efficient and effective recovery. Depending on the sport and the individual match, a player may finish one event with depleted muscle and liver carbohydrate stores, a substantial fluid deficit, and muscle damage or breakdown. Optimal performance in the next match will require a reversal of the first two factors, and for long-term goals, the player will also want to ensure adequate protein repair and adaptation and immune system function. The principles and guidelines for achieving recovery involving these various factors were covered in chapter 6 (second practical issue). These guidelines include consuming carbohydrate to achieve maximal rates of glycogen storage, drinking a volume of fluid in excess of the existing fluid deficit to allow for ongoing sweat and urine losses, and replacing electrolytes to maximize the retention of fluid.

Tournament play in racket sports creates several unique challenges. The first challenge is that there are variable times available for recovery between matches. Depending on the duration of the tournament and the time between rounds, or whether the player has entered into multiple events in the same tournament (e.g., singles and doubles), the recovery period may range from 1 to 48 hr. On some occasions the time interval may be insufficient to allow complete recovery of fluid and fuel stores, and the player will commence the next match with suboptimal preparation. This will create an even greater incentive to refuel and hydrate *during* the next match. To some extent the player may not need to perform optimally during each match but rather will need to beat an opponent who is also facing recovery challenges. However, when players are generally of equal caliber, the player with the superior recovery strategies has a definite advantage.

A tournament timetable, at least in the early phase, is somewhat uncertain. Many matches are scheduled to commence after the completion of a series of other matches on the same court and are dependent on the outcome of these games. In this situation, players may not always know how much time they have for recovery from their last match or when to consume their prematch meal. Generally, to enhance recovery when the interval between matches is less than 6 to 8 hr, the player is advised to consume a source of key nutrients as soon as practical after the completion of the first match. This may cause some practical difficulties when the tournament finishes late at night or is held at a venue that has poor access to catering. Postmatch commitments (e.g., attending press conferences) or travel to distant accommodations may also interfere with recovery eating. When there is uncertainty over the timing of the next match and the potential for a start within hours, the player may be reluctant to consume large amounts of food. The risk of gastrointestinal discomfort or upsets can be reduced by choosing carbohydrate-rich foods, including sport foods such as liquid meal supplements and sport bars, that are low in fiber or easily digested. Foods that have minimal storage or preparation requirements are also useful in that

they allow players to have rapid access to nutrition after the match or to meet their nutrient needs while undertaking other postmatch activities.

The following plan best addresses postexercise recovery meal between close matches, or indeed the preevent meal before any match. When players can be confident of having a 2 to 4 hr gap until their next activity, they should consume a comfortable amount of carbohydrate-rich food and drinks. Thereafter, small snacks can be consumed to continue to fuel and hydrate, or indeed just to avoid hunger, every 20 to 40 min until the start of the warm-up. Light choices include the sport products previously mentioned but can also include fruit, rice cakes, and confectionery items. Fluids such as sport drinks can be consumed during warm-up to continue with recovery and preparation goals.

When a player is preparing for an open-ended match, a proactive attitude is to assume that the match will last for its potential. For example, a male tennis player should prepare for the possibility of a 4 hr match in a five-set tournament; when the best of three sets is contested by men or women, a 2 to 3 hr match should be assumed. Proactive preparation includes the consumption of a substantial amount of carbohydrate in the preevent meal (see table 1.2). However, additional fueling and rehydration can also be achieved during the match as long as the player has organized a supply of sport drinks courtside and has practiced drinking to ensure that this is well tolerated.

When players are involved in a prolonged competition season, with short intervals from one tournament to the next, competition eating is likely to make a significant contribution to overall nutrition status. In such a scenario, the player needs to consider total nutrient needs (e.g., protein and micronutrients) in addition to carbohydrate fuel requirements and to achieve an energy balance consistent with long-term physique goals. Although it is tempting and sometimes convenient to choose recovery foods based only on carbohydrate content, the player should consider the potential benefits of making more nutrient-rich choices—to aid both short-term recovery goals and long-term nutritional balance. There is already evidence that a protein–carbohydrate combination promotes better recovery than a postexercise snack providing carbohydrate alone, because the combination may enhance protein repair and adaptation (see chapter 6, the second research topic 2 and practical issue). It is also possible that the early intake of other nutrients such as key vitamins and minerals may enhance recovery processes in ways that are not yet understood.

Players with lower energy needs, or a desire to reduce body weight or fat, may find it difficult to reconcile aggressive fueling strategies for competition with their true energy requirements. Repeated incidences of increased carbohydrate intake in anticipation of a lengthy match may lead to a chronic energy intake surplus, particularly when the actual match is decided quickly and with modest energy expenditure. This outcome is most likely to be experienced by female players, because their matches are of shorter duration and because they are more likely to be concerned about weight control. It may be necessary for these individuals to take a less aggressive approach to competition fueling: for example, to consume carbohydrate within their true energy budget for most situations and save carbohydrate-loading techniques (higher carbohydrate and energy intakes) for key tournaments or key matches.

Eating on the Circuit

Because competition plays an important role in the development of the racket sport player, the committed athlete is soon enveloped by the circuit of regional, national, or international tournament play. Depending on the level of the tournament and the player, accommodations may range from homestay programs to hostels and to five-star hotels. Eating on the road creates nutritional challenges. These challenges are compounded when the travel is so constant and when the player is on the bottom rung of the competition ladder with a tight budget and little assistance. Even at the top levels, with an entourage that includes specialists to deal with the various aspects of competition preparation, the player can still expect to face difficulties that are not experienced at home. The challenges of nutrition for the traveling athlete are outlined in the first practical issue, and guidelines are provided to assist the athlete to develop sound eating practices away from home.

Sport Foods and Supplements

At the beginning of 2004, the issue of supplements in tennis hit the headlines with the announcement of a doping case against top player Greg Rusedski. In the subsequent hearing of this case, the positive test for the steroid nandrolone was deemed to have occurred as a result of the intake of contaminated supplements, and sanctions were dismissed. Additional publicity surrounding this case suggested that Greg was one of a large number of tennis players who had recorded an inadvertent doping finding. Initially, a particular electrolyte supplement that had been provided to players by ATP-endorsed trainers was suspected to be the contaminated product. Later this supplement was exonerated, and the cause of all of the positive doping offences remains unknown. The fierce discussion that ensued during the Australian Open, when the positive doping outcome was first announced, polarized opinion on two issues—Do elite tennis players need to take supplements to compete optimally? And what is the risk of a positive drug test arising from supplement use? The opinions of many top players were that supplements played a critical role in achieving the unique nutritional needs of elite level tennis but that players were now paranoid about using any such products. It was hard to settle the debate, because of confusion over the definition of a supplement and because many of those involved in the debate seemed to have rigid opinions that covered all products.

In this book, we have taken the view that specialized sport foods and supplements can play a valuable role in the achievement of sports nutrition goals and optimal performance. However, the value of any product lies first in how it addresses specific needs of an individual athlete or the nutritional issues in the sport and second in how it is used by the athlete. This assessment can only really be made on a case-by-case basis, and in most instances the answer is not absolute. Rather, it is a matter of weighing the potential positive outcomes against the potential negatives associated with the use of a product. The risk of an inadvertent doping outcome has been identified as one of the possible disadvantages of the use of supplements, with evidence that some products are contaminated with compounds such as prohormones that are banned by many sporting organizations (see chapter 3, first practical issue). Because strict liability is usually applied in doping cases—in other words, athletes are deemed guilty regardless of the source or motive behind their ingestion of a banned substance—this outcome can be career ending. However, there are steps that athletes can take to reduce their risk of this serious outcome. See chapter 3 for further information on this issue as well as a general perspective on the pros and cons regarding the use of supplements and sports foods.

It is difficult to provide well-supported advice on the supplements and sport foods that might be valuable to racket sport players. There is little scientific study involving racket sport players or racket sport performance from which direct answers can be found. The few studies that are available involve fluid and carbohydrate replacement (see tables 9.e and 9.f) and supplementation with creatine and caffeine (table 10.c in appendix). Even these studies need to be interpreted with care, because the results are not always consistent with each other or the general literature. This is often the case when dealing with a complex activity such as racket sports where it is difficult to measure a change in performance (see the first research topic). In the case of tennis, a specific test of stroke performance, called the Leuven Tennis Performance Test, has been developed to measure ball velocity and precision. This test has been used in two studies involving nutritional interventions to see whether an effect on some of the skill aspects of the game could be detected (Op 't Eijnde et al. 2001; Vergauwen et al. 1998).

The summary in table 10.1 provides suggestions of typical situations faced by racket sport athletes where sport foods can be valuable. In some scenarios, such as match play and training sessions, there is good evidence that the use of a specialized sport food (i.e., a sport drink) can directly enhance performance. In other cases, the rewards are more indirect and relate to assisting players to achieve their nutrient needs or nutrition goals. The list of supplements for which there is evidence of a direct performance benefit to racket sports is very short—limited, at the present time, to a reasonable level of support for the use of caffeine and creatine. This judgment has been made not just from the results of the few studies presented in table 10.c but from the general literature regarding prolonged exercise and intermittent high-intensity sports. The issue of creatine supplementation in team and racket sports is discussed in the third research topic. Although new information on bicarbonate loading for repeated sprint efforts has been briefly studied in relation to team sports (see chapter 8), it has not yet been considered in relation to racket sports. Further studies on these supplements and other purported ergogenic aids are warranted so that advice to racket sport athletes can be made with greater confidence.

Research Priorities

Future research in racket sports should include the following hot topics:

- Dietary practices of top players, with a focus on eating on the circuit and integrating long-term nutrition goals within a lengthy competition season
- Development of valid and reliable protocols to monitor performance
- The effect of muscle mass and body fat levels on performance
- Carbohydrate utilization during training and competition; guidelines for carbohydrate intake in the preevent meal and during play and recovery between matches
- Fluid and electrolyte losses during match play and practice
- The role of fluid and electrolyte losses in heat cramps
- Supplement use by racket sport players
- Effect of creatine, caffeine, and other ergogenic aids on performance in racket sports

RESEARCH TOPIC

Measuring Effects of Nutrition Interaction on an Unpredictable Sport

A new diet, supplement, piece of equipment, or training strategy emerges as the hot new thing in sport. Athletes and coaches want to know if it enhances sporting performance, and they are impressed by the testimonials and hypothetical claims. In contrast, sport scientists hold up the scientific trial as the only way to assess the efficacy of a new intervention. In chapter 3 we discussed the challenge of measuring changes in athletic performance, with a focus on simple activities such as a running, cycling, or swimming race. We saw that detecting changes is not as easy as it might appear. In fact, few scientific studies are capable of detecting the small but real changes in performance that can move an athlete from fourth place to a medal. But what methods are available to tackle the complex issue of performance in team sports?

Performance in team and racket sports is determined by a complicated mixture of physical and mental skills. Players must be able not only to run to the ball or scene of play but to execute skills involving cognitive function (e.g., reading the play, make tactical decisions) and motor control. Nutritional strategies can create an impact, both by sustaining the optimal running ability of players and maintaining optimal function of the central nervous system. Fatigue may be manifested in terms of reduced distance covered or a decrease in the number or duration of high-intensity activities as well as an increased number of mistakes and decision errors.

In many simple sports, the best tests of performance are actual competition outcomes. This is because the conditions are real, and the outcome is absolute—the athlete achieves a measure of time, distance, or mass that can be directly compared between a control trial and an intervention trial. However, team and racket sports involve competition between two opponents where the game characteristics are unique and unpredictable and performance is relative. It is more difficult to make precise judgments about performance, because each team or player reacts to the other and is being compared with the other rather than to a set standard. Sport scientists generally use three different approaches to monitor the outcome of a performance intervention in team and racket sports. All methodologies have limitations, especially in achieving the ideals of reliability and validity discussed in chapter 3.

Method 1. Isolation of Characteristic Movement Patterns and Skills

- Overview: Time–motion studies can allow the performance of a team or racket sport to be broken into a series of skills and movement patterns. Furthermore, these studies can identify the characteristics of winning outcomes or the top athletes in the sport. Protocols can then be designed to investigate the performance of these isolated characteristics—for example, the ability to undertake repeated high-intensity running tasks with brief recovery time, or perhaps the completion of a task involving reaction time or decision making. In this method, it is assumed that if an intervention such as a nutrition strategy improves the performance of this isolated task in comparison to a placebo treatment, the strategy will also enhance the performance of the team or racket sport per se. Additional strategies to enhance the reliability of such methodologies include providing participants with the opportunity to become familiarized with the test protocols, so that all learning effects are minimized. This is especially important when the performance tests involve novel protocols.

- Advantages of methodology: The results of well-conducted studies using this design may provide some insight into factors that limit performance in team sport or interventions that may enhance performance.

- Disadvantages of methodology: The major limitation of such studies lies in the validity of performance measures: whether changes in an isolated physical or cognitive task

Table 10.1 Sport Foods and Supplements That Are of Likely Benefit to Racket Sport Players

	Product	Comment
Use in achieving documented nutrition goals	Sport drinks	• Use to refuel and rehydrate during prolonged training sessions and matches and to rehydrate after the session. Contain some electrolytes to help replace sweat losses and increase voluntary intake of fluid.
	Sport gels	• Convenient and compact carbohydrate source that can be used for additional refueling during matches and prolonged training sessions, especially if water is used for hydration goals.
	Sport bars	• Convenient, portable, and easy-to-consume source of carbohydrate, protein, and micronutrients for prematch meal or postexercise recovery. Especially useful for tournament situations when match times are not well known and may finish very late at night. • Low-bulk and portable form of energy and nutrients that can contribute to high energy needs, especially to support resistance training program or growth. • Convenient and compact source of energy and nutrients for the traveling athlete.
	Liquid meal supplements	• Well-tolerated preevent meal that can be consumed to provide a source of carbohydrate quite close to the start of a match or workout; seems to be better tolerated than solid food by some athletes with high risk of gastrointestinal problems. Especially useful for tournament situations when exact time of commencement of match is not known. • Convenient, portable, and easy-to-consume source of carbohydrate, protein, and micronutrients for postexercise recovery. • Low-bulk and practical form of energy and nutrients that can contribute to high energy needs, especially to support resistance training program or growth. • Convenient and compact source of energy and nutrients for the traveling athlete.
	Multivitamin and mineral supplement	• Supplemental source of micronutrients for traveling when food supply is less reliable. Especially useful for athletes on the circuit. • Supplemental source of micronutrients during prolonged periods of energy restriction (female athletes).
	Electrolyte supplements	• May provide additional source of sodium for replacement during exercise by cramp-prone players with heavy sweat and electrolyte losses.
Some potential for ergogenic benefit	Creatine	• Creatine phosphate serves a number of important roles in exercise metabolism; the most well-known role is the rapid regeneration of adenosine triphosphate by the phosphagen power system. Studies show that creatine loading enhances the performance of exercise involving repeated high-intensity work bouts with short recovery intervals (<2 min recovery). Chronic creatine supplementation may be valuable in enhancing the response of racket sport players to various training protocols—interval training undertaken to enhance anaerobic fitness, match-specific play, and for some players, resistance training undertaken to enhance muscle mass and strength. Studies are needed to examine the effect of acute supplementation with creatine on the performance of match-simulation protocols or movement patterns within actual field play, to investigate whether creatine can be seen as a competition aid. The two available investigations of creatine supplementation in tennis did not find an ergogenic benefit; however, another study involving squash players reported enhancement of an on-court routine involving repeated sprints. Further studies are needed. Typical protocols for creatine use: loading dose of 20-30 g in multiple doses (e.g., 4 × 5 g) for 5 days followed by maintenance dose of 2-5 g/day. Uptake appears to be enhanced by consuming creatine with carbohydrate-rich meal or snack. Acute weight gain of about 1 kg occurs with creatine loading, presumably attributable to fluid retention.

(continued)

Table 10.1   (continued)

Product	Comment
Caffeine	• May enhance performance of prolonged exercise (e.g., matches) by reducing perception of fatigue. The two available studies of caffeine supplementation and tennis performance show conflicting evident of benefits; additional studies need to be undertaken in racket sports to further investigate the potential for enhancement of movement patterns or attenuation of decline in skills and concentration over match. Caffeine may be consumed in cola and energy drinks or as an ingredient in some sport products (e.g., some gels). There is conflicting evidence over the efficacy of coffee as a source of caffeine, because it contains other chemicals that might impair performance.

translate into on-field performance. Although characteristics such as concentration, reaction time, or the ability to recover between repeated sprints may be important features in a game, it is difficult to extrapolate from an isolated feature to the total game performance. We might see single effects being either overridden or exaggerated when they are integrated into the complex context of a match. For example, in the laboratory setting, a cognitive skill may be clearly impaired by a factor such as dehydration. However, performance deterioration may not be as evident in a game situation where the athlete is receiving optimal psychological arousal. Alternatively, the overlay of the number of factors involved in performance may exacerbate any deterioration in each. For example, the need to simultaneously control a ball or withstand tackles may exacerbate the deterioration in running ability in the fatigued athlete. Or the need to concentrate to recruit the motor units involved in running may detract from the focus needed to make tactical decisions.

Method 2. Simulation of the Team or Racket Sport

• Overview. This method involves the development of a test protocol that mimics the team game—either in a laboratory setting or in a field setting with some control over environmental conditions. The simulated game may be played on a treadmill according to the typical work characteristics undertaken by players or undertaken as drill involving real play and game skills that achieve similar physiological and psychological stresses to those occurring in a real game. Different types of performance tests may be monitored at set intervals; for example, before and after the match simulation, or at various time points throughout the simulated match. The training and nutritional preparation of participants should be standardized between trials and chosen to represent the real-life conditions of competitive play. For example, participants should be fed a standard prematch meal and undertake supervised workouts on the days between trials or before a trial.

• Advantages of methodology: With good control, this type of design allows a simulated match to be played twice, and the investigator can record changes in selected performance parameters over time and between treatments.

• Disadvantages of methodology: There are still some issues regarding the validity of performance measures. Inevitably, the performance tasks that are monitored are not integrated into game play and may not reflect true on-field performance. See comments for method 1.

Method 3. Observation of Real Match Performance

• Overview: The final method involves observation of a real match performance. The first challenge of this approach to undertaking a comparative study of team and racket sports is that the same match can't be played twice. In other words, even with the same two teams playing each other, it is impossible to have an identical match played with and without the treatment. However, one way around this in team sports or doubles tennis is to subdivide each team into two groups. The match is then undertaken with one of each of the groups on the treatment and the other group on the placebo. The groups should be matched for important characteristics such as game position or style of play. If a repeated-measures or crossover design is to be used, the researchers should have the same two teams play each other on a number of occasions, matching the conditions of the match and prematch preparation as closely as possible to try to produce an even match stimulus. Again, half of each team should be assigned to the treatment or placebo group. The next challenge of this method is to design a quantitative way of measuring the performance of individual players. This can vary from time–motion analyses that estimate the duration and intensity of game activities to various strategies that monitor the number of errors and successful plays made by each participant.

• Advantages of methodology: This type of study is likely to have the highest validity.

• Disadvantages of methodology. It may be difficult to find performance measures that are reliable and can be accurately measured. Match-to-match variability or differences between the two groups may also mask real differences in the outcome to a treatment.

RESEARCH TOPIC
Cramping in Team and Racket Sports

Most people can recall a tennis or football match that has dramatically changed as a result of heat cramps. One moment the play is intense and the scores are close; the next moment, a player cramps and the game is over. Either the player has to forfeit the match or leave the field or his or her performance crumbles and the opponent takes control. At various times, players have gobbled salt tablets, drunk pickle juice, and eaten bananas on their field of play to combat the risk of cramps. Each of these therapies has generally been discredited, as has the general theory that cramps are caused by an electrolyte deficiency. However, recent work including input from experts in tennis (Dr. Michael Bergeron) and American football (Dr. Randy Eichner) has revived the interest in the electrolyte hypothesis, at least in susceptible individuals.

One feature of this renewed interest is the proposal that athletes can experience different types of muscular cramps during exercise with different etiologies. Many athletes experience localized muscle cramps during activities attributable to fatigue and general lack of conditioning (Schwellnus et al. 1997). These cramps can be relieved by stretching, ice, and massage. Bergeron suggests that heat-associated muscle cramps have a different presentation and cause, with the affected muscle groups being more widespread and failing to respond to local treatment. These cramps occur during prolonged exercise in hot conditions and progress from an annoying sensation to a debilitating pain. Bergeron (2003) described the onset of heat cramps as being a sensation of twitching or fasciculation in voluntary muscle groups such as the calf or quadriceps, often first noticed when the player is stationary during a break in play. Within 20 to 30 min, these symptoms increase to full-blown and widespread cramps, in which a few muscle bundles contract at a time and then spread to adjacent muscle fibers. The sensation of the "wandering" cramp has been confirmed by electromyography.

According to one group of researchers, cross-sectional studies of athletes who have a history of these heat cramps have found that athletes experience extreme losses of fluid and sodium during exercise in the heat (Bergeron 1996, 2003; Stofan et al. 2005), with some studies showing that such losses are significantly greater than in a cohort of athletes who do not have such a history. Losses of other electrolytes (calcium, magnesium, and potassium) are not elevated (Bergeron 2003). The sweating profiles of 17 male tennis players with a history of heat cramps

during tournament have been presented as evidence that sodium and fluid deficits may be a potential cause of the problem (Bergeron 2003). These players were observed in tournament play during hot conditions (around 32°C and 55% relative humidity) and were reported to have a mean sweat rate of 2.6 L/hr (range = 2.0-3.4 L/hr). Sweat sodium concentrations in this group ranged from 23 to 61 mmol/L (mean = 45 mmol/L), leading to a total sodium sweat loss of 118 mmol/hr (2.7 g/hr). The range of hourly sweat sodium losses in these players was 1.4 to 4.8 g/hr.

Clearly, a player who has high sweat sodium concentrations can expect to incur substantial sodium losses with prolonged sweating. However, even with the lower sweat sodium concentrations typically seen in well-trained and acclimatized individuals, a large sodium deficit can accrue given high sweat rates and prolonged exercise times. In the Bergeron study (2003) a voluntary fluid intake of 1.6 L/hr was observed by the group of tennis players, which represents the high end of the range of reported drinking rates during real-life sporting activities (Broad et al. 1996; Noakes et al. 1988). Even when a sport drink (10-20 mmol/L sodium) is consumed at such aggressive rates of intake, replacement of sodium will only occur at rates of 0.37-0.74 g/hr. Thus, prolonged exercise will lead to a substantial sodium deficit during the session or over the day. Such a scenario has also been reported in groups of American football players (Godek, Godek, et al. 2005; Stofan et al. 2005) and soccer players (Maughan et al. 2004).

Repeated sessions of exercise in the heat can lead to chronic dehydration and sodium deficit unless aggressive rehydration strategies are undertaken. This exercise pattern is seen in tournament play or the two-a-day practices undertaken in the training camps of many team sports. Strategies to rehydrate after exercise have been previously discussed (chapter 1, goal 6) and include the replacement of sodium losses. The Western diet is generally considered to provide adequate, if not excessive, levels of sodium—through manufactured foods such as deliberately salted snacks and processed meals, takeaway foods, and the salt added in meal preparation or consumption. Many staple foods that are otherwise considered to be healthy, such as breakfast cereals or bread, also provide a substantial level of salt to dietary intakes. However, it is possible for athletes to fail to consume sufficient sodium in their everyday eating to replace very high sodium losses, especially if they deliberately choose heart-healthy or low-sodium eating. A case history of a tennis player with a 2-year account of heat cramps during prolonged matches in the heat reported that this athlete was consuming a low-sodium diet in response to a family history of high blood pressure (Bergeron 1996). Calculations of sodium balance found that it was possible for sweat sodium losses during play (sweat rates of 2.5 L/hr, moderate sweat sodium concentrations) to exceed dietary intake.

Replacement of sodium may be particularly difficult in the acute situation of recovery between two practices or tournament matches, where the athlete may not be able to consume everyday foods and balanced meals. Many sport foods such as sport bars and gels, or snacks such as bananas and confectionary items, are low in sodium content. A sodium deficit will not necessarily be detected through plasma sodium levels, because plasma homeostasis will be defended in the short-term by the reequilibration of body fluid compartments. In fact, according to Bergeron (2003), many cramping players present with normal or even slightly elevated plasma sodium concentrations because of the hemoconcentration from sweating. This may also explain why other researchers refute the involvement of sodium or other electrolytes in the etiology of cramps. Indeed, studies of sporting events fail to find differences in the hydration status and serum concentrations of electrolytes between athletes who report cramps and "noncrampers" (Schwellnus et al. 2004). Nevertheless, the observations of some clinicians working with players at risk of cramping are that sodium replacement during and after exercise is effective in preventing and treating this problem (Bergeron 1996, 2003). These observations need to be investigated further with controlled intervention studies.

Until more information is available, athletes with extreme sweat losses or high sweat sodium and a history of cramping might experiment with the following strategies (Bergeron 2003):

- Be aware of fluid losses during exercise by monitoring changes in body mass over the exercise session.

- Be aware of high concentrations of sodium in sweat via the detection of dried salt on the skin after the evaporation of sweat.

- Where these risk factors are present, develop strategies to rehydrate over the 2 to 6 hr after each exercise session by replacing fluid in volumes of ~150% of postexercise fluid deficit and by consuming sodium in fluids, foods, and meals.

- Achieve sodium replacement after exercise by consuming sport drinks and oral rehydration solutions, by eating salty foods (e.g., bread, breakfast cereals, pretzels, cheese, and processed meats), and by adding salt to cooking and meal preparation.

- During an exercise session, add extra sodium to fluids consumed on the field or court—for example, add 1.5 g of salt to each liter of water or sport drink. Although salt tablets are useful, they should be dissolved in fluid to ensure that fluid losses are also addressed. Specialized electrolyte replacement products (e.g., oral rehydration solutions) are valuable in providing a standardized sodium replacement regimen.

- At the first sign of heat cramps, consume a higher salt solution—for example, 3 g of salt (half a teaspoon) in a 600 ml drink bottle. In urgent situations, consider intravenous rehydration with normal saline.

RESEARCH TOPIC

Creatine Supplementation in Team and Racket Sports

When creatine supplements first hit the world of sport in 1992, the publicity was focused on sprint athletes and the success of certain British track-and-field athletes at the Barcelona Olympic Games (see chapter 7). Since then, creatine has caught the interest of both scientists and athletes. It is still one of the best-selling supplements in the sports world. But unlike most of the products on the market, it has been the subject of more than 200 studies on its effect on exercise performance (Rawson and Volek 2003). Sprint and power athletes continue to be the major consumers of this supplement. However, athletes in team and racket sports are also considered to be a target group for the benefits of creatine use.

As summarized in chapter 3, an increase in muscle stores of creatine may enhance the performance of exercise that is dependent on the creatine phosphate energy system—that is, brief high-intensity activity. Creatine supplementation does not appear to provide clear benefits to the performance of a single bout or the first of a bout of sprints. Rather, it is of most value to the performance of repeated exercise bouts or sprints (6-30 s) separated by a short recovery interval (20 s to 5 min). Proposed mechanisms to explain the benefit are an increased starting phosphocreatine content in the muscle or an increased rate of phosphocreatine resynthesis during the recovery period, producing higher phosphocreatine levels at the start of the next exercise bout and reducing the decrease in force or power production that would otherwise occur (for review, see Casey and Greenhaff 2000). Because the activity patterns in racket and team sports involve repeated short sprints interspersed with brief recovery periods, these sports appear to be a good candidate for creatine supplementation trials.

Theoretically, creatine supplementation could offer a range of benefits to team and racket sport players.

- Acute supplementation before a match could help the athlete perform the movement patterns and meet the activity demands of competition in team and racket sports, because these are undertaken in a repetitive manner with brief recovery periods.

- Chronic supplementation could allow the athlete to train harder and gain greater adaptations to training activities based on repeated high-intensity exercise. This includes resistance training, interval training, and simulated match play. Superior training could ultimately leave the athlete better prepared for competition.

Although the hypotheses underpinning creatine supplementation for team and racket sports are sound, several steps or hurdles must be overcome before we can be certain that the enhancement of muscle creatine stores in players involved in these sports translates into improved game outcomes. It is difficult to undertake studies that can adequately measure performance in team and racket games to allow the effects of an intervention such as creatine supplementation to be properly investigated (see the first research topic). Ultimately, team and racket sports are won by the execution of a skill—for example, a well-directed pass, a goal, or an unplayable shot. Creatine supplementation can only be of value if the enhancement of physical activity assists in the execution of this skill. This may occur if greater strength or endurance achieved through enhanced training increases the power of a shot or kick or attenuates the fatigue that would otherwise occur during a game. Alternatively, greater speed achieved through the training process, or via an attenuation of fatigue toward the end of a game, might allow a player to beat an opponent to the ball or to reach a better position from which to execute the skill.

Several studies have been undertaken involving creatine supplementation and racket or team sports. Details of these studies are summarized in tables 8.d, 9.d, and 10.c. Briefly, acute supplementation studies have reported positive outcomes to the movement patterns of soccer players (Cox, Mujika, et al. 2002; Mujika et al. 2000; Ostojic 2004), handball players (Aaserud et al. 1998; Izquierdo et al. 2002), ice hockey players (Jones et al. 1999), squash players (Romer et al. 2001), and a group of mixed team sport players (Ziegenfuss et al. 2002). Only four studies of creatine supplementation and activity patterns in team and racket sports—rugby (Ahmun et al. 2005), soccer (Biwer et al. 2003), and tennis (Op 't Eijnde et al. 2001; Pluim et al. 2006)—have failed to detect a performance benefit. A range of studies have examined chronic supplementation with creatine on the outcomes of the specialized training programs undertaken by team sport players. The most commonly studied scenario has been the resistance training programs undertaken by American football or other field sport players, with most (Bemben et al. 2001; Brenner et al. 2000; Kreider et al. 1998; Noonan et al. 1998; Pearson et al. 1999; Stone et al. 1999) but not all (Larsen-Meyer et al. 2000; Stout et al. 1999; Wilder et al. 2002) studies reporting that creatine supplementation enhanced the results compared with training with a placebo. The effects of chronic creatine supplementation on the interval training programs undertaken by football players from various codes has been less convincing (Kreider et al. 1998; O'Connor and Crowe 2003; Stone et al. 1999). Overall, although these results cannot be directly translated into enhanced match performance, they help to explain why surveys of team and racket sport players show that many experiment with creatine use. Creatine supplementation appears to be a popular practice among football players at elite and collegiate levels, with several studies reporting that more than two thirds of their sample of players used creatine (Greenwood et al. 2000; LaBotz and Smith 1999). However, even adolescent athletes appear to be significant consum-

ers of these supplements; 20% to 30% of respondents to surveys of large numbers of high school football players in the United States reported creatine use (McGuine et al. 2001; Smith and Dahm 2000).

Because chapter 3 encourages athletes to weigh the potential pros and cons of supplement use before deciding to use a particular product, athletes should consider the possibility of side effects from creatine use in team and racket sports. The risk of inadvertent doping was discussed in chapter 3. In general, there is no evidence of systematic side effects from creatine use, apart from a gain in body mass and a risk of gastrointestinal symptoms that most participants consider tolerable. Studies specific to team sport players include a longitudinal study reporting that three seasons of creatine supplementation by collegiate American football players, according to the accepted doses for loading and maintenance, did not appear to adversely affect markers of health status (Kreider, Melton, Greenwood, et al. 2003). A retrospective study of college football players found no difference in parameters related to kidney and liver function between players who reported creatine use (mean duration = 3 years) and a control group who used no supplements (Mayhew et al. 2002).

There have been anecdotal reports of an increased prevalence of muscle cramps, strains, and injury associated with creatine supplementation (Juhn et al. 1999). Several hypotheses have been proposed to explain such outcomes including musculotendinous stiffness and a disturbed cellular environment, secondary to fluid retention and dry matter growth in the muscle cell. An increased risk of heat injury when training in hot environments has also been proposed, resulting from the increased ability to undertake high-intensity exercise as well as fluid retention in the muscle. An increased exercise capacity and suddenly enhanced muscle strength could also be a cause of muscular and tendinous injuries. Although these theories sound plausible, evidence for an increased prevalence of muscle-related problems needs to be carefully examined.

A prospective study over three seasons of collegiate football tracked the number of injuries sustained in practice and games over a variety of weather conditions (Greenwood et al. 2003). The incidences of cramping, heat illness or dehydration, muscle strains, muscle tightness, and noncontact joint injuries among creatine users were reported to be lower or proportional to the rate of creatine use among players. The authors concluded that creatine supplementation did not appear to increase the incidence of muscle injury or cramping in American football players (Greenwood et al. 2003). A separate study using the same methodology tracked another group of American football players over a season (Greenwood et al. 2004), where roughly half of the 72 players volunteered to take creatine. In this group, the creatine users were observed to have a significantly lower incidence of muscle cramps and strains, heat illness and dehydration, and total injuries than the nonusers. Finally, a study exposed participants to creatine supplementation or a placebo for 4 weeks, reporting an increase in body mass and improvement in performance of a countermovement jump and drop jump in the posttrial testing in the creatine group (Watsford et al. 2003). Despite this evidence of functional changes in the muscle resulting from creatine use, there was no increase in musculotendinous stiffness in the triceps surae musculature. Therefore, there are no data to support an increased risk of muscle problems or injuries arising from creatine use.

Several studies have examined the effect of creatine supplementation on thermoregulatory responses to exercise in the heat. In one investigation, participants undertook a heat stress test that involved cycling for 40 min in a hot environment (39°C), before and after a 5-day supplementation period in which half the group received creatine and the other half received a placebo treatment. Participants were able to complete the work with a lower core temperature after supplementation in both groups, with differences between the groups being nonsignificant but showing a trend to a lower temperature in the creatine group (Mendel et al. 2005). In another study, a 28-day supplementation with creatine was associated with an attenuated increase in rectal temperature during 60 min of cycling in the heat compared with a placebo group (Kern et al. 2001). Finally, endurance-trained participants completed a time to exhaustion cycling protocol in the heat (30°C), before and after a creatine or placebo loading protocol (Kilduff et al. 2004). The creatine group showed evidence of hyperhydration as a result of their supplementation: increased intracellular water and reduced thermoregulatory and cardiovascular responses to the exercise. Although there was no change in endurance for the whole creatine group, participants were divided into responders and responders based on the uptake of the supplementary creatine estimated from urine creatine levels. Examination of performance changes in the responders subgroup showed a significant increase in time to exhaustion in the postsupplementation trial. Therefore, this study suggests that creatine supplementation may offer a benefit to thermoregulatory responses to exercise in the heat as a result of cellular hyperhydration.

In conclusion, despite caution from expert bodies regarding creatine use, especially in young athletes (American College of Sports Medicine 2000), there does not seem to be any evidence of long-term side effects arising from creatine use in otherwise healthy team and racket sport players. However, the current studies have tracked creatine users for relatively short periods (<5 years) who are using accepted loading and maintenance doses. Players contemplating creatine use should make an informed decision about this supplement. In general, groups with specialized health and nutritional needs such as adolescents are cautioned against the chronic ingestion of unusual products. However, the major reason for recommending against creatine supplementation in young players would be that against the improvements achieved through maturation and training processes, the benefits of creatine would seem unnecessary.

PRACTICAL ISSUE

The Traveling Athlete

A modern athlete is faced with an increasing set of opportunities to become an accidental tourist. It is becoming more common to travel nationally and internationally to compete and train. Many sports have national and continental competition structures, and the international calendar is filled with World Championships, World Cup events, and Grand Prix series in addition to Olympic Games. A modern athlete travels more often and for lengthier trips to find competition overseas and to take part in special training camps (such as heat training or altitude training). Although this trend is crucial to improving the standard of sport in a country and for the individual athlete, it raises a whole new set of nutritional challenges for the traveling athlete and the team management. To ensure that they optimize the gains from the experience and maximize the value of the large financial commitment, athletes need to recognize the following challenges of travel (Burke, Bell, et al. 2004):

• Being on the move interrupts the normal training routine and changes energy needs.

• Changing time zones creates jet lag and the need to adjust one's eating schedule.

• A change in environment—sudden exposure to altitude or a different climate—alters nutritional needs and goals.

• The new environment is often associated with reduced access to food and food preparation opportunities compared with the flexibility of one's own kitchen and routine. Leaving home also means leaving behind many important foods and favorite foods.

• The catering plan or expense account may not cover usual eating habits and nutritional needs, especially snacks and sport foods.

• A new food culture and different foods can be overwhelming to young athletes and those with fussy palates.

• Differences in hygiene standards with food and water in different countries exposes the athlete to the risk of gastrointestinal pathogens.

• Reading food labels or asking for food may involve mastery of a new language.

• A substantial part of an athlete's new food intake may be coming from hotels, restaurants, and takeaway outlets rather than being tailored to the special needs of athletes.

• The excitement and distractions of being away make it easy to lose the plot—with common challenges being "all you can eat" buffets and athlete dining halls, being away from Mum's supervision, and being confronted with a whole new array of food temptations.

Strategies to deal with these challenges are discussed in table 10.2 and should provide a blueprint for the athlete or manager who is organizing team travel.

Table 10.2   Issues and Strategies for the Traveling Athlete

Background	Guidelines
PLANNING AHEAD	
Good preparation solves many of the challenges of travel. The athlete will need to follow a good plan while away, but many elements of this plan will need to be organized ahead of time.	• Well before leaving home, take time to consider the issues likely to be faced on the upcoming trip. • Locate good sources of information about what to expect, including people who have previously ventured to the same destination or competition. • Consider issues such as travel itself, the general food supply at your destination, specific catering plans that are in place, and special nutritional needs arising from training and competition goals or from the new environment.
EATING AND DRINKING ON THE MOVE	
The challenge starts even before you arrive at your destination! Travel itself is stressful, changing both your nutritional needs (changes in activity levels, increased fluid losses in artificial environments) and your opportunities to eat. Changes in time zones must be taken into account. The air-conditioned environments of trains and buses and the pressurized cabins in planes increase the loss of fluid from the skin and lungs. Although fluid is provided regularly when flying, the small serving sizes are usually insufficient to maintain hydration. When you travel by road or rail, hydration is entirely your responsibility. A travel eating plan that matches new nutritional goals to food availability will help you to arrive at your destination in the best shape possible. This is especially important for the athlete who is constantly on the road.	• Contact your airline in advance of departure to find out what special meals consist of (e.g., low-fat, vegetarian, sport meals) and the timing of food service during the flight. • Plan food intake in advance and decide which meals you need and whether your own snacks are also required. Remember that inactivity during travel will reduce energy needs—you may not need to consume all the food on offer. • On long-haul flights, try to adopt the meal pattern you will have at your destination. This will help to reduce jet lag and adjust your body clock. • Travel is often boring. To avoid eating for entertainment, pack plenty of activities to keep yourself occupied. Reading material, travel games, playing cards, music CDs, and audiotaped books can all help to fill in the hours of unaccustomed "down time." • Chew sugar-free gum to decrease the temptation to eat unnecessary amounts or inappropriate choices of snacks during flights. Alternatively, pack your own snacks and decline the in-flight service. • When fuel needs are high, supplement the food provided in-flight with your own carbohydrate-rich snacks (fruit, rice cakes, sandwiches, bars). When traveling by road, pack your own supplies to avoid being tempted to stop at shops along the way. • Pack an additional supply of snacks in case unexpected delays cause you to miss meals. However, don't be tempted to eat them just because they are there. • Minimize the risk of constipation by choosing high-fiber foods in snacks and meals and by staying well hydrated. • Take your own fluid supplies when traveling and drink in appropriate amounts to avoid over- or underhydration. -Water reduces the risk of unnecessary energy intake from soft drinks, juice, or sport drinks when inactive. -Carbohydrate-containing fluids assist with fueling-up. -Electrolyte-containing drinks (sport drinks or oral rehydration solutions) assist fluid balance by promoting thirst and maximizing the retention of ingested fluid. -Although caffeine-containing drinks may cause a small increase in urine production, this has a minimal effect in habitual consumers.
THE TRAVEL FOOD SUPPLY	
Foods that are important to everyday eating are likely to be absent or in short supply at your destination. It is not always necessary to disrupt your familiar and successful eating patterns or risk missing out on important nutrients.	There are a number of foods and special sports products that can travel with you, or ahead of you, to establish a supplementary food supply. Depending on the travel destination, this may consist of the following: • Favorite foods that are unlikely to be available at the destination • Supplies to compensate for poor nutritional quality or unsafe meals • Snacks to supplement shortfalls in organized catering • Special sport foods or supplements that are a regular part of your nutritional regime or competition preparation

(continued)

Table 10.2 *(continued)*

Background	Guidelines
THE TRAVEL FOOD SUPPLY *(cont'd)*	

Background	Guidelines
Useful traveling supplies *General snacks* • Cereal bars • Dried fruit and nut mixes • Breakfast cereal + powdered milk • Dried biscuits, crackers, or rice cakes • Spreads: jam, honey (and Vegemite for Australians!) *When food availability or food safety is an issue* • Dehydrated meals (e.g., low-fat 2 min noodles, flavored rice) • Canned meals (e.g., spaghetti, baked beans) • Snack packs of fruit • Juice concentrate • Foil sachets of tuna or salmon • Long-life cheese (e.g., cheese sticks) • Powdered liquid meal supplements *Sport foods* • Powdered sport drink • Powdered liquid meal supplements • Sport bars • Gels *Useful equipment* • Cup and immersion heater to boil water • Snap-lock bags or plastic containers • Large plastic bowl and cutlery • Herbs and spices stored in film canisters to jazz up "ordinary" tasting meals	Tips for organizing a travel food supply include these: • Research the food availability at your destination as thoroughly as possible to avoid taking unnecessary supplies. Consider the weight of food supplies, especially if flying. • Reduce weight by choosing powdered or concentrated products where possible (e.g., powdered milk, concentrated juice, dried fruit). • Remove any excess packaging from products—snap-lock bags are a lightweight alternative to tins, jars, and boxes. • To avoid excess baggage on a flight, divide supplies among team members or freight supplies ahead of the team. • Check with customs and quarantine regarding foods restrictions in certain countries or states. Check to see if any taxes will be applied.

| **ACCOMODATE A NEW FOOD CULTURE** | |

Background	Guidelines
The fun side of travel is immersing yourself in a new culture. Of course, the priority is to find local ways of achieving your nutritional goals, balancing enough of the "tried and true" with the adjustments that a new country will require. You will need to identify new foods and eating styles that are compatible with your goals and how to tap into the best of what will be on offer. Eating is associated with a vast range of customs and cultural norms, and an athlete will need to understand these to avoid culture shock.	Issues that may need to be addressed in different countries: • Not all cultures consider the evening meal to be the most substantial meal of the day. • Siestas and long lunches or late evening meals may conflict with athlete's training timetable and desired meal schedule. • Eating utensils may include hands, chopsticks, or fork and spoon, with different etiquette regarding the serving of foods. • A shared style of eating may be expected in some cultures with norms regarding who serves, who eats first, and who receives the prize food. • Different staple foods are used to provide the main sources of carbohydrate, protein, fruits, and vegetables in the diet. These should be investigated before leaving home, with a visit to a relevant ethnic restaurant. • Language barriers provide a major challenge in foreign countries and interfere with understanding food labels, menu reading, and ordering in restaurants. It helps to understand a few key food terms and phrases, as well as general terms and phrases such as "please," "thank you," "I would like . . . ," and "what is . . .?"

Background	Guidelines
ESTABLISHING A NEW ROUTINE QUICKLY	
Hit the ground running, by adjusting your body clock and eating habits to the needs of your destination as soon as possible—even while traveling to get there.	• Move meal times as quickly as possible to the new time frame, including meals eaten while traveling to your new location. • Factor in not only the general adjustment to a new time zone but also the timetable of training and meals that your new environment requires. It may be quite different to the way you do things at home. • Enhance the adaptation to a new time zone and sleep patterns by a smart pattern of light exposure. Although special diets have been suggested to reduce the effects of jet lag and enhance body clock adjustment, the timing of meals, light exposure, and sleep is probably the most important factor in beating jet lag. • Remember that you may have different nutritional needs at your destination, resulting from a change in climate or altitude or a change in the energy expenditure of your training and competition program. Adjust your meal and snack routine immediately, rather than waiting for problems to occur.
FOOD AND WATER HYGIENE	
Even in safe-sounding destinations, you are exposing yourself to a new set of "bugs" and new routines of personal and food hygiene. Communal living, the stress of travel, and a new training and competition program may reduce resistance to illness. Being aware of the risks and behaving responsibly will improve your chances of an illness-free trip.	Minimize your risk of succumbing to gastrointestinal upsets or other easily spread illnesses: • Wash hands with soap thoroughly before eating or after blowing your nose or using the restroom, and dry with a clean towel or air-dryer. Antibacterial towel wipes are a handy aid. • If the local water supply is unsafe, drink only water that has been boiled or that comes from sealed bottles. If bottled or canned juice and soft drinks are used to provide fluid needs, the energy content will need to be taken into account. Make sure the seal of the bottle or can is opened in your presence, and wash the external surface of the container before drinking. • Avoid ice in drinks. • Avoid drinking water from the shower or pools. Clean teeth using safe water. • Food should be either steaming hot or refrigerated. It can be better to order à la carte from a restaurant so that the food is cooked to order. If buffet food service is used, ensure that the food is well cooked and kept steaming. All dishes should have their own serving utensil, and food should be protected from coughs and sneezes by a guard or lid. • Avoid salad and raw vegetables unless confident that these foods have been washed in bottled or boiled water. • Take care, and perhaps avoid, foods that are common sources of contamination: fish and shellfish, soft poached eggs, rare meats, hamburgers, stuffed meats, and pastries with cream fillings. • Eat only fruit that can be peeled, and avoid any fruit with damaged skin. • Avoid buying food from hawker stalls and street vendors. Choose food premises that look clean and busy and where staff use serving utensils to handle food. • Eat food bought from takeaway outlets immediately. • Do not share drink bottles, eating utensils or food, or towels with other people.

Table 10.2   (continued)

Background	Guidelines
FOOD AND WATER HYGIENE *(cont'd)*	
	If you do become sick: • Notify the manager or coach and isolate yourself from teammates. • See a team doctor or local doctor for treatment. • Drink fluids to combat losses from vomiting or diarrhea. Use an oral rehydration solution to compensate for lost electrolytes from severe diarrhea. • Stick to a bland diet during recovery. Avoid milk, ice cream, and other foods containing lactose, at least in large quantities for a day or two—this includes most liquid meal supplements. • Think about what foods or drinks you have consumed in the last 2 days to determine what may have caused the problem. Avoid and warn others about risky items. • Avoid handling or preparing food for others while sick. Take extra care not to share materials such as clothing or food and drink utensils.
ORGANIZING CATERING AHEAD OF TIME	
Let airplanes, hotels, or host families know about your catering needs in plenty of time to adjust. Special menus and special food needs may take time to organize, and in cases where your requests can't be met, advance warning will provide time to consider a "plan B." It takes time to look after the needs of a large group.	• Organize meal times and menus in restaurants and hotels ahead of time, especially if you have a large group or special needs. Buffet service generally provides more flexibility with food choices and quantities, as well as providing a faster service. • See chapter 9, practical issue 2, for a discussion of menu planning for athletes.
MASTERING RESTAURANTS, TAKEAWAY, AND DINING HALLS	
"All you can eat" and buffet-style eating provide many challenges, even when it is within an athlete village. A new style of eating requires a new style of behavior.	• Recognize the challenges of buffet style eating and athlete dining halls and adopt eating behaviors that allow you to eat what you need, rather than what is on offer (see chapter 9, practical issue 2). • Be proactive when ordering in restaurants and takeaways to choose meals and food items that suit the goals of sports nutrition. Extra attention to fluid needs, carbohydrate needs, and low-fat cooking styles may be needed.
DEBRIEFING FOR THE FUTURE AND FOR OTHERS	
Don't consider the trip to be over until you've had time to "debrief."	• Write all down your experiences while they are fresh in your mind—your memories will fade over time. • Review what you learned on your travels—what worked, what didn't work, what challenges still need a good solution. • Be prepared to share this information with other traveling athletes.

PRACTICAL ISSUE

Working With Tennis Players: An Interview With Dr. Michael Bergeron, Medical College of Georgia

Michael, let me start by asking how you developed a special interest in the physiology and nutrition of tennis, and to what level you have been involved in working with tennis players?

Twenty-five years ago, I was teaching and coaching tennis for a living. It became increasingly apparent, particularly with the more advanced players, that I was not able to provide sufficient information in response to their questions and needs specific to training and nutrition. For example, "How much and what kind of running or weight lifting should I be doing?" and "What should I be eating and drinking before, during, and after play?" were questions that I believed I was not prepared to adequately answer. As I inquired around, it was readily apparent that few others had any definitive information on these issues either. This is what actually prompted me to return to school. Tennis seemed like a great model to study physiology and nutrition because no one had done so to any great extent, but also because of my own personal passion for the game. Since obtaining my doctorate and completing a fellowship in sport nutrition, I have been involved with many levels of tennis, from juniors to top-ranked international players. Through working with the United States Tennis Association (USTA) and other international tennis governing bodies (i.e., ITF, ATP, WTA), I have been fortunate to have established a niche in the area of tennis physiology and nutrition with a particular focus on the demands of playing in the heat and managing fluid and electrolyte balance to optimize performance and reduce the risk for heat illness.

What sort of activities have you undertaken to investigate the specific nutritional issues of tennis, and what education strategies are effective in working with tennis players?

Most of my research studies using tennis players have been specific to examining issues related to fluid electrolyte balance (i.e., preexercise hydration status, fluid intake, sweat fluid and electrolyte losses, and perceptual measures) during training and competition and often the consequent effect on core body temperature. I have also done a little work looking at reported calcium intake and the effect of training on markers of bone turnover in young female players. Through the assessment of many individual players with heat illness history (particularly heat cramps), I have been able to obtain a much better understanding of dietary habits related to fluid and electrolyte intake but also with respect to other dietary factors such as carbohydrate and supplement intake for example. At certain tournaments, I've met one-on-one with a number of players (particularly from the women's tour) who have sought overall nutrition information as well as particular guidance on managing fluid balance in the heat. Tennis players are like most athletes. They pay attention to a variety of resources (e.g., coaches, trainers, other players) regarding nutrition information and recommendations and are willing to try almost anything if there is at least a purported positive effect on performance. However, like with most athletes, if you are able to measure and identify a player's own individual nutritional needs and subsequently demonstrate an immediate positive performance effect, then the athlete is a practicing believer. Relieving a player completely from the burden of heat cramps through an individual strategy of managing fluid and electrolyte intake is a powerful education tool. Visual aids work well too. No one really appreciates what losing 3.5 L/hr during a 4 hr match really means until you line up the bottles.

It seems to be that almost every year the media make a high-profile story about a top-level female player struggling with her body weight (accompanied by an unflat-tering photo and often some unsympathetic comments from male players). From time to time we see female players with a lean and athletic build who dominate play—the Williams sisters and Martina Navratilova spring to mind. How important are body fat levels in tennis performance? Do you think there is too much emphasis on body fat levels in female players?

Martina set the standard years ago, and even the other top players such as Chris Evert soon realized that they needed to adjust their own training regimen and goals if they wanted to be competitive. The Williams sisters raised the bar even further to a level that few have matched to date. Overall, it seems that the female players on tour are fitter and much leaner than before and certainly not fairly portrayed by selected unflattering photos that periodically appear in the media. However, it seems as though a female player can still be quite successful, even if she is carrying a little (or a bit more) extra fat, so long as she is strong and talented. Jennifer Capriati would be a good example. But again, this does not seem to be the trend. More and more you see the women participating in supplemental conditioning in the gym (even during tournaments) right alongside the men. This may be, in part, to help manage their weight, but it's also because the women recognize the value of fitness in preventing injuries and enhancing performance. Whatever the motivation, the net effect has been more lean and athletic female players.

Let's take the position that female tennis players appear to have more problems than their male counterparts in maintaining a level of body fat level that keeps them and their coaches happy and that some players are clearly "overfat." I can see several tennis-specific issues that could contribute to the problem: The lifestyle on the circuit, with its constant travel, takes players away from home at an early age and makes it hard to develop a sound eating routine. In addition, with so much competition play and so little time for background conditioning, it must be easy to get into a mindset of aggressively "fueling up" for matches that are actually quite brief and modest in energy expenditure. In your experience, how important are these factors, and what other issues can lead to chronic energy imbalances?

I'm not so sure that, except for early round matches against the top players, most matches are brief and modest in energy expenditure, especially on the clay courts. Moreover, many women are playing singles and doubles and even mixed doubles too at the Grand Slam events. So the volume of activity is often quite high for some players. But, yes, it is difficult to regularly fuel up and maintain energy intake on-court through consumption of a sport drink and not run at least a little bit of a risk for gaining weight. For a player who is trying to eat sufficiently but not consume too much food too close to the start of competition, delayed starting times also present problems. Through the educational efforts of the women's tour medical staff (and others), competitive female players are realizing that they can't diet extremely and compete successfully on the tour at the same time.

Strategies have been promoted to assist players in wise food selections to manage energy balance but also to provide sufficient nutrient intake to optimize on-court performance and avert premature fatigue, as well as to maintain health. If one is looking to lose weight or body fat, the recommended strategy typically involves small to modest reductions in calorie intake, improved food selections, increased supplemental conditioning, but also sufficient preplay and on-court nutrient intake to perform well.

Tennis is also famous for producing extreme environments in which players do battle. Our Australian Open has seen players taking center court in temperatures of up to 40 °C (even hotter on the court surface). What sort of sweat losses occur with such high-intensity games, often played to five sets, and how should a player try to combat such conditions?

Adult male and female players (and even many older adolescents) are typically capable of sweating at rates anywhere from 1.5 to 3.5 L/hr. The highest sweat rate that I have ever measured in a male pro player was 4.3 L/hr. With a match going three to five sets, it's easy to imagine the potential for extraordinary fluid losses and body weight deficits. Of course, most adults cannot tolerate consuming much more than 2 L/hr on-court. Moreover, even if they could consume more, the limitation in intestinal absorption rate would readily make them feel bloated. However, most players can match sweat losses with fluid intake up to almost 2 L/hr. If the sweat rate is higher than this, then the player can expect to incur a measurable fluid deficit that is proportional to the length of play. In these situations it's even more important for the player to come into the match well hydrated. However, one of the biggest problems is that many players do not sufficiently recover from the sweat-induced fluid deficits incurred during the previous matches. Consequently, one will develop an increasingly larger fluid deficit as the tournament continues and the player has to keep playing. Therefore, weighing oneself before and after a match would at least provide some insight into how much fluid needs to be consumed over the period of time before walking out on the court again (e.g., a 2 kg postmatch body weight deficit would require up to 3 L of appropriate fluid intake over the course of the evening and early the next day to restore the previous preplay level of hydration).

The television coverage of major tournaments often focuses on players taking drinks at the change of ends or between sets. Often the fluid is clear—it looks like water. What drinks would you advise players to consume during matches, and would you change your recommendation for various situations?

During any match, even if preplay meals are appropriate and sufficient, I think that most players would benefit from some level of regular carbohydrate intake. This is even more evident during intense matches in the heat, as an increase in core temperature will cause the body to use more car-

bohydrate at a faster rate. Sport drinks work well because the carbohydrate tends to readily absorbed (and the players need the fluid anyway). Moreover, the electrolyte content can help to prompt greater fluid intake and can be part of a player's overall management of sweat electrolyte losses. However, some players find it helpful to periodically ingest a little extra easily digested and absorbed (high glycemic index) carbohydrate between sets or in the later stages of a match.

Some players seem to have a problem with cramps in long matches in hot conditions. Do you have any personal experiences with this issue, and have you found any strategies that help these players?

More than for any other reason, a history of heat-related muscle cramps (heat cramps) has prompted numerous players (juniors through touring professionals) to seek advice from me. Quite simply, players who have experienced heat cramps tend not to match sweat electrolyte loss (particularly sodium and chloride—salt) with intake. The thought is that insufficient sodium intake, in response to extensive and repeated sweat losses, will prompt contraction of the interstitial fluid compartment, which causes selected neuromuscular junctions to become hypersensitive and seemingly spontaneously fire—often yielding painful and debilitating widespread muscle cramps. This scenario can develop even if a player is aggressively consuming fluid (without sufficient sodium). In fact, too much water intake can enhance the risk for developing heat cramps. Notably, at all levels of tennis, almost all players that I have worked with have been able to avert further incidence of heat cramps by consuming an appropriate amount of fluid and salt, based on an assessment of their individual needs, during periods of extensive play and training.

Finally, tournament tennis provides a grueling match schedule, with many top players also playing in doubles matches as well as their singles program. What are the secrets to recovery between matches, especially when there may be only hours or a day between contests?

The primary nutrients a player needs to consume between matches are water, carbohydrates, and electrolytes (primarily sodium and chloride). The less time a player has between matches, the more focus there has to be on these nutrients alone. With more time (e.g., several hours or more), a player can ingest greater quantities of other nutrients such as protein and fat that not only will assist in quelling hunger but will also play a role in more complete muscle recovery. Of course, there are tradeoffs. A player can often get away with consuming more fat and protein closer to playing doubles, for example, or even before another singles match, in an effort to reduce hunger and meet other daily nutrient requirements. It's sometimes individually quite variable, with respect to what a player can tolerate being in the stomach during competition.

chapter 11

Strength and Power Sports

Strength and power are important characteristics in the performance of many sports. This is most apparent in lifting and throwing events where the athlete produces a single effort to lift the heaviest weight possible or throw an object as far as possible. The ability to produce explosive bursts of power is also important in sprints and jumping as well as in the intermittent passages of play in team sports. American football, rugby league and union, and even Australian football (for some positions) require players to be highly muscled and powerful in order to generate speed and momentum. Bodybuilders also strive to be highly muscled, although the emphasis for competition is on appearance rather than function. Resistance training plays a varying role in the preparation of all these sports, from a supportive and periodized role in team games and sprint events to the major training focus in lifting events and bodybuilding. Although many strength and power sports are dominated by the male competition, in most sports there are now opportunities for females to train and compete at a high level.

Because of the number and diversity of sports that rely on strength and power, this chapter does not attempt to describe the characteristics of individual sports in great depth. Rather, the discussion is directed to the major nutritional issues underpinning resistance training and a brief consideration of the needs of athletes in lifting and throwing sports. In addition, because the culture of bodybuilding is so striking and focused on nutrition, some attention is paid to the beliefs and practices of athletes in this sport.

Competition

In lifting and throwing events, performance is based on the generation of explosive power for a couple of seconds, relying almost completely on anaerobic energy. Muscle stores of adenosine triphosphate and phosphocreatine are used to supply the energy for a single effort and are quickly regenerated between efforts. In the throwing events of javelin, shot put, discus, and hammer, athletes compete against each other in open competition. By contrast, in the sports of powerlifting and weightlifting (an Olympic sport), athletes are grouped together according to body mass, and in the case of subelite competition according to age. In each of these sports, athletes complete a number of separate lift categories—the snatch and the clean and jerk in Olympic weightlifting, and the bench press, squat, and deadlift in powerlifting. In weightlifting there is an outcome for each lift category as well as the total of both lifts, whereas powerlifting recognizes the total of all lifts. Depending on the event within lifting and throwing sports, the overlay of technique or skill involved in completing the required task ranges from small to complex.

During competition, the athlete is provided with a prescribed number of opportunities to achieve a maximum weight or distance. Typically, throwing events allow three opportunities per competitor, with the leading eight athletes having another three throws to decide the final placings of the event. The competition is usually conducted without a break and may take a couple of hours to complete. In large international competitions, a qualifying round may be held on the day before the final, with a qualifying distance being set for entry into the final. In the lifting events, each lift category is undertaken separately, with athletes attempting to lift a series of gradually increasing weights. Each competitor can nominate the mass of the weight at which he or she wishes to enter the competition, then continues with three attempts to lift each weight until eliminated. There is a weigh-in before the competition, usually 2 hr beforehand, and a short break between each lifting category. In the case where two lifters achieve the same final weight, the athlete with the lowest body mass is designated the winner, on a count-back. Typically, competitions in the lifting sports are conducted indoors in an air-conditioned arena. The throwing events are generally conducted as outdoor field events and may expose competitors to a range of environmental conditions.

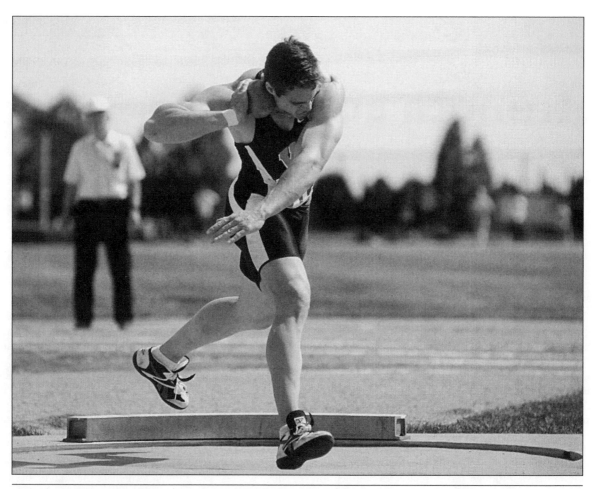

Whereas the lifts in powerlifting involve simple movements, Olympic weightlifting and the throwing sports are more technical sports, requiring greater flexibility and control of movement.

There is little evidence that acute nutritional strategies can benefit or hinder competition performance in these sports. First, muscle fuel stores are unlikely to be limiting for the performance of a single effort. Dehydration may be experienced by some lifters and throwers during competition; in the case where field events are conducted over hours in hot conditions without shelter, a mild fluid deficit can occur if sweat losses are not replaced while the athlete is waiting for their turn to throw. Lifters are even more likely to undertake their event with moderate to substantial levels of fluid loss, because many use dehydration techniques in the days before competition to make weight to reach their competition weight division (Burke and Read 1988a). However, although data concerning the specific performance of throwing and lifting events are not available, dehydration is not considered to impair maximal strength and power (for review, see Sawka and Pandolf 1990). In general, lifters and throwers are able to take a more relaxed approach to the nutritional preparation for their competition than endurance and team athletes, because their major nutritional challenges occur during the training phase. Nevertheless, strength and power athletes should be aware of the general principles of competition nutrition (chapter 1), and, in the case of lifting sports with weight divisions, the issues regarding weight making (chapter 12).

Training

Strength and power athletes undertake various types of training according to the demands of their event. Resistance training, whether undertaken as a small component of the overall training program or as its main focus, is a highly periodized activity. Components of the program are carefully planned within each session, within a week or microcycle, and within the longer training macrocycles. Specific activities are undertaken using free weights and resistance machines but may also include plyometrics and speed loading. Variations in programs include the duration and frequency of resistance training sessions, the number of sets of each exercise, and the number of repetitions and the load applied. The outcomes of resistance training that lead to an increase in muscle size or strength include neural adaptations, enhanced net protein balance (increased synthesis and reduced breakdown), and a hormonal environment that favors muscle anabolism. The contributions of these factors vary according to the stage of the resistance training program. Nutritional strategies for such training programs should both assist the athlete to train hard (optimizing the training stimulus) and provide a well-timed supply of the nutrients needed for the manufacture of new tissues (optimizing the training adaptations).

Although the phosphagen energy systems (adenosine triphosphate and phosphocreatine) supply the main fuel source for a single resistance effort, there is evidence that repetitive lifting in a training set also uses significant amounts of glycogen (Haff et al. 2003). Most of the available literature on glycogen utilization during resistance training has targeted sessions involving high repetitions (e.g., 8-12 repetitions) of moderate loads, such as those used during the hypertrophy phases of programs by bodybuilders and strength training athletes. Various studies have reported a 20% to 40% reduction in glycogen from the relevant muscles with as little as three to five sets of such training. In one study, five sets of 10 repetitions of knee extensions performed at a weight equal to 60% of one-repetition maximum (1RM) caused a 40% reduction in muscle glycogen content, whereas sets performed at 45% 1RM caused a 20% decrease (Tesch et al. 1998). Another investigation noted that six sets of six repetitions at 35% and 70% of 1RM resulted in 38% and 39% reductions in muscle glycogen (Robergs et al. 1991). Glycogen depletion was greater in the type II fibers than type I fibers in this study. Further research needs to be undertaken on glycogen depletion patterns in low-volume heavy-load resistance training protocols. Because low glycogen content has been shown to reduce strength in isometric exercise (Hepburn and Maughan 1982) and decrease isokinetic force production (Jacobs et al. 1981), it is possible that the depletion of this substrate can limit the performance of training sessions.

Other possible causes of fatigue or suboptimal completion of a resistance workout include depletion of phosphocreatine stores and intramuscular acidosis (Lambert and Flynn 2002). There is a substantial reduction in phosphocreatine content in muscles following multiple repetitions of high-intensity resistance exercise (Tesch et al. 1986). A well-constructed training program should provide sufficient recovery between sets for almost complete recovery of the phosphagen pool. Furthermore, increased muscle creatine and creatine phosphate stores may enhance recovery within and between sets, allowing the athlete to complete more work in the training session.

Physique and Physiology

The most obvious physical characteristic of strength and power athletes is a high level of muscularity; in some cases, this is accentuated for the esthetics of competition. Because lifting events are conducted in weight divisions (e.g., classes in Olympic weightlifting range from <46 kg to >83 kg for females and <54 kg to >108 kg for men), absolute levels of lean body mass and body mass vary across such power and strength athletes. However, most power and strength athletes aim for a large body mass and muscle mass.

In throwing events where there are no weight limits, athletes can carry high levels of body fat, by both community standards and athletic norms. Unless body fat levels become so high that they interfere with the athlete's health or body shape is changed so that it impairs technique, there seems little penalty for throwers to carry body fat. The exception to this is the javelin thrower, who has a longer run-up before throwing and needs to generate as much speed as possible. As a result, javelin throwers carry the lowest body fat levels among throwers. Where weight divisions exist, we might expect athletes to try to maximize lean body mass and restrict body fat levels within their weight category. This seems to be in evidence in the lower weight divisions of lifting sports; however, as the weight class increases, there is an increase in relative body fat levels along with absolute muscle mass. In comparison with other athletes in weight division sports, lifters seem less concerned about the need to achieve very low levels of body fat (Burke and Read 1988a). Heavyweight and super-heavyweight lifters may be justified in being concerned with absolute power rather than power-to-weight ratios.

Lifestyle and Culture

The world of muscle building is unique and insular. Resistance training athletes spend many hours in the gym in contact with other like-minded athletes, creating the potential for the exchange of ideas within and between sports. Typically, the nutrition beliefs and practices of strength and power athletes are based on trial and error, observations of top athletes within the sport, and sporting folklore, rather than scientific studies. These beliefs are largely shaped by a lucrative industry that produces magazines, supplements, and other training merchandise and often also owns or controls gyms and professional sporting competitions. Many strength and power athletes believe that mainstream sport science is focused on endurance sports and that conventional sports nutrition experts do not understand their needs and issues. Nevertheless, some supplement companies employ exercise physiologists to undertake research and education programs. The culture of strength and power sports is examined in this chapter from two angles: an examination of the world of bodybuilding (second practical issue), and a brief survey of the content of muscle magazines (third practical issue). It will be seen that word of mouth and word of magazine are very influential in spreading ideas within such a close-knit sports community. Although the Internet has the potential to increase the exposure of athletes to a greater range of information sources, in the case of strength and power sports it has probably simply reinforced the same messages. The most visible change associated with the growth of Internet has been to provide resistance-trained athletes with another forum to purchase supplements.

Dietary Surveys

A reasonable number of dietary surveys have been undertaken on male lifters, throwers, and bodybuilders, including national- and international-caliber athletes representing a variety of countries. Unfortunately, there is little information on the practices of contemporary athletes and world-class performers; the majority of published studies, summarized in table 11.a in the appendix to this chapter, are at least a decade old. Given the speed and enthusiasm with which strength and power athletes appear to embrace new science as well as fads, it is disappointing that recent information does not exist. Data on dietary practices of female athletes are less common, reflecting the smaller number of female competitors in most strength and power sports (table 11.b).

The available data show that the typical daily energy intakes reported by male strength and power athletes during normal training phases is ~15 to 20 MJ (3,500-4,800 kcal). Such intakes are similar to the absolute intakes reported by endurance athletes in heavy training. However, when expressed relative to body mass, the daily energy intakes of strength and power athletes are generally below 200 kJ (48 kcal) per kilogram and are lower than those of cyclists and distance runners (see chapters 4 and 5). Protein intake is a striking feature of the dietary intakes reported by strength and power athlete, typically providing ~18% to 20% of total dietary energy intake and reaching absolute intakes in excess of 150 g or $2 \text{ g} \cdot \text{kg}^{-1} \cdot \text{day}^{-1}$. Of course, these figures are mean values, and within these surveys are examples of groups who report daily protein intakes in excess of 3 $\text{g} \cdot \text{kg}^{-1} \cdot \text{day}^{-1}$ (Chen et al. 1989; Heinemann and Zerbes 1989; Kleiner et al. 1989) or above 20% of dietary energy intake (Baldo-Enzi et al. 1990; Bazzarre et al. 1990; Faber et al. 1986; Heyward et al. 1989; Keith et al. 1996; Kleiner et al. 1989; Van Erp-Baart et al. 1989a). The surveys of female strength and power athletes show a less consistent picture of dietary intake (table 11.b). As expected, intakes of energy and protein are lower than in male strength and power athletes, on the basis of both absolute intake and intake relative to body mass.

There are different patterns in the intake of other macronutrients with different groups of strength and power athletes; alternatively, changes have occurred over time. In the case of the dietary surveys of lifters and throwers, fat intake typically accounts for around 40% of total dietary energy intake, with carbohydrate intake providing a similar contribution to energy (Burke et al. 1991; Chen et al. 1989; Faber et al. 1990; Grandjean 1989; Grandjean and Ruud 1994a; Heinemann and Zerbes 1989; Van Erp-Baart et al. 1989a; Ward et al. 1976). Daily carbohydrate intake, expressed relative to body mass, is reported to be about 3 to 5 g/kg in these surveys. In contrast, some dietary surveys of bodybuilders report higher carbohydrate consumption at the expense of fat intake, with carbohydrate providing around 50% of dietary energy intake during training (Baldo-Enzi et al. 1990; Heyward et al. 1989; Keith et al. 1996; Tarnopolsky et al. 1988; Van Erp-Baart et al. 1989a; Zuliani et al. 1996). Among these athletes, daily intakes

equivalent to 4 to 7 g/kg carbohydrate are more typical, although there may be a variation in dietary intakes and macronutrient ratios in the different phases of the training and competition year (Heyward et al. 1989; Steen 1991); this is discussed in greater detail in the second practical issue. The low to moderate intakes of carbohydrate reported by strength and power athletes in the older surveys probably reflect leftover energy after protein foods have been consumed rather than a deliberate dietary choice. The available studies are unlikely to include groups of strength and power athletes who have been exposed to the recent resurgence of interest in diets that purposely avoid carbohydrate intake. New studies are needed to see how far programs such as the Zone diet and Atkins or ketogenic diets have infiltrated the dietary intakes of strength and power athletes.

Reported intakes of micronutrients appear also to differ between groups of strength and power athletes. Some studies of throwers and lifters have found reported intakes of vitamins and minerals from dietary sources that exceed the relevant recommended dietary intakes (Burke et al. 1991). By contrast, other studies have reported that although mean intakes for the group meet such standards, significant numbers of individual athletes reported intakes that were considered marginal—for example, less than two thirds of the recommended intake (Faber and Spinnler-Benade 1991). Nutrients most at risk of suboptimal intakes include iron, calcium, magnesium, and vitamins B_6 and C (Faber and Spinnler-Benade 1991), and the main cause was reported to be a reliance on processed and convenience food. Among surveys of female bodybuilders there are also reports that dietary intake fails to achieve two thirds of recommended intakes for minerals such as zinc (Bazzarre et al. 1990; Heyward et al. 1989) and calcium (Bazzarre et al. 1990). However, this outcome is considered to result from restricted energy intake. Further studies examining the nutritional status of these athletes, including biochemical and hematological results, are needed to investigate the adequacy of intakes of vitamins and minerals. Of course, the dietary intakes of micronutrients of strength and power athletes may not represent the final picture, because most of these athletes consume significant numbers of dietary supplements. How much these supplements contribute to total macro- and micronutrient intake, and how well total needs for these nutrients are met, are topics that merit investigation. In summary, although the present dietary literature on strength and power athletes provides interesting descriptive data, there is a clear need for further studies on contemporary athletes and the latest dietary practices.

Nutritional Issues and Challenges

A number of nutritional issues and challenges can be identified for the training and competition programs of strength and power athletes. Major issues are summarized in the highlight box on page 269, and they address concerns that are shared by lifters, throwers, and other athletes undertaking resistance training to increase muscle size and mass. It is probably fair to note that this assessment and the advice provided in this chapter may not be accepted by hard-core bodybuilders and other resistance-trained athletes. Although this textbook attempts to provide nutrition advice that is both state of the art and sympathetic to the athlete's perspective, it is anchored to guidelines and dietary strategies that can be reasonably supported by scientific studies. Many of the beliefs of serious strength and power athletes, and the ideas promoted to these groups, are different and even diametrically opposed to such nutrition advice. It may not be possible to achieve middle ground between conventional sport science and some of the extreme ideas from the flamboyant world of bodybuilding (see the second practical issue). On some occasions, the sports dietitian or nutritionist and the athlete will have to agree to disagree.

Because the competition nutrition needs of lifters and throwers can be achieved within the general guidelines for sport nutrition provided in chapter 1, the remainder of this chapter focuses on issues of nutrition for resistance training. Weightlifters are directed also to chapter 12 for discussion of the issues involved in making weight for competition.

Optimizing the Gain of Lean Body Mass

The overall success of a resistance training program is underpinned by the characteristics of the workouts and the athlete's training experience, gender, and genetic predisposition. To maximize the outcome, the athlete should practice dietary strategies that will support hard training, provide a hormonal environment favoring anabolism and reducing catabolism, and supply the nutrients needed to

Common Nutritional Issues Arising in Strength and Power Sports

Physique Issues

- Increasing and maintaining high levels of lean body mass for strength and power and, in some cases, appearance
- In weightlifting and powerlifting (weight-division sports): maintaining moderately low body fat to optimize lean body mass within weight category
- In bodybuilding: achieving low body fat level during period of competition to enhance appearance
- In other power and strength sports: maintaining body fat levels at a level consistent with good health

Training Issues

- Consuming adequate energy to maintain high level of body mass and lean body mass and to optimize gains in lean body mass achieved through resistance training
- Consuming optimal amount of protein at strategic times to meet increased requirements attributable to heavy training and to promote maximal gains in lean body mass achieved through resistance training
- Achieving adequate carbohydrate at strategic times to provide fuel for resistance training sessions and to optimize net protein synthesis response to training
- Achieving variety and moderation in food choices to achieve a healthful and nutrient-dense diet—being neither restrictive and overzealous (e.g., some bodybuilders) or undiscerning about food choices (e.g., some lifters and throwers)
- Considering creatine supplementation to optimize the response to resistance training
- Judiciously using supplements and sports food that have proven benefits or an ability to assist the athlete to meet nutritional goals
- In sports with an antidoping code, avoiding supplements with high risk of contamination with banned substances

Competition Issues

- In weightlifting and powerlifting (weight-division sports): achieving weight division with minimal impact on health or performance
- Preevent meal and intake during an event: following general strategies to keep the athlete well hydrated, well fueled, and comfortable.

build new tissues. Despite the history and popularity of muscle building, few studies have attempted to integrate the various nutritional strategies proposed to increase muscle mass in order to determine the optimal plan. Nutritional factors of interest include a positive energy balance, protein intake, and the frequency and timing of intake of key nutrients. Total protein intake and the strategic intake of protein and carbohydrate in relation to a workout are discussed in separate sections of this chapter.

A positive energy balance promotes a gain in body mass partitioned into lean body mass and body fat. Even in the absence of a training stimulus, a positive energy balance is associated with a gain in lean body mass, perhaps because of the elevation of anabolic hormones such as insulin, insulin-like growth factors, and testosterone (Forbes et al. 1989). Unfortunately, most studies have been undertaken with sedentary participants, and the interaction of overfeeding and resistance training has not been well characterized. Nevertheless, there is a considerable variation in the amount and distribution of the weight gain achieved by individuals, even when exposed to the same strategies (Bouchard et al. 1990).

At the onset of a resistance training program aimed at increasing body mass and lean body mass, the athlete will have increased energy requirements to cover the fuel cost of the training program and the energy cost of new tissue. The extent of this increase in energy need and the degree of positive energy balance needed to maximize the gain in lean body mass have not been studied systematically in athletes. Although it is possible to calculate the energy cost of a training program and new tissue—both for body fat and for muscle—this doesn't take into account the intricate nature of energy and protein metabolism. For example, Bouchard and colleagues (1990) noted that overfeeding is associated with a highly variable thermic response to food that significantly affects the partitioning of energy available for the development of new tissues. For most strength and power athletes, and particularly bodybuilders, a gain in fat mass is undesirable. Therefore, the aim of most resistance training programs is to maximize the gain in lean body mass and minimize the increase in body fat. The role of positive energy balance in achieving such a goal is debated by various experts. For example, in separate reviews, Grandjean considered that overfeeding is an important factor underpinning for the gain of lean body mass (Grandjean 1999), whereas Kreider concluded that overfeeding shouldn't be recommended to athletes because of the potential gain of body fat (Kreider 1999). The literature is surprisingly sparse in terms of investigations that address the dilemma. One study compared the results achieved with either an amino acid supplement, nutritional supplementation that achieved a positive energy balance, or resistance training alone. At the end of 10 weeks, the energy-supplemented group showed a greater gain in lean body mass than the other treatments (3.6 kg vs. 2.1 and 2.1 kg). However, there was no apparent advantage in terms of a superior improvement in strength (Gater et al. 1992b). Further studies are needed to determine optimal energy balance for gain of lean body mass without signifi-

cant gain in body fat. Interactive factors include the amount of protein consumed and the timing and distribution of energy intake over the day. In particular, investigations need to confirm whether there is a greater long-term gain in muscle mass and strength following strategic intake of protein and carbohydrate before, during, and after a resistance workout compared with the generic intake of these same nutrients over the day. In the meantime, some general strategies and the practical implications that underpin them are presented in the first practical issue.

Protein Needs

Strength and power athletes typically believe that a high intake of protein is required to promote optimal returns from training and to maximize their muscle mass and strength. Dietary surveys summarized early in this chapter found that such athletes typically report protein intakes of at least $2 \text{ g} \cdot \text{kg}^{-1} \cdot \text{day}^{-1}$ with some habitually consuming in excess of 3 g/kg of protein each day. As discussed in chapter 7, a belief in the benefits of a high-protein diet has been held by athletes for more than 2,000 years. Milos, a Greek wrestler from the sixth century BC, was revered as a strong man after winning the wrestling events at five Olympic Games (Ryan 1981). According to legend, his training and nutrition were intimately linked. He used to carry a calf around each day—her gradual growth probably provided the first progressive-overload resistance training program. When she turned 4 years old he carried her for the length of the Olympian stadium and then killed, roasted, and ate her. His typical daily intake of meat was reported to be about 10 kg! The high protein intakes of early athletes were probably underpinned by beliefs that the characteristics of animals that were strong and fast might be conferred by eating their flesh or by beliefs that muscles were fueled by protein.

The philosophies of exercise scientists concerning protein needs for strength and power athletes have varied over time and between groups. The view of the 1970s was that protein requirements are not increased by exercise (Durnin 1982). In fact, to this day, the dietary reference standards of the overwhelming majority of countries do not make any allowance for individuals who undertake habitual prolonged exercise; recommended protein intakes are typically set at $\sim 0.8 \text{ g} \cdot \text{kg}^{-1} \cdot \text{day}^{-1}$. The most notable dissenters of this view were scientists and coaches from Eastern European countries who promoted protein intakes of $3 \text{ g} \cdot \text{kg}^{-1} \cdot \text{day}^{-1}$. Athletes from these countries dominated sports such as Olympic weightlifting for many decades, providing a dimension of credibility to these guidelines. Nevertheless, there is little evidence from the peer-reviewed literature that such intakes enhance muscle mass and strength (for review, see Lemon 1991b).

The consensus statements on nutrition for sport produced during the 1990s, by bodies such as the International Olympic Committee (IOC), appeared to make some concessions to the special needs of athletes (Lemon 1991a). Increases in protein needs were recognized both for strength and endurance athletes, to account for the oxidation of amino acids as a fuel during prolonged exercise sessions as well as to allow for the production of new proteins in enzymes, hormones, and tissues as a response to the exercise stimulus. Strength and speed athletes were recommended to consume daily protein intakes of 1.2 to 1.7 $g \cdot kg^{-1} \cdot day^{-1}$, at least during the beginning phases of a new training block (Lemon 1991a). These recommendations were based on nitrogen balance studies that appeared to show increased protein requirements given habitual exercise of sufficient duration and intensity. The most recent reviews of the protein needs of athletes have returned to a more cautious approach to protein and exercise, acknowledging that much of the confusion and disagreement between experts stem from technical difficulties with protein research (Tipton and Wolfe 2004). Various interpretations of the outcomes of this protein research also cloud the picture.

Nitrogen balance studies, which monitor the balance between the nitrogen consumed (from dietary protein) and the nitrogen excreted (mostly in urine), have been the backbone of the research used to set requirements for protein intake. Such investigations have been undertaken in strength athletes by measuring protein balance in participants consuming various intakes of protein and then extrapolating to the zero line (Tarnopolsky et al. 1988, 1992). These nitrogen balance studies are notoriously difficult and expensive to conduct and carry various methodological limitations. Artifacts may arise because of the failure to account for energy balance, carbohydrate intake, and adaptations both to protein intake and a training program. The short-term nature of most studies means that they can fail to account for the increase in the efficiency of protein utilization and reduction in protein requirements after a period of training or the increase in protein utilization that accompanies a high protein intake (Millward et al. 1994). Both factors would lead to an overestimation of true protein requirement. On the other hand, strength athletes do not desire to be in nitrogen balance; rather, a positive nitrogen balance leading to an increase in lean body mass is the target.

The most important limitation of nitrogen balance studies is that they fail to directly address the questions asked by coaches and athletes—does a certain intake of protein enhance training adaptations and performance? Studies that track longitudinal changes in body composition and strength resulting from changes in dietary protein intake are surprisingly rare. Many of the available studies are of limited value; they were undertaken on noncomparable populations or conducted for short periods in which a detectable change in body composition would be unlikely (for review, see Tipton and Wolfe 2004). One investigation that supported the benefits of a protein intake in excess of the dietary reference standards monitored changes in lean body mass over 6 weeks of resistance training in experienced weightlifters (Burke, Chilibeck, et al. 2001). Participants consumed a daily protein intake of either 1.2 g/kg or 2.1 g/kg, with only the higher protein diet resulting in a significant gain in lean tissue mass over the training period. By contrast, however, a meta-analysis of studies of

various dietary supplements and their impact on muscle mass and strength changes with resistance training found that additional protein intake does not have a significant effect (Nissen and Sharp 2003).

Although the lack of systematic investigations is disappointing, the debate regarding the need for protein intakes higher than dietary reference intakes may be considered moot for the majority of athletes, especially those involved in strength and power sports. As shown in tables 11.a and 11.b (appendix), typical protein intakes reported by strength and power athletes are at least double the levels recommended in most population nutrition guidelines. Most male athletes report intakes of protein that are within or above the ranges suggested by sources such as the 1991 consensus statement of the IOC (see table 1.1). Female athletes and others who restrict dietary energy intake consume lower intakes of protein; typically, their reported intakes fall into the low end of the ranges of such guidelines. Strength and power athletes who fall into such a category may benefit from an increase in protein intake, but this can be achieved simply as a by-product of an increased energy intake. An additional benefit of a higher energy intake is that protein balance can be achieved at a lower intake of protein.

A potentially exciting chapter in the protein story is currently emerging from studies that use tracer techniques, often in conjunction with muscle biopsies, to monitor the acute effects of diet and exercise on protein synthesis and breakdown rates. Although there are still many questions to be answered before specific nutritional guidelines for resistance training can be finalized, the implication of these studies is that strategic patterns of protein intake may be more important than total dietary protein (see the first research topic).

Carbohydrate Needs

Many strength and power athletes do not see any role for carbohydrates in their diet. Indeed, the carbohydrate needs of strength and power athletes have not been systematically studied. However, carbohydrate intake could play a direct role in optimizing the gains achieved by a resistance training program in two separate ways. First, data from repeated sets of resistance exercise (Robergs et al. 1991; Tesch et al. 1998) indicate that glycogen is likely to provide an important fuel source for prolonged training sessions and that its depletion may be a limiting factor in the completion of the session. Strategies to ensure an adequate supply of carbohydrate substrate for the muscle may allow the strength or power athlete to train harder or to maintain better technique for the session. Second, the hormonal and cellular environment associated with high glycogen levels or following the intake of carbohydrate may be valuable if it increases net protein balance or enhances other aspects of recovery and adaptation, especially if the effect is additive to that of resistance training. Although these outcomes have been the subject of several studies, the results are hard to extrapolate into specific guidelines for carbohydrate intakes by strength and power athletes.

There have been no longitudinal investigations of the effect of total dietary carbohydrate intake on the outcomes of a resistance training program. However, several studies have examined the effect of acute supplementation with carbohydrate before and during a training bout on aspects of performance of that session. The results of these investigations are conflicting, with some studies reporting performance enhancement following acute carbohydrate intake (Haff et al. 1999, 2001; Lambert et al. 1991) but others failing to detect any benefits (Haff et al. 2000). A number of factors can explain this apparent lack of consistency, with the most important of these being related to the amount of glycogen used during the bout (Haff et al. 2003). An ergogenic effect is more likely when the training session is prolonged and involves a high volume of work; studies that report benefits of carbohydrate supplementation on resistance training involve sessions of ~60 min or longer in duration (Haff et al. 1999, 2001; Lambert et al. 1991). Carbohydrate intake before and during the session can allow strength and power athletes to do more work in a repetition set (Haff et al. 2001) or increase the number of sets and repetitions lifted before muscular failure is reached (Lambert et al. 1991). Carbohydrate intake during and after a session has also been shown to enhance the performance of a second bout of resistance training undertaken after a 4 hr recovery period, allowing participants to exercise for a longer duration and complete more repetitions and sets in the subsequent training session (Haff et al. 1999).

The effect of carbohydrate intake on the anabolic environment during and following a resistance training session has also received some attention. Specifically, the ingestion of carbohydrate increases insulin secretion, attenuating the muscle protein breakdown that normally occurs with resistance training (Biolo et al. 1999). In one study where carbohydrate was fed after a resistance workout, participants excreted less urea nitrogen and 3-methylhistidine—a marker of muscle protein breakdown—during the recovery phase and showed a slight increase in fractional protein synthetic rate (Roy et al. 1997). There is evidence that the postexercise stimulation of insulin by carbohydrate intake is later followed by increased blood concentrations of growth hormone (Chandler et al. 1994). Carbohydrate supplementation has also been shown to suppress blood cortisol levels in participants undertaking resistance training (Kraemer et al. 1998), presumably reducing the catabolic effects of this hormone. In prolonged endurance exercise protocols, a suppression of the cortisol response to exercise has been shown to counteract negative effects on the athlete's immune system (for review, see Gleeson et al. 2004). This has yet to be adequately tested during prolonged resistance training.

Finally, an understanding of nutrient–gene interactions and the cellular signaling pathways that promote muscle adaptations to exercise has created a new angle with which to consider the role of dietary carbohydrate. Commencing exercise with low compared with normal or elevated muscle glycogen content may enhance the transcription of a number of genes involved in training adaptations (Febbraio et al. 2003; Pilegaard et al. 2005). This is probably because several transcription factors have glycogen-binding domains, and when muscle glycogen is low, these factors are released and become free to associate with different targeting proteins. This information underpins the recent hypothesis that alternating muscle glycogen stores may be desirable to optimize the training response and adaptation—"train low, compete high." Indeed, a unique study of a 10-week endurance training protocol undertaken by previously untrained men has received recent publicity. This study required participants to cycle with one leg at a time, so that each leg could be trained separately. Although each leg did the same number of training sessions, these sessions were spaced differently to manipulate glycogen content in the muscle. The investigators found that the leg that trained with low muscle glycogen levels (two training sessions undertaken every second day, with the second training session being undertaken with minimal refueling) had a more pronounced increase in resting glycogen content and citrate synthase activity than the leg that trained with normal glycogen concentrations (one training session every day, with opportunity for refueling between sessions). Such adaptations would be favorable for endurance performance, and, indeed, exercise time to fatigue was more than doubled in the leg doing the two-a-day training. These results suggest that under certain conditions, a lack of muscle substrate might be desirable for optimizing the training response. If so, there might be value in implementing diets and training programs that intentionally deplete muscle fuel stores, at least in the short term. Of course, this needs to be balanced against the effect on the athlete's capacity to train and other negative side effects (see the second research topic in chapter 4 on high-fat diets for endurance athletes).

Whatever promise this unproven theory holds for aerobic exercise, it appears to have little benefit for increasing muscular size and strength. ERK 1/2 and Akt represent two of the signaling pathways that have been implicated in cellular growth and development in response to resistance training. In a recent study, a bout of resistance exercise was undertaken with high or low glycogen levels by trained cyclists. There was no change in the activation of the ERK 1/2 pathway; however, stimulation of the Akt pathway was greater in the high-carbohydrate trial than the low-glycogen trial, suggesting a more favorable response to training in a well-fueled state. Further investigation of the responses of specific cellular signaling pathways is warranted but should be coupled with studies that assess the outcomes of such responses on real-life training adaptations in athletes.

The improvement in net protein balance when carbohydrate is consumed after resistance training (Borsheim, Cree, et al. 2004) is minor compared with the response to postexercise intake of amino acids. In fact, the effect of carbohydrate intake on postexercise protein metabolism may be delayed. For example, in a recent study in which participants consumed 100 g of carbohydrate after a resistance workout, the improvement in breakdown in muscle protein did not reach a positive net balance (i.e., synthesis exceeding breakdown) until 3 hr after intake of the drink (Borsheim, Cree, et al. 2004). Because most studies of protein balance following exercise only last for 3 to 4 hr, it is possible that they fail to detect any delayed or longer lasting effects of carbohydrate intake. Therefore, the real effects of carbohydrate on protein synthesis after resistance training may be underestimated. Theoretically, the co-ingestion of carbohydrate and protein in conjunction with resistance training should enhance net muscle protein synthesis compared with protein alone. However, the available research suggests that the addition of carbohydrate to protein enhances net protein synthesis in a manner that is numerically, but not always significantly, greater than that achieved by the intake of a source of amino acids alone (Miller et al. 2003). The effects of protein intake after resistance training and its interaction with carbohydrate consumption are discussed in more detail in the first research topic in this chapter. This discussion includes a theory that there may be benefits in delaying the intake of protein after resistance training so that it coincides with the timing of peak insulin action from carbohydrate ingestion.

Further studies are needed to investigate the optimal amount of timing of carbohydrate intake in relation to resistance training and recovery and whether enhances training response. One study has examined the effect of 10 weeks of carbohydrate and amino acid ingestion following a bout of resistance exercise on the training responses achieved by previously untrained participants (Williams et al. 2001). This study used a one-leg design in which resistance training was undertaken on alternate legs on successive days, with a supplement supplying carbohydrate (0.8 g/kg) and amino acids (0.2 g/kg) being ingested after training one leg, whereas a placebo was received on training sessions involving the other leg. Although the supplement caused a substantial and sustained increase in the postexercise insulin response compared with the placebo condition, there were no differences in the improvements in strength between the supplement leg and the placebo leg.

Overall, the current literature fails to provide sufficient evidence to make definitive guidelines about carbohydrate intake for strength and power athletes. However, it is reasonable to encourage athletes to consume carbohydrate strategically in relation to training sessions so that carbohydrate availability is maintained during prolonged workouts involving a heavy volume of work. Consuming carbohydrate immediately before and during a workout may allow the athlete to train harder or better. Furthermore, postexercise refueling will assist with recovery of glycogen stores for a subsequent bout, even if it has only a small impact on the net protein synthesis rates arising from the stimulus achieved by the first workout. Strategic timing of carbohydrate consumption in conjunction with workouts may help to compensate for moderate intakes of total carbohydrate over the day. There do not appear to be any reasons to justify deliberate carbohydrate restriction by strength and power athletes, particularly in the form of very low (ketogenic) carbohydrate diets such as the Atkins regimen. Further studies need to be conducted to investigate the long-term effects of various patterns of carbohydrate intake on the performance of workouts and the overall outcomes of resistance training programs in well-trained athletes.

Lipid Levels

The 1980s saw the publication of a body of literature on the blood lipid profiles of strength and power athletes. This interest arose for a number of reasons. First, the high prevalence of the (illegal) use of anabolic steroids by strength and power athletes allowed the investigation of possibly deleterious effects of these medications on lipid subfractions. Second, although physical activity is believed to improve lipid levels and the ratios of subfractions, the early literature was limited to studies of aerobic exercise. Third, several characteristics associated with some strength and power athletes were considered to be atherogenic risk factors or, at least, contraindicated in the guidelines for a healthy lifestyle. These factors included having a high body fat content and consuming a large amount of saturated fat associated with protein-rich foods. The regular intake of large numbers of eggs, a well-known practice among muscle-building athletes during the 1970s and 1980s (Faber et al. 1986), was also targeted as a high-risk practice because of its impact on dietary cholesterol intake. Of course, these characteristics are not uniformly seen across all groups of strength and power athletes and may not be a contemporary concern.

The negative effects of steroid use on blood lipids were confirmed in one longitudinal study where bodybuilders were screened once during a period of self-administration of steroids and again after 3 months following the cessation of this treatment (Baldo-Enzi et al. 1990). A control group of bodybuilders who had never taken steroids was included to differentiate the effects of these drugs from those caused by training changes. Steroid use was associated with markedly lower levels of high-density lipoprotein (HDL) cholesterol, especially the HDL_2 and HDL_3 subfractions, compared with levels of control participants. This disturbance appeared to be transient, because there was a sharp improvement in lipid levels when the drug use was suspended. The lipid profiles of the bodybuilders who had never used steroids were similar to those of a group of sedentary control participants, suggesting that bodybuilding training (and lifestyle) did not have a substantial effect on cholesterol levels. The interaction of diet and steroid use was investigated in another longitudinal study of bodybuilders, which found that although fat intake affected on plasma cholesterol and triglyceride concentrations, self-administration of steroids was a much greater negative influence (Kleiner et al. 1989). A cross-sectional study of bodybuilders at a competition reported that about a third had a blood lipid profile that would be considered borderline to high risk for cardiovascular disease on the basis of elevated total cholesterol and low HDL cholesterol concentrations (Bazzarre et al. 1990).

Non-steroid-using bodybuilders were involved in an investigation that compared their lipid profiles with those of soccer players and age-matched lean sedentary controls, to see if resistance training improved cardiovascular risk factors (Zuliani et al. 1996). The absence of differences in total lipid levels and subfractions between groups suggested that any benefits from the training undertaken by

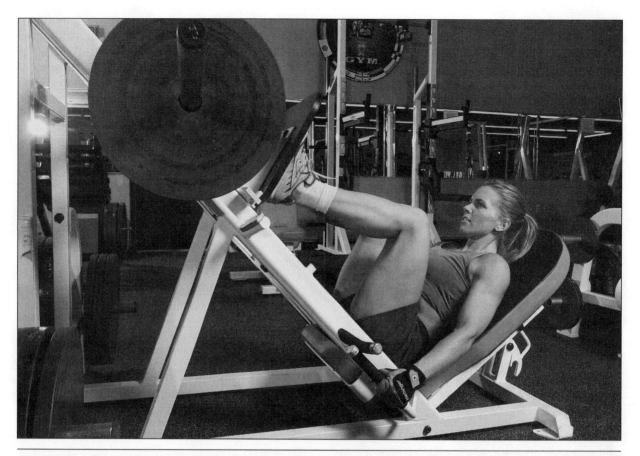

Given the variability in the presence of purported risk factors within and between groups, it is not surprising that the results of the available lipid studies of strength and power athletes show many inconsistencies.

the bodybuilders were counteracted by negative influences such as a higher intake of dietary cholesterol and saturated fats. Another study (Faber et al. 1986) found that despite dietary patterns that would be considered unfavorable in terms of saturated fat and cholesterol intake, lipid levels of a group of bodybuilders were within the normal range. Furthermore, a high intake of eggs (more than six per day) was not associated with a significantly higher total plasma cholesterol concentration; in fact, HDL cholesterol was higher in this group of bodybuilders than those who reported lower egg consumption. Of course, this information may be irrelevant to modern bodybuilders who, at least from anecdotal reports, choose low-fat versions of animal protein foods and consume only the whites of eggs to achieve their protein intake goals. Finally, a study of throwers found that a significant number of participants were hypercholesterolemic or had poor plasma ratios of HDL to total cholesterol (Faber et al. 1990). In this study, high levels of body fat were determined to be a major factor underpinning this problem.

It is uncertain whether the diets and training practices of contemporary strength and power athletes are associated with abnormal or suboptimal blood lipid profiles. Given the background from these older studies, it would be useful for future dietary studies of strength and power athletes to

include lipid status measurements as part of the nutritional assessment package.

Sport Foods and Supplements

It is hard to think of a sporting group that is more associated with the use of supplements than strength and power athletes. The history of sport supplements can be traced back to the earliest days of muscle building, and the contemporary sport supplement industry is particularly sensitive to the interests of gym-based athletes. A survey of the contents of four popular muscle-building magazines undertaken in preparation for writing this chapter revealed that 30% to 40% of the page space was taken up by advertisements for supplements and sport foods. In addition, supplements were one of the most popular issues covered in articles and columns. A study of five issues of similar magazines conducted a decade ago counted 624 different supplement products within advertisements (Grunewald and Bailey 1993). Although supplements targeted at strength and power athletes may have initially focused on products purported to increase muscle mass and strength or reduce body fat, the current range of products includes compounds and ingredients that are claimed to allow athletes to train harder, recover faster, reduce muscle injury, and increase their sexual function.

Not surprisingly, most sports dietitians and nutritionists find it hard to keep pace with the range and turnover of products promoted to strength and power athletes. It is challenging to keep up with the sheer numbers of products and to address the aggressive marketing campaigns prepared by supplement companies. Marketing tactics include testimonials from successful or satisfied consumers, including impressive before-and-after photos and accounts of the improvements achieved in conjunction with the use of the product. Sometimes these anecdotes are accompanied by disclaimers that the results are not necessarily representative of typical outcomes or that the participants received financial reward for their stories. However, this information is displayed in fine print. Although such endorsements and testimonials have a powerful influence on lay consumers, most sport scientists are aware of the limitations of this type of information and can educate athletes on such matters. It is more problematic for the sports dietitian or nutritionist to address the use of scientific claims and charges that products have been clinically proven to achieve various benefits. Many supplement advertisements include the endorsement of people who are claimed to be medical and scientific experts, provide written and graphic forms of data from studies, and cite references from peer-reviewed journals. This information is not merely an invention of the marketing arms of supplement companies; many of these organizations employ exercise scientists and sports nutrition professionals to undertake or coordinate the outsourcing of scientific trials and to prepare communications about the science behind supplements and sports foods. Although only a few of the studies of the efficacy of sport foods and supplements are directly undertaken by the companies that manufacture or market them, a larger number of studies undertaken in independent laboratories are funded by the companies. Unlike the case for pharmaceutical products, there is no compulsion for companies to undertake premarket testing of the efficacy of supplements and sport foods. However, many companies have realized that when undertaken well, research can enhance credibility and sales.

This textbook has promoted the well-controlled scientific trial as the best option for testing the value of sport supplements and foods and has encouraged athletes to seek the expertise of a sports dietitian or nutritionist on the use of these products (see chapter 3). Unfortunately, this may not always be sage advice. There is some debate within sport science circles about the credibility of research related to the supplement industry and the role of scientists who are directly employed by supplement companies. Clearly, many of these scientists work ethically toward goals that enhance sports nutrition science and practice. In fact, some are critical of the general sports nutrition profession, claiming that they are conservative and unwilling to provide proactive advice that is sympathetic to the real-life needs of athletes. On the other side, critics within the general community of sports nutrition and exercise science accuse the supplement industry of exaggerating the results of studies and suppressing negative findings in its product development and marketing. Other tactics that have been criticized include citing studies that are not directly relevant to the product involved—for example, animal studies or studies of ingredients that are present in the product rather than the product itself, without regard to the doses involved.

In finishing this chapter with a discussion of the supplements and sport foods that may be of documented benefit to strength and power athletes, we acknowledge that the majority of the products marketed to, and used by, these athletes lack proof of efficacy. Table 11.1, which provides a summary of sport foods and supplements with likely benefits for strength and power athletes, is dominated by products providing energy and nutrients in a convenient form to address everyday nutrition goals. Products such as sport drinks, sport bars, and liquid meal supplements may be used by the strength and power athlete before, during, or after a workout to meet needs for key nutrients and thus enhance performance and recovery in such a session. Logically, this should assist strength and power athletes to achieve optimal outcomes from their training programs. Such products may also increase energy intake and thus contribute to the positive energy balance needed to promote an increase in muscle mass and strength in conjunction with resistance training. Creatine was identified as the only product with strong scientific support for ergogenic benefits to resistance training programs (see table 11.c in the appendix to this chapter) and is discussed in greater detail subsequently. The use of caffeine or bicarbonate/citrate to enhance the ability to train harder is also a possibility, but has not been tested in the context of resistance training or overall gains in muscle mass and strength.

There is insufficient evidence to support the claims made for other products promoted to strength and power athletes. A brief overview of popular compounds such as β-hydroxy β-methylbutyrate (HMB), colostrum, chromium picolinate, ribose, *tribulus terrestris*, and free-form amino acids is provided in chapter 3, with table 11.d (see appendix) summarizing the results of studies of these products in relation to resistance training. In each case, the available data fail to provide substantial proof that these products provide either direct or indirect benefits to resistance training or performance. The majority of other supplements promoted to strength and power athletes and most of their individual ingredients have not been submitted to the scrutiny of a randomized controlled trial—at least, in the form of studies that have been published in the peer-reviewed literature. This list includes compounds that may have potential value—for example, caffeine taken as a training aid, with the intention of reducing fatigue and increasing the volume of work achieved in a resistance session. Although this theory has some merit based on results of caffeine studies of other prolonged exercise protocols, it

Table 11.1   Sports Foods and Supplements That Are of Likely Benefit to Resistance Training

	Product	Comment
Use in achieving documented nutrition goals	Sport drinks	• Use to refuel and rehydrate during prolonged training sessions and to rehydrate after the session. Contain some electrolytes to help replace sweat losses and increase voluntary intake of fluid.
	Sport bars	• Convenient, portable, and easy-to-consume source of carbohydrate, protein, and micronutrients for pre- or postexercise intake to aid recovery. • Low-bulk and practical form of energy and nutrients that can contribute to high energy intake and promote positive energy balance. • Convenient and compact source of energy and nutrients for the traveling athlete.
	Liquid meal supplements	• Convenient, portable, and easy-to-consume source of carbohydrate, protein, and micronutrients for pre- or postexercise intake to aid recovery. • Low-bulk and practical form of energy and nutrients that can contribute to high energy intake and promote positive energy balance. • Convenient and compact source of energy and nutrients for the traveling athlete.
	Multivitamin and mineral supplement	• Supplemental source of micronutrients for traveling when food supply is unreliable. • Supplemental source of micronutrients during prolonged periods of energy restriction (female athletes and bodybuilders during precompetition phase).
Strong potential for ergogenic benefit	Creatine	• Meta-analyses show that creatine loading is associated with enhanced response to resistance training programs. Evidence of direct stimulation of protein synthesis is equivocal. Effect is probably achieved as a result of increased training capacity—that is, enhanced ability to undertake repeated high-intensity bouts with short recovery intervals, such as resistance training. More sport-specific research is needed to ensure that this translates into better performance of events such as lifting and throwing sports. Typical protocols for creatine use: loading dose, 20-30 g in multiple doses (e.g., 4 × 5 g) for 5 days followed by maintenance dose of 2-5 g/day. Uptake appears to be enhanced by consuming creatine with carbohydrate-rich meal or snack. Acute weight gain of about 1 kg occurs with creatine loading, presumably as a result of fluid retention.

has not been directly applied to resistance training and the overall outcomes of a resistance training program.

Many of the more exotic supplements appear to have been manufactured purely on the basis of hypotheses. For example, several products promoted in muscle magazines purport to be nitric oxide (NO) promoters and are marketed with claims including vasodilation and enhanced blood flow to the muscle "a perpetual pump". The advertisements for such products note that they contain the amino acid arginine and related compounds such as arginine α-ketoglutarate or arginine ketoisocaproate. Other components include ornithine and citrulline. The many and diverse roles of NO in the body are a hot topic for many physiologists and medical researchers, and there is some emerging evidence that oral or intravenous supplementation with the amino acid arginine can increase NO production. However, at the time of writing of this book, there were no studies of long-term supplementation with arginine, or related compounds found in bodybuilding supplements, on NO production and its effects on training capacity in healthy resistance trained athletes. There was certainly no evidence

to support claims found in bodybuilding magazines that these supplements are "the greatest thing since creatine." It is not possible to make further comment about these and other unstudied supplements.

Creatine

Creatine supplementation has been enthusiastically embraced by many strength and power athletes, and there is a sizable body of literature from which to draw information about its benefits to the outcomes of resistance training programs. Studies of creatine supplementation and resistance training in previously trained participants are summarized in various chapters of this book. In this chapter, table 11.c presents the results of studies undertaken on strength and power athletes, whereas other studies of interest can be found in the appendixes to chapter 7 (table 7.b summarizing investigations of creatine supplementation and resistance training with sprint athletes) and chapter 8 (table 8.d, resistance training undertaken by team athletes). Many but not all these studies report that supplementation with creatine produces a greater response to resistance training than a placebo supplement, at least by producing a greater increase in strength measurements. Typically, studies also report an increase in body mass following acute supplementation and, in some cases, a greater increase in body mass following chronic creatine supplementation in conjunction with a resistance training program. It is uncertain if these outcomes translate into better sport performance—for example, superior performance in throwing and lifting events. The reader is directed to these tables to review the results of the various studies.

Several groups have attempted to summarize this literature by undertaking meta-analyses (Branch 2003; Dempsey et al. 2002; Nissen and Sharp 2003) or other forms of review (Rawson and Volek 2003). One meta-analyses of the literature involving a variety of supplements promoted to strength and power athletes concluded that creatine has a positive effect on the gains in lean body mass and strength associated with resistance training, with the effect sizes being small but significant (Nissen and Sharp 2003). A 2002 meta-analysis of the literature involving creatine supplementation and strength and power outcomes in healthy adults located 16 studies that met the authors' inclusion criteria (Dempsey et al. 2002). The authors noted that general flaws in the design of most studies included in the meta-analyses would tend to overestimate the benefit of creatine supplementation. They concluded that creatine supplementation improves the performance of absolute strength measures, such as 1RM to 3RM lifts, in resistance-training males. However, no overall benefits were apparent in females or in the performance of other measures such as cycle ergometer sprint peak power or isokinetic peak torque. Another meta-analysis with a 2003 publication found 96 publications (100 studies) that met its criteria of being double-blind studies of creatine supplementation with randomized group formation and a placebo control (Branch 2003). This meta-analysis examined effects of a range of creatine supplementation protocols (e.g., acute and chronic, with and without previous training) on a variety of performance outcomes. The author reported small but significant effect sizes for changes in body composition with creatine supplementation, with the effect sizes being greater for an acute protocol compared with a chronic or maintenance regimen. Specifically, creatine was found to have an overall effect on increasing body mass and lean body mass compared with a placebo, with minimal effect on body fat levels. Performance of brief bouts of resistance exercise (<30 s) was enhanced with creatine supplementation, with larger effect sizes being seen for repetitive bouts of exercise compared with single bout tasks and for upper-body exercise rather than lower-body or total-body tasks. No evidence of an overall effect of gender or training status on effect sizes was found in this meta-analysis (Branch 2003).

Finally, a 2003 review of the effects of creatine supplementation and resistance training on muscle strength and weightlifting performance included a total of 22 studies, ranging in duration from 7 to 91 days (Rawson and Volek 2003). Performance outcomes included 1RM testing of both large and small muscle groups as well as assessment of the number of repetitions performed in a resistance set using a standard weight. This review attempted a simple pooling of the results of these studies rather than undertaking a true meta-analysis. The authors noted that 16 of the 22 studies found that creatine supplementation produced a significantly greater improvement in strength or repetitive lifting performance compared with the gains achieve by the placebo group. The average increase in muscle strength in the creatine group was 20%, whereas the placebo group improved by a mean of 12%. Relative improvements in weightlifting performance (number of repetitions of a set weight) were 26% for the creatine group and 12% for placebo. Untrained participants appeared to make greater gains with creatine and resistance training than trained participants: The mean increases in muscle strength following creatine supplementation were 31% and 14%, respectively. Females were considered to respond similarly to males (Rawson and Volek 2003).

The mechanism of the enhanced gains in body mass and muscle strength with creatine supplementation remains speculative. Possible explanations include direct effects on protein transcription and expression (for review, see Hespel et al. 2001) or increased protein synthesis secondary to cellular swelling (Haussinger et al. 1993). However, because resistance training fits the criterion of repetitive high-intensity exercise with brief recovery intervals, it is also likely that creatine acts as a training aid, allowing athletes to train harder. In one study in which training volume was standardized for the duration of the 37-day protocol, there was no difference in the gains in strength achieved by the creatine and placebo groups. The authors concluded that in the absence of a potential for a greater training volume to be achieved, the main stimulus for the benefits of creatine was removed (Syrotuik et al. 2000). Further studies are needed to explain the apparent benefits of creatine supplementation for resistance training.

Amino Acids

Free-form, or individual, amino acids are a popular supplement for strength and power athletes and are available in tablet or powder form or as an additive to drinks and bars. A range of benefits have been claimed, including the stimulation of protein synthesis after a workout. The benefits of timely intake of amino acids in relation to a bout of resistance training are covered in greater detail in the first research topic. There is insufficient information to provide guidelines for the amount, type, and timing of amino acids to optimize this effect. In addition, there is no evidence that free-form amino acids alone achieve a superior effect to amino acids provided from the intake of food. Further research is needed to address this issue. This section deals with possible effects of amino acids that are separate from their role as building blocks of proteins.

Some amino acids, particularly arginine, ornithine, and lysine, have been claimed individually, and in combinations, to promote the release of growth hormone, leading to an increase in muscle mass and a decrease in body fat.

Arginine and ornithine are also purported to stimulate insulin release when consumed in combination with carbohydrate, enhancing anabolic activities including glycogen storage. These amino acids have been marketed as legal anabolic compounds, recovery agents, and stimulators of muscle growth. Two studies (Elam 1988; Elam et al. 1989) are often cited as supporting gains in muscle size and strength in participants undertaking bodybuilding training while supplementing with 2 g/day of arginine and ornithine (see table 11.d). However, these studies are considered to have an inadequate design, in one case lacking appropriate pre- and postintervention measures in the control group (Elam et al. 1989). Therefore, it is not possible to demonstrate whether the superior features of the treatment group in this study are attributable to the amino acid supplementation.

Data supporting the stimulation of growth hormone following oral intake of amino acids are sketchy and inconsistent. One investigation found only modest changes in growth hormone release following ingestion of large amounts (up to 20 g/day) of arginine and ornithine (Lemon 1991b). Furthermore, growth hormone release was found to be greater following heavy resistance training and was not further stimulated by the addition of these amino acids. Studies at the Australian Institute of Sport also failed to find improvements in growth hormone release following intake of 3 to 4 g/day of these amino acids (Fricker et al. 1988, 1991). In a series of studies investigating the interaction of training, food, and supplements on acute or late-night release of growth hormone, these researchers found that exercising in a fasted state produced the greatest growth hormone stimulus (Fricker et al. 1988, 1991). Inconsistent effects on growth hormone release were observed over 3 hr following the intake of ~2 g of arginine–lysine and ornithine–tyrosine amino acid combinations by bodybuilders (Lambert et al. 1993), while a twice daily supplementation with 3 g of a combination of ornithine, arginine, and lysine failed to produce any effect on growth hormone or insulin concentrations (Fogelholm, Naveri, et al. 1993). Finally, Collier and colleagues (2006) found that the oral intake of 7 g of arginine found that *attenuated* the growth hormone response during the 3 hr after a resistance training session. In this study, plasma growth hormone concentra-

tions were tracked at rest and after exercise, and with and without the arginine supplement. The total area under the curve of plasma growth hormone concentrations was largest in response to exercise alone, and while arginine supplementation also stimulated growth hormone release, the response to arginine + exercise was lower than exercise alone (Collier, Collins, and Kanaley 2006).

Other studies of the effects of oral amino acid supplementation on insulin responses are equally unconvincing. Ornithine supplementation (170 mg/kg) and postexercise arginine supplementation ($80 \text{ mg} \cdot \text{kg}^{-1} \cdot \text{hr}^{-1}$) in combination with carbohydrate feedings were not associated with an enhanced insulin response (Bucci et al. 1992; Yaspelkis and Ivy 1999). Chronic intake of arginine–lysine supplements (132 mg/kg LBM) for 10 weeks failed to change oral glucose tolerance test parameters in inactive participants or participants undertaking resistance training (Gater et al. 1992a). These supplements also failed to alter body composition or strength changes (Gater et al. 1992b). Finally, the potential role of arginine supplementation in enhancing the production of nitric oxide was mentioned briefly in an earlier part of this section. There are no studies in which oral arginine supplementation has been examined in healthy athletes to see if training capacity and performance benefit from the enhancement of this pathway.

In summary, it appears that the oral intake of amino acids fails to achieve the hormonal stimulation seen when amino acids are intravenously administered in clinical situations. Furthermore, very high intakes of some amino acids are associated with cramping and diarrhea (Yaspelkis and Ivy 1999). There is no convincing evidence to prove that amino acid supplements per se enhance hormonal response or increase the response to resistance training. Furthermore, the 2,000 to 3,000 mg doses recommended by many amino acid manufacturers can easily be obtained by eating common foods. Table 11.2 provides a few examples of food portions that are needed to provide 2,000 mg of branched chain amino acids, including leucine. Most athletes are unaware of the potential of their everyday eating patterns to provide the doses of individual amino acids or amino acid classes that are used in many research protocols.

Table 11.2   Sources of Branched-Chain Amino Acids (BCAA) in Foods and Sport Foods

Type of food or supplement	Amount of product needed to provide 2,000 mg of BCAA
Lean grilled steak	40 g (1.3 oz) cooked weight
Eggs	1.5 eggs
Low-fat milk	260 ml (1 cup)
Low-fat fruit yoghurt	170 g (2/3 cup)
Almonds	65 g (2 oz)
Whole-grain bread	145 g (5 slices)
Liquid meal supplement	45 g (1.5 oz) powder

Research Priorities

There is a gulf between the beliefs and practices of many power and strength athletes and the current sports nutrition guidelines. It may not be possible for sports dietitians and nutritionists to bridge this gulf. However, the priorities for sports nutrition research related to strength and power athletes are as follows:

- Dietary practices of elite strength and power athletes, including popular carbohydrate-restricted diets and supplement use

- Optimal intakes of energy and protein to maximize increases in lean body mass accompanying a resistance training program

- Carbohydrate requirements for optimal training outcomes, including the ingestion of carbohydrate before and during workouts to provide fuel for the session

- The amount, type, and timing of protein intake before and after resistance training sessions to promote optimal net protein balance; the value of co-ingesting carbohydrate to promote this outcome; the translation of improvements in net protein balance into enhancement of gains in muscle mass and strength

- The efficacy of various supplements and their ingredients on resistance training outcomes

- The prevalence of disordered eating among bodybuilders and the harmful effects of extreme dietary practices on health

RESEARCH TOPIC

Protein Needs for the Athlete: Timing and Type of Protein Intake May Be Important

The body protein pool is highly dynamic, undergoing constant synthesis from, and breakdown to, free amino acids that exchange between intracellular and plasma pools. To achieve an increase in muscle mass, or any other form of increase in net protein balance over any period of time, the instances of positive protein balance must outweigh those of negative protein status. This can occur through increases in protein synthesis, decreases in protein breakdown, or a combination of both (for review, see Tipton and Wolfe 2001). The specific study of muscle protein balance is complex and relatively new. Typically, expense and practicality limit the duration of these studies to periods of several hours; thus, measurements have been limited to the immediate response to exercise and dietary interventions. However, one investigation tracking net muscle protein balance over 3 hr following exercise and amino acid intake found that the improvement in protein balance compared with rest was maintained over a 24 hr period (Tipton et al. 2003). In other words, the immediate response to such interventions appears to be additive to 24 hr muscle protein balance rather than lost in a later counterbalance. Further support that acute measurements of protein balance can track the long-term outcome of interventions come from studies on muscle loss during bed rest (Paddon-Jones et al. 2004) and muscle gain during resistance exercise (Phillips et al. 2005). Taken together, these investigations provide some confidence in conducting and interpreting the results of acute interventions of diet and resistance training. This emerging research suggests that the timing and type of feedings consumed in relation to resistance training may have substantial effects on net protein balance. Further

improvements in knowledge may be made when future technology allows the measurement of the synthesis of protein subfractions rather than mixed muscle protein. In the absence of a direct measure of functional outcomes such as changes in muscle size and strength, this information would at least pinpoint that increases in protein balance occurred in protein subfractions of particular interest, such as the myofibrillar protein.

At rest, elevated blood concentrations of amino acids, resulting from either oral intake (Tipton et al. 1999) or infusion (Biolo et al. 1997), stimulate muscle protein synthesis and result in net muscle protein synthesis. The effects of resistance exercise and amino acid intake appear to be additive because the combination of these strategies results in a greater positive protein balance (Biolo et al. 1997). This outcome results mostly from changes in muscle protein synthesis rather than muscle protein breakdown (Biolo et al. 1997; Tipton et al. 2001). It has been hypothesized that the increase in muscle protein synthesis following ingestion of amino acids results from an increase in intracellular amino acid concentrations (Wolfe and Miller 1999). The increase in muscle blood flow associated with exercise would be expected to increase both the delivery of amino acids to the muscle and their subsequent uptake, explaining the additive effects of amino acid intake and a resistance workout. However, the results of other studies suggest that it is the extracellular concentration of amino acids within the normal diurnal range that regulates muscle synthesis, and that the effect becomes saturated at high amino acid concentrations (Bohe et al. 2003).

The response of muscle protein balance following resistance exercise appears to be influenced by the type of amino acids ingested. Several studies, including data summarized in figure 11.1, show that muscle protein synthesis is stimulated by essential amino acids only; the nonessential amino acids are not necessary for this process (Borsheim et al. 2002; Tipton et al. 2001, 2003). Individual essential amino acids, particularly leucine, are thought to stimulate protein synthesis, with this outcome arising from activity as a regulator as well as the direct supply of substrate for protein synthesis (Tipton and Wolfe 2004). The dose of amino acids needed to achieve a substantial increase in muscle protein synthesis appears to be small—as shown in figure 11.1, there are large responses to the intake of as little as 3 to 6 g of essential amino acids, which equates to 10 to 20 g of high-quality protein (Borsheim et al. 2002; Miller et al. 2003; Tipton et al. 2001). There is evidence of a dose response to amino acid intake; the results of several studies combined indicate that the intake of two 6 g doses of essential amino acids results in a response that is twice as large as that seen following the dose of two 6 g doses of mixed amino acids, each containing about 3 g of essential amino acids (Borsheim et al. 2002; Miller et al. 2003). It also appears that there is continued response to repeated intake of recovery snacks (Miller et al. 2003) but an upper threshold above which no further stimulation occurs. At present, the minimal dose of amino acids needed to produce a worthwhile response and the smallest dose needed to produce the maximum response are unknown.

The consumption of carbohydrate stimulates insulin secretion and decreases the normal stimulation of muscle protein breakdown (Biolo et al. 1999). The combined intake of carbohydrate and amino acids after exercise appears to optimize net muscle protein synthesis, by increasing synthesis and reducing breakdown. However, the available studies show that the additional effect of carbohydrate intake is small (Miller et al. 2003). This finding is displayed in figure 11.1.

The timing of intake of the recovery feeding in relation to resistance training has been explored in several studies. In one study, participants ingested 6 g of essential amino acids plus 35 g of carbohydrate either immediately before or immediately after an acute bout of resistance exercise (Tipton et al. 2001). The response of net muscle protein

balance, indicated by phenylalanine uptake, was considerably greater when the solution was ingested immediately before exercise. Another study using a similar methodology found no difference in net muscle protein balance when this amino acid–carbohydrate mixture was consumed either 1 or 3 hr following resistance exercise (Rasmussen et al. 2000). Comparison of the combined results of the two studies indicates that the response of net muscle protein balance was greatest when amino acids are provided immediately before exercise (see figure 11.2). This effect is most likely explained by the enhanced delivery of amino acids to the muscle by the increased blood flow that occurs during exercise. A longitudinal investigation of resistance training in elderly participants provides some evidence of the benefits of exploiting this outcome. In this study, participants who received a protein supplement immediately after weight training achieved greater improvements in muscle mass and strength over 12 weeks of their program than a group who received the same supplement 2 hr after each session (Esmarck et al. 2001).

There is preliminary support for manipulating the timing of carbohydrate ingestion relative to amino acid ingestion. The uptake of amino acids ingested immediately after a resistance training session is greatest in the first hour following ingestion and declines in the subsequent 2 hr (Miller et al. 2003). On the other hand, the major effect of carbohydrate intake on protein synthesis is delayed for several hours (Borsheim, Aarsland, et al. 2004; Borsheim, Cree, et al. 2004). This suggests that muscle protein balance may best respond by staggering or mixing the ingestion of these nutrients so that the responses are superimposed and maximized. Indeed, when a mixture of amino acids, carbohydrate, and whey protein was consumed after resistance training, there was evidence of two distinct peaks in net protein balance (Borsheim, Aarsland, et al. 2004). One, deemed to be a response to the free amino acids, occurred

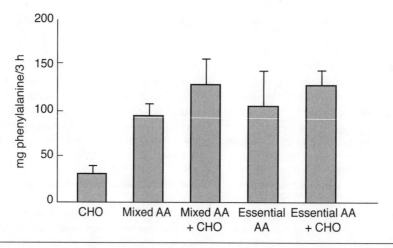

Figure 11.1 Effect of intake of amino acids (AA) and carbohydrate (CHO) following a resistance training bout on muscle protein synthesis.

Various feedings were provided to healthy participants over 3 hr of recovery from a resistance workout. CHO = 100 g sucrose; mixed AA = 2 × 6 g of mixed amino acids, including 3 g of essential AA in each dose, consumed at 1 and 2 hr postexercise; essential AA = 2 × 6 g of essential amino acids at 1 and 2 hr postexercise. Carbohydrate added to amino acid feedings = 35 g sucrose.

Reprinted from Tipton and Wolfe 2004.

within the first 30 min after ingestion, whereas the other occurred after 90 min, consistent with the delayed effect of insulin. Net protein balance following this mixed nutrient drink was directly compared with that achieved by an energy-matched carbohydrate drink and was, predictably, greater. But, compared with the findings of other studies using similar methodology, the presence of the whey protein in the drink appeared to prolong the effect on net protein balance typically seen with the intake of free-form amino acids. The authors suggested that this effect occurred because the slower digestion of the protein sustained amino acid availability for a longer period Another study reported that fractional synthetic rates of protein in the muscle were greatest over the 6 hr following resistance training when a mixture of free leucine, carbohydrate, and whey protein was ingested, compared with carbohydrate only and carbohydrate plus protein supplements (Koopman et al. 2005). Future studies are needed to test the timing and mixture of nutrients to optimize the total protein response to exercise.

One of the limitations of the studies discussed here is that they have involved healthy but sedentary participants undertaking a single bout of resistance exercise. Whether the same impact is seen with repetitive exercise—that is, training—is important. One study to address the issue tested previously untrained participants before and after an 8-week resistance training program (Phillips et al. 2002). A resistance bout involving only one leg was monitored, with protein synthesis and breakdown being measured separately across the exercised leg and rested leg while participants consumed a supplement providing carbohydrate and protein during the recovery period. Before training, the resistance bout increased rates of muscle protein synthesis and breakdown across the exercised leg, with the overall effect being a greater positive net balance across this leg than the rested leg (see figure 11.3). After training, a session conducted at the same absolute workload was associated with increased synthesis and breakdown rates in the rested leg but no further increase in the exercised leg. As a result, there was no longer any enhancement of net protein balance in the exercised leg. Because the exercise test in this study was conducted at the same absolute workload, it remains to be seen how training affects protein turnover when adjusted to the same relative intensity (Phillips et al. 2002).

It is challenging to set practical guidelines for recovery eating for resistance training based on the present literature. In addition to failing to address the timing and amounts of protein and other nutrients needed to promote optimal returns from resistance training, most of the present studies have focused on feedings of nutrients in elemental form—for example, free-form amino acids and glucose. Despite the marketing hype from the manufacturers of supplements, in real life, athletes receive the majority of their protein intake from foods providing a range of amino acids in combination with varying amounts of other nutrients in a unique food matrix. It is likely that just as carbohydrate-rich foods are known to produce their own effect on blood glucose, hormonal responses, and metabolism, foods providing a substantial source of amino acids also will also produce a specific postprandial amino acid and metabolic response. Knowledge about the digestibility and amino acid content

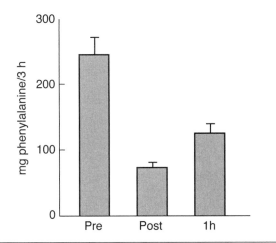

Figure 11.2   Effect of timing of intake of carbohydrate and amino acids after resistance training on muscle protein synthesis. Phenylalanine uptake, signifying muscle protein synthesis, over 3 hr following a resistance training session when 6 g of essential amino acids and 35 g of carbohydrate are consumed immediately before the workout (PRE), immediately after the workout (POST), and after 1 hr of recovery (1 H).

Reprinted from Tipton and Wolfe 2004. Data from Tipton et al. 2001 and Rasmussen et al. 2000.

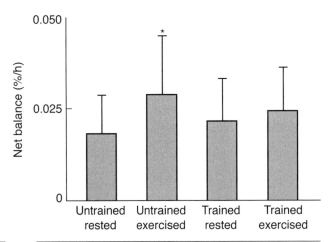

Figure 11.3   Effect of training on net muscle protein balance following a bout of resistance training and postexercise intake of carbohydrate and protein. A single session of resistance training acutely increased net protein balance compared with nutrient intake alone. Following training, the response to resistance exercise at the same absolute workload was attenuated.

* = P<0.05 greater than rested.

Reprinted from Phillips et al. 2002.

of protein-rich foods could be used to provide information to athletes with regard to the following:

- Sources of protein that deliver useful amounts of essential amino acids or specific amino acids believed to be important in enhancing net protein balance

- Sources of protein or other nutrients that might achieve a specific metabolic or hormonal profile that maximizes the effect on muscle protein synthesis

- The timing of intake that could allow peak amino acid levels to coincide with the timing of a desirable effect on protein metabolism (e.g., when to consume a protein source before a resistance training session to promote increased net protein balance during postexercise recovery)

Preliminary data from studies of sedentary participants have shown that the specific amino acid response to different protein sources has a differential effect on protein metabolism. Whey protein has been identified as a "fast protein" with a rapid, high, and short-lived amino acid response to its ingestion, whereas casein has been termed a "slow protein" because it produces a slower and more sustained amino acid response (Boirie et al. 1997). Different metabolic consequences of ingesting similar amounts of these two protein sources have been reported; whereas whey protein intake stimulated protein synthesis and oxidation, with no change to protein breakdown, casein intake produced a smaller increase in protein synthesis and oxidation and a marked inhibition of protein breakdown (Boirie et al. 1997). This latter profile resulted in better net leucine balance. Other studies have confirmed that protein digestion rate is an independent factor modulating protein deposition (Dangin et al. 2001, 2003).

Few studies of muscle protein metabolism in response to resistance training have used real foods or food proteins in their design. Although the anabolic responses to the intake of food proteins or whole foods in relation to resistance training have not been directly compared with those following free-form amino acids, it appears that they are similarly substantial (Tipton et al. 2004). It is tempting to suggest that that different muscle outcomes may be achieved by protein that provides a sustained amino acid response compared with protein that achieves a large but short-lived response, or that an optimal response might be achieved by a mixture of a quickly available amino acid source consumed in combination with a more slowly digested protein (Borsheim, Arsland, et al. 2004; Koopman et al. 2005). However, the literature is brief and unclear. One study compared amino acid balance across the muscle for 3 hr when solutions containing a placebo, 20 g of casein, or 20 g of whey protein were consumed 1 hr after a resistance exercise bout (Tipton et al. 2004). The plasma amino acid response to whey protein was larger and more transient than with casein. Muscle uptake of leucine, which reflects the sum of leucine utilized for muscle protein synthesis and oxidation, was greater from whey than casein. However, the uptake of phenylalanine, which has the sole fate of

protein synthesis, was apparently similar for both proteins. The authors concluded that despite differences in amino acid responses to the ingestion of these food proteins, the protein synthesis response related to the amount of amino acid ingested was similar.

Another investigation to involve protein sources or real foods reported that uptake of amino acids into muscle following resistance exercise was greater from milk proteins than from soy protein (Phillips et al. 2005). This study found that even when balanced quantities of total protein and energy were consumed, milk proteins were more effective in stimulating amino acid uptake and net protein deposition in the muscle after the workout than hydrolyzed soy proteins. This finding was independent of the differences in amino acid composition of the two proteins, and the authors proposed in contrast to the findings of Tipton et al. (2004) that it might be due to a different pattern of amino acid delivery. A follow-up investigation in young men who completed 12 weeks of resistance training (5 day/week) found that this difference resulted in a tendency (P = 0.11) for greater gains in whole body lean mass and muscle fiber hypertrophy with consumption of milk, although this didn't translate into differences in strength gain over this time.

Whether altering the timing of the intake of whole proteins mimics the results seen in studies of amino acids has also been studied (Tipton et al. 2006). A study compared muscle amino acid uptake in one group consuming whey protein immediately before resistance training, to another group who consumed the protein immediately after the workout. Both treatments increased net amino acid balance, and produced similar results whether the results were measured from the time of ingestion of the protein or from the time of the start of exercise. The authors concluded that the response of net muscle protein balance to timing of intact protein ingestion does not respond as does that of the combination of free amino acids and carbohydrate. Finally, a study comparing nonfat milk and whole milk found that amino acids may be utilized to a greater extent when fat is ingested at the same time as protein (Elliot et al. 2006). In this study, different groups of subjects consumed a cup of whole milk, a cup of fat-free milk, and a larger volume of fat-free milk that was an energy match for the whole milk. When the uptake of phenylalanine by the muscle was compared with the intake of this amino acid, there was a trend for a larger result with the whole milk. The authors suggested that the presence of the fat in whole milk may have increased utilization of available amino acids for protein synthesis.

We look forward to future studies of protein balance that confirm and refine our knowledge of dietary strategies that can enhance the net protein response to resistance training. In the meantime, it is premature to provide definitive guidelines for eating practices for strength and power athletes, other than to provide a good source of protein and carbohydrate before and after a workout and to support the fuel needs of a prolonged resistance bout. These guidelines are integrated into the advice offered in the first practical issue, "Eating to Bulk Up."

PRACTICAL ISSUE

Eating to Bulk Up

Gaining muscle mass and strength is one of the most common goals in sports nutrition. Therefore, it is both surprising and frustrating that guidelines for eating strategies to optimize this goal cannot be provided in the precise detail that other issues of sports nutrition enjoy. In this section, the best advice based on current evidence is provided. Two overlapping nutrition philosophies are offered to enhance the outcomes of a well-designed resistance training project:

- Achieving a modest positive energy balance over a sustained period
- Providing a timely intake of key nutrients before, during, and after a resistance workout to enhance the volume of training and promote maximal recovery

The increase in energy intake needed to promote an increase in muscle mass with minimal impact on body fat content is unknown. Typically, a daily energy surplus of about 2 MJ or 500 kcal over requirements for energy balance is considered a sensible starting point for a weight gain program. The athlete should also take into account the energy requirements of additional training sessions undertaken to promote muscle gain, increasing his energy intake to also cover these costs. Monitoring results over a sustained period should allow the athlete to fine-tune his intake, increasing energy further if weight gain is insufficient or reducing intake if gain in body fat is unacceptable.

In some cases, the total energy requirements of the athlete become difficult to achieve without a careful plan. The challenges of sustaining a high intake of energy were discussed in chapter 6 (first practical issue) and include issues related to poor access to food, gastrointestinal discomfort, appetite disturbances, and inadequate time to prepare and eat food in a busy lifestyle. Strategies to address these challenges were presented in table 6.h and include tactics related to organizing optimal spacing of meals and snacks, enhancing food availability, and managing appetite and gastrointestinal comfort.

Strength and power athletes are often concerned that a large intake of protein-rich foods is central to a gain in lean body mass and that protein supplements are also needed to reach protein intake goals. However, table 11.3, which provides the protein content of a range of common foods, shows that it is relatively easy to achieve daily intakes in excess of 2 g/kg BM (e.g., 120-200 g protein per day for the 60-100 kg athlete) when a variety of foods are consumed in a high-energy budget. For example, a meal plan providing 15 MJ (3,500 kcal) of energy contributes 140 g of protein, when protein is consumed at the level of 15% of dietary energy that is typical of most Western eating patterns. An intake of 20 to 25 MJ (4,700-6,000 kcal) per day, as is often required by large athletes with high energy requirements, would provide 180 to 225 g of protein even without a special focus on protein-rich foods.

Protein supplements, at least those providing a dedicated source of protein, are considered unnecessary by most sports nutrition experts—because of their expense and the current lack of evidence for a specialized role for protein hydrolysates, most free-form amino acids, isolated whey protein, or other fancy forms of protein. Further research is needed to investigate whether particular types or forms of protein and amino acid further enhance the outcomes of resistance training programs and whether these benefits can be duplicated through food forms of protein.

Many strength and power athletes become consumers of these protein supplements because it is part of the culture of resistance training groups and because foods are not marketed with the same hyperbole. Whereas the content of protein bars and powers is clearly labeled, it can often be difficult for an athlete to obtain information on the protein content of fresh foods and mixed dishes. Specialized information such as the type of protein found in foods (e.g., soy, casein, whey, gluten) or the amino acid profile is even harder to source. Athletes may be impressed by the purchase of a supersized sport bar that promises to deliver 35,000 mg of amino acids. However, they may not be aware that this translates to 35 g of protein, which can be provided in a small serving of meat (120-150 g cooked weight) or a range of meals or substantial snacks containing a variety of foods. Nutrition education is needed to assist athletes to use everyday goods to meet their nutritional goals.

Of course, there are occasions and situations when everyday foods are not a convenient form of protein—because of problems related to portability, perishability, preparation needs, or gastrointestinal comfort. Solutions to these problems can be found via packaged sport foods and drinks that provide a known amount of protein in a compact form. Sport bars and liquid meal supplements that provide a range of macronutrients and micronutrients in addition to protein are the products preferred by most sports nutrition experts. These products are less expensive than the protein-only choices and have the potential to address a number of the athlete's nutrition goals. When practicality is important, the athlete may decide that the additional expense of these purpose-built foods is warranted. However, the athlete can often find a homemade and lower-cost alternative to sport foods—for example, table 11.3 provides ideas for fortified milk drinks that provide an easily consumed form of energy, protein, and carbohydrate.

One strategy that the strength and power athlete may use to increase total energy intake is to provide nutrient support for resistance workouts. In particular, the athlete should fuel a prolonged session by consuming carbohydrate before and during the workout and a combination of protein and carbohydrate before and after the workout to enhance the muscle protein response. These strategies will help the athlete to achieve a positive energy balance over the day but may also promote better training and enhanced adaptation to the training stimulus. The strategic timing of key nutrients is a new interest in sports nutrition that offers the potential for enhanced competition performance through more effective training. This integrated approach to eating for recovery was discussed in chapter 6 (second practical

Table 11.3 Protein Content of Everyday Foods and Specialized Sport Foods and Supplements

Type of protein source	Amount of product needed to provide 10 g of protein
Animal foods	• 2 small eggs • 300 ml (10 oz) of reduced- or low-fat milk • 30 g (1 oz) of reduced-fat cheese—1.5 slices • 70 g (2.5 oz) of cottage cheese • 200 g (carton) of low-fat fruit yoghurt • 250 ml (cup) of low-fat custard • 35 g (oz) of lean beef, lamb, or pork, cooked weight • 40 g (1.5 oz) of lean chicken, cooked weight • 50 g (2 oz) of grilled fish • 50 g (2 oz) of canned tuna or salmon
Vegetable foods	• 4 slices (120 g) of whole-meal bread • 3 cups (90 g) of whole-grain cereal • 2 cups (300 g) of cooked pasta • 3 cups (400 g) of cooked rice • 3/4 cup (150 g) of lentils or kidney beans • 200 g (small tin) of baked beans • 120 g (4 oz) of tofu or soy meat • 400 ml (13 oz) of soy milk • 60 g (2 oz) of nuts or seeds
Supplements and sport foods	• 10,000 mg of free-form amino acids • 15-20 g (tablespoon) of high-protein powder or protein hydrolysate • 120-150 ml (3-4 oz) of liquid meal supplement • 60 g (2 oz) sport bar • 20-30 g (1 oz) high-protein sport bar
Less expensive alternatives to sport foods and supplements	• 25 g (1 oz) of nonfat milk powder • 250 ml (8 oz) of homemade fruit smoothie (Recipe for 600 ml = 250 ml of low-fat milk, 200 g of fruit yogurt, 1 banana or cup berries) • 150 ml (5 oz) fortified milkshake (Recipe for 600 ml = 500 ml of low-fat flavored milk + 4 tablespoons of ice cream + 1/4 cup of nonfat milk powder)

Research Priorities

Further research is needed to determine whether certain types of protein, including free-form amino acids, are superior to others in promoting the gains in muscle mass and strength following resistance training. Until such investigations are completed, the following simplified advice is offered:

- The strength and power athlete should consume a protein–carbohydrate meal or snack providing at least 1 g of carbohydrate per kilogram of BM and 10 to 20 g of high-quality protein just before and soon after the resistance workout. This is likely to make a worthwhile contribution to fuel needs and to provide at least 3 g of essential amino acids as used in research protocols to achieve a significant enhancement of protein synthesis.

- Everyday meals are likely to provide intakes of protein and carbohydrate that easily achieve these nutrient goals, but the athlete may not find it practical to consume meals so close to a session of resistance training. A well-chosen snack may also be able to meet these nutrient targets—table 6.h provides examples of suitable food combinations. Nutrient-rich drinks such as liquid meal supplements and fruit smoothies or purpose-built sport bars provide compact and portable snack options that are particularly suited to recovery eating in the training arena. The additional expense of specialized products such as liquid meal supplements and sport bars may be warranted when there are few opportunities for the preparation and storage of food at a training venue or when the athlete has gastrointestinal discomfort or loss of appetite in conjunction with high-intensity training.

issue), with table 6.h providing a summary of the principles of consuming a source of protein and carbohydrate before and after a resistance training session.

PRACTICAL ISSUE
The Culture of Nutrition for Bodybuilding

Bodybuilding is a sport, an art, and a culture. Bodybuilders sculpt their own bodies to challenge the limits of muscularity and definition. Although many bodybuilders compete in posing competitions and for titles, the goal for most devotees is simply to train to achieve their desired physique and appearance. It is a flamboyant and close-knit world that can only be fully understood from within. Nutrition and training fads change regularly and often dramatically. Ideas come from the hyped claims and testimonials spread by word of mouth in gyms or from publications such as muscle magazines and, more recently, the Internet. Most bodybuilders believe that conventional sport science and medicine do not address their needs and practices. This is probably true. However, it is also probably true that hard-core bodybuilders push the limits of what is ethical, safe, or scientifically supported in terms of their training and nutrition. Many sports dietitians and nutritionists who have tried to counsel bodybuilders find it hard to establish common ground with the extreme beliefs and practices of hard-core bodybuilders.

The bodybuilder's year is divided into three distinct phases: the training phase, cutting for competition, and competition itself. The training and nutrition practices of bodybuilders vary dramatically between these phases. Although there are variations between bodybuilders and new fads that appear and disappear, the following description provides an overview of the key nutritional issues and patterns during each of these phases:

- During the training phase or off-season, the main goal is to gain muscle size. Bodybuilders support their training outcomes by consuming high intakes of energy and protein, with a pattern of multiple meals and snacks over a day.

- Bodybuilders typically show a rigid attitude to food patterns, even during this hypertrophy phase. Examples of extreme and rigid practices include scheduling meals every 2 to 3 hr (even through the night) and limiting food choices to a small range. Typically, meals are based on protein-rich, low-fat food choices, and although attitudes to carbohydrate-rich foods appear to change from time to time, there is a general focus on choices that are low in glycemic index, low in fat, and high in fiber and micronutrients. Although these food choices are embraced by the principles of healthy eating and sports nutrition guidelines, the routine of many bodybuilders is to follow the same food plan, involving a small rotation of foods, for periods of months. An example of such a plan is provided in table 11.4.

- Although dietary choices are heavily focused on protein-rich foods, bodybuilders perceive that protein

supplements, including powders, bars, and free-form amino acids, are also necessary. Total protein intakes of bodybuilders from foods and supplements during this phase typically exceed 2 to 3 g·kg^{-1}·day^{-1}.

- In general, bodybuilders consume a large number of other supplements, including products providing prohormones that are claimed to provide steroid-like activity. Although these compounds are banned by antidoping agencies such as the World Anti-Doping Agency (WADA), a range of products containing prohormones can be purchased over the counter or by Internet and mail order in many countries. Use of anabolic steroids and other banned or illegal substances is rife among bodybuilders. The culture of cycling and stacking drugs also spills over into the use of legal supplements.

- Preparation for competition typically begins 6 to 16 weeks out from the event and involves energy restriction to reduce body fat levels and increase muscular definition. Typically, there is a substantial reduction in energy intake—for example, a reduction to 50% to 60% of usual intake during the training phase (Heyward et al. 1989; Steen 1991). Such extreme energy restriction produces a large and sustained loss of weight of up to ~1 kg/week (Heyward et al. 1989; Lamar-Hildebrand et al. 1989; Walberg-Rankin et al. 1993). Most of this weight loss appears to come from a reduction in body fat, even when body fat levels were already considered to be low.

- During this cutting phase, a further restriction on food range and intakes of fat and carbohydrate is often achieved. Many studies show that intakes of micronutrients drop below dietary reference intakes during this phase (Heyward et al. 1989; Kleiner et al. 1990, 1994; Sandoval et al. 1989), and although most bodybuilders consume large numbers of supplements, there is an ad hoc approach to supplement choices such that there is no guarantee that micronutrient intakes will meet recommended intakes.

- During the final competition phase, bodybuilders follow bizarre regimens designed to achieve final loss of body fat and cosmetic changes such as skin dehydration, muscle pump, and reduction of gastrointestinal contents. Such changes are undertaken to achieve the desired look of muscularity, vascularity, and definition. Some bodybuilders have experimented with carbohydrate loading to expand muscle pump, although one study has reported that this practice failed to achieve a measurable change in muscle girth (Balon et al. 1992). More typically, drastic alterations to fluid and electrolyte intake (Kleiner et al. 1990), and the use of dehydrating techniques including drugs such as diuretics, are used to alter muscle and skin hydration status. For example, one bodybuilder reported restricting his fluid intake to two cups of distilled water and eventually one cup a day during the week before a contest (Steen 1991). Another report noted that one bodybuilder did not consume any fluid for 3 days before a contest, in concert with other strategies to induce dehydration. This athlete died of a heart attack shortly after winning the contest (Balik 1993).

- The postcompetition period is often characterized by binge eating as bodybuilders relax after months of restricted eating, compounded by fasting and other extreme dietary practices in the period immediately before the contest. A case history has documented that a bodybuilder consumed 5,000 kcal (20 MJ) of energy on the day after the contest, compared with the mean intake of less than 2,000 kcal (8 MJ) of energy from the previous week (Steen 1991). Other studies have reported that bodybuilders double (Walberg-Rankin et al. 1993) or more than triple (Hickson et al. 1990) their intake of energy and increase fat intake by tenfold (Walberg-Rankin et al. 1993) during this postcontest binge. An example of this postevent eating is provided in table 11.4. This pattern suggests that some bodybuilders have problems with disordered eating and at the very least can expect to experience rapid weight gain after competition. In one study, bodybuilders reported a gain of 4 kg in 3 weeks after a contest (Walberg-Rankin et al. 1993), and another study reported a gain of nearly 9 kg in 4 weeks (Lamar-Hildebrand et al. 1989).

PRACTICAL ISSUE
Making Sense of Bodybuilding Magazines

Before the Internet, magazines provided the major forum for dissemination of information to strength and power athletes. Magazines continue to be an important influence today. Muscle magazines are often published by companies that manufacture and market supplements, own gym franchises, or organize bodybuilding competitions. Depending on your perspective, these magazines either reflect or direct the belief and practices of many athletes. A large readership and the involvement of top bodybuilders in articles and advertisements underpin the power of these publications to spread ideas around gyms and within the resistance training community. A number of exercise scientists and sports dietitians, usually on the scientific advisory boards or in the direct employment of supplement companies, are involved with some publications.

The sports dietitian or nutritionist who wishes to work with bodybuilders and other resistance training athletes should consider bodybuilding magazines as a useful resource. It is important to keep abreast of the latest ideas and products presented to readers of these publications. They often provide the first sighting of a new supplement and the rationale for its use or expose a radical dietary strategy endorsed by a successful athlete. Some of the material presented in these magazines is scientifically credible, and may provide the reader with up-to-date information on performance-enhancing nutrition strategies. Other information does not have sound scientific support—ranging from supplement advertorials (material written in the guise of an article that really serves as an advertisement for a supplement) to the paid or unpaid testimonial from an athlete. In between these extremes are articles that praise the benefits of supplements or eating strategies that have not yet been tested but which seem, on the basis of sophisticated hypoth-

Table 11.4 Example of food patterns of bodybuilders

Sample day for training phase	Postcontest binge (Walberg-Rankin et al. 1993)

Breakfast:
    Rolled oats and nonfat milk
    Omelet made with 10 egg whites
    Unsweetened apple juice
Morning snack:
    200 g of tuna in spring water
    Protein shake
Lunch:
    200 g of chicken breast
    2 cups of broccoli
Afternoon snack:
    Protein shake
    100 g of rice cakes
Dinner:
    200 g of grilled chicken breast
    1 cup of brown rice
    2 oranges
Evening snack:
    Protein bar
    Protein shake
	1 brownie
	2 cups of 2% milk
	2 chocolate doughnuts
	360 ml of beer
	1 cream popsicle
	2 cups of potato chips
	30 g of dip
	1 Hardees biscuit (bacon, egg, cheese)
	1 cup of hash browns
	1 cinnamon and raisin biscuit
	2 cups of Mountain Dew
	2 cups of Dr. Pepper
	1 Big Mac hamburger
	3 biscuits
	1 brownie
	1 piece of pineapple cake
	60 g of barbeque ribs
	9 scallops
	1 cup of steamed shrimp
	4 crab legs
	1.2 cup of seafood casserole
	1/2 cup of corn
	1 piece of strawberry shortcake
	1 piece of cheesecake

eses, to offer benefits to resistance exercise or recovery. Of course, these articles do not acknowledge the lack of controlled scientific trials on the effects of these interventions on actual outcomes in strength and power athletes. These authors of these features may be ahead of their time in predicting the next big thing in sports nutrition. On the other hand, they may simply be contributing to a short-lived interest in a strategy that will ultimately disappear. In any case, these publications offer an insight into the culture of bodybuilding and resistance training that may help the sports dietitian or nutritionist to develop rapport with and empathy for athletes with whom they are working.

An examination of popular bodybuilding magazines, undertaken at the time of writing this book, revealed the following findings:

• There appears to be a hierarchy within magazines, with a range in both the content and presentation style. At one end of the spectrum are science-focused publications presumably targeted at mainstream resistance training athletes. These magazines feature an editorial advisory board of exercise scientists and sports nutritionists with master's- and doctoral-level qualifications and often a track record in research. These scientists contribute articles on training, nutrition, and supplements and coordinate columns in which peer-reviewed research of interest to resistance training is summarized. Although many of the nutrition articles provide information that is consistent with the guidelines and research presented in this textbook, other material appears to go beyond what is scientifically defensible. Many such articles are written using a blend of scientific language and bodybuilding jargon and extrapolate from studies undertaken in animals or humans with diseases. It is likely to be difficult for the lay athlete to distinguish between credible and unsubstantiated information, because both may be presented with the same format including a sophisticated discussion of biochemistry and exercise metabolism and lists of scientific citations.

• At the other end of the spectrum are magazines targeted at hard-core bodybuilders with a greater emphasis

on competition reports, coverage of training routines of well-known bodybuilders, and advice columns provided by athletes. Nutrition articles in these publications tend to be shorter and less sophisticated.

• Supplements are the overwhelming nutrition interest of all the publications. Typically, more than one third of the pages in bodybuilding magazines are taken up by advertisements for supplements. The most highly promoted supplements are those promoted for fat loss and those containing prohormones. Prohormone-containing supplements, which are banned under most antidoping codes including the World Anti-Doping Agency, receive greater amounts of advertising space in publications targeted at hard-core bodybuilders. These magazines also encouraged readers to lobby against potential changes to government regulations regarding supplement manufacture and sale. Among supplements that could be considered sport foods (e.g., energy-containing bars and powders), whey-containing powders received most advertising attention.

• Supplement advertisements are constructed using emotive language, testimonials with exaggerated success stories, and hyperbolic use of scientific data. Other common marketing devices include claims that supplement formulas are associated with secret patents, scientific breakthroughs, and unprecedented delivery systems. "Advertorials" consist of 4- to 6-page articles that purport to give training and nutrition advice but focus heavily on the use of specific supplements. Claims of benefits from supplements are made as a statement of fact; there is no indication that a particular product may not actually have been studied.

• There is a small amount of nutrition advice that involves food use. Common themes include fat loss, low- or restricted-carbohydrate diets, nutritional characteristics of specific food items, and recipe columns.

• Question-and-answer columns are a popular inclusion in magazines. Readers' queries are addressed by a variety of experts ranging from successful bodybuilders to medical professionals and exercise scientists. Advice ranges from personal experience to evidence-based practice.

chapter 12

Weight-Making Sports

There are a number of sports in which competition is conducted with weight limits or weight classes. In some cases, such as lightweight rowing or sprint football, this is to provide a separate competition division for smaller athletes who would not be competitive in the normal or heavyweight version of their sport. In other cases, such as combative and lifting sports, weight classes are designed to promote competition between athletes of roughly equal size. Typically, body mass is considered a proxy for lean body mass or muscle mass and, therefore, the athlete's strength and power. However, in some sports limb length and body size are also an important determinant of performance—for example, the lever length of limbs is important in the biomechanics of rowing performance, and in combative sports, limb length influences the athlete's reach and leverage. In this case, body mass is meant to correlate to body size. In the final example, horse racing, the jockey's body mass is used to provide a handicap for the horse.

The intention of weight classes in sport is to promote fair and interesting competition by matching opponents of equal size and capability. However, the prevailing attitude in these sports is that the athlete will gain a performance advantage by competing against smaller and lighter opponents in a weight class that is lower than his natural training weight. Typically, the athlete aims to reduce his body mass to the lowest level possible, with much of this effort taking place in the days before competition. The rapid weight loss tactics used by athletes to successfully weigh in at a lower weight class are given various names in each sport. These terms include *making weight*, *cutting weight*, and *wasting*. In this chapter we refer to all techniques as *making weight*, and because *weight* is the term used in these sports in place of *body mass*, we will also use this term.

A number of the strategies used by athletes to make weight. These include mild to moderate food restriction as well as techniques to induce dehydration such as fluid restriction, exercise- and sauna-induced sweating, and the use of diuretics. Such techniques are diametrically opposed to the sports nutrition guidelines for competition preparation described in chapter 1 and are claimed to threaten the health and performance of the athletes involved. Sports nutrition professionals who work with these athletes are often troubled by the ethics of weight-making itself or the ethics of assisting athletes to undertake potentially harmful practices. It is easy to condemn weight-making practices—even if only on the grounds that they try to cheat the original goal of achieving fair competition. However, they persist despite the continued attention of medical, educational, and research bodies, because they have been internalized and even romanticized within the cultures of the sports involved. It is hard to shift beliefs and practices that have been ingrained for such long periods, but it is particularly hard to shift something that works. From the performance view, the penalties of replacing sound sports nutrition guidelines with weight-making are not as black and white as nutritionists and scientists outside these sports might first think. A number of arguments from within weight-making sports are offered in defense of their practices:

- The performance impairments caused by dehydration and energy depletion vary according to the type of activity, the frequency of the activity, and the environment in which it is performed. Sports that may incur fewer effects from weight-making are those of brief duration that are based on strength, performed in a cool environment, and performed infrequently. For example, a weightlifter who makes weight for an annual competition conducted in an air-conditioned arena may detect minimal impact on his lifting performance and overall health.

- In a few sports there is considerable opportunity for recovery after the weigh-in. For example, in some sports such as professional boxing, contestants weigh in on the day before the title match and have 24 hr to refuel and rehydrate.

- In most of these sports, absolute performance is not the issue. Rather, success is judged in comparison to other competitors. Although weight-making strategies may reduce athletes' performance, they may still be successful relative to their opponents. This is particularly relevant to combative sports. The culture of those involved in wrestling, judo, and other one-on-one competitions is that a larger person will

other one-on-one competitions is that a larger person will

maintain an advantage in terms of strength and reach over a smaller opponent despite performance losses resulting from making weight. In addition, the nature of the event allows a stronger competitor to play to this advantage rather than his weakness. For example, athletes may use their superiority to force an early end to the match with a fall or knockout, rather than allow the effects of dehydration to gradually eke away at their endurance over the full time limit.

• In some sports there are few weight divisions. Athletes in these sports will find it harder to find a weight class suited to their true body weight. In sports with a simple light versus heavyweight category (e.g., rowing), there will be a number of borderline cases who are too small for an open category but significantly heavier than the lower division. For these athletes the choice is to "size down" or not to compete at all.

• Finally, case histories sometimes show that the most successful athletes "make" considerable amounts of weight. It is possible that there is individual tolerance to the detrimental effects of weight-making techniques and at the high levels of sport a selection process takes place so that penalty-resistant athletes advance.

The goal of this chapter is to examine current weight loss practices by weight division athletes, within the context of the special characteristics of their sport. The evidence for deleterious effects on health and performance is presented, along with a discussion of programs that some sports have undertaken to reduce the severity of weight-making practices among athletes. Because this chapter attempts to discuss other nutrition issues related to training and competition in these sports, a different format is followed from other chapters in this book.

Defining Characteristics

Although each of these sports shares the characteristic that athletes must qualify for competition by weighing in at a designated weight class or division, a range of other features of a sport define and differentiate weight-making practices. These characteristics determine issues such as the type and extent of weight-making practices and what level of effect this might have on the athlete's performance and health. Such issues include the following:

• The number of weight divisions or weight classes in a sport, which provides flexibility for the athlete to choose a competition weight suited to his training weight

• The frequency of competition

• The physiological basis of competition (intensity and duration of the event)

• The environment in which competition is held: heat, humidity, altitude

• The competition schedule—single event versus series of bouts, heats or finals

• The timing of the weigh-in in relation to the start of competition (providing opportunity for recovery after the weigh-in)

• The requirement to weigh in before every event or bout within a competition, particularly when competition is conducted over several days

• Regulations within the sport regarding weight-making

Table 12.1 provides a summary of a range of weight-making sports and the characteristics that apply in each sport. Some of these features are discussed in greater detail in the following sections.

Horse Racing

Last week (jockey) Shane Scriven had to drop from about 56 kg to 53.5 kg to ride Opressor. This is what he ate: Monday—one meal of brown rice; Tuesday: an apple and an orange; Wednesday: one cob of corn; Thursday: a muesli bar; Friday: nothing; Saturday: nothing until after the races. "Saturday night had a good meal after a good day at the races. I didn't eat a lot though, because your stomach feels contracted after all that wasting.". . . Scriven says that he feels so much better since he has sworn off the weight reducing pills, which he depended on for some years. "My doctor said that if I keep doing that to my body I am not going to live long.". . . This week, Scriven has been giving the plastic bags a workout and on Sunday he walked for two hours. . . . This exercise if wearing plastic and wetsuits and then walking for such a period of time can result in a loss of about 2 kg.

Andrew Eddy, "The wasting game,"
The Age newspaper, Melbourne, Australia,
October 20, 1995, p. 28

Retired Hall of Fame jockey Angel Cordero Jr., winner of more than 7,000 races and three Kentucky Derby features, subsisted on a starvation diet. . . . "I only ate one meal a day for 34 years," he said. "It's very uncomfortable when you make all that money and can't eat like a person. Sometimes you let yourself go and have a pizza, but I had to pay the price the next day and I'd hate everybody who was with me." Cordero was so thin, when his spleen was removed after a riding accident that ended his career; the stitches couldn't hold the wound together. There was just no body fat. . . . "The scale of weights is killing a lot of kids," Cordero said. "You sacrifice so much it makes you weak. First you work in the morning, exercising horses. Then you have to pull weight without eating. Then you ride all day. Then you come home and can only eat a little bit. Then the next morning you do the same routine. It wears you out, mentally and physically."

Andre Baptiste, "Health problems in racing,"
The Independent newspaper, London
April 14, 2000, p. 30

Table 12.1   Characteristics of Sports With Weight Divisions

Sport	Weight categories	Description of competition	Rules and recovery
Horse racing—jockeys	Horses are handicapped according to age or ability, with handicap weight including saddle and riding accessories. Flat races are handicapped at lower weights than jump races. Minimum and maximum weight categories vary between countries and states and even within states (city vs. country race meets). Minimum weight in some races can be as low as 46.5 kg. In other races, weight handicaps vary between 51 and 57 kg.	Jockeys may compete in 2-4 race meets per week during season, with up to 8 rides during each meet, lasting more than 6 hr. Races are conducted over varying distances from 1,000 to 2,000 m (1-2 min) to special events such as the Melbourne cup (3,200 m). Riding involves controlling a horse weighing ~500 kg.	Jockeys weigh in 30 min before each race in which they compete. Jockeys of horses that earn prize money (plus next best finisher) must weigh in after the race to allow final placings to be confirmed.
Lightweight rowing	**Males:** • Average weight of crew shall not exceed 70 kg and no individual rower shall weigh more than 72.5 kg. • A single sculler shall not weigh more than 72.5 kg. **Females:** • Average weight of crew shall not exceed 57 kg and no individual rower shall weigh more than 59 kg. • A single sculler shall not weigh more than 59 kg. **Coxswain:** • Minimum weight is 55 kg for men and 50 kg for women and mixed crews. • Coxswain may carry up to 10 kg of dead weight to achieve this weight.	Elite-level regattas generally last 4-7 days with boat classes competing in heats, repechages, and finals. Each boat may expect to race each 1-2 days. Race over 2,000 m typically lasts 6-8 min.	Rowers are expected to weigh in on morning of each race for each boat class in which they compete. Weigh-in is conducted 2 hr before start of day's competition and lasts for 1 hr.
Olympic weightlifting	Male <56 kg <62 kg <69 kg <77 kg <85 kg <94 kg <105 kg 105+ kg Female <48 kg <53 kg <58 kg <63 kg <69 kg <75 kg 75+ kg	Competition is carried out over single session lasting several hours, with competitors competing in separate divisions of clean and jerk and snatch lifts. In each division, competitors nominate weight at which they wish to enter the competition and continue with 3 attempts to lift each weight, until they are eliminated. In case of a tie, competitor with lowest body weight is deemed the winner.	Weigh-in is conducted 2 hr before start of day's competition and lasts for 1 hr.

(continued)

Table 12.1 (continued)

Sport	Weight categories		Description of competition	Rules and recovery
Lightweight or sprint American football	A separate lightweight competition of American football is played at a small number of U.S. colleges to allow participation of players who are too light to be competitive in regular football teams. Weight limit = 75.4 kg (165.9 lb)		Separate teams of offensive and defensive players undertake game of 4 × 15 min quarters plus substantial time on (clock stopped for time outs and interval between plays).	Weigh-in is conducted 48 hr before game. Players must be <165.9 lb (75.4 kg).
Amateur boxing—male	Division Light fly Fly Bantam Feather Light Light welter Welter Middle Light heavy Heavy Superheavy	Weight <48 kg 48-51 kg 51-54 kg 54-57 kg 57-60 kg 60-64 kg 64-69 69-75 kg 75-81 kg 81-91 kg >91 kg	Competition conducted as tournament with successful boxers fighting every second day for up to 6 bouts over 10-14 days. Each bout = 4 × 2 min rounds.	All competitors weigh in on the first day of competition at an appointed hour between 8 and 10 a.m. to qualify for tournament. Boxers are required to weigh in again on mornings on which they are drawn to box, between 8 and 9 a.m. Boxing commences no earlier than 3 hr after the time appointed for the close of weigh-in.
Professional boxing—male	17 weight classes according to WBA Minimum or straw Light fly Fly Superfly Bantam Superbantam Feather Superfeather Light Superlight Welter Superwelter Middle Supermiddle Lightheavy Cruiser Heavy	<47.63 <48.99 <50.80 <52.16 <53.52 <55.34 <57.15 <58.97 <61.23 <63.50 <66.68 <69.85 <72.57 <76.20 <79.38 <90.72 90.72+	Numerous national and international professional boxing organizations with different rules. Rules are presented for WBA. Competition conducted as fight between two competitors over 4 × 3 min to 12 × 3 min rounds (1 min between rounds).	Weigh-in occurs between 4 and 8 p.m. the day before the fight. If boxer is overweight, an additional 2 hr is allowed to meet prescribed weight.

Sport	Weight divisions	Competition	Weigh-in
Judo	**Male** <60 kg, <66 kg, <73 kg, <81 kg, <90, 100 kg **Female** <48 kg, <52 kg, <57 kg, <63 kg, <70 kg, 78 kg	Tournament conducted over a single day with draw requiring competitors to contest 4 or 5 bouts to decide winner. Each bout = 4 min (females) and 5 min (males). Minimum of 10 minutes between bouts.	Minimum time between weigh-in and start of competition is 2 hr. Weigh-in conducted as trial period (1 hr) followed by official period (1 hr).
Karate	Weight divisions only in individual competition **Male** <60 kg, <65 kg, <70 kg, <75 kg, 80 kg **Female** <53 kg, 60 kg	Tournament over a single day with 6-8 bouts according to number of competitors in draw. Bout = 3 min (males) and 2 min (females),	Weigh-in at international competition conducted day before competition.
Taekwando	4 divisions at Olympic competition and 8 divisions at World Championships Division / Male / Female: Fly <58 kg / <49 kg; Feather 58-68 kg / 49-57 kg; Welter 68-80 kg / 57-67 kg; Heavy >80 kg / >67 kg	Competition is conducted as a single-day tournament with competitors undertaking 5-8 bouts. Each bout = 3 × 3 min rounds with 1 min between rounds.	Weigh-in on morning of competition. Weigh-in lasts 1 hr, usually 1-2 hr before start of competition.
International wrestling—Greco-Roman and freestyle	Olympic competition now recognizes male and female competition with weight divisions **Male** 55 kg, 60 kg, 66 kg, 74 kg, 84 kg, 96 kg, 120 kg **Female** 48 kg, 55 kg, 63 kg, 72 kg	Competition for each weight category is conducted over a single day with competitors undertaking up to 4 bouts. Bout = 2 × 3 min + 30 s rest period. Additional 3 min may be required in international competition if match is tied or inadequate points are scored.	Weigh-in is conducted the day before competition.

(continued)

Table 12.1 (continued)

Sport	Weight categories	Description of competition	Rules and recovery
Collegiate wrestling (NCAA rules, 2004)	10 weight classes 56.8 kg (125 lb) 60.4 kg (133 lb) 64.1 kg (141 lb) 67.7 kg (149 lb) 71.4 kg (157 lb) 75 kg (165 lb) 79.1 kg (174 lb) 83.6 kg (184 lb) 89.5 kg (197 lb) 83-129.5 kg (183-285 lb)	Competitions are held between teams with one wrestler in each weight class: Matches are 7 min long divided into 3 periods: 3 min, 2 min, 2 min. Competition can be undertaken as single day meets between 2 and 4 teams or tournaments lasting 1 or several days.	Dual–triangular–quadrangular meets: Weigh-in begins 1 hr before meet starts. Order of competition is randomly selected after weigh-in so time to event varies from meet to meet. Tournaments: weigh-in is conducted 2 hr or less before first matches on first day and 1 hr or less before matches on subsequent days. Competition is held with lightest weight classes first

WBA = World Boxing Association; NCAA = National Collegiate Athletic Association.

The circumstances underpinning the weight-making practices of jockeys are perhaps the most severe of all weight division sports. First, the weight targets that jockeys must reach are substantially below the weight for height norms of the general population, with handicap weights (jockey's weight plus riding tack) typically being within the range of 47 to 56 kg for flat racing. It is likely that a large number of jockeys, particularly older riders who have reached physical maturity, will have a true body weight that is well above these ranges. Second, the jockey is required to make weight frequently and for prolonged durations, with riders typically racing at least twice a week during the season and often riding a number of races over the ~6 hr of a race meet. For the duration of the racing season, weight-making is a constant cycle in the jockey's life, with a small respite on the night after a race meet, generally followed by wasting practices leading up to the next meet.

Although several studies have reported on weight-making practices of jockeys, total numbers who have participated in such studies remain low. Fourteen male jockeys undertook a survey distributed to 48 stables in England (King and Mezey 1987). The mean weight of the group was 13% below the population norm for weight for height,

with the lightest jockey being 21% below this norm. Weight control was a priority over most other aspects of the jockeys' lives during the racing season. A variety of methods were reportedly used to further reduce their low body weight. Food restriction was a popular practice, with one jockey reporting a fast of 6 days. Other methods included the use of laxatives (reported by 70% of group), diuretics (60%), and appetite suppressants (20%). Sweating in saunas was common; jockeys spent up to 4 hr in the sauna in a single session. Sweating via exercise was universally practiced. The use of a combination of techniques to make weight was also found in a larger study of 93 South African jockeys (Labadarosius et al. 1993). In this study, the common weight-making practices were food restriction (77%), saunas (70%), exercise (80%), diuretics (70%), laxatives (27%), and appetite suppressants (48%). Drugs such as diuretics and appetite suppressants are typically banned by antidoping codes of most sports. However, in the case of horse racing, it is the horse rather than the jockey that is the target of doping tests.

A comprehensive investigation of 20 New Zealand jockeys included senior and apprentice jockeys of both genders (Leydon and Wall 2002). Jockeys reported the current use of

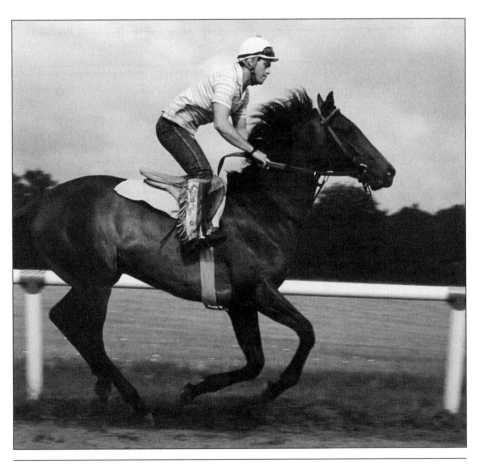

Unlike other weight-making sports, there is no opportunity for recovery between the weigh-in and the event; riders of place-getters are required to weigh in after the race. Furthermore, the jockey is likely to have other races in the same meet for which he or she must remain at weight (see table 12.1).

restriction of fluids (56%) and food (67%), saunas (56%), hot baths (28%), and diuretics (17%). Only 22% of jockeys used exercise for weight control because it was believed to add muscle mass, countering weight loss goals. Past practices included fasting (61%) and laxative use (28%); however these practices were reportedly discontinued. The EAT-26 Eating Attitude Test, a self-reported measure of weight and eating concerns, revealed that 20% of the group scored values indicative of disturbed eating patterns, with scores being similar between male and female jockeys. Mean energy intake, estimated from a 7-day food diary, was reported to be 6.8 MJ and 6.2 MJ for male and female jockeys, respectively. However, wide fluctuations in daily intake suggested a cycle of food restriction, with daily energy intake ranging from a group mean of 3.4 MJ to 10.2 MJ, and between individuals from 0 MJ to 15.5 MJ per day. Assessment of bone mineral density at four sites classified 44% of the jockeys as being osteopenic (i.e., bone density was between 1 and 2.5 standard deviations below population mean).

A final survey involved 116 jockeys, representing 55% of the total population of senior-grade and apprentice jockeys registered to ride in the Australian state of Victoria (Moore et al. 2002). These jockeys reporting riding an average of three race meetings per week (range = 1-5) and 3.2 races per meeting (range = 1-6). The most common weight-making strategies reported by the group were exercise (78% of group) and skipping meals (75%). The use of saunas was reported by 59% of the group, with half this number confining the use to race days and the others using saunas on multiple occasions during the week. Laxatives and diuretics were reportedly used by 23% and 37% of the group, respectively, and again a substantial number of users reported that their practices were not confined only to race day. Male riders and A-grade riders were more likely to use saunas than female riders and B-grade or apprentice jockeys. Otherwise, techniques for weight-making were reported equally among the different groups represented in the survey. Self-induced vomiting was reported by 9% of the group, and nearly half of the jockeys reported smoking cigarettes as a means of weight control. High rates of smoking, and the specific use of cigarettes to replace food intake, were also reported in the other studies of the weight control practices of jockeys (Labadarosius et al. 1993; Leydon and Wall 2002).

High School and College Wrestling

During November 7-December 9, 1997, three previously healthy collegiate wrestlers in different states died while each was engaged in a program of rapid weight loss to qualify for competition. In the hours preceding the official weigh-in, all three wrestlers engaged in a similar rapid weight-loss regimen that promoted dehydration through perspiration and resulted in hyperthermia. The wrestlers restricted food and fluid intake and attempted to maximize sweat losses by wearing vapor-impermeable suits under cotton warm-up suits and exercising vigorously in hot environments....

(Centers for Disease Control and Prevention 1998). Hyperthermia and dehydration-related deaths associated with intentional rapid weight loss in three collegiate wrestlers—North Carolina, Wisconsin, and Michigan, November-December 1997

Wrestling is a popular sport for male athletes in high school and colleges in the United States. School wrestling teams, comprising one representative in each of 10 to 13 weight classes, compete in various tournaments and competitions against other schools, with each wrestler undertaking at least 10 and up to 40 events per season. The frequency of competition (and therefore weight-making practices) is a defining issue in this sport, as is the involvement of wrestlers at a serious level at a time when the adolescent growth spurt should lead to significant weight gain. Concern about weight-making in this sport has a long history, with reports dating back to the 1940s (see review by Steen and Brownell 1990). A survey of more than 700 high school wrestlers conducted in the late 1960s found a mean loss of 3.1 kg (~5% of body mass) over the 17-day period before certification for the season, with most of this loss occurring during the last 10 days (Tipton and Tcheng 1970). Information on techniques to make weight was typically provided by coaches and other wrestlers and included decreased intake of food (16% of the group) and fluid (14%), increased exercise (31%), and sweating in a hot environment (23%) or rubber suits (5%).

From the large number of more recent studies of weight-making practices of wrestlers, two representative investigations have been chosen for greater comment. These studies both involved large sample sizes and survey instruments for which considerable effort had been undertaken to determine the reliability and content validity. A 1990 study surveyed 368 high school and 63 college wrestlers at training camps or tournaments (Steen and Brownell 1990). These wrestlers began making weight at a mean age of 14 years and typically undertook such practices 15 times and 9 times a season at the college and high school level, respectively. At the extreme level, however, weight-making occurred 41 to 60 times in the season. The magnitude of the weekly weight fluctuations achieved by college wrestlers was equally spread between 5 to 9 kg (41% of group) and 2.7 to 4.5 kg (44%), whereas high school wrestlers weight cycled at a lower differential (49% of group cycled between 1.4 and 2.3 kg). Overall, 35% of the college group reported losing up to 4.5 kg more than 100 times in their life, and 22% reported losing 5 to 9 kg between 20 and 50 times. At the extreme end of the range, the most weight loss in the present season was 20.5 kg for college and 22.7 kg for high school wrestlers. The restriction of food and fluid was almost universally used to make weight; half the college wrestlers and a quarter of the high school cohort reported that they fasted once a week. Sweating techniques were widely used, especially among college athletes. Small numbers of wrestlers reported the use of laxatives, vomiting, and diuretics. The weight-making practices of these wrestlers appeared to be confined to the season, with ~80% of both groups reporting that they never or rarely dieted during the off-season. These results and other surveys undertaken over the past 30 years suggest that weight-making practices are rife among wrestlers, that these practices are more extreme in collegiate competition than among high school athletes, and that little change occurred as a result of a range of education strategies (see practical issue)

The most recent comprehensive study of weight-making practices of collegiate wrestlers was undertaken in 1999, following the implementation of new rules within the NCAA designed to curb excessive weight loss (Oppliger et al. 2003). The survey sampled 741 wrestlers from a total of 43 colleges representing each of the three NCAA divisions and included athletes from the 4 years of college and the nine weight-restricted classes (heavyweight wrestlers were excluded). The wrestlers were questioned about their practices over the previous season (1998-1999), which was the first year of implementation of new NCAA rules (see practical issue), but included replies from freshmen wrestlers about their season as high school seniors. These wrestlers, with a mean age of 20 years, competed in an average of 28 matches over the season, with the high school seniors fighting more matches (mean = 38 per season) than at collegiate level. Overall, the mean weekly weight loss was reported to be 2.9 kg (4.3% body mass), with the mean value for the highest weight loss for any one weigh-in during the season being 5.3 kg. Gradual dieting and increased exercise were the major techniques used by the group, with more than 75% of athletes reporting these practices. A differential analysis of the amount of weight loss and the techniques used by wrestlers revealed that collegiate wrestlers were more extreme than the high school athletes but appeared to use less severe techniques than the collegiate wrestlers interviewed in the 1990 survey of Steen and Brownell. Although restriction of fluid and food was still commonly practiced by the modern wrestlers, there was a lower prevalence of reports of fasting and vomiting, and the use of diuretics, laxatives, and sweat suits was apparently lower. On the other hand, the high school wrestlers were considered to be more extreme in their practices than high school wrestlers involved in previous studies. Within the present groups, freshmen were considered to be more extreme than upperclassmen, and wrestlers in the lower weight divisions were more extreme than those in higher weight divisions (Oppliger et al. 2003). Forty percent of the group reported that they had curbed their practices because of the new NCAA rules (see practical issue).

Boxing and Other Combat Sports

Jeff Fenech is on a diet that would kill a lesser man. The boxing star is so hungry for another world title that he has launched himself into a punishing seven-day-a-week program of strict dieting and exercise . . . before he can step into the ring, Jeff must lose more than 13 kg to trim himself down to his fighting weight of 59 kg. . . . Jeff wears a plastic suit when training and can lose nearly 3 kg in one session. . . . "The morning of the weigh-in," he says, "I'll wake up with cracked lips and my tongue will be stuck to the roof of my mouth because I am so dry.". . . A day on Jeff's routine: Breakfast: one bowl of porridge, smoothie and/or juice. . . . Dinner: steamed fish with vegetables, or a rice dish or pasta with seafood sauce.

Annette Allison "Down for the count," Woman's Day *magazine, Sydney, Australia, January 18, 2003, p. 45*

I was waiting for the weigh-in, because I had to drop to such a low-weight category. Mentally, that was incredibly hard—it was probably one of the hardest things I've ever done in my life. I'm normally fit at 55 kilos and I fight at 51 and that's pretty challenging, but 49 was the Olympic weight category. The dining hall was just absolute torture, filled with an abundance of every kind of food you could possibly imagine, and it was the only place I could get food because it was such a hassle to go out of the village. I was starving hungry. The day before competition, I only had half a glass of Sustagen.

"Milestones: Lauren Burns, talks about her gold medal in taekwando at the Sydney 2000 Olympic Games," The Sunday Age, Melbourne, Australia, July 11, Agenda, p. 35

Table 12.1 summarizes the weight-making characteristics of boxing and other combat sports. There is little information on weight-making practices of athletes in these sports. A survey of 16 experienced Irish amateur boxers (Hall and Lane 2001) identified four phases to weight-making practices, with mean values of self-reported weights being natural weight (74.5 kg), training weight (71.9 kg), weight for interclub competition (70 kg), and championship weight (67.9 kg). The boxers reported a mean weight loss of 2 to 3 kg in the week before a championship, achieved by dieting and restricted fluid intake. In some cases, no fluid was consumed for the 24 hr period before the weigh-in. Exercise was undertaken on the day of competition (73% of group) to promote further dehydration. In a separate part of this study, when boxers were asked to achieve their championship weight by their preferred techniques, actual weight loss over the week was 5.3% body mass (range = 3.6-7.3%).

The other investigation compared 11 French judo athletes of regional and national caliber during habitual training and 2 months later in the week before a competition. Body mass decreased by 4.9% between periods, with food records indicating a ~30% reduction in energy, carbohydrate, and fluid intake during the precompetition period (Filaire et al. 2000).

Lightweight Rowing

Lightweight rowing places weight restrictions on individual competitors as well as the crew average (see table 12.1). Under the regatta style of competition, the successful rower or crew must race three to four times to decide the final outcome, and weigh-ins must be undertaken 1 to 2 hr before each race. Weight-making practices add another layer to the physiological demands of rowing (see chapter 6), as does the potential for competition to be undertaken in hot summer conditions.

Over a season, 18 Australian lightweight rowers (6 female, 12 male) were found to reduce body mass by a mean of 5.9% for the women and 7.8% for the men (Morris and Payne 1996). Chronic weight changes were underpinned by loss of body fat rather than lean mass and were achieved by reductions in energy and fat intake. Common acute weight-making practices included additional exercise (73%), food restriction (71%), and fluid restriction (63%). This research team reported a 5.8 kg (9.3%) loss of body weight over the competitive season in another group of 12 lightweight female rowers (Morris et al. 1999). Another study found that, on average, lightweight athletes report making weight almost five times over season, with males reporting a greater frequency of these practices than females (Sykora et al. 1993). The most popular strategies were fasting (68%), restrictive diets (58%), and strenuous exercise (70%).

A survey of 100 lightweight rowers, representing about 75% of the lightweight race field at the 2003 Australian national rowing championships (Slater, Rice, Sharpe, Mujika, et al. 2005), found that rowers reported the use of acute and chronic weight loss strategies to reduce from a peak off-season weight of ~76 kg (males) and ~62 kg (females). Most rowers lost weight over 4 weeks before the regatta using two or more techniques, most popularly gradual dieting, fluid restriction, and increased training. Typical weight lost on the day of race was ~0.5 kg, and serum osmolality from blood samples taken immediately after weigh-in revealed that about 80% and 90% of males and females were dehydrated. Rowers consumed food and drinks to replace carbohydrate, fluid, and sodium in the 1 to 2 hr period between weigh-in and race, with reported strategies meeting current guidelines for carbohydrate only.

Lightweight American Football

Because lightweight or sprint football is played only at a small number of U.S. colleges, it has drawn little attention from sport scientists (see table 12.1 for characteristics). A sample of 131 players from four U.S. schools with a lightweight football program participated in a survey of weight loss practices (Depalma et al. 1993). Sixty-six percent admitted to fasting during the previous month, with 26% fasting once per week and almost 20% fasting more than once per week. Seventeen percent used vomiting, 4% laxatives, and 2.5% diet pills, diuretics, or enemas for weight loss. These efforts to lose weight were perceived

to often or always interfere with their mental health and extracurricular activities.

Weightlifting

Sydney's little weightlifting champion Mehmet Yagci found the perfect cure for making the weight for the Commonwealth trials by covering himself in salt. Yagci had to lose 6 kg in four days to make the 56 kg body-weight class by the 9.30 am weigh-in on Saturday. . . . "I spent 15 hours in the sauna. I have never done it this hard," said Yagci. "I was in there wearing a jumper for 40 minutes before the weigh-in and I was still 300 grams overweight. . . . I had kilos of table salt poured over me. I looked like a pillar of salt, but it worked just in time." The draining effort left the reigning Games gold medallist disorientated and "talking nonsense" which may have been a factor in his missing his first two attempts at his opening snatch lift of 105 kg.

Mike Hurst, "Mehmet's salty solution."
Daily Telegraph *newspaper, Sydney, Australia,*
May 6, 2002, p. 30

Only one study of weight-making practices of weightlifters could be located, an investigation of 19 elite Australian lifters undertaken during the 1980s (Burke and Read 1988a). Half the lifters regularly endeavored to lose weight in the 48 hr before a competition to qualify for a weight division below their normal training weight. The usual method of making weight was to reduce intake of food and fluid over these days (55% of group), whereas two athletes reported fasting and another two depended on total fluid deprivation. The estimated body fat levels of these male athletes were relatively high (16% body mass), but little was done in the months of training between competitions to lose weight permanently by reducing body fat.

Common Threads of Weight-Making Practices in Sport

As shown by the anecdotes throughout this chapter, many athletes choose their competition class because of culture or circumstances rather than to suit their true physical characteristics. In many sports the prevailing attitude is to compete at the lowest class possible to gain a competitive edge; in others, the available weight classes or targets are so few or so far spread that the natural weight of the majority of athletes sits well above them. In situations where a better athlete has already qualified for a team, or where a class is not represented in a particular competition, an athlete will have to manipulate her weight to permit involvement in a sport.

Typically, athletes in weight-making sports use a combination of acute and chronic techniques to reduce body weight to their required weight class or target, although the contribution and extent of each technique to overall weight loss vary between sports and between individual athletes. In general, chronic techniques of weight loss rely on long-term energy restriction (reduction of food intake) to reduce body fat. In some but not all sports, the athlete strives to achieve the lowest body fat levels possible and is often prepared to sacrifice muscle mass. Athletes vary in their use of additional exercise to contribute to the achievement of a long-term energy deficit. In some sports, athletes are prepared to undertake aerobic exercise in addition to their specific training to increase energy expenditure, whereas others perceive that unnecessary exercise will lead to a weight increase attributable to an increase in muscle mass. In some sports, athletes try to achieve loss of weight and body fat over a prolonged period in anticipation of, or at the start of, the competition season. For other athletes, the culture of the sport is that large amounts of body weight can be reduced over shorter periods with more dramatic energy restriction.

The acute weight-making strategies that are imposed against this background of chronic weight loss reduce body weight at the expense of body fluid, glycogen stores, and gastrointestinal contents. The major component of the weight loss is a reduction in body fluid levels, achieved by intentional sweating (saunas, exercise, sweat suits), failure to replace normal daily body fluid losses, or diuretic or laxative purging. The reduction in gastrointestinal content can also be achieved by restricted intake or by purging (vomiting and laxatives).

Performance and Health

Because of the factors outlined in the introduction to this chapter, it is hard to make definitive statements about the effect of weight-making techniques on performance and health. This section attempts to provide an overview of possible outcomes of the restriction of fluid and food, both in the acute situation and as a chronic pattern of behavior.

Perceived Effort, Cognitive Function, and Psychological Status

Acute dehydration is known to impair cognitive skills and concentration, especially when the athlete is exposed to a hot environment (Gopinathan et al. 1988). As well as impairing the cognitive aspects of performance, weight-making techniques are expected to increase the perception of effort. For example, the loss of weight over 4 days before a test simulating wrestling performance was associated with a 7% increase in perceived exertion (Horswill, Hickner, et al. 1990). Because weight-making techniques typically also involve food restriction, at least some of the potential cognitive and mood disturbances could be mediated by lower blood glucose concentrations (Choma et al. 1998).

The Profile of Mood States (POMS) has been used in a number of studies to monitor the psychological status

of athletes as they undertake weight-making practices. Collegiate wrestlers were tested for mood and cognitive ability after a mean loss of 6.2% of body mass and after a 72 hr recovery period (Choma et al. 1998). Compared with baseline levels, four of the five subscales of the POMS test were increased after the weight loss, indicating a more negative mood. In addition, the wrestlers had poorer short-term memory ability after weight loss. After 72 hr of recovery, all changes returned to pre–weight loss levels. Similar mood changes were reported when amateur boxers reduced weight by ~5% of body mass over a week. These boxers reported increased levels of anger, fatigue, and tension and a decrease in vigor on the POMS scale after making weight (Hall and Lane 2001). The same increases in tension, anger, and fatigue and reduction in vigor were found after judo athletes achieved a ~5% decrease in body mass over 7 days (Degoutte et al. 2006; Filaire et al. 2000).

Several studies have presented evidence that athletes in weight-making sports have a greater risk or higher prevalence of disordered eating behaviors and disturbed relationships with food and body image than other athletes or sedentary controls. For example, lightweight rowers reported more dietary restraint and a greater use of diuretics than runners and controls (Karlson et al. 2001). Use of the Eating Disorder Inventory (EDI) with a group of male lightweight rowers and wrestlers suggested that 11% of the athletes fit the profile for a subclinical eating disorder (Thiel, Gottfried, and Hesse 1993). Preoccupation with food was often or always experienced by two thirds of a group of collegiate wrestlers, with 40% of wrestlers feeling out of control with their eating during the period after a match (Steen and Brownell 1990).

Whether the use of pathological weight loss practices by weight-making athletes is a symptom of an underlying eating disorder or simply an occupational hazard cannot always be distinguished by questionnaires and eating inventories. Indeed, it is possible that disordered eating behaviors such as fasting and purging are simply a means to an end for many athletes in weight-making sports, because the practices and the perceived lack of control with food stop during the off-season (Steen and Brownell 1990). A study of high school wrestlers (Dale and Landers 1999) tried to distinguish disordered eating practices that are transient and vocational from the true psychopathology of an eating disorder. Wrestlers completed the Eating Disorder Inventory on two occasions (during the season and during the off-season), whereas another group of high school students undertook the survey on a single occasion as a comparison. All participants classified as at risk were further assessed by interview. In contrast to the hypothesis, the in-season wrestlers were not at greater risk for bulimia nervosa than nonwrestlers, and high scores on the EDI for concepts such as Drive for Thinness disappeared in the off-season. Despite the limitations of applying eating disorder questionnaires to the specific issues of wrestling, it was concluded that weight loss concerns arising from a sport do not reach the severity required for the classification of an eating disorder and do not represent a central psychopathology (Dale and

Landers 1999). Therefore, although it is possible that some weight-making athletes will go on to develop more serious and long-lasting disturbances to their eating attitudes and practices, the greatest concern is the immediate impact on health and performance.

Acute Effects of Dehydration and Food Restriction on Health

Severe dehydration is considered to pose a series of risks to an athlete's health (for review, see American College of Sports Medicine 1996). The risk is related to both the extent of fluid loss and methods used to achieve it. For example, dehydration induced by diuretic use increases the loss of electrolytes compared with sweat-induced dehydration (Caldwell et al. 1984). Substantial loss of fluid and electrolytes can impair cardiovascular and thermoregulatory function and, as the most severe outcome, cause death. This outcome was well described in case reports at the beginning of this chapter of three wrestlers who died following extreme weight-making practices (Centers for Disease Control and Prevention 1998). The consequences of making weight in dangerous sports such as horse racing has not been well documented. However, jockeys experience an average of 2.4 fractures over their career because of falls (De Benedette 1987) and it is possible that weight-making techniques interfere with the jockey's physical and mental capacity to control their horses.

Acute Effects of Dehydration and Food Restriction on Performance

The acute outcomes of weight-making include dehydration, depletion of body carbohydrate stores, and loss of lean body mass. Other chapters of this book have discussed the effects of suboptimal fuel and fluid status on the performance of various types of exercise. This section focuses on studies with specific relevance to weight-making sports. Physiological characteristics that are important to the outcomes of these sports include strength, speed, and anaerobic power. The ability to undertake repeated high-intensity efforts is also required in some sports.

A range of methodologies has been used in studies of the effects of weight-making practices on such sport-specific performance. Performance outcomes have included actual competition, protocols simulating competition, or isolated tasks with relevance to competition outcomes. In some studies, absolute outcomes were measured; in others, performance measurements were adjusted to body weight. Strategies used to make weight have differed not only between studies but, in some cases, within the same study. Whereas some investigations have compared performance before and after a standardized technique of dehydration or food restriction, in other studies, participants have been permitted to reduce their body weight to a prescribed level, using techniques of their

own choosing. Acute weight losses have been undertaken over hours or several weeks and have ranged from 1% to 10% of body mass. In some studies performance has been monitored after a prescribed recovery period after weigh-in. Recovery nutrition strategies have involved standardized protocols of refueling and rehydration or have been undertaken according to the individual athlete's usual practices. Although this variation in methodology increases the challenge of interpreting the overall effect of weight-making techniques on performance, it reflects the diversity of issues that exist in real-life practice. A brief overview of studies where weight-making has been achieved over 1 week or less is presented next.

• Amateur boxers were involved in the design of a sport-specific boxing task (Hall and Lane 2001). Performance was measured as repetitions of a burpee drill during four 2 min bouts, separated by 1 min of recovery. Sixteen male boxers performed twice: at training weight and after self-chosen weight-making practices to achieve a mean loss of 5.2% body mass followed by 2 hr of unsupervised recovery with food and fluids. Although there was no difference in the performance of this task between trials, the boxers failed to achieve their expected performance levels at their lower (championship) weight.

• Seven amateur boxers undertook a boxing protocol using an ergometer developed to analyze punches delivered to a target area (Smith et al. 2000). Performance was measured as the force of punches delivered during three 3 min rounds interspersed by 1 min of recovery. Boxers undertook two bouts: in a euhydrated state and after sweating by low-intensity cycling in a hot environment for ~2 hr to lose a mean of 3.8% body mass. Changes in plasma volume and performance as a result of this exercise-induced sweating were variable. One boxer improved punching performance while dehydrated, whereas the mean effect on other participants was a 27% decrease in performance ($p < .05$). The authors noted that some individuals may be physiologically predisposed to cope more effectively with the effects of dehydration.

• Serial weight-making efforts, as experienced in a boxing tournament, were investigated in eight amateur boxes (Smith et al. 2001). Performance was measured as the force of punches delivered to an ergometer during three 3 min rounds interspersed by 1 min of recovery. Each boxer was monitored over a 5-day period with bouts undertaken on days 3 and 5. Trials were undertaken both at normal weight and nutrition patterns and following weight-making with energy and fluid intake restricted to 1,000 kcal (4.2 MJ) and 1 L, respectively. This restriction resulted in a ~3% loss of body mass, with most of this loss occurring in the first 3 days. Blood glucose concentrations were significantly lower on completion of each of the boxing bouts in the weight-making trial compared with control, reflecting the carbohydrate intake of <2 $g \cdot kg^{-1} \cdot day^{-1}$. Total punching force was consistently lower in both bouts during weight-making compared with the control trial, but differences were not statistically significant because of large interindividual differences.

• Eight elite lightweight rowers performed a rowing ergometer trial while euhydrated and after a weight-making and rehydration protocol (Burge et al. 1993). This protocol involved 24 hr of fluid and food restriction to reduce weight by a mean of 5.2% followed by a 2 hr recovery period in which 1.5 L of water was consumed. The time trial was slower with weight-making compared with control (7.38 vs. 7.02 min, $p < .05$), which equated to a performance impairment of ∼100 m in a 2,000 m race. This impairment was attributed to a lower plasma volume (6% lower despite the rehydration protocol) and a 30% reduction in glycogen utilization. Post-time-trial concentrations of plasma lactate were lower in the weight-making trial (6.8 vs. 8.8 mmol/L, $p < .05$).

• Ten male judo athletes who lost 5% of body mass over a 7-day period of energy and carbohydrate restriction were found to have reduced handgrip strength and maximal strength during a 30 s rowing task compared with a group of judo athletes who did not practice dietary restriction. A similar reduction in physical performance was found at the end of a simulated competition involving five 5 min bouts in both groups (Degoutte et al. 2006).

• Rowers who reduced body mass by ∼4% over 24 hr and then aggressively refueled and hydrated during a 2 hr recovery period between weigh-in and their event experienced only a small and nonsignificant increase in time (∼2 s) to complete a 2,000 m rowing ergometer time trial (Slater, Rice, Sharpe, Tanner, et al. 2005). In a separate study, a similar acute weight loss and recovery strategy resulted in an even smaller decrement (∼1 s) in time to complete an on-water 1,800 m time trial in cool conditions (Slater et al. 2006b). The repetition of acute weight-making to simulate a multiday regatta also resulted in a small and decreasing performance decrement when aggressive recovery was undertaken between weight loss efforts (Slater et al. 2006a) (see research topic).

• Athletes from open-weight sports were recruited for a study designed to eliminate the effect of habituation to acute weight loss practices (Gutierrez et al. 2003). Six male and six female athletes from various endurance and team sports performed a battery of strength tests for upper and lower limbs. Tests were performed at baseline, after three 20 min exposures to a sauna to induce a mean weight loss of 1.8% body mass in males and 1.4% body mass in females, and after consuming 10 ml/kg of a carbohydrate–electrolyte drink over 1 hr. This rehydration protocol only partially reversed the fluid deficit. There were no differences in upper-limb tests and a countermovement jump test in either gender as a result of dehydration or partial rehydration. Performance of a squat jump was unchanged in male athletes. However, performance of the females was significantly improved after rehydration compared with the baseline performance and attributed to the lower body weight.

• The effects of three weight-making techniques on maximal strength, rate of force development, vertical jumping height, and mechanical power were studied in track-and-field athletes and volleyball players (Viitasalo et al. 1987). The methods were sauna (weight loss = 3.4% body mass), very low energy diet of 600 kJ (150 kcal)/day for 60 hr followed by a diuretic (5.8% body mass), and diuretic alone (3.8% body mass). The sauna and diet and diuretic treatments were both associated with a decrease in maximal isometric leg strength and rate of force development. Dehydration by diuretic alone did not impair neuromuscular performances. The hypothesis that weight loss would improve vertical jump via a rise in the body center of gravity was confirmed. All three treatments were associated with an improvement in jumping performance, with the greatest improvement following the diuretic treatment. However, when work was extended to 15 s, an improved power output was observed only with the diet and diuretic treatment.

• Seven men were tested after exposure to a sauna on two occasions: with a fluid deficit of 4% body mass and when fluid was consumed to replace all sweat losses (Greiwe et al. 1998). Compared with baseline testing, there was no difference in isometric muscular strength or endurance at the knee or elbow for either treatment. These authors concluded that isometric strength and endurance are unaffected 3.5 hr after dehydration of approximately 4% body mass.

• Twelve collegiate wrestlers consumed an energy-restricted diet (18 kcal [76 kJ]/kg body mass/day) for 72 hr without dehydration. Tests undertaken with an arm ergometer before and after the intervention showed no difference in peak power but an 8% reduction in work done. Lactate accumulation was reduced following the weight loss diet (Walberg-Rankin et al. 1996).

• Twelve well-trained wrestlers lost 6% of body mass over 4 days on two occasions: with an energy-restricted with low carbohydrate intake or matched energy diet with higher carbohydrate (Horswill et al. 1990). Performance testing (6 min of high-intensity arm cranking) was undertaken before and after the weight loss. Total sprint work was maintained with the high-carbohydrate weight loss diet; however, the low-carbohydrate diet was associated with a reduction in sprint work. Lactate accumulation was reduced following both diets.

• Wrestlers ranked a 6 min variable-intensity test using an arm crank ergometer as a suitable simulation for the physical demands of a wrestling match (Hickner et al. 1991). Five other athletes with upper-body training undertook this testing protocol before and after rapid weight loss of 4.5% body mass over a 3-day period. The work performed at baseline testing was greater ($p < .05$) than that performed after weight loss.

• Two-well trained wrestlers were monitored before and after rapid weight loss of 5% to 6% body mass over 3 days (Oopik et al. 1996). Plasma volume was reduced by 7% and 15% by this weight loss. Peak torque, time to peak torque, rate of peak torque development, and maximal power output measured during a single maximal contraction of the quadriceps femoris muscle, as well as muscle working ability measured during a 5 min isokinetic performance test, were all impaired by weight reduction. Body weight, plasma volume, and muscle isokinetic performance characteristics did not return to the initial levels even after 16.5 hr of ad libitum food and drink intake.

• Nineteen experienced weightlifters were assigned for 1 week to a control diet or energy-matched weight loss diets (18 kcal [76 kJ] $\cdot$ kg^{-1} $\cdot$ day^{-1}) that were either moderate protein and high carbohydrate or high protein and moderate carbohydrate (Walberg et al. 1988). A loss of ~3.8 kg was recorded over the 7 days. According to hydrostatic weighing, the energy deficit achieved similar loss of body fat and fat-free mass regardless of the composition of the diet. However, the high-protein diet conserved nitrogen balance. Biceps endurance was unchanged after the week, but quadriceps endurance declined for the high-protein diet. The authors concluded that an energy-restricted diet providing twice the recommended daily allowance for protein was more effective in retaining body protein than a diet with higher carbohydrate but lower protein content. However, the lower-carbohydrate diet contributed to reduced muscular endurance in these athletes.

The evidence for acute impairment of performance following weight-making techniques is not consistent. Dehydration does not appear to affect maximal muscular strength and power, and there may even be an enhancement of power applied against gravity (e.g., jumps) or expressed relative to body mass following dehydration-induced weight loss. By contrast, muscular endurance and prolonged anaerobic or aerobic performance are more likely to be impaired by weight loss, especially when energy restriction is undertaken or added to dehydration. There appears to be some individual tolerance to the effects of dehydration.

Effects of Longer Term Strategies for Weight-Making on Performance

Most athletes in weight-making sports undertake prolonged periods of energy deficit to reduce body weight via the loss of body fat and lean body mass. The relative loss of these tissues is determined by factors including the severity of the energy restriction and the athlete's preexisting fat stores. Several studies have investigated the effect of longer weight loss efforts on performance; again, a range of methodologies has been used in these investigations. The following studies involve a weight-making attempt lasting greater than 7 days, where a true change in body composition has been achieved via chronic energy deficit:

• A case study followed two elite wrestlers over the 22-day preparation for European Championships (Maffulli 1992). The athletes lost 8% of their initial body mass via intensive training coupled with a hypocaloric diet. Maximum oxygen uptake, anaerobic threshold, and maximum isometric strength were maintained at absolute levels. Therefore, these variables increased when expressed relative to the lower body weight. By contrast, isometric

endurance and short-term sprinting ability were impaired by the weight-loss regimen, decreasing by up to 7% and 13%, respectively.

• Judo athletes decreased body mass by 4.9% over a 2-month period with a self-selected diet, with food records indicating a ~30% reduction of energy, carbohydrate, and fluid intake during the 7-day period before competition (Filaire et al. 2000). Competitors were shown to have a reduction in left-hand grip strength and 30 s jumping performance at the end of this period but no difference in 7 s jump test and right-hand strength.

• Muscle dynamic strength of the quadriceps and biceps brachii was reduced about 8% in athletes who lost 3.3 kg over a 10-day period of a low-energy diet (18 kcal (75 kJ). kg^{-1} $\cdot$ day^{-1}) and was not attenuated by the intake of arginine supplements (Walberg-Rankin et al. 1994).

• Ten male athletes (seven wrestlers and three judo athletes) undertook two different weight loss protocols to lose 5% to 6% body mass (Fogelholm, Naveri, et al. 1993). The rapid protocol achieved a 6% loss of body mass over 2.4 days by fluid and diet restriction and forced sweating, followed by a 5 hr recovery with ad libitum food and drinks. In the gradual procedure, a 5% loss was achieved in 3 weeks by energy restriction. The net weight change after weight loss and recovery was 2.7% BM. Sprint (30 m run) and anaerobic (1 min Wingate test) performance was similar throughout the study. Jumping results were not changed by the rapid protocol, but the gradual protocol was associated with a 6% to 8% increase in vertical jump height with extra load ($p < .05$). The authors concluded that a weight loss of 5% body mass by either rapid or gradual protocols did not impair the performance of experienced athletes.

• The effects of losing similar amounts of weight over either 2 or 4 months were studied in six national-caliber lightweight rowers (Koutedakis et al. 1994). In the first year, a rapid weight loss strategy (3.8 kg over 2 months) was implemented, whereas a gradual approach (4.7 kg over 4 months) was undertaken in the next year. Neither method exclusively caused fat loss; about 50% of the weight lost with both strategies was a reduction in fat-free mass. However, the rapid weight loss was associated with a decline in lactate threshold and leg strength, whereas the slower weight loss was associated with an increase in these measures as well as aerobic capacity and anaerobic power. This study suggests that a more gradual weight loss is superior for maintaining or increasing performance but does not affect body composition change.

• Twenty-four recreationally trained men and women were assigned to either a control (energy-matched) diet or 2 weeks of energy restriction (to produce an energy deficit of 750 kcal/day) while undertaking a running program (Zachwieja et al. 2001). A mean weight loss of 1.3 kg was achieved, mostly from a reduction in lean body mass. Muscle strength (1 RM leg press), 5-mile run time, and muscle endurance (squatting repetitions to fatigue) were enhanced in both groups after the training intervention. Anaerobic capacity (work done during 30 s cycling Wingate test) increased in the energy restriction group after the

2-week period, whereas a decrease was seen in the control group. The authors concluded that a short-term moderate energy deficit did not impair training adaptation and performance.

There are few good studies of the effects of prolonged weight loss on performance; however, the evidence for impairment of performance following prolonged weight loss techniques is inconsistent. Further studies are required to better study the outcomes of the various weight loss practices observed among athletes. These investigations should also include monitoring the combination and repetition of the weight-making practices, because this may not be appreciated from the results of studies of single methods.

Chronic Effects of Weight-Making on Health

A number of potential negative outcomes are associated with chronic episodes of weight-making. These are most likely to occur when athletes are in a pattern of weight cycling attributable to the frequent nature of their competition and when there is a substantial difference between their true weight and their competition weight class. Chronic effects on psychological well-being have already been discussed; this section focuses on the effects of chronic episodes of restricted energy intake on physiology and long-term health. Energy restriction is likely to be compounded by inadequate intake of carbohydrate, protein, and micronutrients. Some studies have noted that athletes report intakes of calcium, iron, and other micronutrients that are below daily recommended intakes when these athletes are in the active phase of weight-making or energy restriction (Filaire et al. 2000; Steen and McKinney 1986). Although a short-term weight loss effort is unlikely to cause problems in nutrient status, prolonged or repeated periods of weight loss with suboptimal intakes of micronutrients are likely to cause a deterioration of vitamin and mineral status (Fogelholm, Naveri, et al. 1993). Repeated dieting by wrestlers has been associated with a significant reduction in prealbumin and retinol-binding protein, plasma indicators of protein status (Horswill, Park, and Roemmich 1990). Similarly, low serum prealbumin levels were seen in adolescent wrestlers during their season, with an increase in these levels when dietary intake improved at the end of the season (Roemmich and Sinning 1997b).

Energy restriction lowers resting metabolic rate (RMR) in normal-weight and obese persons. Early studies found that wrestlers who reported repeated weight loss and gain, termed *weight cyclers*, had a lower metabolic rate than those who were not cyclers. For example, 27 wrestlers classified as cyclers or noncyclers based on their weight loss history were found to be similar in age, weight, height, surface area, lean body mass, and percent body fat (Steen et al. 1988). However, cyclers had a significantly lower mean RMR than noncyclers (4.6 vs. 5.5 kJ per kilogram of lean body mass per hour), and a 14% difference in resting energy expenditure (6,632 vs. 7,703 kJ/day). Such data suggested that weight cycling caused metabolic rate to decrease.

Longitudinal studies undertaken to test this theory have failed to find evidence of long-term changes to RMR in weight cyclers. Examination of a group of wrestlers in the preseason, peak season, and off-season failed to find differences in resting energy expenditure between or within groups labeled as cyclers or noncyclers based on their reported dieting history (McCargar and Crawford 1992). Another study followed a group of weight-cycling college wrestlers and a sedentary control group of similar weight and body composition over a 6-month wrestling season (Melby et al. 1990). Resting metabolic rate was significantly higher in the wrestlers than the control group at baseline but was reduced by almost 18% over the season as the wrestlers lost weight. After a season of weight cycling and the final weight regain, the wrestler's postseason RMR was similar to preseason values and higher than the postseason RMR of the control participants ($p < .05$). The authors concluded that participation in numerous cycles of weight loss and regain did not permanently lower RMR in the athletes. Finally, a group of weight-cycling collegiate wrestlers and a control group of sedentary students matched for body composition were monitored over 2 years, with a group of noncycling wrestlers added in the second year of the investigation (Schmidt et al. 1993). Resting metabolic rate was measured before and after each of the 6-month seasons. The wrestlers were found to have higher pre- and postseason measures of RMR compared with the control group, and there was no difference between the cyclers and noncyclers in the second year. In summary, the literature suggests that resting metabolic rate may decrease significantly during the wrestling season and will alter the energy intake prescription for weight loss. However, evidence that these metabolic changes continue after the season is not strong.

Studies have reported depression of sex hormone concentrations in athletes who undertake weight-making. Significant reductions in progesterone and strong trends to reductions in estrogen levels were observed over a season of weight loss in female lightweight rowers (Morris et al. 1999). Changes in testosterone and other growth-related hormones have been monitored in adolescent male wrestlers over the season and in the off-season (Roemmich and Sinning 1997a). Preseason and late season, wrestlers had significant elevations of growth hormone (GH) and significant reductions in GH-binding protein, insulin-like growth factor 1 (IGF-1), testosterone (T), and free testosterone. There were significant postseason reductions in GH but elevations in GH-binding protein, IGF-1, T, and free T. Concentrations of other hormones including cortisol, insulin, and thyroid hormones did not differ. The in-season changes in hormones were consistent with an impairment of the normal function of the sex hormone cycle; however, this impairment was quickly reversed in the off-season. The authors called for further studies to address hormonal responses to several years of wrestling and weight loss.

Dietary energy intake per se appears to have a role in regulating bone turnover, because a restriction in energy intake interferes with the complex nature of bone metabolism. A study using healthy females showed that 4 days of fasting was associated with 40% to 50% reduction in markers of bone synthesis and resorption (Grinspoon et al. 1995). The negative effects of fasting on bone appear to occur in even shorter time periods. Male lightweight rowers who fasted for a 24 hr period to cause a 1.7 kg decrease in body weight were found to have a 20% reduction in serum osteocalcin (marker of bone synthesis) and reductions in urinary pyridinoline and deoxypyridinoline cross-links, indicative of bone resorption, of 27% and 22%, respectively (Talbott and Shapses 1998). Nonfasting participants in the same study showed evidence of a relationship between dietary energy intake and bone turnover, where partial energy restriction appeared to promote bone resorption and suppress bone formation. Because a reduction in bone turnover is likely to reduce bone mass over time, follow-up studies should be undertaken with athletes who undertake weight-making practices frequently. Female athletes with menstrual disturbances, who already have an elevated risk of reduced bone mass, should be particularly concerned about the additional effect of repeated episodes of severe energy restriction on bone. There may be some protection to bone provided by the mode of exercise undertaken by weight-making athletes. For example, a study of male and female judo athletes found that the elevated bone formation resulting from the biomechanical characteristics of judo activities lent protection from alterations in bone metabolic balance associated with weight-cycling (Prouteau et al. 2006).

Finally, there is some concern that weight-making is associated with a loss of muscle mass and impairment of growth in adolescent athletes. For example, one study reported a reduction in fat-free mass of female lightweight rowers over a season compared with preseason measurements (McCargar et al. 1993). Several studies on high school wrestlers (15-16 years) found lower increases in arm and thigh muscle cross-sectional area over the wrestling season compared with nonwrestling classmates (Roemmich and Sinning 1996, 1997b). Fortunately, no effect on linear growth and maturation was seen, because the wrestlers showed a rebound in muscle growth during the off-season to bring them up to the average for controls. A cross-sectional study of high school wrestlers compared anthropometric characteristics of 477 athletes with values from a national representative sample of adolescent males (Housh et al. 1993). The results indicated that there were few differences between the wrestlers and the national sample for yearly changes in the anthropometric dimensions. The authors concluded that participation in high school wrestling, which typically includes repeated bouts of weight cycling, does not adversely affect normal anthropometric growth patterns. In summary, athletes practicing repeated weight loss over a season are likely to inhibit lean tissue growth. In older athletes at least, there appears to be catch-up of lean growth during the off-season. Further study on this important area is warranted. In the meantime, to ensure that there is minimal impact on long-term growth, athletes who practice energy restriction should ensure that adequate intakes of energy, protein, and other important nutrients are maintained.

Weight-Making Advantages to Competitive Outcomes

Despite the negative effects on mood or absolute performance, many athletes who make weight consider that it has a positive outcome. A group of boxers reported that weight-making is a necessary part of boxing competition and that they perform better having reduced weight (Hall and Lane 2001). The authors of this study explained the apparent paradox, in which boxers made such claims despite performing below expectations in a simulated boxing protocol, in terms of the interactive nature of a tournament. In such a scenario, a boxer can perform below a baseline level or benchmark but still win the contest by being relatively better than opponents. Additionally, wrestlers have claimed that weight-making increases their anger, making them more aggressive and competitive (Steen and McKinney 1986).

The concept of relative performance has not been well studied. The performances of 159 high school wrestlers from schools providing education programs relating to the minimum wrestling weight (MWW—see practical issue) were tracked at a postseason tournament (Wroble and

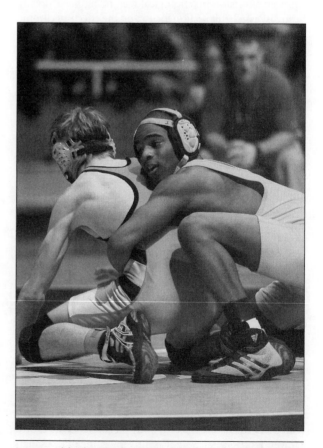

It is possible that the best wrestlers are more likely to take risks to wrestle at a lower weight or are more tolerant to the effects of the strategies used to make weight.

Moxley 1998). The study found that 33% of the wrestlers chose to compete in a class that was below their MWW. These wrestlers were more likely to place in the tournament (57% of this group placed) than the wrestlers who competed in weight classes above MWW (33% of this group placed). These differences were more pronounced in the lighter weight classes. A study of 2,638 competitors in international-style wrestling in the United States reported that the mean weight gain between weigh-in and wrestling, said to reflect the extent of weight-making, was greater in place-getters in the competition (3.8 kg) compared with the nonplacers (3.0 kg, $p < .05$). Again, this discrepancy was more noticeable in the lower weight classes (Alderman et al. 2004). Although the results suggest that wrestling below MWW or losing greater amounts of weight loss was associated with greater success, cause and effect cannot be ensured.

Further studies are needed to investigate the intriguing issue of weight-making and relative performance, particularly in tournament-style sports. In the meantime, it has been noted that performance-based arguments should not be used in the justification or education surrounding minimum weight programs (Wroble and Moxley 1998). Athletes and coaches intuitively know of the benefits of reducing weight to compete in a lower weight division.

Strategies for Recovery After Weigh-In

Many variables are involved in recovery after weigh-in in a weight classification sport. The potential for recovery depends not only on the extent of weight loss and the methods used to make weight but also on the period of time between the weigh-in and the start of the event. This can vary from 1 to 24 hr. The acute needs of most weight-making athletes following a weigh-in are restoration of fluid balance following moderate to severe levels of dehydration and intake of carbohydrate to provide a fuel source for the upcoming event. Practical considerations underpinning refueling and rehydrating strategies during the recovery period include the potential for gastrointestinal discomfort and upset in the subsequent event resulting from the timing and amount of fluids and foods consumed.

Depending on the duration of the recovery period and the nature of food restriction and exercise undertaken to make weight, carbohydrate consumed after weigh-in may contribute to muscle glycogen stores or liver glycogen or may simply provide a source of glucose released from the gastrointestinal tract during the event. The principles and strategies for optimal storage of muscle and liver glycogen are presented in chapter 1 (goal 6). The storage of substantial amounts of glycogen is a lengthy process, taking up to 24 hr to normalize muscle stores when they have been substantially depleted. In the case where weight-making has involved fasting or extreme dietary restriction

in concert with exercise, it is unlikely that there will be sufficient time for a worthwhile restoration of glycogen stores. For example, studies have shown that wrestlers who lost 5% body mass with food and fluid restriction had a 54% decline in muscle glycogen (Tarnopolsky et al. 1996), whereas rowers who lost a similar amount of weight in 24 hr incurred a 30% decrease in muscle glycogen content (Burge et al. 1993).

The failure to restore muscle glycogen content after weigh-in may not be problematic in brief, high-intensity sports where high-energy phosphates provide the main source of fuel (e.g., weightlifting). However, athletes in sports that depend heavily on carbohydrate utilization (e.g., rowing) should undertake strategies to promote glycogen storage during the recovery period. The main factor in determining glycogen storage is the amount of carbohydrate consumed, although there may be some merit in consuming carbohydrate in small, frequent snacks rather than large meals in the first hours of recovery after exercise (Burke, Kiens, et al. 2004). These strategies are outlined in greater detail in the following section (table 12.2). Carbohydrate restoration practices during the recovery period may enhance but not necessarily restore performance in subsequent events. For example, when wrestlers made weight by energy restriction, an 8% reduction in the work done on an arm ergometer was found immediately after weigh-in (Walberg-Rankin et al. 1996). In the 5 hr recovery period following weigh-in, refeeding was undertaken with either a high-carbohydrate (75% of energy) or moderate-carbohydrate (47% of energy) diet with matched energy content of 21 kcal (88 kJ)/kg. Work done after recovery on the high-carbohydrate diet was 99% of the baseline test, whereas the moderate-carbohydrate group achieved 91.5% of their initial work ($p = .1$). Although these results failed to reach statistical significance, they suggest that the high-carbohydrate refeeding diet was superior in restoring performance compared with the moderate-carbohydrate diet.

The restoration of a severe fluid deficit incurred through weight-making may also require a recovery period of 6 to 24 hr. Principles and strategies for rehydration are presented in chapter 1 (goal 6) and include the restoration of electrolyte losses, particularly sodium, as well as the consumption of a volume of fluid that compensates for continuing urine and sweat losses (Shirreffs et al. 2004). The pattern of fluid intake may be determined by the duration of the recovery period and the risk of gastrointestinal discomfort. The consumption of a large amount of fluid immediately after the weigh-in will more rapidly restore plasma volume but will be associated with larger urine losses and less overall retention of this fluid. A pattern of small, frequent intake of fluid is likely to be better at restoring the fluid deficit over a longer time period (Kovacs et al. 2002). These strategies are outlined in greater detail in the highlight box on page 307.

A recent issue of interest to weight-making and post-weigh-in recovery is the effect of creatine supplementation strategies. One investigation examined the effects of creatine

Table 12.2   Weight-Making Practices of College and High School Wrestlers

	College (n = 63)	High School (n = 368)
Age (years)	20 (18-23)	16.1 (13-19)
Age began wrestling (years)	10.8 (5-16)	12.3 (6 -16)
Age began weight-making (years)	14.0 (7-18)	13.7 (8-18)
Times of making weight this season (times)	15>0 (0-60)	8.8 (0-41)
Most weight lost this season (kg)	7.2 (1.4-20.5)	5.4 (0-22.7)
Weekly weight fluctuation (% of group) • 0-1 kg • 1.4-2.3 kg • 2.7-4.5 kg • 5-9.1 kg • >9.5 kg	0 13 44 41 2	21 49 23 6 1
Weight gain postseason (kg)	7.6 (1.8-20.5)	
Weight-making techniques undertaken at least a fortnight (% of group) • Sauna • Rubber suit • Fluid restriction • Food restriction • Fasting • Vomiting • Laxatives • Diuretics	55 88 92 92 68 2 5 3	28 42 75 79 50 7 7 4

Data from Steen and Brownell 1990.

supplementation during rapid weight loss on muscle creatine, performance of repeated sprints (10 bouts of 6 s, with 30 s rest), nitrogen balance, and body composition in male resistance trainers. Athletes consumed an energy-restricted diet (18 kcal or 75 kJ · kg^{-1} · day^{-1}) for 4 days, supplemented with either creatine (20 g/day) or a placebo. Results of the sprint test showed a 3.8% increase in work done by the creatine group, whereas the placebo group showed a reduction of 0.5% following energy restriction ($p = .058$). Creatine supplementation increased muscle creatine during short-term energy restriction without changing protein or fat losses and produced a trend for higher total sprint work (Rockwell et al. 2001). Benefits to maximal intensity efforts were also seen in a crossover study on five male wrestlers who reduced their body mass by ~5% in two series of investigations separated by 1 month (Oopik et al. 2002). During the 17 hr recovery period, participants consumed a controlled diet supplemented with glucose or with glucose plus creatine. There was no effect of treatment on regain of body mass during 17 hr of recovery. A 19% increase in maximal work from weight loss to recovery was seen with glucose and creatine, whereas no change was evident with glucose treatment ($p < .05$).

By contrast, creatine supplementation during a 5-day period of weight loss was associated with maintenance of some performance parameters and a decrement in others (Oopik et al. 1998). Well-trained participants were studied before and after losing 3% to 4% body mass, supplemented with either creatine or placebo. A knee extensor test was undertaken for 3 min, with measurements of both maximal and submaximal work. The results indicated that creatine supplementation did not influence maximal work or the rate of fatigue development during maximal work but adversely affected submaximal work. The reasons for the detrimental effect of creatine supplementation on submaximal work were unclear.

Safer Approaches to Making Weight

It is difficult to provide detailed guidelines for weight-making practices in sport. This is partially because of the diversity of factors that are involved in weight-making sports. More important, many sports nutrition professionals are troubled by the ethics of assisting athletes to undertake practices that are potentially detrimental to health or performance or that violate the intention of the rules of sport. Although the situation usually provides an opportunity to assist athletes to undertake safer practices than they are currently using, there is still some hesitation in promoting practices related to intentional dehydration

Guidelines for Safer Practice in Weight-Making Sports

Understand the Requirements and Practices of a Sport

- Investigate the rules of a sport regarding weight classes, weight-making practices, and weigh-ins before competition. Know these issues thoroughly for your sport, including variations occurring at different levels or competition.
- Understand the physiological basis of performance in the sport, including the issues of repeating performance in a tournament or multievent competition, and the effect of physique characteristics on performance outcomes.
- Investigate the culture of athletes within the sport regarding choosing competition weight classes and manipulating body weight to successfully meet weight targets.
- Investigate other weight-making sports to see if there are lessons that can cross over, but be prepared to accept the specificity and nuances of each sport.

Develop Rapport and Understanding With the Weight-Making Athlete

- Take a thorough history of the athlete's weight history and weight loss practices, including the type and frequency of practices and the weight losses achieved.
- Find objective and subjective data describing the athlete's performance history, particularly in relation to weight-making practices.
- Be nonjudgmental as you collect information.

Develop a Long-Term Weight Management Program With the Athlete That Includes a Sensible Choice of Weight Class

- Encourage the athlete to choose a competition weight class that is within 2% to 3% of a body mass that is suitable for long-term training. This weight should be consistent with good eating and hydration patters, effective training, and a comfortable relationship with food and body image.
- Develop weight targets that are safe, realistic, and effective for the individual athlete to suit various times of the competition calendar. These might encompass goals for off-season, heavy training, competition preparation, competition period, weigh-in, and actual competition.
- Undertake any weight loss to achieve the weight goals of training through long-term moderate energy restriction and appropriate exercise. Achieve this weight loss well in advance of the competition period.
- In the case of young adults and adolescents, be prepared to alter weight targets to accommodate growth and maturation. This should include a gradual move across weight classes, and in the case where qualification for a major tournament (e.g., Olympics or World Championships) or competition season takes place well in advance of the event, seek to qualify at a higher weight class that can take into account the need for growth.
- Use objective anthropometric data (lean body mass, body fat, height, growth changes) in setting competition weight classes rather than subjective information.
- Consider the option for the athlete to gain weight to move up a weight division as an alternative to continuing to make weight for a lower weight class.
- Maximize training adaptations through good nutritional status and attention to fueling and hydration strategies for workouts.

Fine-Tune Body Weight by 2% to 3% in the Days or Week Before Competition

- Manipulations to reduce body weight by 2% to 3% may be tolerated in some sports, particularly if undertaken against a background of good nutrition and hydration practices.
- Consider a small reduction in energy intake, particularly against a background of reduced training load or competition taper, to assist with a small weight loss in the final preevent period.
- Achieve an acute loss (typically 0.5 to 1.0 kg) by manipulating the residue content of a varied diet. The athlete should experiment with switching from a normal dietary intake of moderate to high levels of fiber to

(continued)

(continued)

a low-residue menu for 12 to 24 hr before a competition (e.g., replacing whole-grain cereals and fruits and vegetables with white cereals, liquid meal supplements, canned fruit, and jelly). This allows the athlete to maintain energy and nutrient intake while reducing body weight via a reduction in the weight of gastrointestinal contents.

- Consider mild restriction of fluid and salt intake over a period of up to 24 hr before weigh-in, in conjunction with appropriate training, to achieve a small level of dehydration.

Recover Well During the Period Between Weigh-In and Competition

- Use the time between weigh-in and competition to complete the athlete's hydration and fueling goals, especially if intake of fluid and carbohydrate has been less than optimal in the days leading up to the weigh-in.

- Ideally, restore fluid balance by replacing 150% of the volume of any fluid deficit incurred to make the weigh-in target. Sodium replacement should occur simultaneously with fluid intake, either through the use of specialized rehydration products (e.g., oral rehydration solutions or electrolyte supplements) or through the intake of sodium-rich foods and salting of foods in the recovery meal.

- Top up fuel stores by the intake of readily available sources of carbohydrate. Intake of fluids and foods in the hours before competition should achieve a target of at least 1 g of carbohydrate/kg BM. Greater amounts may be needed when fuel status is suboptimal and where there is opportunity between weigh-in for substantial amounts of glycogen storage (e.g., >4 hr).

- Be practical with fluid and food intake. It may not be possible to consume large amounts in the 1 to 2 hr between the weigh-in and competition in some sports. In this case, the athlete should consume as much as is possible and comfortable.

- Ensure that the type and amount of foods and drinks consumed during the recovery period are chosen with attention to the risk of gastrointestinal discomfort in the subsequent event.

- Experiment with consuming recovery fluids and foods as a series of small snacks, rather than one large meal, to enhance the effectiveness of recovery and avoid the gastrointestinal discomfort associated with overeating.

Seek and Consolidate Expertise

- Be confident of the expertise that a sports nutrition expert can provide in the development of a weight loss plan. Consider enlisting the involvement of other professionals such as an exercise scientist, sport psychologist, and sports physician so that physiological, medical, psychological, and performance changes associated with weight-making can be monitored objectively.

- Keep an objective account of all strategies and outcomes of competition weight-making should be kept, so that practices can be fine-tuned in the light of experience.

- Rather than implementing new practices in competition, encourage the athlete to experiment with fine-tuning techniques, such as the effects of the low-residue diet, during a phase of training.

or moderate to severe energy restriction. General and purposely conservative guidelines are summarized below, with the caveat that they should not be used in situations where they are expressly against the rules of a sport.

RESEARCH TOPIC

Making Weight in Lightweight Rowing

The following is an interview with Dr. Gary Slater, Sports Dietitian, about his doctoral work undertaken at the Australian Institute of Sport.

Gary, lightweight rowing was devised to allow competition among rowers with a smaller physique. It's different to other sports in that there is both a weight limit for each competitor as well as a limit on the crew average. How does this work in real life?—How does a multiseat boat organize weight targets within the crew? The lightweight category is defined by maximal weights of 59 kg (crew average 57 kg) and 72.5 kg (crew average 70 kg) for females and males, respectively. Take for example a boat with two male rowers: If one oarsman weights in at the maximal weight (72.5 kg), his partner would have to "spot him" and weigh in at 67.5 kg.

Until now, the decision to spot a partner has been somewhat ad hoc and dictated primarily by the beliefs of the coach.

Research Priorities

The effects of weight-making techniques on health and performance range from benign to serious, but the results are inconsistent and specific to the sport and the individual athlete. The following priorities for research are suggested:

- Techniques of weight-making in various sports, including the frequency of use and typical weight losses achieved
- Effect of various techniques of rapid weight loss, individually and combined, on performance in sport-specific protocols
- Effect of various techniques of recovery after rapid weight loss, individually and combined, on performance in sport-specific protocols
- Effect of weight-making practices on relative performance and overall competitive success in various sports
- Comparison of chronic weight loss involving loss of body fat and lean body mass in already lean athletes versus acute weight loss involving dehydration
- Effect of repeated episodes of weight-making on performance in sport-specific protocols
- Effects of chronic participation in a weight-making sport, including years of rapid weight loss practices, on indexes of health, nutritional status, and growth
- Efficacy of various education and regulation programs in weight-making sports on changing practices of weight loss

There are those who insist all athletes must weigh in at the designated boat average weight with no allowance made for bigger athletes in a crew. However, other coaches and athletes acknowledge the value of a bigger, more powerful crew member in a boat and are willing to make body mass allowances accordingly. I've been able to work with some coaches with such beliefs who plan the body mass management strategies of their athletes well in advance of a regatta. Armed with relevant information (body mass and body composition both past and present, personal experience with acute weight loss), regular assessments (of performance, physique traits, and dietary intake), and the support of relevant staff (exercise physiologist, sports dietitian), individual body mass targets are devised that have the entire crew collectively in their best shape for a regatta.

Your doctoral studies involved investigations on Australian lightweight rowers. What have you observed about their weight-making practices—acute and chronic? How often do these athletes compete? How much weight do they typically need to drop for each regatta? What techniques do they use?

The Australian domestic rowing season is very much focused on the selection of national crews for major international regattas such as World Championships and Olympic Games. Selection is heavily focused on the outcome of two or three regattas (including the Australian Rowing Championships) that are scheduled within a few months of each other. In an attempt to encourage athletes to avoid acute weight loss and focus more on chronic manipulation of mass over a season, allowances are made for progressive loss in body mass over the season. At the first two regattas, athletes can be above their final weight targets—4% above the FISA (Federation Internationale des Sociétés d'Aviron)

specified crew average limits for the first regatta (i.e., 59.3 kg and 72.8 kg for males and females, respectively) and 2% (58.1 kg and 71.4 kg) at the second regatta. It's only the final selection regatta in which the full FISA weight limits are enforced.

In reality, the athletes still use acute weight loss tactics (in addition to chronic strategies) to reach the specified weight limits throughout the season, including those regattas in which weight allowances are made. Acute weight loss remains very common among Australian lightweight rowers.

During the 2003 Australian Rowing Championships, we sought information (via questionnaire) on the weight-making and recovery practices of lightweight competitors. The majority of athletes competing in the regatta acknowledged they had to reduce their body mass in the 4 weeks prior to competition, averaging 2 to 2.5 kg, irrespective of gender or age. One week out from competition athletes reported being just 1 kg above weight. While maximum weight loss in the week prior to previous regattas averaged 2 kg, some athletes acknowledged losses as high as 4 to 6 kg.

Dietary and fluid restriction plus an increased training load are the most popular self-reported methods of body mass management. The uses of saunas and sweat suits are less common but remain a strategy common to one third of respondents in the day prior to weigh-in. Of athletes acknowledging some form of weight loss prior to a regatta, the majority made use of two or more weight loss practices. Among athletes acknowledging some form of dietary restriction, the majority (83%) also conceded the use of fluid restriction.

Monitoring the physique traits of lightweight rowers has revealed some interesting information on the body composition changes of these athletes over a season. Despite athletes typically presenting several kilograms above weight at the start of the preseason, their body fat stores are low. With limited potential for further reductions in fat mass, much of the weight loss that occurs during the ensuing season is derived from fat-free mass. We have little idea of the performance implications of such losses in lean body mass.

What evidence is there that weight-making practices impair rowing performance—either in the laboratory or on the water?

The impact of acute weight loss on rowing performance has received little attention despite the majority of lightweight rowers acknowledging the use of acute weight loss techniques. Aside from the work we've undertaken in the last few years, the only other study that has assessed the impact of acute weight loss on rowing performance reported a substantial performance decrement. After inducing a 5% reduction in body mass over 24 hr, Caroline Burge and associates observed a 22 s increase in time to complete a simulated 2,000 m time trial on an ergometer. However, recovery strategies between weigh-in and racing were less than optimal, with total nutritional intake limited to just 1.5 L of water.

These data contrast markedly with our own. In three investigations assessing the impact of acute weight loss (4-5% over a 24 hr period) on ergometer performance, we have found that when aggressive nutritional recovery strategies are enforced following weigh-in, the overall decrement to time trial performance is small, typically less than 1 to 2 s. Furthermore, this effect is not exaggerated when sustained for several days, as occurs during a multiday regatta. The performance implications of acute weight loss appear to be even smaller for time trials conducted on water, possibly because absolute physical exertion in a boat is somewhat limited by the need to maintain biomechanical efficiency.

In the past, most nutritionists have proposed the loss of body mass to reach specified weight limits should be achieved via chronic manipulation of diet or training. However, we really don't know what impact chronic manipulation of body mass has on performance, especially among very lean individuals for whom much of the body mass reduction is derived from fat-free mass. Our data suggest that the acute loss of moderate amounts of body mass (up to 5% body mass), when matched with aggressive nutritional recovery techniques, is an effective method of achieving specified weight limits among lightweight rowers, especially those larger individuals who would otherwise struggle to make weight if they relied solely on more traditional, chronic weight loss techniques.

What is the typical time period between weigh-in and the race? What do rowers typically do to recover during this period? Do you have any thoughts on the best way to approach this recovery?

Rowers are required to weigh in not less than 1 hr and no more than 2 hr prior to the start of each race during a regatta. While lightweight rowers acknowledge the importance of food and fluid intake during the recovery period between weigh-in and racing, their self-reported practices do not conform to current recovery guidelines; it's very ad hoc. Fluid and sodium intakes in particular are low, only reaching ~50% of recommendations.

In the investigations we have conducted to date, aggressive nutritional recovery strategies have been enforced following weigh-in. We have set particular guidelines for intakes of fluid (28 ml/kg), sodium (34 mg/kg), and carbohydrate (2.3 g/kg). To assist with restoration of plasma volume and maximize gastrointestinal tract comfort, we have prescribed a certain pattern of fluid intake—larger volumes of fluid ingested initially, followed by progressively smaller volumes as the warm-up and race approach. Despite the volume of food and fluid ingested, the recovery formula has been extremely well received with only one report of nausea across almost 150 ergometer time trials.

We recently compared a number of different nutritional recovery strategies—fluid only, carbohydrate and sodium together, or a combination of carbohydrate, sodium and fluid. While the combination of all nutrients was the most effective, the fluid-only formula resulted in similar performance outcomes and was far superior to carbohydrate, suggesting rehydration remains critical following weigh-in. However, it may well be that the optimal nutritional recovery formula varies depending on the method of acute weight loss undertaken to make weight.

During a regatta, lightweight rowers need to weigh in each day that they race. How often will they race and what weight management strategies do they use—do they make weight for each occasion, or make weight once and then stay down for the rest of the regatta? Do you have any feeling for which tactic is more successful?

Depending on the number of athletes competing in a regatta, competitors may have to race several times. During major international, multiday regattas, athletes are required to race every 24 to 48 hr, depending on previous race results. Two different body mass management strategies (between days of racing) are common among athletes who make use of acute weight loss strategies. Rowers are either conservative with food and fluid intake following the first race and remain "at weight" for most of the regatta, or they implement aggressive nutritional recovery strategies for each race, with an associated rebound in body mass that must be lost again prior to the next weigh-in. There doesn't appear to be a clear preference in weight management strategies among athletes. However, it is plausible that these strategies may impact differently on performance, especially for the later and most important races of a regatta.

We addressed this issue among a group of 16 lightweight oarsmen during a simulated regatta. One group "got down to weight" (losing 4-5% body mass loss over 24 hr) and remained near this specified body mass for two subsequent races, while another group dropped a similar amount of weight then restored most of it between weigh in and the first race, repeating this process for subsequent races. Body mass management practices over the 24 hr following the first race seemed to favor the better recovery technique; in fact, there was less of an impairment of performance of ergometer time trials as weight-making was repeated. Again the benefits of aggressive recovery were seen, but there may also have been an adaptation to repeated bouts of acute weight loss.

What appears to be the optimal physique for a lightweight rower? Are successful rowers truly lightweights or are they heavyweights who make weight?

Theoretically, taller athletes are at a biomechanical advantage over their smaller counterparts. Research undertaken at the world rowing championships in the mid-1980s indicated that larger lightweight rowers were more successful than those with a smaller body size. We recently confirmed a competitive advantage among rowers with lower body fat and greater muscle mass. The ideal physique for a lightweight rower is therefore likely to include long levers and low body fat levels, allowing a moderate degree of muscularity. Possession of these traits inevitably ensures the athlete is not a true lightweight—that is, they are not naturally at or below the specified crew average. Certainly most of the athletes I've worked with in recent years follow the pattern of commencing the preseason several kilograms above their designated weight requirement despite already low body fat stores and then gradually reducing their mass to within 2 to 3 kg of the specified limit as the season progresses. These athletes may only be at weight at the time of weigh-in, with their prerace recovery strategies increasing their body mass 1 to 2 kg by the start of a race.

However, physique traits are only one of the factors that contribute to overall competitive success; technical excellence, a large aerobic capacity, and sound psychological skills remain critical.

Publications from doctoral studies: Slater, Rice, Sharpe, Mujika, et al. (2005); Slater, Rice, Mujika, et al. (2005); Slater, Rice, Sharpe, Tanner, et al. 2005; Slater et al. (2006a, 2006b)

PRACTICAL ISSUE

Programs to Limit the Damage Caused by Weight-Making: The Wrestling Experience

Concerns about the weight-making practices of high school and college wrestlers in the United States date back more than 60 years. In 1944 it was observed that "purposely shedding a number of pounds of body weight and then engaging in very strenuous combat is not a normal procedure . . . done obviously to increase a competitor's chance of winning a match. However, because a reduction on weight usually involves either one or three of the following—interference with the laws of good nutrition, excessive exercise, artificial methods of dehydration—many interested persons question the effect of rigorous procedures on performance

and health of the athlete" (Doscher 1944, cited in Steen and Brownell 1990, p. 762).

In the 1960s and 1970s, the American Medical Association and the American College of Sports Medicine produced position statements condemning the rapid weight loss techniques observed among interscholastic wrestlers (American College of Sports Medicine 1976; American Medical Association 1967). These papers noted that already lean wrestlers further reduced their body mass for competition, with the primary methods of weight loss affecting body water, glycogen, and lean body mass. They pointed out a variety of health and performance issues associated with dehydration and severe food restriction and called for coaches and athletes to abandon practices aimed at competing in weight classes significantly lighter than a natural or healthy training weight. This position was reaffirmed by the ACSM in 1996 (American College of Sports Medicine 1996). Despite these pronouncements and education messages, surveys of the weight-making practices of college and high school wrestlers suggest that little change occurred over the next 30 to 40 years. A landmark 1990 study provided clear documentation that the tradition of making weight was still integral to the interscholastic sport of wrestling, with practices being more severe at college level than among high school wrestlers (Steen and Brownell 1990). The authors concluded that a more aggressive approach was needed to eradicate such weight control practices.

In 1989, the Wisconsin Interscholastic Athletic Association embarked on a project aimed at reducing unhealthy weight loss practices in wrestlers. This Wrestling Minimum Weight Project involved a double-pronged approach: targeting changes in the rules governing high school wrestling competition and providing education programs for athletes and coaches (Oppliger et al. 1995). Rule changes included setting a minimum competition weight for each individual wrestler (set at 7% body fat), and minimizing weight loss to 3 lb (1.4 kg) per week. The implementation of the project over a 3-year period involved considerable effort to research, develop, and pilot test the components of the program. For example, an army of testers were trained to perform a validated skinfold assessment on each high school wrestler and certify his minimum wrestling weight before the start of the competitive season. The nutrition education programs involved the development of visual aids, including a booklet titled *The Wrestlers' Diet*.

During the first years, the program was undertaken on a voluntary basis by schools within the state of Wisconsin. In 1991, the program became a mandatory implementation and continues to be self-evaluated and modified on an annual basis. According to one evaluation, during the voluntary phase, 80% of participants adhered to the MWW recommendation. More than 60% of wrestling coaches were initially opposed to the project in 1989, but by 1993, positive responses were received from more than 95% (Oppliger et al. 1995). This turnaround apparently occurred when coaches realized that the program relieved them of the burden of selecting weight classes for wrestlers and worrying about weight control, freeing up time to concentrate on conditioning and technique. Acceptance of the program by wrestlers was also reported to be high (>75%), and surveys reported a reduction in the amount of weight cycled, the frequency of weight-making episodes during a season, and the duration of fasting prior to a weigh-in (Oppliger et al. 1995, 1998). Following this success, other wrestling organizations have instigated or mandated programs based on similar models. Although progress appears to have been made, the difficulty in making change is noted. For example, although an MWW program was in place among a group of high schools, substantial numbers of the wrestlers involved in a survey (33%) reported ignoring the guidelines (Wroble and Moxley 1998).

The National Collegiate Athletic Associated responded to the 1997 deaths of three collegiate wrestlers by making a number of rule changes to curb excessive weight cutting. The regulations, introduced at the beginning of the 1998-1999 season, included the following features (NCAA 2003):

- The weight limits for the 10 weight classes were adjusted to add ~10 lb (~5 kg). For example, the old 119 lb class was increased to 125 lb.

- Weigh-ins were moved closer to competition (1-2 hr) instead of the previous typical 5 hr recovery period. This reduction in the opportunity for refeeding and rehydration after the weigh-in was undertaken to reduce the temptation to cut weight.

- Body fat is now assessed at the beginning of the season by a physician or athletic trainer to certify each wrestler at a minimum competitive weight, equivalent to a body fat level of 5% body mass.

- Measurement of urinary specific gravity is undertaken at the time of weight certification, and a reading of <1.020 must be achieved to demonstrate adequate hydration.

- Wrestlers are given a time period to reach this competitive weight, and no more than 1.5% body mass can be lost on average per week to achieve this loss.

- Weight loss practices including excessive food restriction and dehydration, saunas, hot boxes, steam rooms, sweat suits used for the purposes of dehydration, self-induced vomiting, and the use of emetics, laxatives, and diuretics are banned. One violation will lead to suspension for the competition in which the weigh-in was targeted, whereas a second violation will lead to suspension for the whole season.

A short report (Scott et al. 2000) of the mat-side weight gain of wrestlers (weight replaced after the weigh-in) found that results from the 1999 NCAA championship (mean gain = 0.66 kg) were significantly lower than results reported in 1992 (mean gain = 3.73 kg). Because mat-side weight gain was said to reflect rapid weight lost before weigh-in, the reduction in opportunity for recovery appeared to have a major effect on the wrestlers' willingness to cut weight. A large study of weight making practices across tournaments at the three divisions of collegiate wrestling from 1999-2004, collected data on the difference between the pre- and postseason body composition of wrestlers, as well as rapid weight loss over the day leading into a competition weigh-in and rapid weight gain between the weigh-in and the end of the first day of a competition (Oppliger et al. 2006). This study found that there was a significant loss of weight and body fat over the season. However, the average body fat level of wrestlers at postseason testing was 9.5%, well above the minimum level. Very few wrestlers were estimated to have body fat levels below 7%, even at the lighter division where lower body fat levels are expected. These authors concluded that few wrestlers were constrained by their weights since they were not required to reach the minimum weight of 5% body fat. Furthermore, the average values seen for rapid weight loss and gain over the day of competition were ~1 kg or ~1.2% BM (Oppliger et al. 2006). Other recent surveys concluded that the weight-making strategies of collegiate wrestlers are less extreme than those reported in the previous decade, however, banned practices and large weight losses still persist among some individuals (Oppliger et al. 2003).

Clearly, substantial effort and resources are required to combat the ingrained traditions and practices of athletes in weight-making sports. The importance of enforcing rule changes was highlighted by a study of high school wrestlers who engaged in freestyle and Greco-Roman wrestling in an amateur competition outside the scholastic system (Alderman et al. 2004). In this competition, although rapid weight loss practices are banned, regulations are not well enforced and strategies such as reducing the period between weigh-in and the event are not in place. This study reported that large amounts of weight were gained after weigh-in (~5% body mass), similar to the practices of high school wrestlers before the implementation of the new rules in their competition. The authors concluded that unless rules are imposed and enforced, wrestlers will continue to believe in the benefits of weight-making and will engage in these practices according to the opportunities provided.

chapter 13

Gymnastics

In a number of activities, participants perform skills requiring exceptional development of power, strength, flexibility, and agility. Typically, participants complete a series of standard routines or skills, with a subjective evaluation of the outcome. In the case of competitive sports—for example, rhythmic and artistic gymnastics, figure skating, synchronized swimming, trampoline, and diving—a panel of judges award points for the performance of each competitor according to their perception of technical or artistic merit. Although participants in activities such as dancing, ballet, and cheerleading share common issues and challenges as these "aesthetic" athletes, the former compete for selection in a company or show rather than for medals.

In aesthetic sports and activities, appearance is a factor in either the judging of competition or the perception of coaches and selectors. This is particularly the case for female athletes. There is considerable pressure for athletes to conform to a homogeneous physique: a small and light frame, with low levels of subcutaneous body fat but some muscular development, particularly in males. Height limits are prevalent in some sports or activities. This chapter focuses on the nutritional needs of elite-level artistic and rhythmic gymnastics because these sport has received most attention. Nevertheless, participants in other aesthetic activities may be able to benefit from the guidelines developed for gymnasts.

Competition

The Federation Internationale de Gymnastique (FIG) is the international governing body for the elite sports of artistic and rhythmic gymnastics. Within these sports there are four disciplines: women's artistic gymnastics, men's artistic gymnastics, women's rhythmic gymnastics, and women's group rhythmic gymnastics. Competition in each of these sports involves between two and six separate apparatuses, with the duration of a routine in each apparatus lasting from around 6 s up to 150 s (see table 13.1). Female artistic gymnasts undertake four apparatuses in

competition, whereas males perform on six apparatuses. For each apparatus there are compulsory routines set on a cycle by the FIG as well as optional routines selected by the gymnast. There are separate competitions for teams and for individual performers, with individual prizes being awarded for each apparatus as well as the overall (known as all-around) score. In rhythmic gymnastics, individual competitors undertake separate floor routines with four different apparatuses, whereas group rhythmic gymnastics involves a team of six gymnasts who perform two different floor exercises. In these disciplines, the competition program is chosen every two years with different apparatuses being involved.

The major competitions in elite gymnastics are the Olympics Games, World Championships, and World Cup–ranked events such as continental championships, category A and B tournaments, and the World Cup Final. A competition program generally takes place over a number of days, with a variety of performance demands depending on the gymnast's involvement in individual or team sessions and all-round or individual apparatuses. Anaerobic energy sources underpin the performance of a gymnastics routine; the creatine phosphate system and anaerobic glycolysis is most important for the apparatuses involving the shortest duration (e.g., vault, lasting 6-8 s, including the approach run, and bar routines, lasting 15-30 s). Aerobic energy production has a more prominent role in the longer floor routines. Even when the gymnast is required to perform more than once in a day or over successive days, there is ample time for the recovery of muscle fuel sources. Of course, the recovery of muscle glycogen stores may be compromised in athletes who restrict food intake because of weight concerns.

The competitive peak in gymnastics occurs at a younger age than seen in many sports, particularly for female competitors. Top-class male gymnasts achieve their peak performances in their late teens to early 20s. By contrast, there has been a decrease in the age of elite female gymnasts; for example, the mean age of gymnasts in the U.S. Olympic team dropped from 18.5 years in 1960 to 16

Table 13.1   Components of Elite Competition in Gymnastics

MEN'S ARTISTIC		WOMEN'S ARTISTIC		WOMEN'S RHYTHMIC		WOMEN'S GROUP RHYTHMIC	
Apparatus	Duration (s)	Apparatus	Duration (s)	Apparatus	Duration (s)	Apparatus	Duration (s)
Floor exercise	50-70	Floor exercise	60-90	4 different floor exercise routines with various appara- tuses[a]	75-90	2 different floor exercise routines with combination of apparatuses[b]	135-150
High bar	15-30	Balance beam	70-90	Ribbon		Ribbon	
Parallel bars	20-30	Uneven bars	20-30	Rope		Rope	
Pommel horse	20-30	Vault	6-8	Ball		Ball	
Vault	6-8			Hoop		Hoop	
Rings	20-30			Clubs		Clubs	

[a]After each World Championships, the Federation Internationale de Gymnastique (FIG) announces 4 apparatuses from these 5 choices for competition program over subsequent 2 years; [b]after each World Championships, FIG announces which combination of apparatus from these 5 choices will be used in competition program over subsequent 2 years.

years in 1992 (Nattiv and Mendelbaum 1993). This trend appears to be related to the value placed on a prepubertal physique over the recent decades (see section on physique characteristics). To counteract this trend, which encourages young girls to participate at high-level competition involving highly skilled (and dangerous) routines and a lengthy training history, the FIG has introduced an age limit for elite competition. Female participants are now required to be aged 16 in the year that they are involved in elite events such as the Olympic Games. Nevertheless, young gymnasts from 10 to 16 years can be heavily involved in demanding junior-level competitions.

Training

Achievement of the increasingly complex skills involved in elite gymnastics takes years of intense practice and requires the gymnast to commit her lifestyle to the sport. Because it is estimated that 7 to 10 years of such training is required to master these skills, gymnasts may enter an elite development program with a training schedule of 10 to 25 hr/week before they reach their teenage years (Weimann et al. 2000).

In the noncompetitive season, or in the early development of a gymnast, much of the training program is spent on acquiring skills through technique work and body conditioning. Supplementary resistance training is undertaken by some gymnasts, typically male performers, although a gymnastics workout also involves strength-based routines against the resistance of the athlete's own body mass. Typically, elite gymnasts train twice per day, with one rest day each week. Sessions usually last 1 to 4 hr.

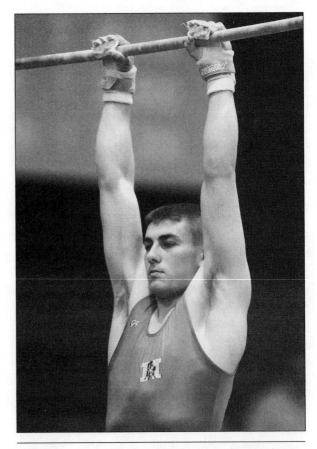

Preparation for a specific event, for example, an Olympic Games, now begins 4 to 8 years in advance of the competition, and the athletes gradually build up to a full training load of 30 to 40 hr/week.

Although the training commitments of the elite gymnast are lengthy, the energy expenditure of skill and conditioning activities within a session is quite modest. A warm-up is undertaken at the beginning of the session, involving stretches and a set of basic skills on the floor mat. The rest of the session is spent rotating between the apparatuses in groups, with each gymnast taking a turn to perform a skill or part of a skill. The time performing this skill is never longer than the competition piece and is usually a small fraction of this routine (Benardot 2000). Thus, practice is spent undertaking brief but high-intensity bouts, with plenty of rest time between exercises.

Physique and Physiology

Elite male gymnasts are lean with a well-developed musculature of the trunk, shoulder, and arms. Elite male gymnasts show a homogeneous physique, with a typical height of 168 cm, weight of 66.5 kg, and body fat level of 3% to 4% (Bale and Goodway 1990). Even so, there is some specialization of the physiques of particular racial groups and of gymnasts who excel in a particular apparatus. For example, Japanese gymnasts are described as being shorter and stockier than their European and American counterparts, with relatively shorter arms and legs. Such a physique, which positions the center of gravity near to axes of rotation and creates a small moment of inertia, achieves a biomechanical efficiency for apparatuses involving arm support activities. At a subelite level, where athletes can specialize in one apparatus, floor routines that require fast tumbling and rapid aerial rotations are dominated by the shortest and most powerful gymnasts. By contrast, gymnasts who specialize in the pommel horse are taller and leaner, with longer limbs (Bale and Goodway 1990).

Elite female gymnasts have changed in physique over the past decades. Whereas a mature and elegant physique was typical of champions of the 1950s and 1960s, the dominance of champions such as Olga Korbut and Nadia Comaneci in successive decades made a light and prepubertal shape popular. Studies in the 1970s described a short and light body type for the typical female gymnast—mean weight 50 kg, height 158 to 164 cm, and percent body fat 13 to 16% (Bale and Goodway 1990). Today's female athletes are even lighter and smaller, with very low body fat levels (10-12%), some upper muscular development, and relatively broad shoulders and small hips (Bernadot 2000). Changes in the physical characteristics of members of the U.S. Olympic gymnastics team from the 1960s to 1992 exemplify the "downsizing" trend; average heights and weights changed from 157.5 cm and 50 kg to 146 cm and 37.5 kg, respectively (Benardot 2000). Such a body shape provides less resistance to rotation skills, allowing explosive tumbling movements in the air and on the bars (for review, see Bale and Goodway 1990).

A popular perception of aesthetic sports is that the ideal physique is chosen by coaches or judges. Undoubtedly, there is a component of appearance that impresses judges or selectors. Nevertheless, the benefits of a light and lean body shape in aesthetic sports are real rather than arbitrary. Physique is a major factor in the ability to perform certain physical skills and movements. A short stature and small frame are of benefit where athletes must rotate and twist their bodies in a small space (e.g., diving and gymnastics). Being light is an advantage when body mass must be moved against gravity by the individual (i.e., gymnastics) or a partner (i.e., ballet). Because the skills required of athletes at high levels of competition are predetermined, those who conform to the ideal shape will be at a performance advantage. Conversely, a sudden gain in weight will change important characteristics such as power-to-weight ratio and the body's center of gravity, not only reducing performance but making it dangerous to attempt many of the previously mastered skills. A gain in height will also change aspects of the biomechanics that underpin the performance of various skills.

There is evidence that changes in weight and height have different effects on various movement skills. A longitudinal study on the effects of body size on gymnastics performance tracked 10- to 12-year-old national and state level female gymnasts for just over 3 years (Ackland et al. 2003). Participants were tested at 4-month intervals and were divided into "high growers" and "low growers" based on changes in height (increase over the 37 months of >18 cm or <14) and body mass (>15 kg or <12 kg). Smaller gymnasts, with a high power-to-weight ratio, had greater potential for performing skills involving whole-body rotations. Larger gymnasts, although able to produce more power and greater angular momentum, could not match such performances. The magnitude of growth experienced by the gymnast over this period had a varying effect on performance. Although some activities were greatly influenced by rapid increases in whole-body moment of inertia (e.g., back rotation), the performance of others (e.g., the front rotation and vertical jump) was less affected by the physical and mechanical changes associated with growth. There are practical observations to match these findings; many young gymnasts who grow beyond the physique dimensions considered ideal for their sport switch to activities such as diving, trampolining, or aerial skiing. It appears they are able to transfer the skills achieved in an early career in gymnastics to activities that are more tolerant of a larger body size.

In an ideal world, performance expectations in aesthetic sports would reflect appearance and skills commensurate with a healthy physique and a reasonable training load. Furthermore, talent identification processes would direct only athletes who are genetically suited to attain the necessary physical characteristics toward an elite career in these sports. In reality, serious training begins at a young age in gymnastics, and many of the athletes who show early promise outgrow an ideal physique as they reach adolescence or maturation. It can be hard to let go of dreams of a successful career when so much time has been invested and talent has been previously rewarded. Many gymnasts resort to unhealthy dietary restrictions, trying to whittle themselves into the required shape and size or to prevent further growth. The importance of nutrition in health and performance is often misunderstood or ignored.

Lifestyle and Culture

Gymnastics is practiced around the world, with more than 80 member nations of FIG. In some countries (e.g., Australia, United States), gymnastics is essentially an amateur sport, although it is a popular spectator event at competitions such as the Olympics Games. In other countries (e.g., China, former states of the USSR, other Eastern European countries), gymnastics is a state-sponsored sport, with well-developed programs for talent identification and progressive training in special sport schools and institutes. There are clear differences between these systems in the social and cultural approaches to the training of elite gymnasts. This often leads to a clash of cultures when coaches from the more regimented systems are imported to programs in Western countries.

Female gymnasts reach their peak in their mid- to late teens, with males peaking in their teens to early 20s. However, because of the intensive training required to master the skills of elite competition, gymnasts undertake adult training commitments of 10 to 20 hr/week when they are as young as 10 years of age. This commitment is made not only in terms of the hours of training undertaken each week but also in the exclusion of many physical, recreational, and social activities that are typical for children and adolescents. Some gymnasts suffer frustration or unhappiness because of the level of sacrifice required by their sport—particularly their inability to enjoy the growing independence and freedom with food intake that is part of a normal adolescence. At the day-to-day level, gymnasts and their parents are challenged by the difficulty of juggling training sessions and school commitments, as well as travel, special nutritional needs, and the medical or physiotherapy appointments that are part of a sport with a high rate of injury.

It is tempting to blame coaches, judges, and parents for the nutrition problems that occur in gymnastics, citing the emphasis on physique and an environment of restrictiveness and discipline as the cause of the problems. Ideally, a gymnast's environment would be constructed to support the legitimate need for these factors yet provide an atmosphere that is positive and nurturing for all participants. Undoubtedly, this does not always happen and some gymnasts will find themselves at odds with an individual or a system that does not recognize their specific needs. However, it is also important to recognize that elite gymnastics is selective for a certain personality type, just as it selects for physical characteristics and talent. The contribution of personality traits to the development of disordered eating is discussed in more detail subsequently.

Finally, the education of gymnasts must include resources and activities that are appropriate for children and adolescents while meeting the specific needs for high-level participation in a sport. Of course, nutrition educators need also to be aware that many gymnasts continue their career into their 20s. It is a trap to treat all small gymnasts as young and naive. Counseling techniques, education activities, levels of responsibility, and other attributes of a gymnastics program need to be relevant to the real age of the athlete rather than skewed by his or her appearance.

The importance of appropriate nutrition tools was discussed by Dan Benardot (1996), in reflections on his work as nutritionist for the U.S. national gymnastics team. He found that traditional tools for collecting data on food intake were impractical for his interaction with gymnasts at national camps, competitions, and laboratory visits. For example, he found that the high participant burden caused poor compliance in keeping 3-day food records, whereas 24 hr recalls were reliant on memory and unrepresentative of normal intake, especially when taken at camps. In addition, the focus on food intake was often threatening to the gymnast. He developed a new tool, Computerized Time-Line Energy Analysis (CTLEA), in an attempt to overcome these weaknesses and provide information that his athlete population found interesting. CTLEA requires the athlete to account for every activity done from waking until going to bed over a typical training day. It then estimates the energy expenditure associated with each activity, including, where available, real measurements of energy expenditure from the individual athlete. Once a time line of activities is created, the athlete describes the food and fluids consumed during the various time points. The output from the analysis is a series of activity periods defined by a calculation of energy balance—achieved by comparing energy intake and energy expenditure during each period, plus the carryover from the previous period. CTLEA provides the gymnast with a reportedly valid estimate of energy and macronutrient intake for the day but also identifies the periods during which there are large deficits and surpluses of energy. According to the author, this new style of information not only highlights periods in the day that could benefit from dietary change but also promotes rapport between the gymnast and nutritionist (Benardot 1996).

Dietary Surveys

The literature on dietary patterns of gymnasts is limited by the scarcity of surveys of males in general and recent surveys of groups of elite female performers. The results of available studies are summarized in tables in the appendix to this chapter (tables 13.a and 13.b). Although it is not possible to comment on the few studies of males, the data from a variety of groups of female gymnasts surveyed over the past 20 years show a striking similarity in their findings of apparently modest energy intakes (6-8 MJ or 1,200-1,900 kcal/day). When the small body size of these athletes is taken into account, reported energy intakes are typically ~150 to 170 kJ $\cdot$ kg^{-1} $\cdot$ day^{-1} (36-40 kcal $\cdot$ kg^{-1} $\cdot$ day^{-1}), with levels of <130 kJ $\cdot$ kg^{-1} $\cdot$ day^{-1} (31 kcal $\cdot$ kg^{-1} $\cdot$ day^{-1}) being reported by groups of older gymnasts (Gropper et al. 2003; Hickson et al. 1986; Kirchner et al. 1995). In reviewing this same literature, Benardot (2000) compared reported energy intakes of groups of female gymnasts with either a prediction of their energy requirements or the country-specific

Recommended Daily Allowances for energy intake. His analysis found that reported intakes were typically between 47% and 99% of the recommended level, with gymnasts involved in the highest levels of competition being the most likely to have a differential between energy intake and energy requirement. Age was identified as a factor predicting a reduced energy intake; gymnasts from a 15- to 18-year age group reported an energy intake that was 24% below their estimated energy requirement, whereas 11- to 14-year-old gymnasts appeared to consume within 10% of their estimated energy requirements. Other studies have commented on a mismatch between the energy intakes and expenditure of gymnasts. Gymnasts reported a daily energy intake (food records) that was 3.2 MJ (760 kcal) lower than estimated energy expenditure (activity diaries); this difference was significantly greater than the near energy balance reported by a group of non-weight-conscious female athletes (soccer players) and sedentary controls (Fogelholm et al. 1995).

Typically, carbohydrate intake contributes ~50% to 55% of energy to the typical eating patterns of female gymnasts, achieving a daily carbohydrate intake of ~5 to 6 g/kg body mass (Benson et al. 1990; Jonnalagadda et al. 1998; Loosli et al. 1986; Reggiani et al. 1989; Van Erp-Baart et al. 1989a; Weimann et al. 2000). There are no studies of the specific fuel requirements of gymnastics training, although high-intensity activities within each session are characterized as being carbohydrate-dependent. However, this literature suggests that it is possible for gymnasts to consume carbohydrate intakes within the range generally promoted for nonendurance athletes (table 1.2), even in a modest-energy diet. However, some studies have found reported carbohydrate intakes by gymnasts that are below these targets (Kirchner et al. 1995; Moffatt 1984), and even when mean intakes of a group appear suitable, there are individual gymnasts within the group whose intake is considerably lower.

Protein is an important nutrient for growth and repair, factors that are important during childhood and adolescence and for the intensive training programs undertaken by elite gymnasts. The dietary surveys of female gymnasts report that protein intake typically accounts for 15% of energy intake in the typical training diet, providing a daily intake of 1.4 to 2.0 $g \cdot kg^{-1} \cdot day^{-1}$ (Benardot et al. 1989; Jonnalagadda et al. 1998; Loosli et al. 1986; Moffatt 1984; Reggiani et al. 1989; Van Erp-Baart et al. 1989a). Thus, gymnasts who have been included in dietary surveys appear to meet general guidelines protein intake for athletic populations. Again, there are groups of gymnasts (Gropper et al. 2003; Kirchner et al. 1995) and individuals who are likely to consume intakes below this range. Sport-specific studies are needed to detail protein requirements for gymnasts and to investigate whether current athletes achieve the amount and timing of optimal protein intake. Dietary fat currently appears to provide ~30% of the energy intake of the training diets of gymnasts.

According to dietary surveys of gymnasts that have estimated intakes of micronutrients (Benardot et al. 1989; Hickson et al. 1986; Jonnalagadda et al. 1998; Moffatt 1984; Short and Short 1983), mean reported intakes of most vitamins are typically around the level of the relevant dietary reference standards, particularly when B vitamins are assessed in relation to energy intake. However, even when mean intakes appear appropriate, substantial numbers of gymnasts within the group report intakes of less than 70% to 75% of the recommended daily allowance for a number of vitamins (Hickson et al. 1986; Moffatt 1984); this is the level at which there is a high risk of inadequate intakes by individuals. Minerals appear to be at greater risk of suboptimal intakes in the training diets followed by gymnasts. Many studies have reported mean intakes of calcium, zinc, or iron that were below 70% of the allowance for these nutrients, or at least intakes by large numbers of individual participants below this mark (Hickson et al. 1986; Jonnalagadda et al. 1998; Kirchner et al. 1995; Loosli et al. 1986; Moffatt 1984; Weimann et al. 2000). Gymnasts were identified in a study of adolescent athletes as having a higher prevalence of reduced iron status than groups of other athletes (Constantini et al. 2000). Although a reduced energy intake is the major risk factor for suboptimal intakes of micronutrients, this may be partially compensated by careful choices of nutrient-rich foods. Indeed, in one study, the nutrient density of diets chosen by gymnasts was greater than that reported by adolescent athletes in population dietary surveys (Jonnalagadda et al. 1998). However, in another study, dieting behavior was not associated with the low calcium intakes reported by gymnasts (Webster and Barr 1995), suggesting that poor food choice was also involved.

The authors of dietary surveys of gymnasts have commented that the interpretation of their dietary intake data is challenged by the lack of sport-specific guidelines for intakes of macronutrients and micronutrients. However, the problem is further complicated by the likelihood that reported intakes do not represent the true dietary patterns of these athletes. Underreporting of intake appears to be widespread and substantial within gymnastics populations. Jonnalagadda and colleagues (1998) reported that 61% of gymnasts who completed a dietary survey appeared to be underreporters, based on the Goldberg factor of an energy intake to basal metabolic rate ratio of <1.44 (see research topic). In another study in which gymnasts were found to be in energy deficit, estimates of resting energy expenditure adjusted for fat and fat-free mass were not different than those of energy-balanced soccer players and sedentary controls (Fogelholm et al. 1995). The authors of this study concluded that reduced energy metabolism could not explain the apparently lower energy intakes of the gymnasts, and the authors suggested underreporting resulting from issues with diet and body image. More research is needed to determine the extent and impact of this underreporting by gymnasts. In the meantime, care should be taken in interpreting the nutritional status of gymnasts and in choosing strategies for nutritional interventions.

Nutritional Issues and Challenges

Although a variety of nutritional challenges for training and competition in gymnastics can be identified (see highlight box on this page), these issues are heavily skewed by the focus on achieving an ideal physique. Because there is a lack of specialized information on many aspects of the nutrition of gymnasts, this chapter tackles only a small number of topics in some detail, with a particular interest in issues related to restricted energy intakes. For a broader overview of the nutrition strategies that could be applied to gymnastics, both in everyday eating and in specific preparation and recovery during competition, see chapter 1.

The fuel requirements of training have not been systematically investigated in gymnastics, but it is possible that gymnasts who severely restrict carbohydrate or energy intake may fail to replace liver and muscle glycogen stores between training sessions. Further work is needed to better characterize the carbohydrate needs for gymnastics training and methods to easily identify gymnasts who succeed or fail in meeting these needs. Inadequate fuel availability,

through either depleted muscle glycogen stores or suboptimal blood glucose levels, could impair performance during prolonged workouts. Another cause of fatigue during prolonged training may be acute or chronic dehydration, caused by the deliberate restriction of fluid intake to keep body mass artificially low. Whatever the cause, fatigue during the execution of such precise skills may lead to poor practice at the best outcome and, more seriously, to accidents and an increased risk of injury. Therefore, gymnasts would be well advised to pay attention to future research that better defines carbohydrate needs and to undertake appropriate hydration practices, both during a training session and in the everyday diet.

Competition in gymnastics shares some of the characteristics of a track-and-field meet. This includes the underlying physiological issues of brief high-intensity exercise, the need to compete in more than one event in a session or multiday meet, and the demands of the competition timetable. Carbohydrate and fluid status are unlikely to be limiting factors in a single performance, especially if the gymnast has followed a well-chosen meal pattern over the 24 hr period before the event. Competition performance might be compromised if pre- and between-event intake of fluid or carbohydrate is restricted to meet weight goals

Common Nutritional Issues Arising in Gymnastics

Physique Issues

- Optimal body physique: small body size, low body fat levels, and specific muscular development
- High risk of disordered eating and fad diets related to focus on achieving or maintaining small and lean physique
- Effects on chronic energy restriction on immediate and long-term growth of children and adolescents

Training Issues

- Mismatch between training energy expenditure and achievement of low body fat levels, with low energy expenditure in training providing little assistance to achieve energy deficit to reduce body fat levels
- Adequate carbohydrate and protein intake to fuel training and promote recovery and muscle repair
- Adequate micronutrient intake in view of low energy intake and fad diets
- Effects of chronic energy restriction on pubertal development, including attainment of normal menstrual status
- Bone status of female athletes; can exercise stimulus compensate for suboptimal calcium intake and high prevalence of impaired menstrual status?
- Achievement of the nutritional needs of gymnastics during adolescence, a time of changing nutritional needs and the development of social and cultural issues related to eating

Competition Issues

- Adequate preevent eating in view of fears about body weight and appearance
- Strategies to maintain adequate fuel and hydration status over days of competition to promote optimal performance
- Nutrition for traveling

or an issue of appearance, such as achieving a flat stomach. The general principles of the preevent period, including the preevent meal, are outlined in chapter 1, goals 12 and 13, and in table 1.3 However, as discussed in chapter 7 (Sprinting and Jumping), there are often significant practical challenges to eating well in the competition situation. These challenges include the following issues:

• Integrating competition eating (preevent and postevent meals) into a daily meal plan, especially when the event is scheduled at night. Managing fluid and food intake over a prolonged session or day of competition can be complicated when the gymnast has several routines to undertake.

• Access to suitable foods at the competition venue. Being involved in an event, or simply being at the competition venue, can distract the athlete from attending to her dietary needs. In some cases, foods and fluids are not readily available, particularly when the gymnast has traveled away from the familiarity and reliability of her usual food supply.

The guidelines in chapter 7 encouraged the athlete to meet these challenges with good preparation and tracking. Gymnasts should work with their coach and sports nutrition advisor to consider the nutritional needs of their competition program and the likely timetable of events. This should allow each gymnast to develop a rough outline of where fluid and food breaks will be needed—including the preevent meal, fluid top-ups after a warm-up and between apparatuses, and snacks to promote more substantial recovery between bouts that are more widely spaced. In a multiday meet, the gymnast will need to plan for recovery meals at the end of each session or the end of the day.

The availability of foods and drinks within the competition environment should also be considered, including the wider issues of eating away from home. The discussion in chapter 10 (practical issue, "The Traveling Athlete") encouraged athletes or their travel organizers to investigate the general food supply at the competition destination as well as any specific catering plans that are in place. The chief concern of many gymnastics coaches is that a new food environment will cause their athletes to gain weight at a critical time. As a result, many coaches request or implement programs aimed at ensuring that their athletes consume an appropriate energy intake. Ultimately, an athlete needs to take responsibility for his or her own eating patterns and food intake. However, the young age of many gymnasts at high-level competition means that some level of supervision at meals, as would be experienced within the home environment, is reasonable. The team environment should be neither too restrictive nor uncaring about competition eating. Those in charge of young gymnasts during competition should organize a suitable menu and provide positive education regarding strategies to eat well. Catering plans should be considerate of the portion sizes of meals served to athletes with modest energy needs, as well as the fat content of food and the availability of treats. Although it may be appropriate to organize strategies that

limit or discourage inappropriate eating, practices that are overly restrictive or punitive are rarely successful in helping athletes adopt a healthy attitude to food and suitable long-term eating patterns.

Ideal Weight and Body Fat Levels

The lengthy training sessions undertaken by gymnasts are taken up by low energy expenditure activities such as flexibility and agility drills, practicing of portions of skills, or recovery between routines. This factor, coupled with the small size of athletes and their restricted access to sport and recreational activities outside their main activity, predicts modest energy requirements. Restricting energy intake becomes the major route for producing an energy deficit to reduce weight or body fat levels or to avoid rapid growth spurts. According to various studies of populations of female gymnasts, 50% to 100% of individuals within the group report being on a diet, despite their young age and high levels of leanness (Jonnalagadda et al. 2000; Sundgot-Borgen 1996). Problems arise when weight and body fat targets are set at an unhealthily low level or where there are extreme attempts to prevent the gymnast from achieving his or her genetically determined growth rate.

The concern about remaining lean and trim sometimes leads to frequent weight checks by female gymnasts. Sometimes, weighing in is a routine part of each training session or a requirement set by the coach. Other times it is initiated by the gymnast to check her eating for the day. Coaches have valid reasons for fearing sudden and major increases in body mass. It is dangerous for gymnasts to attempt an intricate routine with the sudden addition of a substantial amount of weight; this upsets balance, the center of gravity, and other aspects of their finely tuned skills. Coaches want to know if their gymnasts are at such a risk at any single training session and to be aware of creeping weight gain that might need to be checked. However, scale watching leads to excessive concern about physique and to poor eating patterns based on misconceptions about normal daily fluctuations in body mass. Some athletes (and their coaches) do not realize that it is normal and healthy for weight to fluctuate each day. This is because of weight losses through sweating, the temporary gain in body mass after eating and drinking attributable to the weight of food and fluids consumed, and weight lost after eliminating. In the absence of large sweat losses (not generally encountered in gymnastics training), the gymnast can expect to record her lowest body mass reading in the morning, after voiding.

When weight checks are undertaken at each training session, with implicit or covert expectations that no gain should occur, the gymnast can easily fall into a vicious cycle of poor nutrition practices based on perceived and immediate needs rather than real and long-term issues. Gymnasts have been noted to restrict fluid intake and to eat minimal amounts of food during the day to minimize any changes in their body mass between sessions or from the previous day. Additionally, food eaten during the day may be limited to light and compact foods. For example, the gymnast may choose a chocolate bar (50 g) for lunch

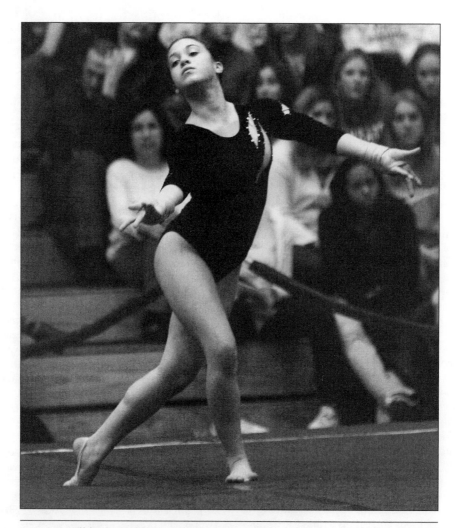

Even in small-bodied athletes, and without the influence of the weight of clothes and shoes, body mass can change by a kilogram each day, without any relationship to changes in physique or body fat levels.

in preference to a salad sandwich (200 g) and a drink (250 g)—because it minimizes the immediate impact on the scales. In many cases, energy restriction during the day is counterbalanced by binge eating at night. Many gymnasts confuse the weight of foods and drinks with their energy content and forget about the overall contribution to nutritional requirements. Unfortunately, size and mass do not correlate with energy value. For example, some small and light foods are also high in fat and kilojoules, low in water content, and poor in micronutrients (e.g., chocolate, potato crisps, and biscuits). Conversely, some heavy foods, such as fruit and vegetables, are low in fat and kilojoules and nutrient-rich. Water is heavy but has no kilojoule value or direct impact on body fat levels.

Clearly, any food pattern based on minimizing the total mass of food and fluid intake or restricting intake during the day is problematic. Immediate issues include the potential risk of inadequate fluid and carbohydrate status for training sessions. Earlier in this chapter, it was suggested that an increased level of fatigue caused by poor nutrition

might reduce the quality of training as well as increase the risk of accidents and injury. Focus on nutrient-poor foods, at least during certain periods of the day, is likely to further compromise the nutritional adequacy of a low energy intake and increase the risk for nutrient deficiencies. A pattern of energy restriction, which is inevitably followed by bingeing, is believed to increase the risk of developing disordered eating. There is also some evidence that an inappropriate spread of energy intake over a day is associated with a higher body fat level. After such results were found during a survey of a small number of gymnasts (Benardot 1996), a study of female gymnasts and runners was undertaken using CTLEA to calculate energy balance (energy intake minus energy expenditure) for 24 × 1 hr blocks of a typical training day (Deutz et al. 2000). This study found differences in energy intake and spread between groups: compared with runners, gymnasts had significantly more hours in the day in which energy deficit was >300 kcal or 1.2 MJ (9.5 vs. 3.7) and fewer hours in which there was an energy surplus of similar magnitude (1.4 vs. 6.2). In both groups, however, there was an inverse correlation between body fat levels and within-day energy deficit, measured either as the frequency of hours of deficit or as the magnitude of the deficit. In other words, the more that these athletes underconsumed their energy needs during at least some portion of the day, the higher their body fat percentage. The authors speculated that this relationship might be explained by an adaptive reduction in resting energy expenditure (Deutz et al. 2000).

It is challenging to provide nutrition education programs to gymnasts or to counsel individual gymnasts on the topic of weight control. Problems that are commonly seen among gymnasts require changes at the organizational level of gymnastics as well as changes to the beliefs and practices of the individual athlete. For example, programs of talent identification and screening of young gymnasts should be undertaken so that athletes who are destined to have a small and lean physique can be channeled into elite programs, whereas those who are unlikely to retain such a physique can reassess their goals or their sport. Ultimately, the aims of individualized nutrition programs should be as follows:

- To assist gymnasts to achieve a body mass and body fat level that can be maintained with healthy eating practices while allowing them to compete at their highest potential
- To allow the growing gymnast to achieve an increase in height and weight within his or her genetic potential, at gradual and steady rates that can be accommodated within the skill demands of the sport
- To teach gymnasts to consume a diet that meets the their requirements for all nutrients, especially nutrients involved in growth (energy, protein, iron, and calcium) and performance (carbohydrate, water)
- To allow the young gymnast to develop independence with food intake and a healthy attitude to body mass and eating
- To retain some opportunities to enjoy the social and enjoyment aspects of food

The individual and specific advice of a sports dietitian is valuable to help gymnasts who desire loss of weight and body fat, or attenuation of a high rate of increase in body mass, to set realistic goals and a suitable time frame in which to achieve these as well as to achieve sound eating practices that encompass all their nutritional goals.

Disordered Eating

Given the pressure within aesthetic sports to maintain a light and lean frame, often in contrast to energy expenditure patterns, it is not surprising that disordered eating and eating disorders might exist. Recent publicity about eating disorders suffered by elite female gymnasts, including the death of top American gymnast Christy Henrich, has increased the awareness of the problem. It was pointed out in chapter 5 that personal characteristics such as perfectionism, dedication, self-criticism, and ability to focus on narrow goals are linked with a high risk of developing eating disorders. These are characteristics that are often linked with success in individual sports, but particularly aesthetic and skill activities that start at a young age. The personality that allows a child or young athlete to dedicate herself to her sport may also predispose the individual to developing disordered eating patterns in a high-pressure environment. A cluster of risk factors may help to explain the observations of disturbed body image and eating patterns among such groups.

It is beyond the scope of this book to provide a comprehensive discussion of the causes, outcomes, and treatments of eating disorders and disordered eating among athletes. Rather, the reader is referred to the excellent text by Beals (2004). A brief overview of information that may assist in the early assessment and intervention of athletes with disordered eating is provided in the practical issue in this chapter. The remainder of this section focuses on studies of eating disorders among gymnasts or studies that have identified key risk factors for the development of these problems.

Several studies of large populations of athletes have noted a high prevalence of disordered eating behaviors in "thin-build" and aesthetic sports including gymnastics (Beals and Manore 2002; Rosen et al. 1986; Sundgot-Borgen 1993). One study (Sundgot-Borgen 1993) involved 500 elite Norwegian athletes in 35 different sports divided into thin-build (including aesthetic, endurance, and weight-dependent sports) and non-thin-build (including power, technical, and ballgame sports) categories. The athletes undertook self-reported questionnaires, physical examination, and clinical interviews to screen for eating disorders (anorexia nervosa and bulimia nervosa) as well as subclinical forms of disordered eating (termed *anorexia athletica* by the author). This study found an overall prevalence of ~1% for anorexia nervosa and ~8% each for bulimia nervosa and anorexia athletica; however, the prevalence of both clinical and subclinical eating disorders was greater in the thin-build groups, with 34% of rhythmic gymnasts meeting the criteria for anorexia nervosa, bulimia nervosa, and anorexia athletica. Another study used questionnaires to investigate the dieting practices and pathogenic weight loss behaviors of 152 female athletes from 10 sports in the U.S. collegiate sports system (Rosen et al. 1986). Overall, just over 30% of females were found to be practicing at least one pathogenic weight loss behavior. However, across all sports, gymnasts reported the highest rate of weight control behaviors, with 74% of these athletes admitting to such activities.

Female athletes (n = 425) from U.S. collegiate sports undertook a survey of weight and dieting history that included several eating disorder inventories (Beals and Manore 2002). Sports were categorized into aesthetic (gymnastics, cheerleading, diving), endurance (middle- and long-distance running, basketball, soccer, rowing, water polo, swimming, field hockey), and anaerobic power (field events, golf, softball, tennis, and volleyball). The study found that a clinical diagnosis of anorexia nervosa could be made in 6%, 3.5%, and 1% of athletes in the aesthetic, endurance, and anaerobic sports, respectively, whereas a diagnosis of bulimia nervosa applied to 6%, 2%, and 2% of the athletes in these groups. Aesthetic athletes also scored significantly higher on the Eating Attitudes Test than athletes in the other groups (13.5 vs. 10 and 10), with a significantly greater number of athletes within the aesthetic group reporting above the cutoff score of 20, which is characteristic of those with an eating disorder (Beals and Manore 2002).

Specific investigations of eating disorders in female gymnasts include studies of 12 members of the Norwegian rhythmic gymnastics team (Sundgot-Borgen 1996) and 25 members of a division I team in the U.S. collegiate system (O'Connor et al. 1995). The results of questionnaires and clinical examination of the rhythmic gymnasts, aged 13 to 20 years, were compared with those collected from a control group matched for age and height (Sundgot-Borgen 1996). All gymnasts were dieting; four met the criteria for anorexia nervosa (n = 2) or anorexia athletica (n = 2) and another two admitted to pathological weight loss techniques. The author noted that the gymnasts had started sport-specific training at a mean age of 9 and suggested that the presence of dieting despite already extreme leanness was a sign that at least some were fighting their natural body weight or attempting to counter the natural physical changes associated with growth and maturity. Although all control participants were regularly menstruating, none of the four gymnasts who had reached menarche reported regular menstrual cycles. Reported energy intake for the gymnasts was below that reported by the control participants, reflecting either underreporting or an adaptation to more efficient metabolism. Two thirds of the gymnasts were injured at the time of the study, mainly from overuse problems (Sundgot-Borgen 1996).

American collegiate gymnasts were compared with a control group of students matched for age, height, and weight over a variety of factors including energy intake, bone density, menstrual history, and responses to the Eating Disorders Inventory-2 (EDI-2) questionnaire (O'Connor et al. 1995). This study tried to account for dishonest answers to the EDI-2 by correcting for fake results defined in a pilot study. Although the groups were matched for body mass, gymnasts had lower body fat than the controls and reported a slightly lower intake of energy. The gymnasts did not report extreme scores on the psychological constructs with relevance to eating disorders. In fact, the gymnasts did not differ from the control group in mean scores for any of the subscales on the EDI-2, and both groups had scores on the Drive for Thinness scale that were above those of norms for female college students. More than half of the participants in both groups reported the lifetime use of at least one pathogenic weight control behavior such as bingeing, vomiting, and the use of laxatives and diuretics. However, the gymnasts reported a greater frequency of menstrual irregularity than the controls, and such irregularity was associated with higher scores on the Drive for Thinness scale. The evidence of disordered eating among gymnasts in this study did not appear to be as severe as reported in other studies or any greater than problems faced by control participants. One explanation for these findings is that the gymnasts involved in the study, although of collegiate standard, were of a lower caliber or had different competition aspirations than those studied in other groups. The height and mean body mass of the group were 159 cm and 55 kg, respectively, meaning that these gymnasts were significantly larger than elite competitors described earlier in this chapter. It is possible that some of the stress involved with physique is removed at lower levels of participation in the sport.

Various authors, across a range of studies, have identified risk factors that are associated with disordered eating in general or the onset of such a problem (see highlight box on this page). In some sports it is impossible to remove these risk factors; indeed, in gymnastics, some are essential for success. However, everyone involved in a sport should work to minimize risk factors that are unnecessary or

Risk Factors Involved in the Development or Onset of Disordered Eating and Eating Disorders in Athletes

- Early onset of sport-specific training (premenarche)
- Dieting and weight cycling
- Emphasis on a low body mass and lean physique—societal pressure for appearance and sport-specific for performance
- Discrepancy between actual body mass or body fat and perceived ideal
- Personality factors: perfectionism, independence, goal orientation, tolerance to pain and discomfort, high expectation, and low self-esteem
- Dysfunctional family life
- Traumatic events: injury, loss or change of coach
- Pressure or advice from parents, coach, or teammate to lose weight

minimize the negative impact of these risk factors. Tactics include implementing programs that teach awareness of, and early intervention into, problems with eating, weight, and body image. The list of people involved in such programs should include coaches, parents, sport scientists, sport physicians, sports nutrition experts, psychologists, and the athletes themselves.

Restrained Eating, the Delay of Puberty, and Impaired Long-Term Growth

A striking characteristic of gymnasts, particularly females, is their short stature. The typical gymnast is significantly smaller than age-matched peers, with size discrepancies becoming more pronounced in older athletes. For example, a cross-sectional study of female gymnasts aged between 7 and 14 years found that although the mean characteristics of the youngest gymnasts were close to population norms for weight and height for their age (48th percentile), percentile rankings decreased dramatically in the older gymnasts, reaching the 26th percentile (Benardot and Czerwinski 1991). Other researchers have noted that gymnasts have a reduced growth spurt during adolescence (Lindholm et al. 1994). Two theories can explain this observation. First, there may be a selection bias, in which individuals who are genetically predisposed to being small are attracted to a sport in which this provides an advantage. According to this theory, as the caliber of participation in the sport increases, smaller athletes would be the most successful and would be retained. The alternative theory is that gymnasts stunt their growth as a deliberate result of their training and nutrition strategies. Of course, these factors may coexist.

Some cross-sectional studies have provided data to examine these theories. Twenty-two female gymnasts and 18 male gymnasts from an elite German training program took part in an assessment of pubertal versus chronological age characteristics (Weimann et al. 2000). The females had been in elite training for a mean of 6.8 years and were training around 22 hr/week. The corresponding values for the male gymnasts were 3.9 years and 16 hr/week. Female gymnasts had low fat mass, bone retardation (chronological age of 13.6 years vs. bone age of 11.9 years), delayed menarche, and reduced height potential (predicted target height of 158 cm vs. familial target height of 161.5 cm). Mean heights and weights were below the 12th percentile of the normal range of age-matched children. The females who were prepubertal based on clinical and hormonal staging showed evidence of greater discrepancies of these indexes (e.g., >2 years for bone age). Reported energy intake of the group was found to be ~60% of daily recommended nutritional intake for females. The authors concluded that in female gymnasts, the combination of intensive training with inadequate energy intake can alter the pattern of pubertal development. By contrast, the male gymnasts displayed unaltered pubertal, height, bone, and growth

development. This was thought to reflect an older age at the onset of intensive training, a lower training demand during the sensitive phase of pubertal development, and a more appropriate energy intake. Plasma levels of the hormone leptin, adjusted for body fat and pubertal state, were found to be inappropriately low, especially in the female gymnasts (Weimann et al. 1999). It was suggested that low concentrations of leptin, resulting from reduced body fat and inadequate energy intake, were associated with failed activation of the sex hormone cycle to induce puberty in a timely manner. The consequence is a delay or impairment of pubertal development and the pubertal growth spurt.

Another investigation followed active female gymnasts, retired gymnasts, and control participants over a 2-year period (Bass et al. 2000). The active gymnasts had delayed bone age and reductions in height, sitting height, and leg length compared with age-specific scores. However, in those training for less than 2 years, the deficit was confined to leg length only. Over 2 years of follow-up, only the discrepancy in sitting height was increased. After 1 year of retirement, there was acceleration in sitting height, and in gymnasts who had been retired for 8 years there was no deficit in sitting height, leg length, or menstrual dysfunction. The authors concluded that the short stature of gymnasts is partly attributable to the specific selection of athletes with preexisting low leg lengths. Reductions in sitting height are likely to be the result of involvement in gymnastics but are reversible on cessation of gymnastics training. Overall, a past history of involvement in gymnastics did not appear to result in reduced stature or menstrual dysfunction.

Several groups have undertaken a thorough review of the literature regarding growth and maturation in female gymnasts. In their review, Caine and colleagues (2001) reported that there is some evidence that females with short stature are attracted to gymnastics. Furthermore, gymnastics training does appear to attenuate growth, although there is a "catch-up" during periods of reduced training or retirement. There is some conflict as to whether this catch-up is complete and how much the effects are attributable to training per se. Unfortunately, most studies fail to partition the effect of training from other aspects of the gymnastics environment such as nutritional factors (Caine et al. 2001).

Roemmich and coworkers (2001) undertook a more global review of the consequences of training during puberty. They noted that growth at puberty depends on genetic potential, nutritional status, and hormonal status, with energy expenditure being able to modify the effects of all three factors on linear growth rate and body composition. Although participation in sports per se does not seem to affect pubertal timing or linear growth rate, the additional burden of a chronic energy deficit in weight-controlled sports may be great enough to slow growth and maturation. Studies of male wrestlers appear to show an altered hormonal picture, which may cause a mild resistance to growth hormone leading to a mild delay in maturation. This is especially apparent among wrestlers in the lower weight classes. However, the effects appear to be rapidly reversed following the end of training and competitive season, with a catch-up of lean body mass and fat mass. By contrast, the situation with female gymnasts involves chronic and marked undernutrition, which can keep adolescent athletes prepubertal for many years. It is unclear whether subsequent growth is disproportionate, but most gymnasts appear to track their genetic potential. There is a need for longitudinal studies of children in energy-restricted sports to better define the mechanisms of growth and maturational delay. It is likely, however, that the major problem associated with delayed puberty in female relates to bone mineralization rather than growth.

Bone Status and Calcium Balance

Achieving a high level of peak bone mass during childhood and early adulthood is an important goal in protecting bone integrity. Peak bone mass determines bone mass and fracture risk in later life, but the athlete's immediate bone mass is also likely to influence her risk of stress fractures and thus her sporting career. Bone is a dynamic tissue that undergoes continual change caused by the addition and resorption functions of osteoblast and osteoclast cells. Barr and McKay (1998) described three distinct processes by which this occurs during childhood and adolescence:

- Growth: a genetically determined, hormonally mediated enlargement of the skeleton that occurs until late adolescence and the cessation of linear growth.
- Modeling: addition of bone, without resorption to surfaces that are undergoing high loading or strain.
- Remodeling: cyclical process in which fatigue-damaged bone experiences bone resorption (activity of osteoclasts) followed by deposition of new bone in the cavity (activity of osteoblasts). Although these processes are usually coupled, over the long term there may be incomplete refilling of bone cavities, leading to net bone loss.

Although the primary determinants of peak bone mass are genetic factors, more than half of the variance of remodeling activities is attributable to factors such as mechanical loading on the bone, the hormonal environment, and calcium homeostasis (for review, see Barr and McKay 1998; Kerr et al. 2000). Suboptimal bone status can occur in some female athletes, with the risk factors being chronic periods of impaired menstrual status and suboptimal calcium intake (see practical issue in this chapter). In chapter 5, female distance runners were identified as one group at risk of suboptimal bone mass because of the interaction of these factors.

Athletes in aesthetic sports are another population in which impaired bone status might be expected. As discussed in the previous section, menstrual disturbances such as primary amenorrhea (absent or delayed onset of periods) and secondary amenorrhea (cessation of periods) are common among females in aesthetic sports. The delayed or impaired menstrual function seen in many female gymnasts reduces the prevailing concentrations of hormones such as estrogen and progesterone, which have a positive effect on bone formation and remodeling. Suboptimal calcium intakes are also frequently reported in dietary surveys of gymnasts, figure skaters, and dancers, usually as a consequence of restricted energy intake. Calcium intake is further compromised by fad diets, disordered eating, and eating disorders. Prejudice about consuming dairy products is a key element in many fad diets; this is a problem because dairy foods provide about 60% of the calcium consumed in a typical Western diet. Table 13.2 summarizes strategies to ensure that calcium needs are met by gymnasts and other athletes.

Because physical activity has a positive influence on bone status, it is hypothesized that gymnastics training can at least partially overcome the negative impact of inadequate calcium intake and menstrual disturbances on bone mass and density. According to the review by Barr and McKay (1998), benefits appear to accrue from the type and frequency of this exercise, as well as the time in the life cycle in which it is undertaken. The most valuable exercise for stimulating bone growth through mechanical loading involves varied and diverse activity that stresses all major muscle groups with large forces. Gymnastics, dance, or other movements continually apply stress across the skeleton with forces that can be up to 10 times body mass during landings. For example, a study of male gymnasts reported that training was associated with a mean of 102 and 217 impacts per session on the upper and lower extremities, respectively, with peak magnitudes of 3.6 and 10.4 times body mass (Daly et al. 1999). This appears to have a greater impact on bone modeling than chronic repetitive movements such as running or walking, which exert a load of 1 to 3 times body mass. In turn, weight-bearing activities such as running and walking are better at loading the skeleton than weight-supported activities such as cycling and swimming. The effects of loading on bone skeleton are greater in the young, growing skeleton than in a mature adult. Thus, exercise undertaken by child and adolescent athletes has a particularly strong role in determining adult bone status.

A variety of studies have examined the bone mineral density (BMD) of female gymnasts across time or compared with other athletic groups to determine the overall impact of the combination of training, hormonal status, and calcium intake. Results of some of these studies are presented next:

- Collegiate gymnasts were found to have greater BMD at various sites including the lumbar spine, femur, femoral neck, and Ward's triangle than controls matched for age, body mass, and height, despite lower intakes of calcium and a greater lifetime prevalence of menstrual dysfunction (Kirchner et al. 1995).
- A study compared BMD in the legs of heavily training rhythmic gymnasts (28 hr/week training), substitute

Table 13.2 Strategies to Assist With Achieving Calcium Balance

Guideline	Practical examples		

Adjust calcium intake goals according to needs for growth and other factors affecting calcium balance.

Compiled guidelines for daily calcium intake across countries
- Children (4-8 years) 800 mg
- Children (8-11 years) 800-900 mg
- Adolescents 1,000-1,300 mg
- Adults 800-1,000 mg
- Pregnant or lactating females 1,000-1,400 mg
- Postmenopausal females 1,000-1,200 mg
- Amenorrheic females 1,200-1,500 mg

Consume enough energy to allow nutrient goals to be met. Avoid chronic periods of energy restriction and severe weight loss.

Adopt food patterns that include regular servings of dairy foods, according to calcium needs.
- Adults: 3 servings a day
- Children and adolescent athletes: 4 servings a day
- Amenorrheic athletes: 5 servings a day

(1 serving = 250 ml of milk, 40 g of cheese, or 200 g of yogurt)

If an athlete is unable or unwilling to consume dairy foods, a calcium-fortified soy alternative should be consumed.

Calcium content of dairy foods and dairy alternatives

Food	Serving	Mg calcium
Dairy		
Nonfat milk	200 ml	250
Calcium-fortified low-fat milk	200 ml	285-350
Flavored low-fat milk	250 ml	280
Reduced-fat cheese	20 g	160
Cottage cheese	100 g (1/2 cup)	80
Low-fat fruit yogurt	200 g	300-350
Light fromage frais	200 g	150-200
Low-fat ice cream	60 g (2 tbsp)	90
Soft-serve yogurt	110 g (single cone)	180
Custard	200 g	200
Soy foods		
Soy milk	200 ml	45
Fortified soy milk	200 ml	290

(continued)

Table 13.2 *(continued)*

Guideline	Practical examples		
	Flavored fortified soy milk	250 ml	280
	Soy cheese	20 g	90
	Soy yogurt	200 g	200
	Soy custard	200 g	200

Integrate dairy (soy) foods into the diet to meet other sports nutrition goals.

Energy restriction goals
- Choose low-fat dairy and soy choices of milk and yogurt.
- If dairy foods are reduced-fat rather than low-fat (e.g., cheese), limit total intake.

Fuel (carbohydrate) intake needs
- Choose sweetened forms of milks and yogurts, including custard, flavored milk, and hot milk drinks (e.g., hot chocolate).
- Choose drinks and desserts made with fruit and dairy combinations (e.g., fruit smoothies, fruit with yogurt or custard).
- Add milk-based white sauces to pasta, make "creamy" soups and curries with milk.
- Add reduced-fat cheese to pasta or sandwiches.

Be aware of other foods that can increase total calcium intake, including fish eaten with bones, green leafy vegetables, and some nuts and legumes.

Be aware that in some countries, everyday foods such as orange juice can be fortified with calcium to provide a substantial and regular source of calcium.

Calcium content of other foods

Foods	Serving	Mg calcium
Salmon with bones	100 g (small tin)	335
Sardines	100 g (drained)	380
Oysters	100 g (n = 10)	155
Tahini	20 g (1 tbsp)	190
Tofu	100 g	130
Soy, kidney, or baked beans	100 g (drained)	35-50 g
Almonds	50 g	125
Spinach	145 g (cup)	70
Broccoli	140 g (cup)	35

If intake of calcium-rich foods is not achieved according to these guidelines, seek the assistance of a sports dietitian to devise a suitable meal plan. When dietary intake of calcium is insufficient, calcium supplements may be prescribed.

rhythmic gymnasts (12 hr/week training), and control participants (Wu et al. 1998). The authors noted that these gymnasts used a different leg in takeoff (left leg) and in landing (right leg), and therefore a different loading was achieved by each leg during training. Vertical ground reaction force were greater during takeoff than during landing, explaining greater BMD in three sites of the left femur of the gymnasts, particularly those with the heavier training loads.

• BMD of female college gymnasts was found to be greater than that of controls over the total body, lumbar spine, arm, and proximal femur (Proctor et al. 2002). Whereas controls showed a greater BMD in their dominant arm, there was no difference between the arms of the gymnasts. Upper-limb BMD tracked use patterns in both gymnasts and controls, demonstrating that the forces imposed on the arms with gymnastics training enhanced BMD and eliminated bilateral differences.

• Longitudinal studies tracked changes in BMD in female college gymnasts, swimmers, runners, and nonathletic controls for 8 to 12 months (Taaffe et al. 1997). The increase in BMD in lumbar spine and femur was greater in gymnasts than in the other groups, despite high initial BMD values. It was also independent of reproductive hormone status because the percent change in BMD at any site did not differ between eumenorrheic and irregularly menstruating athletes.

• Collegiate gymnasts and cross-country runners were tracked over the course of a training season (Bemben et al. 2004). Gymnasts had significantly higher BMD at various body sites than the runners at both preseason and postseason testing. Neither group experienced a significant change in BMD between trials for any site; however, runners showed slight decreases at all BMD sites from baseline to the postseason. There was a higher prevalence of self-reported menstrual cycle disturbances in gymnasts than runners; however, no differences in BMD was found between the eumenorrheic and impaired menstrual function groups.

• Changes in BMD in a group of collegiate gymnasts were followed over 24 months that included two 8-month competitive seasons and two 4-month off-seasons (Snow et al. 2001). There was a clear and consistent pattern of bone density increases over the training seasons followed by clear declines in the off-seasons for total body and specific sites. Increases at the spine were 3.5% and 3.7% followed by declines of 1.5% and 1.3% in the off-seasons. Total hip BMD increased 2.3% and 1.9% during the competitive seasons followed by decreases of 1.5% and 1.2% in the off-seasons. Over the total 2-year period, there was an overall increase of 4.3% in spine BMD but no significant overall change at the hip.

• BMD was measured in prepubertal gymnasts (mean = 10 years), retired gymnasts (mean = 25 years, mean of 8 years of retirement), and controls (Bass et al. 1998). Over a 12-month period, the increase in BMD of the total body, spine, and legs in the active gymnasts was 30% to 85% greater than in prepubertal controls. In the retired gymnasts, the BMD was higher than the predicted mean in controls at all sites except the skull. There was no diminution over the range in years since retirement, despite the lower frequency and intensity of exercise.

• BMD of former gymnasts was compared with that of matched controls (Kirchner et al. 1996). Higher BMD was seen in the total body, lumbar spine, and femur in the gymnasts even when past and present activity levels were taken into account. There were no differences in BMD in the former gymnasts who had always had regular menstrual function compared with those who had had an interruption to their menstrual cycle in the past.

These studies suggest that the bone health of gymnasts is good and even is preserved in the face of risk factors that would normally impair bone status. However, we should not assume that inadequate eating or menstrual dysfunction among gymnasts can be ignored. There is some evidence that gymnast have a reduced BMD in sites that don't receive loading through training (Bass et al. 2000). This may increase the risk of problems at these sites in later life. There is also evidence that increased BMD does not protect gymnasts from injury problems during their career. According to Bernadot (1996), there is a positive correlation between rates of injury in the U.S. gymnastics team and bone mineral density. Gymnasts who have the highest muscle mass appear to increase the loading and bone density response in bones but also increase the potential for fracture. Although there is a positive adaptation to bone as a result of gymnastics training, it may not be able to keep pace with the biomechanical demands of the sport.

Sport Foods and Supplements

There are very few studies of supplement use by gymnasts or the effect of purported ergogenic compounds on the performance of gymnastics. In the case of a subjectively judged sport, there are obvious challenges in developing a test protocol that could detect a direct change in competition performance following the use of a supplement. Rather, sport scientists would have to settle for measuring changes in a factor that is deemed to be important in the performance of a routine—for example, strength or body fat levels. The available published literature on ergogenic aids and gymnasts is limited to a study of soy protein supplementation (Stroescu et al. 2001). Female gymnasts from the Romanian Olympic team undertook a 4-month program of strenuous training and daily supplementation with soy protein (1 g/kg body weight) or identically flavored placebo. Other food and training (4-6 hr/day) were controlled during this period. Results demonstrated that the soy-supplemented group had an increase in lean body mass and serum levels of prolactin and thyroid hormones, whereas the placebo group had a decrease in thyroid hormones. The authors concluded that the consumption of the soy protein led to lower metabolic–hormonal stress in elite female gymnasts undergoing strenuous training. An unpublished thesis, cited by Benardot (2000), provided support for the benefits of creatine monohydrate use by elite female gymnasts, with better maintenance of anaerobic power and endurance over a 3-day intensive training camp.

There are several reasons for gymnasts (or their advisors) to take a cautious approach to the use of ergogenic supplements. In addition to the lack of evidence of benefits to gymnastics performance, there is a need to consider the age of most gymnasts. Although there is no current evidence

of significant side effects from the scientifically supported uses of products such as creatine, there have been no studies related to children and adolescents. Sports nutrition experts caution against the use of unusual products or nutrients in unusual amounts in such special groups (American Academy of Pediatrics 2005).

Products that have a justified role in gymnastics are sport foods and supplements that can be used to achieve a nutritional goal, including the prevention or treatment of a nutrient deficiency (see table 13.3). Even though

Table 13.3   Sports Foods and Supplements That Are of Likely Benefit to Gymnasts

	Product	Comment
Use in achieving documented nutrition goals	Sport drinks	• Use to refuel and rehydrate during prolonged training sessions in the heat or after competition sessions (between apparatus). There may be benefits in refueling during some prolonged sessions; however, the energy cost of sport drinks must be considered by many female gymnasts.
	Sport bars	• Convenient, portable, and easy-to-consume source of carbohydrate, protein, and micronutrients for preevent meal or postevent recovery. • Convenient and compact source of energy and nutrients for the traveling athlete or for competition schedules that conflict with athlete's usual meal pattern. • Micronutrient-rich snack food that can be used to boost intake of nutrients at risk in competition or training diet.
	Liquid meal supplements	• Well-tolerated, low-residue preevent meal that can provide a source of carbohydrate before an event or during gaps of 1-2 hr between events or apparatuses. Some gymnasts may not like to consume solid food before competition in case of gastrointestinal discomfort or because they prefer a compact appearance and light feeling. • Low-bulk and practical form of energy and nutrients that can contribute to high energy needs, especially to support a resistance training program or growth in male gymnasts. • Convenient and compact source of energy and nutrients for the traveling gymnast or for competition schedules that conflict with athlete's usual meal pattern. • Micronutrient-rich drink that can be used to boost intake of nutrients at risk in a low-energy diet.
	Multivitamin and mineral supplements	• Supplemental source of micronutrients during prolonged periods of energy restriction. • Supplemental source of micronutrients for traveling when food supply is less reliable.
	Iron supplements	• Supplemental form of iron for prevention and treatment of diagnosed cases of reduced iron deficiency; should be taken under the supervision of a sports physician or dietitian and in conjunction with dietary intervention.
	Calcium supplements	• Supplemental form of calcium for prevention and treatment of poor bone status when diet is unable to meet calcium requirements; should be taken under the supervision of a sports physician and dietitian and in conjunction with appropriate medical and dietary intervention.

Research Priorities

The nutritional needs of gymnasts are heavily focused on issues of physique: eating strategies that will maintain a small and lean body, and the nutritional consequences of extreme levels of such practices. The result of such a narrow focus of interest means that there are few studies of nutritional strategies for supporting or enhancing training outcomes or competition performance. Future research should examine such issues as well as continue to investigate short- and long-term consequences of the weight loss strategies of gymnasts:

- Eating practices and dietary intake of elite female gymnasts, including strategies to determine the underreporting of intake in self-reported data
- Measures of the nutrient status of gymnasts for at-risk nutrients such as minerals
- Effect of growth in size and weight on gymnastics performance: what can be tolerated?
- Prevalence of eating disorders and disordered eating among female gymnasts and effect of sport-specific strategies to prevent and treat problems
- Short- and long-term effects of restrained eating on health and performance of female gymnasts including injury rates, menstrual status, and bone health
- Eating practices and dietary intake of elite male gymnasts, including prevalence of problems related to restrained eating
- Effect of hydration and fuel status on gymnastics training and competition performance

---

there are situations in which such products may be valuable, the sports dietitian or nutritionist must consider the financial implications of the use of expensive and specialized products and the potential to distract young athletes from learning about making good food choices. The use of multivitamin and mineral supplements should only be considered when it is part of a professionally supervised plan that includes sound dietary patterns and appropriate treatment for any medical issues.

RESEARCH TOPIC

Dietary Causes of Menstrual and Hormonal Disturbances in Athletes: The Energy Drain

The high prevalence of menstrual disturbances among athletes has led to a number of theories to explain the cause of the problem. Potential causes, generally identified from characteristics of females with menstrual irregularities, include (Burke 1994) these:

- Low body mass or levels of body fat below a critical threshold
- Sudden decrease in body mass or body fat levels
- Loss of body fat from specific sites
- Disordered eating
- High volume or intensity of training
- Emotional stress
- Disordered eating
- Low intake of protein or fat, high intake of fiber
- Vegetarian eating practices

Although these factors are often overrepresented in populations of female athletes with menstrual disorders, investigations have failed to find evidence that any of these factors cause menstrual problems per se. Recent work by professor Anne Loucks, from the University of Ohio, has helped to consolidate a theory that explains both the cause of menstrual and other hormonal irregularities in athletes and the frequent coexistence of the factors listed previously. Her theory of energy availability was incorporated into the IOC consensus statement on nutrition for athletes (International Olympic Committee 2004) and presented in more detail in the review papers that accompanied this statement (Loucks 2004).

Amenorrheic athletes display a number of metabolic and hormonal patterns, including low plasma concentrations of glucose, insulin, and leptin; low resting metabolic rates; and elevations of plasma growth hormone and cortisol (Loucks 2004). These patterns are also evident in situations of chronic energy deficiency and among male athletes who restrict energy intake, such as wrestlers in weight classes (Roemmich and Sinning 1997a). Energy-deprived male athletes also show signs of a suppression of their reproductive system, such as a decline in testosterone concentrations below the normal range (Roemmich and Sinning 1997b). Although heavy exercise has been implicated as the cause of such disturbances, a cleverly designed study provided evidence that exercise stress per se has no effect on concentrations or pulsatility (cyclical changes in concentrations) of important hormones (Hilton and Loucks 2000; Loucks et al. 1998). In this study, energy balance was compared with energy deficiency, with separate manipulations of diet and exercise. One group of sedentary female participants were observed for 24 hr after 4 days of an energy-balanced diet (daily intake of 45 kcal/kg fat-free mass— [FFM]) and a restricted energy diet (10 kcal/kg FFM per day). This was compared with group of female exercisers who undertook walking to achieve a daily energy expenditure of 35 kcal/kg FFM. The energy intakes of this group were manipulated so that overall energy availability (energy intake minus the energy cost of exercise) was equivalent to conditions provided to the sedentary group.

The 24 hr observation period involved sampling of blood at 10 min intervals to assess changing concentrations of various hormones and metabolites. A special focus was directed to the pulsatility of the hormones leptin and luteinizing hormone (LH), which are critically involved with ovarian function. The study found that the stress of exercise did not change LH patterns. By contrast, low energy availability suppressed LH pulse frequency, regardless of whether the low energy availability was caused by dietary energy restriction alone or by exercise energy expenditure alone (Loucks et al. 1998). Low energy availability also suppressed leptin, thyroid hormone T3, insulin, and insulin-like growth factor (IGF-I) while increasing growth hormone (GH) and cortisol (Hilton and Loucks, 2000). Such changes in hormone patterns are identical to those seen in athletes with amenorrhea and other menstrual disturbances. An unexpected outcome of the study was the finding that exercise may have a *protective* effect on reproductive function in the face of energy deprivation. In the exercise group, the effects of low energy availability on LH pulse frequency, leptin, and other metabolic hormones were smaller than those in the food-restricted women, even though the study exactly matched energy availability for the balanced and energy-deprived conditions. Further investigation revealed that the exercising women had a higher carbohydrate availability (defined as dietary carbohydrate intake minus carbohydrate oxidation during exercise), because exercise caused glucose sparing during the energy-deficiency treatment. A follow-up to this study found that the response of reproductive hormones and ovarian function to low energy availability is highest is younger females, and that these disturbances disappear in females who have established a menstrual cycle for 14 years (Loucks 2006). This increases the imperative of educating young athletes.

Before additional data on the outcomes of energy deficiency are reviewed, the possible role of leptin in energy availability should be acknowledged. This hormone is synthesized primarily by adipose tissue and secreted into the circulatory system. Circulating leptin levels are correlated with body adipose stores and follow a diurnal rhythm that is partly circadian and partly dictated by metabolic rate and feeding patterns. Various effects of leptin have been noted, including a role as a satiety factor with receptors in the hypothalamus, as well as effects on physiological systems including neuroendocrine and immune function (for review, see Thong and Graham 1999). An investigation comparing leptin concentrations in female recreational runners, elite runners with normal menstrual function, and elite amenorrheic athletes found that elite athletes had reduced leptin levels associated with lower levels of body fat (Thong et al. 2000). However, when leptin levels were normalized for body fat levels, the elite amenorrheic athlete exhibited hypoleptinemia compared with the other groups; reductions in leptin correlated with reductions

in reported energy intake and reduced concentrations of insulin, estradiol, and thyroid hormones (Thong et al. 2000). These findings were confirmed in a study of amenorrheic and eumenorrheic female distance runners showing that the diurnal leptin rhythm was abolished in the group with menstrual dysfunction and was correlated with hypoinsulinemia and elevated cortisol levels (Laughlin and Yen 1997). Although further investigations of the role of leptin are required, it shows promise as a link between energy availability and hormones responsible for reproductive and metabolic function.

Other studies that illustrate the independent or overriding effect of energy deficiency on metabolic and reproductive dysfunction include investigations of the training camps used to selection members of the elite U.S. army group known as the Rangers (Friedl et al. 2000). Selection for this team of combat unit leaders involves an 8-week course, conducted in four consecutive 2-week stages in forest, mountain, desert, and swamp environments. A variety of stresses are experienced by the men who undertake this training, including sustained high levels of activity (daily energy expenditures of 18 MJ/day), sleep deprivation (<4 hr/day), extreme environments of heat and cold, illness and injury, and chronic energy deprivation (mean negative energy balance of 4 MJ [1,000 kcal]/day). Feeding patterns are alternated each week between controlled semistarvation and refeeding. Monitoring of various metabolic and reproductive hormones over the 8-week training schedule showed that a correlation between energy deprivation and reductions in testosterone, IGF-1, thyroid hormones, and LH, despite continued exercise and environmental stresses. These metabolic and reproductive hormones were suppressed during each week of energy deficiency but were fully restored with 1 week of controlled refeeding during the course and 1 week of ad libitum refeeding after the 8-week course.

In summary, studies in both men and women show that low energy availability rather than the stress of exercise disrupts the reproductive system and that this disruption can be prevented by appropriate energy supplementation, without any moderation of the exercise program or other stresses. Evidence for a dose-dependent relationship between energy availability and metabolic substrates and hormones was provided in a study by Loucks and Thuma (2003). In this study, exercising women were exposed to energy availability of 10, 20, 30, and 45 kcal/kg FFM per day—achieved by undertaking an exercise program equivalent to 15 kcal/kg FFM per day (~11 km run) while consuming a daily energy intake of 25, 35, 45, or 60 kcal/kg FFM. Major changes to LH patterns were seen at energy availability between 20 and 30 kcal/kg FFM per day. The effects on the frequency and amplitude of the LH pulse were similar to the effects seen on plasma concentrations of glucose and β-hydroxybutyrate and to the metabolic hormones GH and cortisol. According to the authors, these results support the hypothesis that reproductive function reflects the availability of metabolic fuels, especially glucose, which may be signaled in part by activation of the adrenal axis. They also suggest that athletes may be able to prevent menstrual disorders by maintaining daily energy availabilities above 30 kcal (135 kJ)/kg FFM.

In light of this information, a recommendation to maintain adequate energy availability was included in the education booklet prepared from the IOC consensus statement on nutrition for sports and distributed to athletes at the 2004 Olympic Games in Athens, Greece. Although eating disorders/disordered eating have been previously linked with the Female Athlete Triad or the dietary inadequacies underpinning menstrual dysfunction (Otis et al. 1997; Yeager et al. 1993), newer guidelines for the Female Athlete Triad recognize that low energy availability can occur without the "baggage" of psychological problems with food and body image. Although it may be related to a deliberate and inappropriate restriction of food intake, it may also occur as a spontaneous reaction to an increase in energy expenditure that an athlete is unable to recognize or address. An excerpt from the IOC booklet that includes an example of how energy availability can be calculated is presented in the highlight box on this page.

PRACTICAL ISSUE

Detection and Early Intervention of Problems With Disordered Eating

The size and nature of the problem of disordered eating in sport are hard to define. Studies have variously described almost none or almost all of a group of athletes to be suffering from problems. Apart from the real differences that may occur between sports or groups of individual athletes, there are methodological differences in the way that problems are defined. First, a range of questionnaire and inventory instruments have been used to measure abnormal attitudes and behaviors related to eating, body mass, and body image. These vary in characteristics, particularly in their ability to relate the athlete. The definition of an eating disorder also varies.

Strictly speaking, the term *eating disorder* refers to clinically diagnosable conditions that are recognized by psychiatrists. The *Diagnostic and Statistical Manual of Mental Disorders* (4th ed., *DSM-IV*) of the American Psychiatric Association (1994) is the latest version of the most commonly used reference for such disorders. The criteria for making a diagnosis of the three conditions recognized by *DSM-IV* are summarized in the highlight box on page 332. These descriptions indicate that athletes must exhibit extreme symptoms of problematic eating behavior before such criteria are met. In fact, one of the reasons that the prevalence of these eating disorders is so low among elite athletes is that in many cases it would be difficult for someone suffering from such extreme symptoms to continue to perform at a high level in sport.

Disordered eating is the term generally given to the spectrum of problematic eating behaviors that fall between eating disorders and normal eating. Most experts recognize that eating behavior is a continuum, with a range in frequency and extremity of abnormal or harmful activities or characteristics. Abnormalities of eating behavior, weight control, and body image that fall short of a clinical diagnosis of eating disorder yet cause health and performance problems for an athlete have been described by a number of terms. The most common are *athletica anorexia* (Sundgot-Borgen 1994) or the *subclinical eating disorder* (Beals and Manore 1994). The characteristics ascribed to athletica anorexia are also summarized.

Calculations of Energy Availability

Energy availability = total dietary energy intake – energy used in daily activity/exercise

Example of Low Energy Availability

Low energy = <30 kcal (135 kJ)/kg FFM
- 60 kg female with 20% body fat = 12 kg fat + 48 kg FFM
- Daily energy intake is 1,800 kcal (7,560 kJ)
- Cost of daily exercise (1 hr/day) = 500 kcal (2,100 kJ)
- Energy availability = 1,800 – 500 = 1,300 kcal (5,460 kJ)
- Energy availability = 1,300/48 or 27 kcal/kg FFM (113 kJ/kg FFM)

Example of Adequate Energy Availability

- 50 kg female with 10% body fat = 5 kg fat + 45 kg FFM
- Daily energy intake is 2,200 kcal (9,240 kJ)
- Cost of daily exercise (1 hr/day) = 500 kcal (2,100 kJ)
- Energy availability = 2,200 – 500 = 1,700 kcal (7,140 kJ)
- Energy availability = 1,700/45 or 38 kcal/kg FFM (159 kJ/kJ FFM)

Diagnostic Criteria for Various Eating Disorders and Disordered Eating Syndromes

Diagnostic Criteria for Anorexia Nervosa (American Psychiatric Association 1994)

- Refusal to maintain body mass over a minimal normal weight for age and height (e.g., weight loss leading to maintenance of body mass 15% below expected, or failure to make expected weight gain during growth period leading to body mass 15% below that expected)
- Intense fear of gaining weight or becoming fat even though underweight
- Disturbance in the way that one's body mass, size, or even shape is experienced; undue influence of body weight or shape on self-evaluation, or denial of the seriousness of current low body weight
- In postmenarchal females: amenorrhea (absence of three consecutive menstrual cycles)
- Divided into restricting type and binge eating and purging type

Diagnostic Criteria for Bulimia Nervosa (American Psychiatric Association 1994)

- Recurrent episodes of binge eating characterized by the following:
- Eating in a discrete time an amount of food that is definitely larger than most people would eat under similar circumstances
- A sense of lack of control over eating during the episode
- Recurrent, inappropriate behavior to prevent weight gain, such as self-induced vomiting; misuse of laxatives, diuretics, enemas, or other medication; fasting; or excessive exercise
- Binge eating and compensatory behaviors that both occur, on average, at least twice a week for 3 months
- Self-evaluation unduly influenced by body shape and mass
- Disturbance that does not occur exclusively during episodes of anorexia
- Divided into purging types and nonpurging types

Diagnostic Criteria for Eating Disorders Not Otherwise Specified (American Psychiatric Association 1994)

This category is for disorders of eating that do not meet the criteria for any specific eating disorder. Examples include the following:

- For females, all of the criteria for anorexia nervosa are met except that the individual has regular menses.
- All of the criteria for anorexia nervosa met except that despite significant weight loss the individual's current body mass is in the normal range.
- All of the criteria for bulimia nervosa are met except that the episodes occur less than twice a week for 3 months.
- An individual of normal body mass regularly uses inappropriate compensatory behavior after eating small amounts of food.
- The individual repeatedly chews and spits out, but does not swallow, large amounts of food.
- Binge-eating disorder involves recurrent episodes of binge eating in the absence of the regular use of compensatory behaviors.

Diagnostic Criteria for Anorexia Athletica (Sundgot-Borgen 1994)

- Weight loss >5% expected body weight +
- Delayed menarche (no menstrual bleeding by age 16) (+)
- Menstrual dysfunction (amenorrhea or oligomenorrhea) (+)
- Gastrointestinal complaints (+)
- Absence of medical illness or affective disorder to explain the weight loss +
- Body image distortion +
- Excessive fear of weight gain or becoming obese +
- Restriction of energy intake (<1,200 kcal/day) +
- Use of purging methods (e.g., self-induced vomiting, laxatives, diuretics) (+)
- Binge eating (+)
- Compulsive exercise (+)

Criteria marked + are considered absolute criteria, meaning that they are required for diagnosis, whereas the criteria marked (+) are relative criteria and need not be present to make a diagnosis.

It is beyond the scope of this book to describe the therapy for eating disorders and disordered eating. Instead, the reader is referred to the text *Disordered Eating Among Athletes* (Beals 2004) for a description of multidisciplinary approaches to dealing with the athlete with such problems. Some guidelines for coaches, training partners, and parents are provided here to assist them in dealing with athletes whom they suspect to have problems with disordered eating. Early diagnosis and treatment are important in the successful management of such problems.

• Recognize athletes with compulsive and perfectionist personalities. Although drive and motivation are valuable characteristics, many athletes can benefit from counseling in appropriate goal setting and achievement to ensure that their efforts are positive rather than counterproductive.

• Create an environment that supports healthy nutrition and weight control principles. Allow athletes to set realistic body weight and body fat targets, and make healthy nutrition advice accessible—both at a group and an individual level.

• Be aware of early signs of disordered eating behavior (see table 13.4). Recognize that you may be overreacting, and try to be objective in collecting evidence of a suspected problem.

• If appropriate, confront the athlete carefully. Express concern, and talk only about objective data—such as changes in performance or signs of unhappiness. Do not label the athlete or try to diagnose. The athlete may attempt to deny the problem, so stick to discussing hard evidence.

• If it is not appropriate for you to talk to the athlete, speak to someone who can—perhaps the coach or the team doctor or someone in the athlete's family.

• Seek professional help. You are not trained to deal with disordered eating. You may have the consent of the athlete to organize this step. Alternatively you may have to wait for the right moment before the help is accepted. Sometimes you may need to withdraw your support of the athlete until this step is taken. Make sure the athlete understands that you still care for her but you do not support her behavior.

• Professional assessment and counseling should involve a multidisciplinary team approach—find professionals who specialize in this field.

• Support the professional advice and treatment plan. Try not to become embroiled in the problem, but remain caring, supportive, and objective. Be prepared to be patient and flexible—the athlete may need constant reassessment of her goals.

Table 13.4 Warning Signs of Eating Disorders

Issue	Symptoms
Weight changes	• Sudden loss of weight • Wide fluctuations in weight over a short time
Food behavior	• Consumption of large amounts of food that are inconsistent with the athlete's weight • Evidence of eating in private (food disappearing, empty food wrappers) • Avoidance of eating or refusal to join in social occasions involving eating • Excessive interest in handling food and in preparing food for others • Preoccupation with the dietary patterns and eating behavior of others • Uncomfortable behavior at meals or with food (e.g., movement of food around plate without eating, very fast eating followed by picking at leftovers)
Self-image	• Worry about being too fat • Constant self-examination and comparison with others
Personality	• Withdrawal or anxiety • Mood swings
Evidence of problem behaviors	• Admission or evidence of use of laxatives, diuretics, or diet pills • Admission or evidence that athlete vomits after meals • Excessive exercise in addition to set training program
Physical signs	• Amenorrhea (cessation of periods, or failure to start menstruating at all) • Tooth decay or acid erosion of teeth from vomiting • Gastrointestinal complaints (indigestion, constipation, bloating) • Stress fractures • Cold intolerance • Jaundiced skin (carotenemia) • Lanugo (fine hair on body)

chapter 14

Winter Sports

Nanna L. Meyer, PhD, RD
Research Associate and Sports Dietitian, The Orthopedic Specialty Hospital (TOSH) and Division of Nutrition, University of Utah, Salt Lake City, Utah

Susie Parker-Simmons, MS, RD
Sports Dietitian with the United States Olympic Committee, Colorado Springs, Colorado. Past dietician with the U.S. Ski and Snowboard Team, Park City, Utah

Winter sports are pursuits commonly played during the winter season on snow or ice. Table 14.1 provides a summary of various winter sports, listing the events that are involved in the international competition circuit for each sport. The Winter Olympic Games program includes biathlon, bobsled, curling, ice hockey, luge, skating, skeleton, and the five disciplines of skiing. This chapter concentrates on the sports of Nordic skiing (ski jumping, Nordic Combined, and cross-country), alpine skiing, freestyle skiing (aerials and moguls), snowboarding, and speed skating.

Nordic Skiing

Nordic sports involve the disciplines of ski jumping, cross-country skiing, and the combination of these in Nordic Combined. These sports are popular in many countries located in the northern hemisphere. Ski jumping involves performing a jump with skis from a high ramp overhanging a snow-covered slope; in international competition, these hills are the K90 and K120. Jumpers are able to practice and compete during the summer months using jumping hills with plastic covering and indoor jumping facilities. Originally, cross-country skiing was undertaken using a single technique: a diagonal stride where both skis stay in prepared tracks. However, during the first official International Skiing Federation (FIS) World Cup season in 1982, Bill Koch of the United States popularized the skating technique (freestyle). Modern cross-country skiing competitions are classified into two different styles: classic skiing and freestyle. The evolution of cross-country skiing continues, with new events, new distances, and new venues integrated yearly. In most Nordic Combined events, the ski jumping component of the race is held first, followed by the cross-country skiing. This sport requires physical strength and technical control (ski jumping) and endurance and strength (cross-country skiing).

Competition

Each athlete competes in approximately 30 to 45 events over a 4-month winter season, including 15 to 20 World Cup events. The competition characteristics vary with each event because the terrain, weather, snow conditions, and frequency of competition create a variety of physical challenges for the Nordic athlete.

Ski Jumping

The three main ski jumping events for the Winter Olympic Games and World Championships include the large hill, the normal hill, and the large hill for team competitions. Historically only men competed in the World Cup, at the Winter Olympic Games, and at the World Championships. However, women's ski jumping is an emerging international sport and in 2006 was added to the World Championships, with the first event planned for 2009.

- *Individual normal hill:* A ski jumping event from a hill, which has a k-point (calculation position that determines the hill size and points for jumping distance) between 75 and 99 m. Each athlete takes two jumps. The athlete with the greatest total score (distance and style) from both jumps is the winner. Elite level ski jumpers cover a distance of approximately 100 m from the K90 hill.

- *Individual large hill:* This event is contested from a hill, which has a k-point larger than 100 m. Each athlete takes two jumps. The one with the greatest total score (distance and style) from the two jumps is the winner. The elite ski jumpers cover a distance of approximately 125 m from the K120 hill.

- *Team large hill:* This event is contested on the large hill (K120). There are four members on each team, and each athlete takes two jumps. The team with the highest total score (distance and style) over the eight jumps is the winner.

Table 14.1 Winter Sports and Their Internationally Held Events

Sport	International organization	Summer Grand Prix	World Cup Series	World Champion-ships	Olympic Games
Cross-country skiing	FIS	No	5 km, 10 km, SP, 2 × 10 km, relay, pursuit, 15 km (women), 10 km, 15 km, SP, pursuit, 30 km (men)	1.5 km SP, 10 km, duathlon, 30 km, 4 × 5 km relay (women) 1.5 km SP, 15 km, duathlon, 50 km, 4 × 10 km relay (men)	1.5 km SP, 10 km, duathlon, 30 km, 4 × 5 km relay (women) 1.5 km SP, 15 km, duathlon, 50 km, 4 × 10 km relay (men)
Nordic combined	FIS	Yes	Individual, sprint, team, mass start	Individual, sprint, team	Individual, sprint, team
Ski jumping	FIS	Yes	K-90, K-120, team, ski-flying	K-90, K-120, team	K-90, K-120, team
Alpine skiing	FIS	No	GS, SL, SG, DH, COM	GS, SL, SG, DH, COM	GS, SL, SG, DH, COM
Freestyle skiing	FIS	No	AE, M, DM, FX, FHP	AE, M	AE, M
Snowboarding	FIS	No	PGS, PSL, HP, SBX, BA	PGS, PSL, HP, SBX, BA	PGS, HP
Speed skating	ISU	No	*100 m*, 500 m, 1,000 m, 1,500 m, 3,000 m, 5,000 m, 10,000 m; *team pursuit;*	Sprint: 500 m, 1,000 m All-round: 500 m, 1,000 m, 1,500 m, 3,000 m, 5,000 m, 10,000 m Single distances: all distances	100 m, 500 m, 1,000 m, 1,500 m, 3,000 m, 5,000 m, 10,000 m

FIS = International Skiing Federation; ISU = International Skating Union; GS = giant slalom; SL = slalom; SG = super giant slalom; DH = downhill; COM = SL and DH combined; AE = aerials; M = moguls; DM = dual moguls; FX = freestyle cross; FHP = freestyle halfpipe; PGS = parallel GS; PSL = parallel SL; HP = halfpipe; SBX = snowboard cross; BA = Big air. *Italics* = new and demonstration events.

Ski-flying is an additional event that is only contested in the World Cup series. This type of competition is contested on a hill that has a k-point larger than 185 m. Each athlete takes two jumps, and the one with the greatest total score (distance and style) is the winner. Distances traveled are approximately 200 m.

Scoring is based on distance points and style points. The distance to be awarded is measured from the edge of the takeoff to the athlete's landing point on the slope in increments of 0.5 m. For a perfect jump, an athlete can obtain 20 style points, and points are deducted for faults during flight, landing, and out-run. On competition days, the athletes will arrive 2 hr before competing to wax their skis, run, stretch, and perform simulated jumps with their coach. They have one practice jump on the jump hill before the competition commences.

The winter competition starts at the end of November and concludes in late March (see table 14.2). The Winter Olympic Games and World Championship events are held during February. All competitions occur in the northern hemisphere, because there are no ski-jumping hills in the southern hemisphere.

Cross-Country Skiing

Elite cross-country skiing competitions are performed over distances ranging from 1.5 to 90 km, with international races equally divided into uphill, downhill, and level skiing. At the Winter Olympic Games and World Championships, women compete in the 1.5 km sprint, 10 km, duathlon (2 × 7.5 km), 30 km, and 4 × 5 km relay. Men compete in 1.5 km sprint, 15 km, duathlon (2 × 15 km), 50 km, and 4 × 10 km relay. For the sprint and the 10 km, 15 km, 30 km, and 50 km events, the technique used (classical vs. freestyle skiing) alternates each year. Individual races last 3.30 to 100 min for women and 3.0 to 120 min for men. During the World Championships or Winter Olympic Games, athletes will compete in a number of races, covering a variety of distances over a 2-week period.

Table 14.2　Annual Periodized Training Year

	April	May	June	July	August	September	October	November	December	January	February	March
Ski jumping	Recovery phase	Preparation phase			GP				WC	WC	WC	WC
Cross-country							WC	WC	WC	WC	WC	WC
Nordic Combined					GP			WC	WC	WC	WC	WC
Alpine skiing							WC	WC	WC	WC	WC	WC
Freestyle—moguls							WC	WC	WC	WC	WC	WC
Freestyle—aerials						WC[a]			WC	WC	WC	WC
Snowboarding							WC	WC	WC	WC	WC	WC
Speed skating							WC	WC	WC	WC	WC	WC

GP = Summer Grand Prix; WC = World Cup competition

[a] = World Cup in the southern hemisphere.

• *Classical and freestyle races:* In the classical races, where skiers use the traditional straight-striding technique (called a diagonal stride), a competitive time for women to complete the 10 km race is 30 min whereas men complete a 30 km race in 80 min. The freestyle technique, which is often referred to as "skating," has no restrictions. The athletes do not keep their skis within narrow tracks but instead push off with both legs in a motion that resembles skating. Times for an international skier to complete the 30 km race (women) and 50 km (men) are 95 min and 120 min, respectively.

• *The 1.5 km sprint:* The 1.5 km sprint is the shortest event on the cross-country program, and the technique used alternates each year. The sprint events are different from the other cross-country events in that they are contested in a series of elimination rounds. The approximate time to complete this distance is 3:30 min for women and 3:00 min for men. There are four rounds in the sprinting competition. The time between the preliminary round and the second round is approximately 90 min, whereas the following rounds last only 15 min.

• *The duathlon:* The duathlon is a continuous event that features both the classical and freestyle skiing technique. The first part of the event is a 7.5 or 15 km classical ski race, whereas the second part is a 7.5 or 15 km freestyle race. The athlete who crosses the finish line first is the winner. A competitive time for the 7.5 + 7.5 km event for women is 50 min and the 15 + 15 km for men is 90 min.

• *The relay event:* For the relay event, each team is composed of four skiers, each of whom skis one of the four 5 km or 10 km relay legs. The first two skiers of the relay ski with the classical technique, while the final two athletes ski with the freestyle technique.

Typical routines on competition days begin with the tests of a variety of skis to optimize waxing. It is quite common that skis are rewaxed prior to the start especially when weather and snow conditions are unpredictable. Athletes then conduct a warm-up on the ski course. Ten minutes before race start, the course is closed. During the final 30 min, athletes stretch, communicate with their coaches, rehydrate, and move to the starting area. The winter competition starts at the end of October and concludes in late March. The Winter Olympic Games and World Championship events are held during February.

Nordic Combined

For the World Championships and Winter Olympic Games, the three Nordic Combined events (individual, sprint, and team) consist of a ski-jumping competition followed by a cross-country ski race. There are no international professional circuits, Winter Olympic Games, or World Championship events for women.

• *Individual:* Each competitor in the individual event takes two jumps on the K90 m hill. Each jump is scored for distance and style. Immediately after the ski jumping event or on the following day, each competitor participates in a 15 km cross-country ski race. The start order for this event is determined by the ski-jumping results. The winner of the ski-jumping competition starts in first place, and the points scored in the ski-jumping competition are converted into time differences for the cross-country race starting order. The distance covered in the K90 is approximately 95 m, and the time to complete the cross-country event is 40 min.

• *Sprint:* The sprint event is contested in 1 or 2 days. The athletes initially jump from the K120 m hill and then complete the 7.5 km cross-country race. Unlike in the individual and team events, the jumping portion of the sprint event is performed on the large hill and includes one jump instead of two. The start order for the cross-country race is determined on the basis of the ski-jumping results. The winner of the ski-jumping competition starts in first place, and the points scored in the ski-jumping competition are converted into time differences for the cross-country race starting order. The distance covered on the K120 is approximately 120 m, and the time to complete the cross-country ski race is around 19 min.

• *Team:* Each team consists of four jumpers who each take two jumps off the normal hill (K90) on the first day of competition. The team's score in the jumping portion is the total score of the eight jumps. The same skiers who participate in the jumping event must compete in the 4 × 5 km relay, which is held on the same or following day. As in the individual and sprint events, the winning team of the ski-jumping competition starts in first place, and the points scored in the ski-jumping competition are converted into time differences for the cross-country race starting order. The winner is the team whose final skier crosses the finish line first. Another international Nordic Combined event, which is performed as part of the World Cup series, is the mass start race, which commences with the cross-country ski race, usually 10 km race, followed by two rounds of ski jumping.

Competition days involve a combination of routines previously discussed for ski jumpers and cross-country skiers. Often athletes jump in the morning and cross-country ski in the afternoon.

Physique and Physiology

Before 1987, studies dealing with the kinanthropometry of ski jumpers were rare. In the studies performed, the mean height ranged from 171.9 to 174.1 cm and body mass ranged from 68.2 to 74.0 kg (Orvanova 1987). In the 1990s, new technical rules were introduced that increased the air permeability of the jumping suit and set a maximum length for the skis. These changes reduced the equipment-induced gliding surface and, thus, shifted the focus from equipment to the athlete's body mass (Rankinen et al. 1998). Computer simulation shows that jump length decreases by approximately 1 m for every kilogram of body mass increase (Müller 2002). Rankinen and colleagues (1998) compared the body composition of 21 Finnish elite male ski jumpers and 20 controls of similar age. The results found no significant difference in stature, lean muscle mass, and bone mineral content between athletes and controls.

The ski jumpers, however, had lower mean body mass (61.9 ± 4.8 kg vs. 71.5 ± 9.0 kg) and percent body fat (8.6 ± 1.9% vs. 16.1 ± 7.2%) and higher bone mineral density in the lumbar spine and proximal femur than the controls. In 2002, the relative body weight in terms of body mass index (BMI) was found to be very low for all world-class ski jumpers, with the mean BMI being 19.5 kg/m^2. For instance, an athlete with a BMI of 19.5 would be 1.75 m tall and weigh 59.7 kg (Müller 2002). Many ski jumpers constantly restrict energy intake to keep their weight down, because of their year-round competition. This desire for a low body mass commences at a very young age. There is also a tendency for very young athletes to participate in international competitions because they generally weigh less than older athletes of similar height. Delayed growth and maturation have been observed in ski jumpers as well as extreme weight loss and eating disorders. Because endurance activity is not an option for assisting in weight loss because of its effect on explosive power, athletes only use energy restriction to reduce and maintain weight. Long-term energy restriction and pressure to maintain a low body mass take their toll on the athlete and, at times, are the cause of early retirement, at least in American ski jumpers.

In 1927, cross-country skiers were described as tall and lean individuals, whereas in the 1950s they were reported as muscular and having average height. Skiers who were light were seen to have an advantage on a hilly and poorly gliding course, whereas heavier skiers had an advantage on a flat course with a good gliding track (Bergh 1987; Saltin 1997). The physiques of cross-country skiers have changed over the last 20 years. However, no recent normative data for international and national level cross-country skiers are available. Research is needed to identify the present physique characteristics of cross-country skiers in relation to height, weight, body fat, muscle mass, and bone mass.

Few studies have been published concerning the physique characteristics of Nordic Combined skiers and none since 1987. The findings from 1987 reported height and weight ranging from 172.7 to 181.7 cm and 67.6 to 71.6 kg, respectively (Orvanova 1987). The typical somatotype of Nordic Combined skiers lies between that of a ski jumper and a cross-country skier. These athletes aim to obtain a low enough body mass to aid their ski jumping performance without compromising their cross-country ski capacity. The athletes' desire to achieve and maintain a low body fat level to increase the power-to-mass ratio may elevate their risk of extreme energy restrictions and disordered eating.

Training

For the three Nordic sports, the preparation phase aims to enhance the athletes' physiology, skiing, and jumping technique and to optimize medical, nutritional, and sport psychology practices. The nutrition goals in the preparation phase will aim to optimize nutritional status, physique, recovery techniques, event feeds, hydration practices, and athlete education. A general scheme of the periodization of training and competition for the Nordic sports is provided in table 14.2.

Ski Jumping

Ski jumping is a technical sport whose movement pattern can be divided into several components: in-run, takeoff, flight, and preparation for landing. As the athlete approaches the landing area after the flight phase, he will then include an artistic element, which involves bending the knees to obtain a smooth landing, followed by a transition into the telemark position. To obtain stability, both arms are stretched horizontally and then upward. Finally the ski jumper will ski to the out-run area, which is the breaking zone at the bottom of the landing hill, where skiers slow down and stop (FIS 2003).

Improving the vertical component of jumping is a major area of focus in the dry land training of ski jumpers. Increases in maximal strength and power occur from neural

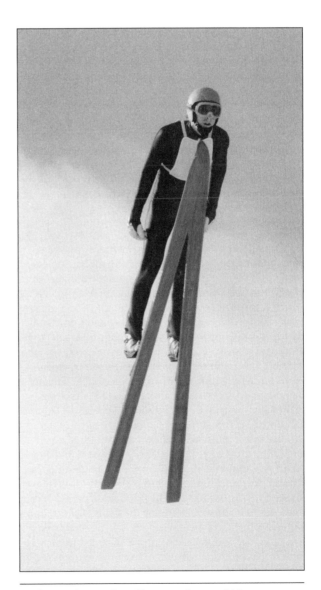

It takes no longer than 12 s to perform a ski jump.

adaptations rather than from alterations in the muscle itself. Any strength and power development in these athletes must occur without increased muscle mass, because increased body mass will decrease jumping length (Hoff et al. 2000). Coaches and athletes perceive that endurance exercise reduces explosive power capacity. Therefore, training consists of ski jumping (in the summer on plastic and winter on snow), strength training, technique-specific strength training, plyometrics, and recovery work. The average number of ski jumps performed during the preparation phase is 600 to 800. Technique-specific strength training involves simulation jumps where the ski jumper is caught or stopped after takeoff (Schwameder et al. 1997). Strength training consists of high-intensity lifts with low repetitions. Plyometric exercise includes bounding activities over boxes and hurdles and recovery includes stretching and short jogs. The preparation phase of the annual year occurs from May to the end of November, with a European Summer Grand Prix held in August each year.

Rankinen and colleagues (1998) used a 4-day activity record to assess the energy expenditure of ski jumpers. The authors demonstrated that the energy expenditure of ski jumpers, adjusted for body mass, was similar to that of normally active controls of comparable age (196 $\pm$ 39 kJ $\cdot$ kg^{-1} $\cdot$ day^{-1} or 47$\pm$ 9 kcal $\cdot$ kg^{-1} $\cdot$ day^{-1} vs. 215 $\pm$ 30 kJ $\cdot$ kg^{-1} $\cdot$ day^{-1} or 51 $\pm$ 7 kcal $\cdot$ kg^{-1} $\cdot$ day^{-1}). Today, there are an increased number of jumping hills with chairlifts, which has probably decreased energy expenditure slightly. Nevertheless, it is estimated that the energy expenditure in ski jumpers is fairly low, because the sport involves the production of only one powerful movement.

Cross-Country Skiing

Different training philosophies and methods are applied in different countries by elite coaches with similarly successful results. In general, training for cross-country skiing consists of activities that aim to improve aerobic power and capacity as well as muscular endurance. The training modes include cross-country skiing, running (endurance and sprint), roller skiing, ski walking, strength and conditioning, and technique work (Rusko 2003a). Arm and upper-body strength and endurance are critical for optimal performance during the freestyle technique and when double poling. Therefore, training now places special attention on the development of upper body strength and muscular endurance (Ekblom and Bergh 2000; Saltin 1997).

Elite male and female skiers train about 650 to 750 and 500 to 700 hr/year, respectively (Ekblom and Bergh 2000). For example, the weekly volume of training for a Finnish skier ranges from 140 to 150 km distributed over 8.5 sessions (Rusko 2003a). The preparation period occurs from May to mid-October. During the summer, the training volume is high and the intensity is low. General strength and muscular endurance training is included to increase muscle mass and strength and to improve neuromuscular determinants of endurance performance. During the late preparation period, the intensity of training increases, and ski-specific muscular endurance training becomes more

important. During the last 20 to 30 years, cross-country skiers have steadily increased the number of their altitude training camps on glaciers during the summer, and the number of World Cup races at altitude has also increased. In addition to providing specific on-snow training in the summer, glacier training also increases athletes' red cell mass and blood volume in order to improve performance. At the end of the preparation period, training focuses on explosive strength and sprint training with distance training sessions performed at an increased intensity. Before the competition period, on-snow skiing is performed at low intensity with a greater focus on volume. The ultimate goal is to peak for two to three races per year (Rusko 2003a).

The recent technical developments of cross-country skiing have made a large impact on physiology of the sport and, therefore, the training regimen. The sport now involves the harmonic interaction of the whole body and not just the contribution from the arms and legs. This movement pattern results in greater energy demands, with a 1 km sprint for men expending approximately 400 kJ (95 kcal), a 10 km race 3,000 kJ (714 kcal), and a 30 km race 9,000 kJ (2,143 kcal) (Rusko 2003b). Ekblom and Bergh (2000) reported an energy yield of 3,975 to 5,020 kJ (950-1,200 kcal) for a 15 km race and 12,970 to 15,062 kJ (3,100-3,600 kcal) for a 50 km race. Corresponding calculations for females indicate that they use about 30% less energy than males, expressed in absolute terms, for a given distance. Sjödin and colleagues (1994) studied the energy balance of cross-country skiers using the doubly-labeled water technique. Their research demonstrated that during intense, on-snow training, daily energy expenditure of elite male and female cross-country skiers was approximately 30.2 MJ/day (7,149 kcal/day) and 18.3 MJ/day (4,357 kcal/day), respectively.

Nordic Combined

The two disciplines involved in Nordic Combined differ in their physiology, biomechanics, and body composition. Ski jumping requires a low body mass, considerable power, and technical control, whereas cross-country skiing demands a muscular body frame and an excellent endurance capacity. Training for Nordic Combined includes ski jumping, cross-country skiing, roller skiing, running, weight training, and plyometrics. The average number of ski jumps performed during the preparation phase is 400 and the average number of hours of cross-country training is 250. The preparation phase occurs from May to the end of November, with the European Summer Grand Prix occurring in August.

Nutritional Issues and Challenges

Nordic skiing athletes are exposed to a wide range of nutritional challenges, which result from the demands of the sport, competition schedules, lifestyle factors, and the environment.

Fluid Requirements

Nordic Combined and ski-jumping athletes compete in the European Summer Grand Prix and perform approximately 400 to 600 jumps during the summer preparation period. These athletes wear their winter suits during summer training and competition. Consequently, fluid requirements are elevated because of a high sweat rate. Recent unpublished data from American Nordic athletes showed a mean sweat loss of 0.85 L (0.26-1.16 L) and a body mass loss of 0.7% (0.1-2.5%) compared with initial values after a 2 hr ski-jumping session at an ambient temperature of 24 °C. Athletes training and competing in ski jumping during the summer are encouraged to determine their individual fluid requirements, commence each session hydrated, drink regularly, and remove part of the ski suit after each jump to facilitate heat dissipation. No data are available on the fluid requirements of ski jumping in the winter.

For cross-country skiers, the period of the highest volume training occurs during the summer. Certain long-distance runs or roller skiing sessions occur over a 2 to 3 hr time period at temperatures of 20 °C to 35 °C. Recent unpublished data from American cross-country skiers showed a mean sweat loss of 1.869 L (0.800-2.925 L) and a body mass loss of 2% (0.9-2.5%) compared with initial values after a 2 hr trail run performed at a temperature of 25 °C, an altitude of 2,200 m, and humidity of 25%. These environmental factors demonstrate the need for a large fluid intake during training. The majority of research involving dehydration and sport has been performed in warm climates.

Heat dissipation is not a primary concern in the cold as it is in warm temperatures. However, maintaining total body water is crucial in minimizing competition for blood flow between active muscle, organs, tissues, and skin during cold exposure (Seifert et al. 1998). Skiers competing in the 15 to 30 km races have been reported to lose 2% to 3% of body mass (Ekblom and Bergh 2000). The impact of dehydration in the cold on performance in cross-country skiing is unknown. Skiing is also performed at medium to high altitudes, and increasing altitude escalates urine output and respiratory water loss. Ingesting fluid and especially sport drinks during training sessions and races lasting longer than 15 km is required to help reduce physiological stress. Seifert and colleagues (1998) investigated the physiological effect of beverage ingestion during cross-country ski training in six elite collegiate skiers. Their results showed that voluntary dehydration may occur when exercise is performed in the cold, which was represented by a 1.8% loss of body mass after a 90 min easy training session. These authors concluded that water was inadequate in maintaining fluid balance. In fact, water led to a significant dilution of the plasma and, therefore, increased urinary output. The ingestion of a carbohydrate–electrolyte solution reduced the disruption in fluid balance by maintaining osmotic balance in the plasma. Transporting a large volume of fluid onto the ski course and keeping the temperature of the beverages at 10 °C to 20 °C are challenges encountered by these skiers and their staff. It is recommended that warm sport drinks

be carried in leak-proof containers that have thermal covers. Hypothermia, breathing problems, and local cold injuries are additional complications of ski racing. Individuals should watch their intense training sessions in the cold, and competitions should be cancelled when temperature is below –20 °C.

Energy Requirements

During intense, on-snow training, the daily energy expenditure of cross-country skiers has been reported to be 20 to 25 MJ/day, and during training camps this can be 4 to 8 MJ higher (Ekblom and Bergh 2000; Sjödin et al. 1994). These are some of the highest measured energy expenditures for athletes ever reported in the literature. Therefore, one of the main nutritional concerns of cross-country skiing is meeting a high energy demand. Energy requirements differ greatly among Nordic sports. Ski jumpers have the lowest daily energy requirements (less than 8.4 MJ or 2,000 kcal), whereas cross-country skiers have the greatest (approximately 29.3 MJ or 7,000 kcal for men). Individually, these high and low energy intakes are difficult to achieve. Furthermore, when the three Nordic teams compete at the Olympics and World Championships, they will reside together at the same hotel. It is a challenge to design a meal plan that caters to all the athletes' needs. In addition, times of competitions range from early morning to late at night, which requires the kitchen to be open from 6 a.m. to 10 p.m.

Carbohydrate Intake

Nordic skiing involves a whole-body movement, which generates sizable energy and carbohydrate requirements (Sjödin et al. 1994). Environmental extremes such as high altitude and cold temperatures as well as dehydration in the heat have the potential to further deplete muscle glycogen stores during exercise (Hargreaves 1995). For cross-country skiers and Nordic Combined athletes, maintaining blood glucose through continuous carbohydrate delivery is vital for optimal health and performance. Carbohydrate ingested during exercise can help maintain blood glucose levels and prevent premature fatigue. Carbohydrate consumed after exercise assists in restoring glycogen stores and the body's ability to recover from training. Carbohydrate not only is crucial for physical performance but also plays an important role in fueling the brain and in protecting the immune system (Welsh et al. 2002). These athletes require excellent food organizational skills, because they may have difficulty consuming sufficient energy and carbohydrate during a busy day of training (see table 14.3. for energy and macronutrient guidelines for the sports involved in Nordic skiing).

Carbohydrate loading is a strategy that cross-country skiers competing in the 30 and 50 km events use to maximize carbohydrate stores and, therefore, attempt to enhance endurance capacity by delaying the onset of fatigue. It is recommended that athletes follow the modified carbohydrate-loading technique, which involves a

Table 14.3 Energy, Macronutrient, and Fluid Guidelines for Intense Training and Recovery for Winter Sport Athletes

Sports	Energy requirements (kJ·kg⁻¹·day⁻¹, kcal·kg⁻¹·day⁻¹)	Carbohydrate requirements (g·kg⁻¹·day⁻¹)	Protein requirements (g·kg⁻¹·day⁻¹)	Fat requirements (g·kg⁻¹·day⁻¹)	During training	Recovery
Ski jumping	113-155 27-37	5-6	0.8-1.0	0.5-1.0	• Water as required	• Water • 0.5-1 g of CHO/kg after weights and plyometrics
Cross-country skiing	230-314 55-75	8-12	1.2-1.6	>0.8-1.5	• Warm sport drink (5-8% CHO with electrolytes) • 30-60 g of CHO/hr • 300-700 ml of fluid per hr	• Sport drink + water • 500-1,000 ml • 1 g of CHO/kg
Nordic Combined	188-230 45-55	7-10	1.2-1.4	0.8-1.0	• Warm sport drink (5-8% CHO with electrolytes) • 300-700 ml of fluid per hr of cross-country training • CHO-containing snacks between sessions	• Sport drink + water • 500-1,000 ml • 1 g of CHO/kg after cross-country training sessions
Alpine skiing, mogul skiing, alpine and free-style snowboarding	188-230 45-55	7-10	1.5-1.8	1-1.2	• Warm sport drink (5-8% CHO with electrolytes) • 250-500 ml of fluid per hr of training • 15-30 g of CHO/hr • CHO-containing snacks during break	• Sport drink • 500-750 ml • 1 g of CHO/kg • ~10-15 g of PRO
Freestyle aerials	146-180 35-43 (increased for water ramping and cold conditions)	5-7 (increased for water ramping and cold conditions)	1.0-1.4	0.8-1.0	• Summer: cold sport drink • 500-750 ml/hr • Winter: warm tea (slightly sweetened); warm sport drink for cold conditions • 250-500 ml/hr	• Water • 500-750 ml • Light snack ~150-200 kcal • 1 g of CHO/kg after training under cold conditions
Speed skating	197-272 47-65	8-12	1.5-2.0	1.0-1.5	• Sport drink (5-8% CHO with electrolytes) • 250-500 ml/hr • ~30 g of CHO per hr • Addition of protein for long workouts	• Sport drink • 500-750 ml • 1 g of CHO/kg • ~10-15 g of PRO

CHO = carbohydrate; PRO = protein.

3- to 4-day exercise taper and a high carbohydrate intake (10-12 g · kg⁻¹ · day⁻¹) for the 3 days leading up to the event (Sherman et al. 1981). Carbohydrate loading is discussed in greater detail in chapter 5 (second practical issue). Furthermore, carbohydrate supplementation during exercise is recommended for cross-country and Nordic Combined athletes training or competing in events lasting longer than 60 min. It is recommended that 30 to 60 g of carbohydrate be consumed for every hour of cross-country skiing, running, and roller skiing performed.

Because glycogen stores in the muscle, liver, and blood are limited, cross-country skiers and Nordic Combined athletes require daily repletion of carbohydrates through dietary means. After cross-country ski sessions, it is recommended that carbohydrate intakes of 1 to 1.5 g/kg body mass be consumed within 1 to 2 hr after exercise if training or competition occurs once per day and within the first 30 min if training or competition occurs twice per day. However, recovery is often delayed for many Nordic athletes, because transportation, weather, drug testing, and press conferences can all delay the athletes' departure from the mountain. Therefore, athletes should be prepared for unexpected delays and have recovery foods and an emergency food kit with them at all times. Adequate postrace recovery between events, especially when traveling to a new location for the next day's competition, is also a challenge. Teams need to be organized in locating ideal restaurants on their travel route and providing appropriate snacks.

Iron Status

Iron deficiency is the most prevalent micronutrient deficiency in athletes competing in Nordic sports. Table 14.a in the appendix provides a summary of studies of the hematological status of athletes in winter sports published over the previous 2 decades. One study of the nutritional status of 21 Finnish elite male ski jumpers and 20 age-matched controls failed to detect differences in biochemical or hematological characteristics of the groups (Rankinen et al. 1998). However, this study was limited by the failure to measure all parameters able to identify depleted iron stores. Another study (Fogelholm et al. 1992) evaluated the effect of different training periods on biochemical indexes of iron, thiamin, and zinc status in elite Nordic skiers. This year-long study did not find any seasonal changes in biochemical indexes with changes in activity levels. The results indicated that nutritional status was similar between skiers and controls.

Ski jumpers may experience iron deficiency attributable to a low energy intake and a diet low in available iron. Nordic Combined athletes and cross-country skiers may experience iron deficiency resulting from personal dietary restrictions or exercise-induced iron loss. These athletes require nutritional education on how to optimize their iron status effectively.

Cross-country skiers are now aware of the importance of striving for optimal hemoglobin levels and red cell mass. Most Nordic skiers experiment with altitude training, sleep-high and train-low strategies, or altitude houses; all methods propose to increase serum erythropoietin (EPO),

hemoglobin, and red blood cell mass, which may increase endurance performance (Levine and Stray-Gundersen 2001). For a more detailed discussion on iron deficiency and hematological manipulation, refer to the second practical issue. Additional information on iron deficiency in athletes is provided in chapter 1 (goal 3) and chapter 5, including table 5.3).

Overtraining

Nordic Combined athletes and cross-country skiers have large training and competition loads. The challenge is to balance these loads with adequate recovery in order to provide adaptation and regeneration. The overtraining syndrome is especially prevalent in the sport of Nordic Combined (unpublished observation). It is recommended that Nordic athletes at risk for the overtraining syndrome be regularly tested, with close monitoring of training programs and nutritional intake. Urinary and blood markers such as white cell count, creatine kinase, and the testosterone-to-cortisol ratio may be tested regularly. Dehydration and deficiencies of energy, carbohydrate, and micronutrients are the main nutritional stressors that may interfere with optimal recovery after training or competition in these athletes.

Alpine Skiing

Alpine skiing events were first introduced at the 1924 Winter Olympics in Chamonix, France. Whereas only the slalom event was held at that time, today all four events, as well as a combined event, are considered Olympic events.

Competition

Alpine skiing events can be divided into slalom, giant slalom, super giant slalom, and downhill (see table 14.1). Slalom and giant slalom are typically referred to as technical events, whereas super giant slalom and downhill are considered speed events. These events are all considered World Cup, Olympic, and World Championship events.

- **Technical events:** Slalom is characterized by a rhythmic succession of tight turns lasting from 40 to 60 s. A slalom competition includes two runs. The giant slalom is also rhythmic; however, distances between turns are longer. The giant slalom event also consists of two runs, each lasting from 60 to 90 s. Although set on similar terrain, the two runs for both slalom and giant slalom are distinct and set by different individuals, typically coaches. For both technical events, the seeding of the second run is based on the top 30 competitors from the first run, which start in reversed order. The total time of the two runs determines the winner (FIS 2003).

- **Speed events:** The super giant slalom is a relatively new event that was introduced in 1981 in La Ville, Italy, and became integrated as a World Cup event in the season of 1982-1983. This event evolved from giant slalom and downhill, combining the technical nuances of giant slalom with the speed of downhill. The Super-G lasts longer than a giant slalom but is typically shorter than a downhill event, ranging from 80 to 100 s. Finally, the downhill event, also thought of as the king of all alpine skiing events, is characterized by fewer turns and greater speeds compared with the Super-G, usually lasting between 90 and 160 s. Speeds incurred in downhill racing often exceed 120 km/hr, particularly for men. Both Super-G and downhill events consist of one run only, and the fastest time determines the winner. Only downhill events are preceded by a 3- to 4-day training period with organized inspection times and timed practice runs (FIS 2003).

• **Combined events:** The most classical event in alpine skiing combines one downhill run with a two-run slalom event. This event is particularly challenging because of the skills required to master both the technical aspects of the slalom and the speed and gliding skills of the downhill. The two events are held on the same day at the same venue and differ from the regular slalom and downhill competition in that they are typically shorter and often somewhat less challenging. Times for both events are added, and the fastest combined time determines the winner (FIS 2003).

Each event in alpine skiing consists of an organized warm-up on snow with free skiing and skiing in practice courses, inspection time of the course, and then the race. An event lasts between 3 and 5 hr, inclusive of warm-up and inspection, with those events consisting of a single run finishing earlier than those with two runs. In the case of slalom and giant slalom, athletes will rest after the first run, inspect the second run, and race again. Under special circumstances, athletes will compete in two events on the same day. Relatively new on the World Cup schedule are events held at night. These events are very popular and attract thousands of spectators. After a competition is over, alpine skiers either return to their hotels or to on-snow training in preparation for the next day's race. In many instances, however, athletes continue their travels to the next venue. World Cup competition begins in late October and finishes in March, after which international and national racing is likely to continue into April. World championships are held every 2 years and the Winter Olympic Games every 4 years.

Training

Training for alpine skiing begins in May after a phase of recovery (see table 14.2). During the preparation phase, initial attention is given to general physical conditioning and high-volume training, including muscular and aerobic endurance, strength, agility, speed, balance, skill development, and flexibility. Athletes, coaches, and service personnel may also focus on boot-fitting and testing of new ski equipment.

Although endurance training is an important part of early season training, it remains unclear to what extent the skier should engage in such training. Endurance activities for the alpine skier are centered on mountain biking, with some road cycling and running. Alpine skiers also participate in cross-training activities. As intensity is increased during the summer months, more emphasis is put on strength and power as well as anaerobic capacity. Strength training emphasizes both concentric and eccentric work. Plyometric exercises mixed with maximal strength using both dynamic and static tension, and eccentric exercises, are very common.

Specific on-snow training begins as early as June or July. Sources of snow during this period include the Southern hemisphere and glacier snow, challenging the athlete with frequent travels and involuntary "sleep high and train high" conditions. On-snow training is performed on glacier snow at moderately high altitude (2,600-3,500 m) in the summer and fall until enough snow has accumulated at lower elevations. Initially, technical skills are emphasized in simple rhythmic courses on easier terrain. On-snow training in the summer begins in the early morning hour because of better snow conditions, with dry land training conducted in the afternoon. On-snow training in the summer generally lasts around 3 hr. The training period from early to late fall (September and October) is characterized by an increase in training intensity, whereas training volume is initially maintained. Courses are set in steeper terrain, are longer, and are often timed. Racers take an average of 10 to 20 runs, although this varies by discipline and snow conditions. Training at this time lasts between 4 and 6 hr. This is considered the most intense training phase for the alpine skier, with energy expenditure estimated between 188 and 230 $kJ \cdot kg^{-1} \cdot day^{-1}$ (45-55 $kcal \cdot kg^{-1} \cdot day^{-1}$) for both men and women. Environmental extremes, such as altitude and cold, however, can increase energy expenditure. Temperatures can drop below −15 °C, with shivering thermogenesis as a frequent side effect. Under shivering conditions, energy expenditure may be greater than 230 kJ (55 $kcal \cdot kg^{-1} \cdot day^{-1}$). Future research should use the doubly-labeled water technique to measure energy expenditure in alpine ski racers.

Race simulation training is the last step before competition begins. If no snow is available at lower elevations, skiers remain dependent on glacier training. Cold exposure can become more critical during this time of the year, and racers tend to be fatigued and ready to train under more normal conditions. The competition phase begins at the end of October with the first World Cup race typically held on glacier terrain. For periodized training and competition phases, see table 14.2.

Physique and Physiology

Successful skiers are tall and heavy with a high lean tissue mass (Andersen and Montgomery 1988). Anthropometric data were recently summarized by Hintermeister and Hagerman (2000) and included data from previous studies (Andersen and Montgomery 1988; Berg and Eiken 1999; Berg et al. 1995; Bosco et al. 1994; Eriksson et al. 1976; Orvanova 1987; Richardson et al. 1993; White and Johnson 1991, 1993). Ranges for age were 17 to 22 years for females and 16 to 24 years for males, whereas heights and body mass ranged from 159.0 to 169.0 cm and 56.7 to 66.1 kg in females and 168.0 to 180.0 cm and 64.0 to 81.0 kg in males, respectively. Mean percent body fat levels in the 1980s assessed with the skinfold technique were 20.6% for female and 10.2% for male skiers (Agostini 2000; Orvanova 1987), although data from the late 1970s using hydrodensitometry in Austrian skiers demonstrated much leaner physiques for female (13.5%) and male (4.7%) (Veitl et al. 1977). As in many other sports, the physique of alpine skiers has changed dramatically over the past decades (Berg and Eiken 1999; Eriksson et al. 1976; Karlsson et al. 1978). Unpublished data of elite North American skiers demonstrate ranges for height and weight from 161.0 to 176.0 cm and 62.0 to 82.7 kg in females and from 174.0 to 189.0 cm and 77.0 to 103.2 kg in males, respectively. Body composition data also show leaner physiques for both genders. The summary reported by Hintermeister and Hagerman (2002) showed body fat percent ranging from 13.1% to 23.8% for females and 6.1% to 11.0% for males, with the lower values reported by White and Johnson (1993). In general, slalom skiers tend to be lighter and leaner than speed skiers, whereas downhill skiers are the heaviest. Increased body mass may be of some benefit in alpine skiing because of gravitational forces that are partly dependent on body mass, regardless of composition. Nevertheless, lean tissue mass has been shown to be a strong predictor of alpine skiing performance (White and Johnson 1991) and, thus, should be emphasized when athletes are encouraged to gain weight.

Nutritional Issues and Challenges

A range of nutritional issues arise from the training and competition requirements of alpine skiing.

Carbohydrate Intake During Glacier Training

A day of giant slalom training has been shown to reduce muscle glycogen content by 50% (Tesch et al. 1978). Resynthesis of muscle glycogen stores after a day of skiing appears essential for repetitive on-snow training days. It has been shown that a diet with moderate carbohydrate content will not replete glycogen stores during one night of rest in alpine skiers. When extra carbohydrate was ingested, however, glycogen stores returned to baseline values (Nygaard et al. 1978). Diets reported by alpine ski racers have been evaluated as poor (Ronsen et al. 1999) and, thus, may not always be adequate in carbohydrate to quickly replenish glycogen lost during intense training. Although no data exist in male athletes, female athletes do not seem to exceed intakes of 6.8 g·kg^{-1}·day^{-1} carbohydrate regardless of training intensity, volume, and environmental factors (Meyer et al. 1999). The predominant use of blood glucose, without a concomitant sparing effect of muscle glycogen (Green et al. 1989), is a challenge for athletes

training for long hours in these environments, because glucose and muscle glycogen quickly become a limited fuel source. Thus, higher amounts of carbohydrate should be consumed during this type of training, particularly during the intense training phase in September and October. Carbohydrate intakes of 7 to 10 g·kg^{-1}·day^{-1} may be needed to replenish glycogen stores during such training, although higher amounts may be required for certain individuals, particularly technical skiers.

Weather changes can often interfere with training schedules on the glacier. Competition simulation time trials require the athlete to train in thin bodysuits at temperatures around –15 °C. Shivering thermogenesis is a common side effect of such training, possibly increasing the rate of glycogen utilization and the onset of fatigue. Indeed, it has been shown that carbohydrate oxidation may be elevated up to sixfold during shivering thermogenesis. This increase in carbohydrate oxidation is provided by greater plasma glucose turnover, muscle glycolysis, and glycogenolysis (Vallerand et al. 1995). Training for racing is highly competitive, and it is quite common for teams to conduct time trials for World Cup qualifications. One concern may be that low glycogen stores predispose an athlete for injury, because many skiing injuries often occur later in the day (Brouns et al. 1986). Depletion of glycogen from muscle fibers that may be recruited to quickly respond to an unusual situation could potentially increase the chance of a fall and an injury (Brouns et al. 1986). It is also well known that carbohydrate is the primary fuel of the brain and has been shown to affect mental performance of skill-based sports, particularly later in the game (Welsh et al. 2002). To date, no data exist in alpine skiers; however, concentration may be, at least in part, dependent on the maintenance of blood glucose.

Coaches and staff should be educated about the physiological effects of cold and altitude during glacier training. Training under such conditions should be well organized with transport of gear in concert with training runs, availability of extra clothing or blankets, and warm, carbohydrate-containing fluids at the start. Although no data are available from studies in alpine skiing, it can be assumed that the ingestion of carbohydrate-containing sport drinks and foods should provide enough fuel to maintain blood glucose levels and delay both mental and physical fatigue during intense training periods. Thus far, data on female alpine ski racers have shown that carbohydrate intake during ski training in the form of sport drinks and bars is fairly low, averaging 60 g of carbohydrates consumed in 6 hr of on-snow glacier training (Meyer et al. 1999). Technical skiers may deplete muscle glycogen stores quicker than speed skiers. Training routines may allow for continuous fueling (every 15-20 min) or fueling during a general training break, when courses are reset by the coaches. Guidelines should include using a sport drink (5-8% carbohydrate) with electrolytes throughout training, in combination with eating a sport bar or carbohydrate-rich snack during the longer break. To date, there are no specific recommendations for carbohydrate ingestion during training in alpine skiers. It may be safe to suggest that intakes should range from 15 to 30 g/hr (250-500 ml of fluid per hour) with the higher end reserved for extreme weather conditions.

One area that presents a particular challenge to timely restoration of muscle glycogen is the fact that descending from glacier environments may take 60 to 120 min. Meals may be further delayed by other factors such as weather. Thus, rapid recovery should be considered via ingestion of recovery foods and fluids while descending from the glacier area to return to accommodation sites. Sport drinks, bars, and snacks may be used as convenient options. Recovery fuels should include fluids and electrolytes to optimize rehydration and carbohydrates as well as small amounts of protein (~10 g) to aid in glycogen repletion, particularly if carbohydrate intake is low, and to help with muscle repair and protein synthesis. The key is to plan ahead and pack foods and fluids in the morning. For many teams, the physical therapist or athletic trainer is responsible for transporting foods and fluids to the glacier environment. Educating athletes about preparing their own drinks and sport foods is an essential component of sports nutrition services provided to alpine ski racers (see table 14.3. for details).

Fluid Intake and Balance During On-Snow Training

Training under winter sport conditions can result in significant shifts in fluid volume and lead to dehydration. A study on alpine skiers showed that environmental factors such as altitude and cold temperatures exacerbate fluid loss (Seifert et al. 2000). Fluid intake at a dose of 2 ml/kg body mass ingested after each training run of slalom training at an altitude of 2,435 to 3,045 m and temperature below 0 °C was compared with no fluid intake in collegiate male and female alpine ski racers. In the fluid trial, total fluid intake was 1.2 L during 2 hr of slalom training, which led to an increase in body mass of 0.2 kg, whereas 0.6 kg was lost in the no-fluid trial. Urine output was significantly lower and plasma volume changes from baseline significantly greater between the two trials. Plasma and urine osmolality were significantly higher in the no-fluid trial. Thus, even in relatively short training sessions, fluid shifts can occur. Fluid intake in Swiss female alpine ski racers was found to be very low (0.2 L) during 5 hr of on-snow training. Although fluid balance was not assessed in these athletes, fluid intake was probably insufficient to prevent dehydration. Factors that may explain minimal rates of voluntary fluid intake include reduced drive to drink (Askew 1995) and the lack of available restrooms, especially in glacier environments. It was only recently that restroom facilities were built at one of the most frequented training areas in Switzerland on glacier ice at an altitude of 3,000 m. Fluid intake since then might have improved, although no data are available to confirm this.

The use of sport drinks in alpine skiing appears to be an optimal strategy to maintain blood glucose and hydration levels during glacier training. Most ski teams should have products available through sponsorships. Although no current guidelines are available for fluid replacement strate-

gies during alpine skiing or any other winter sport, it may be safe to suggest an intake between 250 and 500 ml/hr. However, more individualized guidelines should be based on calculated sweat rates for alpine skiing under various environmental conditions (see table 14.3 for details).

Precompetition and Competition Nutrition

Alpine ski racers stay in one resort area for a few days to 2 weeks depending on the type of competition. It remains a great challenge for teams to set up and receive optimal food service in every country, especially without a sports dietitian on staff to prepare for winter travel. In addition to optimizing food service during the competition phase, alpine skiers need to be educated about the importance of breakfast as a preevent meal. Preevent meals should be similar to those used in other sports, containing easily digestible, carbohydrate-rich foods and adequate fluids. Athletes should be advised to carry with them foods and fluids that can be stored in backpacks for fueling throughout the course of competition. Resorts also offer foods; however, athletes need to be educated about the types of foods and fluids to use on a competition day. Lunch should be delayed until after the second run. Thus, foods and fluids consumed between runs should be easily digestible, carbohydrate-rich, and if possible warm. Inexperienced ski racers often eat heavy meals between runs when competing, which may interfere with concentration and optimal fuel availability for the second run. A World Cup skier usually has acquired a good routine. In addition, World Cup skiers often have foods and fluids available at the event or snacks prepared in advance by the physical therapist or athletic trainer. Attention should be given to the types of foods athletes may be offered at event buffets, because these foods are often high in fat and too heavy to provide quick refueling. In case of a night event, alpine ski racers should eat their last meal 3 to 5 hr prior to the event, with a carbohydrate-rich snack and adequate fluids approximately 1 hr before race start.

Environmental Factors and Antioxidants

Altitude exposure is associated with increased levels of oxidative stress or reactive oxygen species (ROS) generated from a variety of sources, including exercise, ultraviolet radiation, catecholamines, anoxia or reoxygenation, and hypoxanthine and xanthine oxidase (Askew 2002). Thus, winter sport athletes may be at increased risk for ROS because of the considerable amount of time spent training intensely in glacier environments. Subudhi and colleagues (2001) measured antioxidant capacity and oxidative stress markers of U.S. male World Cup skiers during a combined dry-land and on-snow training camp. Dry-land training occurred at near sea level, whereas on-snow training was conducted at an altitude ranging from 2,200 to 2,800 m. Antioxidant status and oxidative stress markers were measured in blood and urine before the dry-land camp, at day 2 during the dry land camp, and at the end of the on-snow portion (day 10) of the camp immediately after the last training run. Results showed no changes in antioxidant status, except for vitamin E levels, which decreased significantly throughout the study. No differences were found in oxidative stress markers before and after the study. The authors concluded that dietary antioxidant intake may be sufficient (diet and supplements) to maintain a high antioxidant defense, and that alpine skiers may be well adapted to training at higher altitudes. Although consuming a diet rich in antioxidant nutrients should be emphasized to maintain a high antioxidant capacity, this may not always be feasible, especially during travel to foreign countries. Thus, antioxidant supplementation may be considered in certain situations, however, at doses within the current Dietary Reference Intakes, because high intakes of certain antioxidant vitamins may result in adverse effects (Coombes et al. 2001).

Iron Deficiency and Hemoglobin Manipulation

There is only one report demonstrating low iron stores and anemia in male alpine skiers, from almost two decades ago (Clement et al. 1987), but our personal observations and several studies in a variety of countries have shown that between 20% and 36% of female alpine skiers are iron depleted or deficient (Clement et al. 1987; Meyer et al. 1999; Ronsen et al. 1999). Low levels of transferrin saturation were found in 35% of French national team female skiers (Couzy et al. 1989). In contrast, Schena and colleagues (1995) demonstrated for the first time that male alpine skiers had the highest hemoglobin and hematocrit values in a sample of endurance and anaerobic sports. The authors concluded that heavy training at altitude and lower red blood cell destruction in alpine skiers compared with cross-country skiers may have been responsible for these high values. More recent observations have shown that male alpine ski racers appear to maximize iron status through supplemental iron, and it is not uncommon to find alpine skiers with hemoglobin values approaching limits established by the FIS. In fact, in a sample of French alpine skiers, mean hemoglobin levels of 16.0 g/100 ml were recently reported. These values were higher than those of cross-country skiers, biathletes, Nordic Combined athletes, and ski jumpers (Videman et al. 2000). Although iron status has been monitored in many teams throughout the past decades, alpine skiers have only recently begun focusing on hemoglobin and hematocrit levels, probably in an attempt to minimize recovery time when training at altitude and improve oxygen delivery during longer events. Monitoring iron status should be an integral part of medical supervision in alpine skiers and should serve two objectives: minimizing low iron stores and iron deficiency in female athletes and preventing iron overload in male athletes. See the second practical issue for more information on iron deficiency and hematological manipulation in winter sport athletes and table 14.a for an overview of studies on winter sports related to hematological indexes.

Freestyle Skiing

The main events staged in World Cup, World Championships, and Winter Olympic Games include aerials and mogul skiing. As an internationally competitive sport, freestyle skiing is very young, with mogul skiing only added to the official Olympic program in 1992 and aerials in 1994.

Competition

Freestyle skiing is divided into aerial and mogul disciplines, with newer disciplines including halfpipe and freestyle ski cross (see table 14.1 for events).

• **Aerials:** Freestyle aerial competitions consist of two different acrobatic jumps, with focus on the takeoff, the height of the jump and its distance (air), proper style, execution, precision of the maneuver performed (form), and the landing of the jump. Freestyle aerials are considered an aesthetic sport and is scored by judges. Scores are a composite of air, form, and landing, and the total score is multiplied by the appropriate degree of difficulty, which is scored separately. Athletes have the choice of single, double, or triple jumps (kicker), during which a variety of maneuvers are created. The three forms must conform with a specific jump height, jump length from the takeoff area (knoll), and degree at takeoff. Jump height ranges from 2.2 to 4.2 m, jump length from 4 to 7.5 m, and degree at take off from 52 to 71° for single to triple kicker, respectively. For international competition, four formats are used: the final, the standard, the championship, and a format that is similar to the standard except that athletes are seeded based on results from previous competitions. In the final, all participants compete in qualification rounds consisting of one jump. After qualification, the top 12 women and 12 men advance to the final round. The finalists will jump one additional time, and the results from the final round will be added to the results of the first round. In the standard, all participants compete in two rounds. The rounds can be mixed according to starting groups or can be run as individual competitions. The results from the two rounds are added and ranked accordingly. If only one round can be completed, the results from the first round are counted. In the championship format, all athletes compete in a two-jump elimination round followed by a two-jump final. The combined scores from the two elimination jumps determine the finalists. Typically in World Cup events, 12 men and 12 women move to the finals. The finalists start in reverse order of the placing in the qualification round. The remainder of the field is ranked according to the results from the qualification round. Finally, the seeded format is similar to the standard format except that athletes are seeded. The field is split into an A and B seed based on the athletes' top two results from the previous 12 months. Each seed completes training and competition separately. Usually, the B seed begins. This format is rarely used anymore, and it appears that the most popular format among organizing committees is the final, with the standard preferred by the athletes (FIS 2003).

• **Moguls:** The mogul event is characterized by a steep, heavily moguled course with two integrated jumps. Mogul events stress technical aspects of skiing and speed as well as aerial maneuvers performed during the jumps. As in freestyle aerials, most of the score is subjective in nature, with judges responsible for scoring. The majority of the score is based on turns (50%), with 25% dedicated to each air and speed. Racers are timed and compared with a pace time, which varies from course to course. The typical format for mogul competition includes one elimination round followed by a one-run final. Typically in World Cup events, 16 men and 16 women move to the final round. Common duration of an international competition ranges from 25 to 35 s. An additional event is the dual mogul event, which consists of a series of one-run duals with the winner advancing to the next round. Ultimately, the last two remaining competitors ski against each other for the first place. The dual mogul event is a World Cup but not an Olympic or World Championship event, whereas the single mogul events are World Cup, World Championships, and Olympic events (FIS 2003).

• **Halfpipe and freestyle ski cross:** The halfpipe and freestyle ski cross events are similar to the halfpipe and snowboard cross events for snowboarding except for the differences in devices used (skis vs. boards). For the halfpipe event, competitors perform jumps, tricks, and maneuvers in the halfpipe that are judged. In the freestyle ski cross, competitors race against each other in groups of four to six skiers, mastering an obstacle course with banked turns, ridges, jumps, waves, a variety of terrain, and degrees of freestyle elements. The freestyle ski cross and halfpipe events are neither Olympic nor World Championship events; however, they are World Cup events (FIS 2003).

For the rest of this discussion, the focus will be on freestyle aerials and moguls. For both events, each competition is preceded by an official training, which lasts 1 to 3 days. On competition days, aerial and mogul skiers are allowed to train on the race course for a limited time. Both events last approximately 3 to 5 hr, including training. It is common for freestyle events to take place in the evening as part of a night show. After the event, aerial and mogul skiers return to their hotels for recovery or travel to the next venue. The freestyle competition season begins with the first events held in the southern hemisphere in August. Preparation continues after the summer events until the main competition season starts in December for mogul skiers (somewhat delayed for aerialists) and lasts through March or April. The World Championships are held every 2 years and the Winter Olympic Games every 4 years.

Training

Freestyle skiers use similar periodized training plans as discussed for alpine skiers, with a recovery phase scheduled for some time in the spring, followed by the preparation and competition phase (see table 14.2 for training and competition phases). Training for both disciplines involves similar dry land activities, starting with muscular endurance and aerobic activities with increasing intensity and greater focus on strength and power as well as anaerobic capacity as the preparation phase continues. Whereas mogul skiers seek higher altitude environments for specific on-snow training, aerialists can perform much of their specific summer training using water ramps (jumping into water). It is also common for mogul skiers to use water ramps for practicing their tricks and jumps in combination with a dry land camp.

Aerials

Specific training for the aerialist can be performed both on snow or using water ramps. In the summer and early fall, athletes use water ramps to jump into pools wearing skis and boots. Most of the energy expended during summer training appears to accumulate from walking, climbing stairs, and moving in water with 15 to 20 kg of extra weight in the form of ski boots, skis, helmet, and a wet suit. To return to the start, athletes climb 80 to 150 stair steps. Athletes complete 10 to 20 jumps per training session and engage in physical conditioning such as muscular endurance and cardiovascular fitness, strength and power training, core stability, and flexibility and agility training using the trampoline and trapeze to practice jumping. The switch to winter sport conditions for the aerialist depends on snowfall at lower elevations. Thus, aerialists maintain their water-ramping schedule as long as needed before jumps can be built of snow.

Freestyle aerial competitions are held in both summer (in the southern hemisphere) and winter, which complicates training schedules and shortens the time for preparation, particularly for summer competition. The sport of freestyle aerials has turned into a year-round sport, considering the high specificity of training using water ramps in the summer.

Moguls

Training of a mogul skier is similar to training of the technical alpine skier (refer to alpine skiing for further detail). In addition to needing muscle strength, power, speed, and a strong anaerobic capacity, the mogul skier requires a great deal of coordination and acrobatic ability because of the integrated jumps and nature of freestyle skiing. Mogul skiers complement much of their training with sports such as trampolining, skateboarding, or wind or kite surfing.

Unfortunately, no data are available to describe energy expenditure during on-snow training in mogul skiers, but it is expected to be similar to that of alpine skiers (see alpine skiing section for further detail). Training on snow generally lasts 3 to 5 hr, although longer training sessions are not uncommon.

Physique and Physiology

Because many aerialists have a gymnastics background, it is expected that physique characteristics are similar to gymnasts, particularly the female athlete, although aerialists appear older and heavier and, thus, it is probable that aerialists have a higher muscle mass than gymnasts. No scientific data are available on freestyle aerialists or on the physique and physiological characteristics of mogul skiers.

Nutritional Issues and Challenges

Aerialists and mogul skiers present different nutritional issues that arise from the training and competition requirements.

Energy, Carbohydrate, and Fluid Needs for Aerialists

Because of the difference between summer and winter training, careful monitoring of energy balance should be considered during both training conditions. Recent data on energy expenditure and dietary intake of aerialists have shown that energy requirements are higher when athletes use water ramps compared with on-snow training (Meyer 2003). Athletes, coaches, and athletic trainers should be educated about the difference between summer and winter training and the potential for greater energy demands from the repetitive climbing of 80 to 150 steps carrying an additional load such as skis and boots. Adequate energy intake should meet carbohydrate requirements during this type of training. Energy requirements may range from 170 to 180 $kJ \cdot kg^{-1} \cdot day^{-1}$ (40-43 $kcal \cdot kg^{-1} \cdot day^{-1}$), with carbohydrate needs probably approaching 7 $g \cdot kg^{-1} \cdot day^{-1}$. Using sport drinks during this type of training is a convenient way to increase energy and carbohydrate intake and maintain fluid balance. During the warmer summer months, cool sport drinks help maintain the athlete's desire to drink and replace sweat loss, which may be higher when wearing wet suits. Fluid replacement during training using water ramps in the summer should be based on the minimal guidelines published by ACSM (Convertino et al. 1996), with intakes ranging from 500 to 600 ml/hr (5-8% carbohydrate concentration). It appears that female athletes easily meet these guidelines during training under warmer conditions (Meyer 2003), whereas fluid intake likely declines when temperatures drop later during the season. Breaks for the use of restroom facilities need to be incorporated during training using water ramps, even though they are viewed as interrupting to the training routine. Providing adequate fluids and carbohydrates may, in the long run, maintain jumping quality and reduce the risk of injury.

Training and competition on snow probably result in similar or slightly lower energy (146-170 $kJ \cdot kg^{-1} \cdot day^{-1}$; 35-40 $kcal \cdot kg^{-1} \cdot day^{-1}$) and carbohydrate requirements. Environmental factors such as altitude and cold exposure need to be considered, because freestyle aerialists are dependent on stable weather conditions, and weather delays frequently expose athletes to cold temperatures (they sometimes compete at night), possibly leading to shivering thermogenesis, increased energy expenditure, and faster use of glycogen stores. Even though aerialists do not train on glaciers, altitude exposure may nevertheless exceed 2,000 m for training or competition. In addition to finding lower energy and macronutrient intakes during on-snow training, Meyer and colleagues (Meyer 2003) demonstrated that fluid intake is markedly reduced in female aerialists during on-snow training compared with training using water ramps in the summer, with some athletes not ingesting any fluid during 3 to 4 hr of on-snow jump training. Athletes should plan ahead and bring warm, carbohydrate-containing fluids. Approximately 250 ml/hr of fluid should be enough to maintain fluid balance under cold conditions in male and female aerialists. The carbohydrate contained in the fluid may improve overall carbohydrate balance, especially in those athletes who do not meet minimal requirements. In addition, carbohydrate-containing fluids help maintain blood glucose levels and may prevent early fatigue and risk of injury during on-snow sessions in the cold and at altitude, which are both concerns when glycogen levels are depleted. If winter sport conditions are less extreme (temperature >0 °C), attention should be focused on a well-balanced diet with sport foods and drinks ingested in small amounts during prolonged training or competition. Freestyle aerials is a high-risk sport for the development of the female athlete triad. This was recently demonstrated, with more than 60% of aerialists having eating behaviors consistent with disordered eating. In addition, one athlete had previously been diagnosed with an eating disorder (Meyer 2003).

Energy and Nutrient Requirements for Mogul Ski Training

For mogul skiers, on-snow training can be highly intense, possibly depleting muscle glycogen stores to a similar extent as in alpine skiers (Nygaard et al. 1978; Tesch et al. 1978). Intense training periods at altitude and in the cold require careful attention to food service and foods and fluids used during glacier training to ensure energy and nutrient adequacy. Energy requirement may range from 188 to 230 $kJ \cdot kg^{-1} \cdot day^{-1}$ (45-55 $kcal \cdot kg^{-1} \cdot day^{-1}$) during intense training, with carbohydrate requirement as high as 7 to 10 $g \cdot kg^{-1} \cdot day^{-1}$. Because of its high impact, mogul skiing may predispose athletes to soft-tissue damage, slow regeneration and repair of tissues, and increased risk for inflammation in previously injured sites, particularly in the knee and back. Focus on foods, fluids, and possibly dietary supplements that may assist in the recovery process should be emphasized. Daily protein intake should target 1.5 to 1.8 $g \cdot kg^{-1} \cdot day^{-1}$. Many athletes have a long history of sport-related injuries and spend much time in the training room after intense on-snow sessions. Dietary strategies may be implemented that can reduce exercise-associated inflammation, ensure quick repletion of muscle glycogen, and repair damaged tissue. Using sport drinks during on-snow training and recovery foods and fluids after training, containing both carbohydrate and protein, should be emphasized, particularly because of the lengthy return from glacier terrain to accommodations sites. Many mogul skiers also have individual sport supplement sponsors that provide an array of recovery options in powder form possibly applicable for this type of training. Athletes who restrict energy intake may run the risk of delayed recovery.

Similar to alpine skiers, mogul skiers train on glaciers, where restroom availabilities are scarce. Fluid recommendations should include 250 to 500 ml/hr in the form of sport drinks. Coaches should incorporate breaks during training on glaciers for athletes to consume food and fluid and use restroom facilities. Refer to the section on alpine skiing for more information. For the mogul skier, training is markedly different from competition, with somewhat lower energy and carbohydrate requirements during competition. Environmental factors such as cold and altitude, however, prevail also during competition and thus need to be considered. Table 14.3. provides more detail on fueling for intense training.

Snowboarding

Snowboard competition began in the 1980s, with the first U.S. National Championships held in 1982 and the first World Championships held in 1983. The World Cup tour was introduced in 1987, 6 years before the FIS instated snowboarding as an official FIS event. Despite its history, snowboarding has only been recognized as an Olympic sport since 1998, with a giant slalom held at the Nagano Winter Olympic Games. The halfpipe and parallel slalom events, today belonging to the main snowboarding events, were first introduced at the 2002 Winter Olympic Games in Salt Lake City. Snowboard cross was added to the official Olympic program in 2006. It is worth mentioning that the most exciting scene of snowboarding, particularly for the halfpipe discipline, does not occur at World Cup and Olympic level but on the pro tour, such as the U.S. Open Snowboarding Championships. For our discussion, however, we will focus on World Cup–level competition.

Competition

Snowboarding is divided into alpine and freestyle events (halfpipe, snowboard cross, big air). Although most snowboarders specialize in alpine or freestyle events, the snowboard cross is an event that brings alpine and freestyle athletes to common grounds (see table 14.1 for events).

- **Alpine snowboarding:** Alpine snowboarding events are similar to the technical events in alpine skiing, with slalom and giant slalom as their main events. However, snowboarding features an interesting, action-packed parallel slalom and giant slalom competition. Each racer is required to qualify for the 16-person finale. In the finale,

racers compete side by side twice, switching courses after the first run. The combined time determines the winner. This competition can be challenging, because it lasts several hours but does not break for those moving into the final rounds. The parallel slalom and giant slalom are similarly set to alpine skiing slalom and giant slalom and are of similar length. The only difference is that two courses are set next to each other for head-to-head competition. Only the parallel giant slalom was held at the 2002 Olympics. The parallel slalom and giant-slalom events are both World Cup and World Championship events (FIS 2003).

- **Halfpipe:** This freestyle event of snowboarding consists of a set of acrobatic aerial tricks, as snowboarders jump from edge to edge in a half-cylinder-shaped course (halfpipe) situated at a grade. Direction change and traverse across the halfpipe are used to augment speed. The FIS's judging criteria include an overall impression addressing variety, difficulty, and execution, in addition to standard airs, rotations, and amplitude. Several qualification and final formats exist. These are single, heat, double-up, and jam session formats. The single format has several categories but refers to two qualifications rounds, either with all participants competing in each round or ranks 4 through 15 for women and 6 through 25 for men from the first qualification round, competing in the second qualification round. The best 3 women and 5 men from each round qualify for the final, with the winner determined by the best of two or three final runs. In the heat format, riders will be grouped into heats of 25 to 35 competitors, with each rider receiving two runs to qualify for the final. Twenty men and 10 women compete in the final, and the best run out of two will determine the winner. The double-up format is used for qualification only and refers to a judging system composed of two groups of three judges (A and B). Riders receive two qualification runs and are judged by the two groups of judges. The best scores of group A and group B are added to determine the results. Twenty men and 10 women advance to the final. Finally, the jam session format is used as a final format only. Competitors ride for a total of 1 hr, during which two groups of judges (A and B) evaluate their performance. The best two scores out of their runs are added together to determine the winner. This format is judged via overall impression only. The length of a typical run in the halfpipe ranges from 15 to 20 s. In addition to appearing at the Olympics, the halfpipe event is also held at the World Championships and on the World Cup tour (FIS 2003).

- **Snowboard cross:** In the snowboard cross event, competitors race against each other in groups of four to six athletes, depending on the type of competition. Boarders attempt to master a challenging course with jumps and obstacles. The fastest two or three racers of each group (two if four race against each other; three if six race against each other) advance to the final. The fastest time in the final determines the winner.

- **Big air:** Big air competitions are jumping events that are judged according to control of the trick performed in the air, amplitude (height and length of the jump), and landing. Two qualification runs precede the final rounds, with the best two of the three final runs determining the winner. Snowboard cross and big air events are not Olympic events; however, they are World Cup and World Championship events (FIS 2003).

Preparation for competition is quite different between alpine and freestyle snowboarders. Alpine snowboarders have similar schedules to alpine skiers, with free-riding and warm-up in gates before course inspection, followed by competition. Freestyle snowboarders may take a few free-ride runs to warm up, followed by a greater focus on the execution of the maneuvers in the halfpipe planned for competition. In addition, halfpipe events are preceded by two training days, whereas snowboard cross events allow for one training day before the event. Unique for the alpine snowboarder is the parallel slalom and giant-slalom disciplines. This is an all-day event with multiple runs taken in the two courses. Each run is skied at maximal intensity because of the one-on-one battle. In contrast, for the freestyle snowboarder, competition is less intense than training because of the lower number of runs taken. After the event, snowboarding athletes typically return to their hotels for

recovery or travel to the next venue. The competition phase typically begins as early as October on glacier snow. The World Cup circuit finishes with the finale in March, after which international and national competition is likely to continue into April or May. World Championships are held every 2 years and the Olympics every 4 years.

Training

Training plans are similarly periodized for snowboarders as they are for alpine skiers. The reader is referred to the alpine skiing section for further detail. Many snowboarders are also avid wave, kite, and wind surfers, with the freestyle athletes also using skate and surfboards. These activities help improve agility, balance, and speed and simulate at least some aspects of sport-specific training independent of snow availability. Sport-specific nuances are nurtured in freestyle snowboarding fairly early during the season with the inclusion of a week in a skateboard camp before on-snow training is initiated.

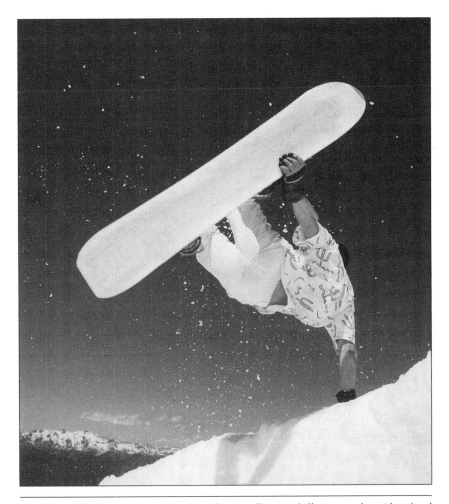

In addition to the rigors of snowboarding, walking uphill at a grade with a load such as the snowboard and heavy gear is cumbersome and will increase energy expenditure.

Energy expenditure for both alpine and freestyle snowboarders is most likely provided through anaerobic means. No data exist on energy contribution, blood lactate response, or glycogen utilization in snowboarders. At least for alpine snowboarders, it may be safe to suggest that lactate responses and glycogen depletion patterns are similar to alpine skiers after a day of intense training. Recent energy expenditure data showed that female freestyle snowboarders expended more energy during on-snow glacier training than did their alpine counterparts (Meyer 2003). This is most likely because freestyle athletes usually hike back to the starting area of the halfpipe. If transportation is available, energy expenditure is expected to be lower and probably similar to that of alpine snowboarders. For further detail on periodized training and competition phases, see table 14.2.

Physique and Physiology

No published data exist on the physique in snowboarders; however, it is expected that alpine snowboarders have similar physique as alpine skiers. The reader is referred to the alpine skiing section for further information. No further data or cross-comparisons exist for freestyle snowboarders. Comparisons may be made with skateboarders and possibly surfers.

Nutritional Issues and Challenges

Energy requirement is probably increased during training on glaciers. Thus, snowboarders should focus primarily on meeting energy requirements (see table 14.3. for recommendations). Predominantly anaerobic activities such as alpine and freestyle snowboarding require moderately high intakes of carbohydrate. If muscle glycogen is similarly depleted in alpine snowboarders as has been shown in alpine skiers (Tesch et al. 1978), intakes of carbohydrates should be high enough to replenish glycogen stores. Daily carbohydrate intake between 7 and 10 g · kg^{-1} · day^{-1} may be recommended for glacier training, with the upper end reserved for intense training. The reason for this requirement is based on the assumption that exposure to environmental extremes may shift fuel use to greater reliance on glucose and glycogen not only when the participant is snowboarding but also when resting, riding the chair, or hiking to return to the start. Similar to alpine and freestyle skiing, snowboarding is a high-risk sport, and low carbohydrate availability may increase the risk for injury. Injury prevention in these sports relies greatly on quick maneuvers and the ability to react to inconsistencies in terrain, possibly recruiting muscle fibers that are depleted of glycogen, particularly late during training (Brouns et al. 1986).

For both alpine and freestyle snowboarders, the use of carbohydrate-containing foods and drinks may help maintain glucose availability when training on glacier snow. In addition, such strategies may also assist in meeting daily carbohydrate requirement. For fluid intake, factors such as

lack of restroom availability, diuresis, and reduced drive to drink (Askew 1995) probably all contribute to difficulty in meeting fluid replacement guidelines when training on snow. Sport drinks provide an optimal combination of fluid, carbohydrates, and electrolytes for snowboarders training on glacier snow. As previously discussed in other sports, training on glacier terrain may delay the restoration of muscle glycogen because of the lengthy descent. Immediate recovery should be considered via recovery foods and fluids ingested while descending from the glacier area to return to accommodation sites. For further details, refer to the alpine skiing section and table 14.3.

Energy, carbohydrate, and fluid requirements may differ between alpine and freestyle snowboarders when training on snow. This is mostly based on the assumption that freestyle snowboarders hike to the start, whereas alpine snowboarders use a chair lift. When hiking is included, energy requirement may exceed 230 kJ · kg^{-1} · day^{-1} (55 kcal · kg^{-1} · day^{-1}). Increased caloric requirement may be met by greater carbohydrate intake during and after training, achieving a total intake of 10 g · kg^{-1} · day^{-1}. Fluid replacement during glacier training should range from 250 to 500 ml/hr, with higher fluids (500-750 ml/hr) required when hiking because sweat rates are probably higher. To individualize fluid replacement during snowboard training, sweat rate should be estimated by weight measurements. Cold temperatures and shivering thermogenesis may lead to a greater energy and carbohydrate requirement in both freestyle and alpine snowboarders, although this is not expected if athletes hike back to the starting area. To evaluate energy, carbohydrate, and fluid needs, careful attention should be given to the number of runs taken, the environmental factors, and dry land activities performed after on-snow training to prevent both under- and overfeeding.

In general, training and competition for snowboarders are markedly different with respect to energy and carbohydrate requirements, as previously discussed in alpine and freestyle skiing, with the exception of the parallel slalom and giant slalom event. This discipline is an all-day event with multiple runs. Top contenders race more than 10 times. If no fluids and carbohydrate-containing foods are available, the athlete may exhaust muscle glycogen stores and may be unable to maintain racing intensity. A mild form of carbohydrate loading may be necessary for these athletes 3 days before competition to prepare for the event. Carbohydrate intake should target 10 g · kg^{-1} · day^{-1}. Pre-event meals (breakfast) should be similar to those used in other sports, containing easily digestible, carbohydrate-rich foods and adequate fluids. Athletes should carry foods and fluids that can be stored in backpacks for fueling throughout the course of competition. Foods consumed between runs should include easily digestible, carbohydrate-rich sources and should provide 30 g of carbohydrate per hour ingested in the form of sport drinks or gels. Fluid intake should be monitored as well, because dehydration may decrease both mental and physical performance. Hourly fluid intake should approximate 250 to 500 ml and should be provided by sport drinks (5-8% carbohydrate concentration) or water, if gels are used for carbohydrate sources.

Recovery foods and fluids should be ingested immediately after racing, because glycogen stores are likely to be low and racing may continue the next day.

Speed Skating

After World War I, speed skating developed into the most important winter sport on the European continent and, thus, became part of the first Winter Olympic Games held in 1924. However, women's events were not introduced until 1960, even though the first speed skating World Championships for females were held in 1936! After World War II, speed skating gradually had to give way to skiing as the number one sport in Scandinavian and alpine countries. The invention of indoor speed skating assisted in rejuvenating the sport to some extent (Bijlsma and van Ingen Schenau 1999).

Important to the competition schedule for international speed skating was the introduction of the World Cup series in 1985-1986 and the World Championships a few years later. Although speed skating competitions were first based on multiple events and an "all-round" champion, today there is also a winner for each event (Bijlsma and van Ingen Schenau 1999).

Competition

Speed skating is generally divided into short- and long-track speed skating as well as marathon skating. This chapter focuses on long-track speed skating, mainly because more data have been collected on long-track speed skating than any of the other events. Long-track events are skated on a 400 m racetrack in the counterclockwise direction. Skaters compete in pairs, with the winner achieving the fastest time skated of all skaters. Skaters prefer to skate in the fastest pair possible, because it increases their chance for achieving faster times. Skaters compete in separate lanes divided by markers. The inside lane is shorter than the outside lane. To skate the same distances, skaters must change lanes during each lap at the crossover point in the backstretch, with the skater crossing the outer lane to the inner lane having the right of way. Any collision or obstruction of an opponent during the crossover or during crossing lanes in the curves can result in disqualification (ISU 2003).

Sprint events are the same for men and women and are divided into 100 m, 500 m, and 1,000 m. The 100 m sprint is the newest event, having debuted as a demonstration event in 2003. The 100 m sprint is now adopted as a World Cup event. The longer events, also called all-round events, include the 1,500 m for both men and women, 3,000 m for women, 5,000 m for both men and women, and 10,000 m for men. Combined events for a sprint champion include 100 m, 500 m, and 1,000 m, whereas all-round champions are determined based on their performances in 500 m, 1,500 m, 3,000 m and 5,000 m for women and 500 m, 1,500 m, 5,000 m, and 10,000 m for men. Recently, new events have been introduced. In the 2004 season, the team pursuit was a new demonstration event that was added to the World Cup program in 2005. All events are skated once only, with the exception of the 500 m race, which is skated twice because there is no lane change during this short race. For each distance, except the 100 m, the skaters compete in two separate divisions, with the currently best ranked skaters competing in division A and the remaining skaters competing in division B. In the case of 500 m, 1,000 m, and events of all-around competitions that do not have World Cup status (500 m and 1,000 m for women and 500 m and 3,000 m for men), all skaters compete against each other, regardless of division A or B. For all other events, separate winners exist for the two divisions (ISU 2003). Currently held world records are shown in table 14.4.

Table 14.4   Current International Speed Skating World Records

Distance (m)	Men (min:s)	Nationality	Venue, year	Women (min:s)	Nationality	Venue, year
500	0:34.30	Japan	SLC, 05	0:37.22	Canada	Calgary, 01
2 × 500	0:68.96	Japan	SLC, 01	0:74.72	Canada	SLC, 01
1,000	1:07.03	USA	SLC, 05	1:13.11	Canada	Calgary, 06
1,500	1:42.68	USA	Calgary, 06	1:51.79	Canada	SLC, 05
3,000	3:37.28	Norway	Calgary, 05	3:53.34	Canada	Calgary, 06
5,000	6:06.78	Netherlands	SLC, 05	6:46.91	Germany	SLC, 02
10,000	12:51.6	Netherlands	Calgary, 06			
Team Pursuit (8 laps for men; 6 laps for women)	3:39:69	Canada	Calgary, 05	2:56:04	Germany	Calgary

SLC = Salt Lake City (1,425 m).

Although speed skating consists of single events, athletes rarely specialize in only one event. Technical skill contributes substantially to success of all distances, decreasing the likelihood of specialization, as seen in other winter sports. In fact, it is not uncommon for the leading skaters in the 1,500 m to also be in the top 10 in shorter and longer distances. Most competitions include more than one event per day, and all-round World Cup events, consisting of four events for both women and men, are completed in a 3-day period, with two events held on 1 day at least once over the 3-day period. In preparation for racing, skaters go through a lengthy ritual of cycling, jogging, and fartlek-type activities before warming up on ice. With races starting around 10 a.m., skaters typically begin their warm-up at 8 a.m. Each event is followed by extensive cool-down procedures on ice followed by cycling, running, and flexibility exercises. Overall, the energy demands of racing are probably lower than those for training, although this is probably different when one is racing in multiple events per day. The World Cup competition season generally begins in late October and early November and concludes in March. World Championships are organized every year for sprint, all-round, and single distances, with the Olympics held every 4 years (see table 14.1. for events).

Training

After a period of recovery in the spring, athletes begin with their general training in May, focusing on endurance and aerobic power, muscular endurance, maximal strength, and explosiveness. Road cycling is probably the most common activity used to build endurance in speed skaters. Longer 100-mile rides and week-long cycling camps focus on building an aerobic base, whereas interval training is used later to increase anaerobic power and capacity. Strength training programs focus on muscular endurance and maximal strength of the hip and knee extensors and stability of the core early during the preparation phase, with transfer to more power-specific models, integrating the velocity of movement and low trunk position specific to speed skating later during the preparation phase. Jumping exercises from the low position, often using sandbags or weight vests and combining strength exercises with forms of plyometrics, are common. Because of the need for a low trunk position to effectively perform the push-off in speed skating, training incorporates many activities to build tolerance for this position. Performing single-leg squats and low walks, using the slide board and jump board, or using turn cables and rubber bands to work on technical aspects of skating the turns are all examples of "dry skating" or skating imitation exercises. In-line skating is also frequently used as a specific training mode, even though not all aspects of in-line skating are optimally transferred to speed skating (de Boer et al. 1987; Nobes et al. 2003). However, a remarkable number of in-line skaters have successfully made the transition to long-track speed skating, and in-line training also appears more specific than cycling as a form of endurance training (Foster et al. 2000).

Specific on-ice training in speed skaters starts as early as July. Training on ice begins with a focus on technique followed by gradual incorporation of more intense sessions as the summer progresses. Training programs incorporate camps in a variety of geographical locations that offer indoor ice-skating rinks, thereby exposing skaters to different environments that influence air density and ice friction.

At the elite level, most training days include two workouts, with one full recovery day per week. The volume of training increases steadily from around 10 hr/week in May to 35 hr/week by August. In early October, training intensity is maintained by the incorporation of time trials and race simulations before the competition phase begins; however, the volume of training decreases substantially. Typically, a 2- to 3-week cycle is used as periodized training plan, with the last week in the cycle used as the recovery week. The most intense phase of training usually begins in late August and lasts through early October and includes more high-intensity training sessions, while maintaining much of the volume. This is also the phase in which athletes more frequently assume a state of overreaching and possibly overtraining.

Energy demands for training in speed skating are high and probably greater than during the competitive season. A recent study in male junior speed skaters (age range 17-20 years; weight 70.4-92.3 kg) assessed endurance training and on-ice technique training early during the preparation phase using the doubly-labeled water technique. Daily energy expenditure ranged from 12.8 to 25.0 MJ/day (169-330 kJ · kg^{-1} · day^{-1}; 40-79 kcal · kg^{-1} · day^{-1}), with an average of 16.8 ± 3.8 MJ/day (221 ± 50 kJ · kg^{-1} · day^{-1}; 53 ± 12 kcal · kg^{-1} · day^{-1}) for this type of training (Ekelund et al. 2002). It is expected that energy expenditure is higher during the most intense training phase. Currently, no data are available on adult speed skaters.

Physique and Physiology

In general, speed skaters are described as short and muscular, with most of the lean tissue mass located in the hip and knee extensors. In addition, speed skaters appear to have shorter legs compared with height with a small upper-to-lower-thigh ratio (Sovak and Hawes 1987), which may be an advantage for the push-off. Although not completely comparable to previous data because of different assessment methods, recent data on Olympic contenders show leaner physiques for both female (age range 19-28 years) and male (age range 21-31 years) skaters, with similar heights and weights, ranging from 162.5 to 175.2 cm and 57.3 to 75 kg for women and 162.5 to 190.5 cm and 64.5 to 95.5 kg for men compared with earlier reports (Sovak and Hawes 1987). The large range is because both sprint and all-round athletes are included. Sprinters are typically heavier with greater lean tissue mass than their all-round counterparts. Body fat percentages assessed by dual energy X-ray absorptiometry (DEXA) from the 2002 U.S. Olympians ranged from 7.1% to 10.5% in males and 12.8% to

16.3% in females (Meyer et al. 2003), which are lower than previously reported data (Snyder and Foster 1994; Sovak and Hawes 1987; van Ingen Schenau and de Koning 1999). Lean tissue mass of speed skaters is remarkable. Comparative studies have shown that both female and male speed skaters have greater thigh diameter and mass than 400 m sprinters (Sovak and Hawes 1987).

Nutritional Issues and Challenges

The requirements of training and competition in speed skating result in a number of common nutrition issues and challenges.

Energy Requirements During Intense Training

To recover from intense training, adequate energy intake is probably the most important factor to consider. In the study by Ekelund and colleagues (2002), exercise-associated energy expenditure ranged from 3.4 to 13 MJ (812-3107 kcal) for high-volume endurance training in early summer and from 4.0 to 12.0 MJ (956-2868 kcal) for on-ice technique training in male speed skaters, with an average for both training conditions of 6.9 MJ (1649 kcal). Especially during intense or high-volume training, energy expenditure is high.

Carbohydrate Intake During Intense Training

Training for speed skating requires a high carbohydrate intake, especially under intense on-ice training conditions in September and October. Data on continuous and intermittent skating have shown that glycogen depletion is high (Green 1978; Green et al. 1978). The low trunk position in speed skating greatly affects blood flow to working muscles (Foster and de Koning 1999), probably further increasing anaerobic energy production and glycogen utilization. Careful attention should be given to the training load within the monthly as well as weekly training cycle. Carbohydrate intake should be adjusted to the intensity and volume of training, with higher intakes ($8\text{-}12\ g \cdot kg^{-1} \cdot day^{-1}$) recommended during high-volume days or weeks using road cycling (summer) and high-intensity and high-volume periods using both on-ice and dry-land training (September and October) and lower intakes ($6\text{-}8\ g \cdot kg^{-1} \cdot day^{-1}$) during on-ice training focusing on technique, on days of recovery, and during the period before competition when training volume is reduced.

Low carbohydrate availability not only affects glycogen stores and recovery but is also associated with a greater stress response and higher immune perturbation (Nieman et al. 2001). Considering the high intensity and volume of training, the frequent cases of upper respiratory illness and mononucleosis (unpublished observation), and the prevalence of a high ratio between rating of perceived

exertion and lactate level when strain is highest (Foster and de Koning 1999), the emphasis should be on adequate carbohydrate intake during this training period. It is also common that this type of training coincides with appetite suppression, which is further exacerbated by the short time available to eat between training sessions. Our observations from a training camp in September 2001 showed that one of the male sprint athletes (age 23 years, weight 93.4 kg), rather than refueling with lunch, skipped lunch and chose to sleep before the second workout held in the afternoon. Average daily energy intake in this athlete was 11.9 MJ (2,844 kcal), with an average carbohydrate intake of $5\ g \cdot kg^{-1} \cdot day^{-1}$ for the training camp. After a tapering week, this athlete showed decreased performance measures at our laboratory's testing session. His lactate response was also markedly reduced (unpublished observation).

In athletes who restrict energy intake or who are too fatigued to prepare and eat a meal, intakes of nutrients other than carbohydrate may also be low (i.e., protein and micronutrients). A simple strategy to increase energy, macronutrients, and micronutrients is to integrate sport drinks, fortified sport foods, nutrient-dense foods, a multivitamin and mineral supplement, and meal replacement drinks, especially when eating becomes too difficult. During intense on-ice training, 30 g of carbohydrate per hour should be consumed, preferably in the form of a sport drink. In addition, for training sessions lasting longer than 3 hr, sport bars and gels in addition to sport drinks may be necessary. Certain sport drinks also contain small amounts of protein and could be used during prolonged training sessions in speed skaters. To ensure quick recovery, carbohydrate sport drinks may be combined with a snack rich in protein, because the addition of protein to carbohydrate has been shown to stimulate protein synthesis (Rasmussen et al. 2000). Recovery should begin early during the skater's cool-down routine, especially if a second training session is planned. In addition to other factors influencing recovery, establishing food service is important in providing adequate and timely fuel for the recovery process and reducing the risk of overtraining. Monitoring training and performance status during this phase is essential. Using training logs with subjective ratings of perceived exertion and other psychological variables, assessing blood biochemistry for endocrine and immunologic indexes, and addressing dietary adequacy are some ways to optimize this challenging training phase. See table 14.3 for guidelines for intense training.

Energy and Carbohydrate Intake During Competition

It is expected that energy requirement in speed skaters is substantially lower during competition compared with training. Thus, energy intake as well as carbohydrate intake should be reduced. High carbohydrate intake and maximized glycogen stores, although important to cover the energy supply during long and intense training sessions, may result in unnecessarily high rates of glycogen breakdown and possibly greater lactate accumulation. This may exacerbate the negative effect of blood occlusion, because the muscle is forced to deal with greater amounts of lactate that cannot be cleared when skating in the low position. Thus, carbohydrate intake, particularly for sprint events, should be lower than during training. A range of 7 to 8 $g \cdot kg^{-1} \cdot day^{-1}$ may be a safe range to support skating in two events, including warm-up and cool-down. All-round skaters, skating multiple events each day over a period of 3 days, should focus on a moderately high carbohydrate intake, although it is not expected that performance will be limited by glycogen availability per se if stores are replenished. Thus, it may be safe to recommend values between 8 and 10 $g \cdot kg^{-1} \cdot day^{-1}$ on the days before and during all-round events.

Fluid Intake

Although only little is known about hydration in speed skaters, it appears that cold exposure in both indoor (5-10 °C) and outdoor (–15-0 °C) environments can equally lead to hypohydration, as seen with other winter sport activities performed in the cold (Rintamäki et al. 1995). Although thermoregulation should not be compromised in these athletes (because of extensive warm-up and cool-down period, indoor environments free of wind and other weather extremes), hypohydration may lead to dehydration in certain individuals and affect performance. In addition to the cold, the low trunk position as well as the inconvenience to interrupt training to use restroom facilities may further keep athletes from drinking when training on ice. Fluid intake during training on the ice may need to range from 250 to 500 ml/hr, although identifying individual sweat rates should be encouraged for optimal fluid replacement. Carbohydrate- and electrolyte-containing sport drinks (5-8%) should be used during intense on-ice training and competition in which two events are scheduled. Compared with water, sport drinks help maintain glucose availability, enhance the palatability of fluids, and assist in fluid retention when one is training and competing in the cold. Sport drinks should also be used for intense dry-land training periods, especially when training occurs twice a day. For this type of training including cycling, standard recommendations for fluid and carbohydrate replacement during exercise presented in earlier chapters of this book should apply. See table 14.3 for guidelines for intense on-ice training.

Iron Status

Throughout the years, the prevalence of iron depletion and deficiency has decreased in speed skaters (Clement et al. 1987; Meyer 2003). The most recent data show that only 11% of female speed skaters had depleted iron stores (serum ferritin <20 ng/ml) in a sample of athletes tested early during the preparation phase before the 2002 Winter Olympic Games (Meyer 2003) (see table 14.a). Because live-high and train-low strategies have been proven effective for sea-level performance of activities lasting between 8 and 20 min (Levine and Stray-Gundersen 2001), speed skating teams have begun to integrate these principles into the daily training plan. Iron supplementation is also commonly used to maximize iron status in combination with live-high and train-low strategies so we may expect to see an improvement of iron status in these athletes in the future. In fact, it is now not uncommon to see that speed skaters exceed hemoglobin limits enforced by the International Skating Union (ISU) and the World Anti-Doping Agency (WADA) (see the second practical issue). Thus, two important areas should be addressed in the sport of speed skating: monitoring female athletes to prevent iron depletion and deficiency and ensuring that no athletes exceed enforced hemoglobin limits. Although an earlier study showed that iron stores of male speed skaters have the potential to be depleted throughout the preparation phase (Roberts and Smith 1990), our recent data do not confirm this (unpublished data).

Nutrition Priorities

The following are major areas of responsibility for a sports dietitian working with winter sport athletes:

- Minimize nutritional risk in individual athletes
- Plan and conduct assessments for anthropometry, disordered eating, the female athlete triad, iron and possibly zinc status, and biochemical indexes for overtraining and altered immune status
- Provide individualized dietary plans specific for dry-land, on-snow, and on-ice training
- Educate athletes and coaches about the importance of nutrition in winter sports, highlighting energy balance, carbohydrate availability, and fluid balance
- Ensure safe supplementation practices, particularly with respect to iron
- Teach planning and food preparation skills
- Organize food service abroad and ensure nutritional adequacy and dietary supplement availability on the road

PRACTICAL ISSUE

Body Composition Challenges in Ski Jumping and Nordic Combined

Body composition requirements differ greatly with each winter sport. The winter sports that require low body mass are Nordic Combined and ski jumping. Nordic Combined athletes are at least 5 kg and ski jumpers 10 kg below the body mass that might be considered their ideal level if they were not Nordic skiers. Therefore, coaches and athletes with the assistance of a sports dietitian or physiologist need to determine the ideal competition and training weight for each competitor.

Ski jumpers are required to keep their body mass low throughout the competitive season and often the year. For these athletes, the length of time at which their competition weight can be maintained before energy levels, nutritional and immune status, and psychological health are affected needs to be individually determined. Regular body composition testing, review of training logs, and experimentation at different weights are required. Ski jumpers generally have a training weight that is 2 kg above their competition weight to help maintain health and performance throughout the year. There are, however, concerns regarding the possible compounding effects of hard training and negative energy balance on growth and development of these young athletes. Unpublished observations have shown that growth and maturation of ski jumpers may be delayed. There is no advantage for an athlete in not reaching peak height, because stature influences the length of the skis that can be used (limitations for ski length are set at a maximum 146% of an athlete's height). Ski length increases the equipment-induced gliding surface. Thus, young ski jumpers need to adopt healthy dietary practices to adequately meet nutritional requirements for growth, maturation, and sport performance. For the athletes who compete internationally at a young age, dietary assistance is strongly advised to safely achieve a healthy training and competition weight.

Difficulty also occurs in determining the ideal body composition for the Nordic combined athlete. Conflict often arises between the ski jumping and cross-country ski coach, because body composition ideals may vary, with a leaner and lighter physique requested by the ski jumping coach and more muscular and powerful body envisioned by the cross-country ski coach. Sports dietitians and physiologists can assist in identifying each athlete's ideal body composition that supports both optimal health and performance in both sports. Ski jumpers and Nordic Combined athletes often try to lose 1 to 2 kg in the few days before major competitions. The effects of rapid weight reduction on muscular strength characteristics are unclear (Viitasalo et al. 1987). A few times per year, certain ski jumpers and Nordic Combined athletes carry out a dietary manipulation diet that has not been shown to impair maximal strength and rate of force production in the athletes (unpublished observation). The aim of the diet is to reduce competitive weight without affecting hydration status, fat, and lean tissue mass. The diet typically used is a calorie-controlled, low-residue, low-sodium diet and, for certain individuals, may also be gluten-free.

The foods the athletes would eliminate from the diet include these:

- Foods high in sodium (salt): processed foods, soy sauce, certain cheeses, and salt added to cooking
- Gluten products: wheat, rye, and oats
- High-fiber foods: beans, nuts, whole grains, vegetables from the cabbage family, and fruit with skin

The foods the athletes would select include these:

- Meats and alternatives: skinless chicken, lean beef, lamb, and pork, fish, tofu, eggs
- Cereals and grains: rice, rice pasta, corn pasta, buckwheat, gluten-free bread
- Fruits and vegetables: watermelon, melons, tinned fruits in natural juices, juices without pulp, lettuce, tomatoes, mushrooms, zucchini, skinless potatoes
- Dairy products and alternatives: low-fat milks, yogurts, and cheeses
- Fats and oils: minimize to aid weight control

PRACTICAL ISSUE

Iron Deficiency and Hematological Manipulation in Winter Sport Athletes

Iron deficiency is a nutritional problem commonly reported in athletes undergoing heavy training (Magnusson et al. 1984; Spodaryk 1993) and has been observed in both male and female winter sport athletes (Clement et al. 1987; Couzy et al. 1989; Fogelholm et al. 1992; Haymes et al. 1986; Meyer 2003; Meyer et al. 1999; Schena et al. 1995). Iron deficiency directly affects aerobic performance and recovery from multiple anaerobic sessions. It also affects active recovery sessions and an athlete's ability to adapt to altitude (Stray-Gundersen et al. 1992). Maintaining iron homeostasis has been and continues to be a major problem for certain winter sport athletes. Athletes are at risk for becoming iron deficient because of an imbalance between intake and absorption of dietary iron, exercise-induced iron loss, and increased need for erythropoiesis.

Table 14.a provides a summary of studies of iron status in winter sport athletes. In the past, iron depletion and deficiency were reported to occur in 30% to 60% of the female winter sport population (Clement et al. 1987; Couzy et al. 1989; Meyer et al. 1999). More current evidence from 135 male and female winter sport athletes during the preparation for the 2002 Winter Olympics shows a decreased prevalence of 20% to 25% in females participating in alpine and Nordic skiing including biathlon, freestyle aerials and moguls, snowboarding, sliding sports (bobsled, skeleton, luge), and speed skating (Meyer 2003). Only one male athlete had low iron stores.

Other recent evidence documents changes in hemoglobin values in cross-country skiers (Videman et al. 2000). A retrospective analysis of the past 12 years showed that in 1987, individual hemoglobin values were just below the population reference value. In 1996, however, the values peaked for both men and women. The fact that these values may not be obtained from simply living or training at altitude appears disturbing (Berglund 1992). In 1997, as a consequence of this dangerous rising trend in hemoglobin levels and to limit further increases in hemoglobin and hematocrit, the FIS issued a new rule to exclude athletes from competition if hemoglobin values exceeded 18.5 g/100 ml and 16.5 g/100 ml for men and women, respectively. After the rule was introduced in 1997, individual maximal values markedly decreased for men, with mean values remaining close to the highest acceptable value (18.5 g/100 ml). For women, mean values dropped slightly after 1997 but individual maximal values increased close to the highest acceptable value (16.5 g/100 ml) (Videman et al. 2000).

Legitimate and frequently used ways of increasing circulating hemoglobin and hematocrit values in winter sport athletes, although artificial, include the use of altitude houses, live-high and train-low strategies, and supplemental iron. Erythropoiesis can be stimulated by living at moderate altitude (2,300-3,000 m) for a 4-week period (Berglund 1992), with increases seen in red cell mass volume, hemoglobin, and oxygen-carrying capacity of the blood as well as aerobic power after return to sea level (Chatard et al. 1999). Strategies of living high (>2,500 m) and training low (<1,500 m) have been shown to improve sea-level performance in events lasting 8 to 20 min (Levine and Stray-Gundersen 2001) and are used by cross-country skiers, Nordic Combined athletes, and speed skaters. Altitude houses, developed in the 1990s with increased concentration of nitrogen and lowered concentration of oxygen, are frequently used by athletes without access to mountainous terrain who like to benefit from such a strategy. Although winter sport athletes use some of these strategies to improve hematological parameters, the training performed on glacier snow provides an additional exposure to a unique environment that may further stimulate EPO if iron stores are adequate. In contrast, illegal ways to increase circulating hemoglobin levels include red blood cell reinfusion and infusion of recombinant EPO. These methods not only impose great concerns of sportsmanship, but may also lead to adverse health effects. If the use of such strategies is detected, an athlete or team may be banned from international competition, in addition to receiving penalties and a shattered reputation within the international community. This was recently encountered at the World Nordic Ski Championships in Lahti, Finland, where the Finnish national cross-country ski team was caught in a drug scandal, which for the interim halted Finnish skiing. Clearly, those working with winter sport athletes must monitor iron status and ensure safe and legal practices to increase and limit hemoglobin values.

There is a trend for winter sport athletes to abuse iron supplementation. Athletes and support staff need to be cautious with large doses of supplemental iron, because excess iron stores (high serum ferritin) are a risk factor for heart disease, stroke, cirrhosis of the liver, and diabetes. In addition, intramuscular injections of iron can also be dangerous because of the risk of potentially fatal anaphylactic shock (see chapter 5). Iron supplementation should also be stopped if it does not affect iron status.

Those working with winter sport athletes should remain informed about the current limits for hemoglobin enforced by sporting organizations such as the FIS, the ISU, and particularly WADA. The IOC and other international federations such as the ISU have adopted the world antidoping code designed by WADA. Hemoglobin cutoff values as well as other hematological procedures to test for artificial means used to increase red blood cell mass are expected to change, and thus, staying informed is key for those working as part of the medical team.

appendix

Table 2.a   Results of Energy Balance Studies in Athletic Groups Using Doubly-Labeled Water

Publication	Study population	Methods	ESTIMATED ENERGY INTAKE IN MJ[a]		ESTIMATED ENERGY EXPENDITURE IN MJ[a]		BALANCE: ENERGY INTAKE AND EXPENDITURE (%)	
			Mean (kcal[a])	Range	Mean (kcal[a])	Range	Mean	Range
Westerterp and Saris 1991	Elite professional cyclists in Tour de France (4 M)	3 periods of doubly labeled water vs. food diary over 22-day race • first 7 days • second 8 days • third 7 days	24.5 (5,835) 26.3 (6,260) 23.2 (5,525)	22.3-26.1 25.2-27.1 21.5-24.5	29.4 (7,000) 36.0 (8,570) 35.7 (8,500)	28.4-30.5 34.2-38.4 33.4-38.0	87 79 65	78-95 89-67 61-71
Schulz et al. 1992	U.S. national- and international-level distance runners (9 F)	6 days doubly labeled water vs. 6-day food diary	9.2 (2,190)	7.7-13.4	11.86 (2,825)	9.87-13.92	78	67-110
Edwards et al. 1993	Highly trained U.S. cross-country runners (9 F)	7 days doubly labeled water vs. 7-day food diary	8.53 (2,030)	6.23-10.03	12.52 (2,980)	10.46-5.63	68	42-96
Hill and Davies 2001	Elite Australian ultra-marathon runner (1 M)	14 days doubly labeled water (during 9-month run around Australia)	26.46 (6,300)					
Fudge et al. 2006	Kenyan national- and international-level distance runners (9 M)	7 days doubly labeled water vs. 7-day food diary	13.2 (3,145)		14.6 (3,475)		90	
Sjödin et al. 1994	International-level Swedish cross-country skiers (4 M and 4 F)	6 or 7 days doubly labeled water vs. 4- or 5-day weighed food diary • Male skiers • Female skiers	30.2 (7,190) 18.2 (4,335)	25.7-36.0 15.7-0.4	30.2 (7,190) 18.3 (4,355)	25.4-34.9 15.1-20.2	100 99	82-119 95-103
Branth et al. 1996	Elite off-shore sailors during Round the World Race (11 M)	13 days doubly labeled water (n = 6) vs. 13-day food inventory averaged for 11 M	17.1 (4,070)		19.3 (4,595)		89	
Jones and Leitch 1993	Canadian collegiate swimmers (5 M and 3 F)	10 days doubly labeled water vs. 10-day food diary kept by trained observers of special test diet fed to estimated energy requirements	14.6 (3,475)		14.51 (3,450)		101	65-110

Trappe et al. 1997	International-level U.S. swimmers (5 F)	5 days doubly labeled water vs. 2-day food diary	13.1 (3,120)	10.6-15.9	23.4 (5,570)	16.7-26.7	56	52-63
Ebine et al. 2000	National-level Japanese junior and senior synchronized swimmers (9 F)	6 days doubly labeled water vs. 7-day food diary	8.9 (2,120)	7.2-12.0	11.5 (2,740)	8.6-16.0	77	52-120
Ebine et al. 2002	Professional Japanese soccer players (7 M)	7 days doubly labeled water vs 7-day food diary	13.0 (3,095)	9.2-16.3	14.8 (3,525)	12.1-17.8	88	
Hill and Davies 2002	National-level Australian lightweight rowers (7 F)	14 days doubly labeled water vs. 4-day food diary	9.27 (2,205)		16.56 (3,945)		56	

M = males; F = females.

[a]MJ can be converted to kcal by dividing by 0.0042.

Table 4.a   Reported Dietary Intakes of Male Cyclists: Training (Mean Daily Intake ± SD)

Publication	Cycling population	Survey method	Age (years)	BM (kg)	ENERGY MJ	ENERGY KJ/kg	CHO g	CHO g/kg	CHO %E	PROTEIN g	PROTEIN g/kg	PROTEIN %E	FAT g	FAT %E
Berry et al. 1949	Luxemburg cyclists at 1948 Olympic Games (n = 2)	4-day duplicate meal collection, chemical assay	18 / 22	78 / 67	19.86 / 14.69	255 / 219	511 / 411	6.6 / 6.1	44 / 47	172 / 137	2.2 / 2.0	14 / 16	223 / 146	42 / 35
Klepping et al. 1984	French national and regional level (n = 32)	7-day food diary (household measures)	23	68	14.48 ± 2.58	214 ± 38	366	5.1	40 ± 6	130	1.9	15 ± 2	158	41 ± 4
Johnson et al. 1985	Irish Olympic team (n = 6)	3-day weighed food diary collected on 2 occasions, 1 year apart	21	71	16.3 ± 0.4 / 16.2 ± 0.4	229 / 226	523 / 483	7.3 / 6.8	54 ± 3 / 50 ± 3	136 / 142	1.9 / 2.0	14 ± 1 / 15 ± 1	143 / 155	33 ± 2 / 36 ± 2
Van Erp-Baart et al. 1989a	Dutch amateur international level (n = 14)	3 × 4-7 day food diary (household measures)	20	72	18.29	253	~663	~9.2	~58	~115	~1.6	~11	~148	~30
Grandjean 1989	U.S. national and collegiate level (n = 18)	3 day food diary (household measures)			17.32 ± 3.67		476		46 ± 5	155		15 ± 2	184	40 ± 5
Heinemann and Zerbes 1989	German national team (n = 9)	3-day semi-weighed food diary	19-26	73	26.5	363	795	10.9	48					
Jensen et al. 1992	U.S. collegiate level (n = 14)	5-day weighed food diary	23	69	17.40 ± 2.9	251	609 ± 114	8.8	58 ± 8	147 ± 38	2.2	14 ± 2	125 ± 49	27 ± 8
Grandjean and Ruud 1994	U.S. Olympic team (n = 9)				17.93	248	471	6.5	43	160	2.2	15	196	41
Schena et al. 1995	Italian national level (n = 18)	7-day food diary (household measures)	30	69	16.26 ± 1.89	240	562 ± 48	8.2	59	94 ± 14	1.4	17	98 ± 12	24
Garcia-Roves et al. 2000	World-class professional level (n = 6)	3-day weighed food diary kept by observer	27	69	22.4 ± 1.7	327 ± 34	770 ± 44	11.3 ± 0.9	58 ± 3	176 ± 16	2.6 ± 0.3	13 ± 0.8	178 ± 31	30 ± 3
Vogt et al. 2005	World-class professional level (n = 11)	6-day weighed food diary kept by dietitian at training camp	29	71	13.5 ± 1.5	190	474 ± 44	6.7	59	150 ± 19	2.1	12	76 ± 18	21

BM = body mass; CHO, carbohydrate; E = energy.

Table 4.b Reported Dietary Intakes of Female Cyclists: Training (Mean Daily Intake ± SD)

Publication	Cycling population	Survey method	Age (years)	BM (kg)	ENERGY		CHO			PROTEIN			FAT	
					MJ	KJ/kg	g	g/kg	%E	g	g/kg	%E	g	%E
Van Erp-Baart et al. 1989a	Dutch national level (n = 21)	3 × 4- to 7-day food diary (household measures)	23	66	10.82	164	~352	~5.3	~52	~86	~1.3	~13	~96	~33
Grandjean 1989	U.S. national and collegiate levels (n = 12)	3-day food diary (household measures)			12.66 ± 3.16		386		51 ± 7	98		13 ± 2	121	36 ± 6
Grandjean and Ruud 1994	U.S. Olympic team (n = 10)				12.64	218	409	7.1	53	100	1.7	13	111	31
Martin et al. 2002	Australian national team (n = 8)	18-day food diary (household measures) • 9 days heavy training	25	59	14.11	210	536	9.1	63	158	2.7	20	65	17
		• 9 days recovery			11.98	179	448	7.6	63	130	2.2	19	59	18

BM = body mass; CHO, carbohydrate; E = energy.

Table 4.c Reported Dietary Intakes of Cyclists: Racing (Mean Daily Intake ± SD)

Publication	Cycling population	Survey method	Age (years)	BM (kg)	ENERGY MJ	ENERGY KJ/kg	CHO g	CHO g/kg	CHO %E	PROTEIN g	PROTEIN g/kg	PROTEIN %E	FAT g	FAT %E
MALE														
General racing														
Jensen et al. 1992	U.S. collegiate level (n = 14)	3-day weighed food diary	23	69	18.67 ± 2.8	270	698 ±166	10.1	61 ±7	149 ±27	2.2	13 ±2	127 ±30	26 ±7
Stage races														
Van Erp-Baart et al. 1989a	Professional cyclists in Tour de l'Avenir (n = 4)	4- to 7-day food diary (household measures)	24	74	23.29	316	~873	~11.8	~60	~207	~2.8	~14	~151	~24
Saris et al. 1989	World-class professional cyclists in Tour de France: 22 days, 4,000 km (n = 5)	22-day food diary (household measures)		69	24.3 ± 5.3	352	849	12.3	61	217 ±47	3.1	15	147 ±37	23
Garcia-Roves et al. 1998	World-class professional cyclists in Tour of Spain, 22 days, 3,600 km (n = 10)	3-day weighed food diary kept by observer	28	71	23.5	352	841 ±66	12.6 ±1.1	60	201 ±17	3.0 ± 0.3	14.5	159 ±16	25.5
Garcia-Roves et al. 2000	World-class professional cyclists in Tour de France: 22 days, 4,000 km (n = 3)	3-day food diary kept by observer	27	69	22.9 ±1.5	334 ±26	831 ±70	12.1 ±1.0	61 ± 3	197 ±19	2.9 ± 0.3	14 ±1	154 ±17	25 ±2
FEMALE														
General racing														
Martin et al. 2002	Australian national team (n = 8)	8-day food diary (household measures)	25	59	14.87	222	588	10.0	67	136	2.3	16	67	17
Stage racing														
Grandjean et al. 1992	Unspecified American cyclists in US Cyclist Federation stage race; 11 days, 497 km (n = 3)	11-day food diary (household measures)	26	60	11.0	183	343	5.7	53	106	1.8	16	96	32

BM = body mass; CHO, carbohydrate; E = energy.

Table 4.d Reported Dietary Intakes of Triathletes: Training (Mean Daily Intake ± SD)

Publication	Triathlete population	Survey method	Age (years)	BM (kg)	ENERGY		CHO			PROTEIN			Fat	
					MJ	KJ/kg	g	g/kg	%E	g	g/kg	%E	g	%E
MALES														
Khoo et al. 1987	International group of Ironman triathletes (n = 19)	3-day food diary (household measures)	44	75	15.14 ± 5.82	202	506 ± 222	6.8	57	124 ± 62	1.7	13	119 ± 66	29
Van Erp-Baart et al. 1989a	Dutch international-level triathletes (n = 33)	4- to 7-day food diary (household measures)	26	70	19.09	272	612	8.7	51	133	1.9	11	186	36
Burke et al. 1991	Australian national-level triathletes (n = 20)	7-day food diary (household measures)	27	69	17.2 ± 3.4	250 ± 50	627 ± 152	9.1	60 ± 8	134 ± 30	2.0 ± 0.5	13 ± 2	127 ± 45	27 ± 7
Brown and Herb 1990	U.S. international triathlete (n = 1)	7-day food diary (household measures)	24	74	28.8	389	1,014	13.7	59	224	3.5	13	215	28
FEMALES														
Khoo et al. 1987	International group of Ironman triathletes (n = 10)	3-day food diary (household measures)	39	57	10.34 ± 4.19	181	351 ± 180	6.2	57	80 ± 34	1.4	12	85 ± 53	30
MIXED GENDER														
Frentsos and Baer 1997	International-level triathletes (4 M, 2 F) • Precounseling	2 × 7-day food diaries (household measures)	31	69	9.69 ± 0.63	138	344 ± 156	4.9 ± 2	59 ± 5	90 ± 25	1.3	15 ± 4	57 ± 7	0.8
	• Postcounseling				16.69 ± 1.78	238	650 ± 118	9.3 ± 2	65 ± 4	166 ± 32	2.4	17 ± 6	79 ± 8	1.1

BM = body mass; CHO, carbohydrate; E = energy.

Table 4.e Relevant Studies of Supplements With Likely Benefit to Cycling and Triathlon Performance

Publication	Participants	Supplement protocol	Exercise protocol	Enhanced performance	Comments
Caffeine					
		Acute supplementation protocol			
Costill et al. 1978	Recreational cyclists (9 M + F) Crossover design	330 mg in decaf coffee at 60 min before exercise (4.4 mg/kg for M, 5.8 mg/kg for F)	Cycling at 80% $\dot{V}O_2$ max to exhaustion	Yes	Increased time to exhaustion compared with placebo trial. Evidence of increased lipolysis. Reduced RPE.
Ivy et al. 1979	Trained cyclists (9 M + F) Crossover design	Total caffeine = 500 mg 250 mg at 60 min before exercise and then 7 doses during exercise	2 hr isokinetic cycling at 80 rpm	Yes	Increase in total work compared with placebo trial. Increased mobilization and utilization of fat. RPE same despite increased work.
Graham and Spriet 1991	Well-trained runners (6 M) Crossover design 2 separate studies in same participants	9 mg/kg at 60 min prerace	Cycling at 85% $\dot{V}O_2$ max to exhaustion (repeated with running protocol at same relative aerobic intensity)	Yes	Caffeine enhanced mean time to exhaustion by ~50%, from ~39 min to ~59 min (individual response = 10-156% enhancement). One nonresponder noted in group and confirmed when same participants repeated test on running treadmill. Some urinary caffeine levels above 12 µg/ml.
Spriet et al. 1992	Recreational cyclists (8 M + F) Crossover design	9 mg/kg at 60 min before exercise	Cycling at 80% $\dot{V}O_2$ max to exhaustion	Yes	Increased time to exhaustion. Glycogen sparing by 55% in the first 15 min of exercise.
Pasman et al. 1995	Well-trained cyclists(9 M) Crossover design with various doses of caffeine	0, 5, 9, and 13 mg/kg 60 min before exercise	Cycling at 80% W_{max} to exhaustion	Yes	Time to exhaustion was 27% longer in caffeine trials. No greater performance benefits with increasing caffeine doses. Large individual variation in urinary caffeine response. Some participants reported urinary caffeine >12 µg/ml with 9 mg/kg caffeine.
Kovacs et al. 1998	Well-trained cyclists (15 M) Crossover design with various doses of caffeine	0, 2.1, 3.2, and 4.5 mg/kg doses (divided into equal doses at 75 min preexercise and at 20 and 40 min of TT)	Cycling TT of about ~1 hr	Yes at all doses	Addition of caffeine to CHO-electrolyte drinks improved 60 min TT performance. Improvement with 3.2 and 4.5 mg/kg caffeine doses equal and greater than improvement with 2.1 mg/kg. Urinary caffeine levels related to total dose, but all below 12 µg/ml.
Van Soeren and Graham 1998	Active participants (6 M) Crossover design	6 mg/kg 60 min before exercise (after 0, 2, and 4 days caffeine withdrawal)	Cycling at 80-85% $\dot{V}O_2$ max to exhaustion	Yes	Increased time to exhaustion in all caffeine trials regardless of period of withdrawal.

Study	Subjects/Design	Supplement protocol	Exercise test	Ergogenic?	Comments
Cox et al. 2002	Well-trained cyclists and triathletes (12 M) Crossover design	6 mg/kg 60 min before exercise; 6 × 1 mg every 20 min during exercise; 10 ml/kg Commercial cola drink in last 50 min (~1-1.5 mg/kg caffeine) or placebo Sport drinks consumed throughout exercise protocol at 30 ml·kg⁻¹·hr⁻¹	2 hr cycling at 70% $\dot{V}O_2$max + 7 kJ/kg TT (~25 min)	Yes at all doses	Compared with placebo, caffeine in large dose (6 mg/kg) provided 3% performance benefit in TT regardless of timing of intake. Commercial Cola drink consumed late in exercise (~1 mg/kg caffeine) produced effect of equal magnitude. Urinary caffeine levels ~4-5 µg/ml for large dose caffeine and <1 µg/ml for cola drink.
Cox et al. 2002	Well-trained cyclists and triathletes (8 M) Crossover design	Sport drink consumed for 80 min of protocol, with switch over last 70 min to 15 ml/kg of a cola flavored drink: • 6% CHO • 11% CHO • 6% CHO +13 mg/100 ml caffeine • 11% CHO +13 mg/100 ml caffeine (=Commercial cola drink)	2 hr cycling at 70% $\dot{V}O_2$max + 7 kJ/kg TT (~25 min)	Yes	Commercial cola drink late in exercise produced 3% performance benefit in TT compared with cola-flavored placebo drink. Benefits attributable to caffeine content (~2%) and increased carbohydrate intake (~1%). Intake of caffeine = ~1.5 g/kg.
Jacobsen et al. 2001	Trained cyclists (8 M) Crossover design	6 mg/kg caffeine 60 min before exercise with 2.6 g/kg CHO, or CHO alone	2 hr cycling at 70% $\dot{V}O_2$max + 7 kJ/kg TT (~30 min)	No	TT performance similar in caffeine + CHO (29.12 min) and CHO (30.12 min).
Hunter et al. 2002	Highly-trained cyclists (8 M) Crossover design	6 mg/kg caffeine 60 min before exercise + 0.33 mg/kg every 15 min vs. CHO and placebo	100 km cycling TT including 5 × 1 km and 4 × 4 km High-intensity efforts	No	No difference between trials with respect to total 100 km time or time to complete high-intensity efforts. No difference between trials in EMG characteristics, although differences within trial attributable to workload
Conway et al. 2003	Trained cyclists and triathletes (9 M) Crossover design	6 mg/kg caffeine 60 min before exercise, or 3 mg/kg before exercise and 3 mg/kg at 45 min during exercise	90 min cycling at 68% $\dot{V}O_2$max + TT (~30 min)	Perhaps	Trend to better performance in TT with caffeine trials (~24.2 and 23.4 min) vs. placebo (28.3 min), $p = .08$. Urinary caffeine concentrations lower with split dose.

(continued)

Table 4.e *(continued)*

Publication	Participants	Supplement protocol	Exercise protocol	Enhanced performance	Comments
Glycerol hyperhydration		**Acute supplementation before exercise in conjunction with fluid**			**The literature suggests that potential benefits may occur in events in the heat, where glycerol hyperhydration is used to increase total body water and provide a substantial reduction in the fluid deficit that is incurred.**
Inder et al. 1998	Highly trained triathletes (8 M) Crossover design	1 g/kg glycerol with 500 ml of water, 4 hr preexercise (compared with 500 ml water)	60 min cycling at 70% $\dot{V}O_2$max + incremental ride to exhaustion	No	Glycerol was consumed with a modest fluid load. No increase in preexercise hydration status, sweat losses, or urine production during exercise. No difference in time to exhaustion or workload reached. 3 participants experienced GI problems with glycerol.
Hitchins et al. 1999	Well-trained cyclists (8 M) Crossover design	1 g/kg glycerol with 22 ml/kg dilute sport drink, 2.5 hr preexercise (compared with sport drink overload)	1 hr cycling TT: 30 min at fixed power + 30 min TT Hot environment (32°C)	Yes	Glycerol treatment expanded body water by 600 ml and increased (5%) work achieved in TT. This was achieved largely by preventing the decrease in power seen at the start of placebo TT. No difference in power profile at end of TT. No difference in cardiovascular or thermoregulatory factors or RPE between trials despite differences in power output.
Anderson et al. 2001	Well-trained cyclists (6 M) Crossover design	1 g/kg glycerol with 20 ml/kg low-joule Kool-Aid, 2 hr before exercise (compared with low-joule Kool-Aid overload)	90 min cycling at 98% LT + 15 min TT Hot environment (35°C)	Yes	Glycerol allowed retention of additional 400 ml of fluid above hyperhydration with cordial alone. 5% improvement in work done in 15 min TT. No change in muscle metabolism. Reduced rectal temperature at 90 min with glycerol trial.
Coutts et al. 2002	Well-trained triathletes (7 M + 3 F) Crossover design Difference in conditions: Hot day (30°C) Warm day (25°C)	1.2 g/kg glycerol + 25 ml/kg sport drink, 2 hr before exercise (compared with sport drink overload)	Olympic distance triathlon (field conditions) Hot conditions 25–30°C	Yes	Decrease in triathlon performance (especially run time) between warm and hot conditions, greater in placebo group (11:40 min) than glycerol group (1:47 min). Greatest difference in times between placebo and glycerol group was found on hot day. Hyperhydration increased fluid retention of drink and reduced diuresis.
(Wingo et al 2004)	Well-trained mountain bike riders (12M) Crossover design	1 g/kg glycerol + fluid equal to 2.8% BM, 2 hr before exercise (compared with water overload and no fluid)	30 mile mountain bike course over rough terrain Hot environment (26°C at start of trial)	Perhaps	Glycerol hyperhydration reduced fluid deficit incurred over trial by increasing fluid retention. Glycerol treatment associated with reduced thirst and scores on an Environmental Symptoms questionnaire. Although performance differences were not statistically significant, glycerol trial showed improvement of 5 minutes on final of 3 loops of course.
Kavouris et al. 2006	Highly trained cyclists (8 M) Crossover design	Participants previously dehydrated by 4% BM: rehydration over 80 min with volume equivalent to 3% BM: 1 g/kg glycerol + fluid, water or no fluid	Cycling at 74%$\dot{V}O_2$max to exhaustion Hot, humid conditions (37°C, 48% rh)	Yes	Greater plasma volume expansion with partial rehydration with glycerol compared with fluid only trial. Increased time to exhaustion with glycerol trial (33 ± 4 min) compared with fluid only (27 ± 3 min, $p < .05$) and no fluid (19 ± 3 min, $p < .05$). No effect on cardiovascular, thermoregulatory, or renal hormone responses to explain the outcomes.

There is equivocal evidence that increased blood buffering may assist performance of high-intensity events of 30-60 min (e.g., time trial or sprint distance triathlon). Further field studies are needed with high-level athletes to confirm benefits.

Bicarbonate and citrate	Acute supplementation protocol				
Potteiger et al. 1996	Trained cyclists (8 M) Crossover design	500 mg/kg sodium citrate	30 km cycling TT	Yes	Reduction in TT time (57:36 vs. 59:22 min). Sodium citrate raised pH values from 10 km onward and improved power output in the initial 25 min.
McNaughton, Dalton, and Palmer 1999	Well-trained cyclists (10 M) Crossover design	300 mg/kg sodium bicarbonate 90 min before exercise	60 min cycling TT	Yes	14% more work completed with bicarbonate.
Schabort et al. 2000	Trained cyclists (8 M) Crossover design	200 mg/kg, 400 mg/kg, and 600 mg/kg sodium citrate 90 min before exercise	40 km cycling TT including 500 m, 1 km, and 2 km sprints	No	Increasing citrate dose increased blood pH but no effect on sprint performances or overall 40 km TT performance (58:46, 60:24, 61:47, and 60:02 min for citrate (200, 400, and 600, mg/kg doses) and placebo.
Stephens et al. 2002	Trained cyclists (8 M) Crossover design	300 mg/kg sodium bicarbonate 2 hr before exercise	30 min cycling at 77% $\dot{V}O_2$max + TT (~30 min)	No	Increase in blood lactate but no difference in muscle glycogen utilization or lactate.

There is new evidence that repeated use of bicarbonate loading before interval training sessions may enhance training adaptations and improve performance of sustained high-intensity exercise, at least in moderately trained individuals. It may also assist the athlete to train harder. Further research is needed to confirm these findings, especially for highly trained athletes.

Chronic supplementation protocol for training					
Bicarbonate and citrate					
Edge at al. 2006	Moderately trained (16 F) Experimental-placebo design	8 wks at 400 mg/kg sodium bicarbonate in a split dose 90 min and 30 min before interval training. Periodized interval training undertaken 3 d/wk: 2 min intervals with 1 min recovery, with 6 to 12 intervals completed at 140-170% of intensity at lactate threshold. Both groups completed the same training load	0 and 8 wks (cycle): • $\dot{V}O_2$peak • lactate threshold • time to exhaustion at 100% pre-trial $\dot{V}O_2$peak	Yes	Both groups increased their $\dot{V}O_2$peak by similar amounts as a result of the 8 wk interval training. Both groups also increased their muscle buffering capacity. This increase in muscle buffering capacity was related to pre-training capacity rather than the treatment (subjects with lower pre-training muscle buffering capacity achieved greater increases as a result of training). Although both groups showed an increase in lactate threshold and time to exhaustion at $\dot{V}O_2$peak, the improvements were greater in the bicarbonate group. The authors speculated that training intensity rather than accumulation of H+ ions is responsible for increasing muscle buffering capacity. Furthermore, inducing alkalosis during exercise may enhance muscle adaptations by reducing the damage to mitochondria or protein synthesis.

M = male; F= female; CHO = carbohydrate; TT = time trial; RPE = rating of perceived exertion; $\dot{V}O_2$max = maximal oxygen uptake; W_{max} = maximal sustained workload; EMG = electromyogram; LT = lactate threshold; BM = body mass; rh = relative humidity.

Table 4.f Relevant Studies of Supplements With Undetermined or Unlikely Benefit to Cycling and Triathlon

Publication	Participants	Supplement protocol	Exercise protocol	Enhanced performance	Comments
Creatine		Acute supplementation protocol for single race, or chronic protocol for training			Most studies suggest that Cr supplementation does not benefit the performance of prolonged aerobic exercise, although it may be of value to the performance of repeated high-intensity sprints within a prolonged event. Most weight-sensitive endurance athletes do not use Cr because of concern over the associated gain of ~0.6 kg BM.
Vandebuerie et al. 1998	Well-trained cyclists (12 M) Crossover design (5-week washout)	4 days at 25 g/day (loading) with or without acute Cr intake 5 g at 0, 60, and 120 min of race protocol vs. placebo (3 trials)	2 hr 30 min cycling + time to exhaustion at workload at 4 mmol/L lactate + 5 × 10 s maximal sprints with 2 min recovery	Yes	No effect of Cr on endurance time to exhaustion at end of 2.5 hr of steady-state cycling. Cr loading improved power output for the 5 × 10 s maximal sprints; however, acute Cr intake during exercise counteracted these improvements so that sprint performance was no different than placebo trial.
Engelhardt et al. 1998	Well-trained triathletes (12 M) Crossover design with order effect (placebo trial first)	5 days at 6 g/day	2 × 30 min submaximal cycling at 3 mmol/L lactate workload, with 2 bouts of up to 10 × 15 s maximal sprints with 45 min recovery in interval between submaximal bouts	No, aerobic Yes, interval	Trend to better performance of endurance bouts following Cr loading: 4 participants who were unable to complete second bout in first placebo trial were able to ride longer on Cr trial. However, hard to separate order effect. Improved performance of intervals with Cr treatment; participants were able to achieve 18% increase in number of intervals performed.
van Schuylenbergh et al. 2003	Well-trained cyclists or triathletes (14 M) Experimental–placebo design	7 days at 7 g/day Cr-pyruvate (~4 g/day Cr)	1 hr cycling TT followed by 5 × 10 s intervals with 2 min rest	No, TT No, intervals	No difference between pre- and postsupplementation trials in either Cr-pyruvate group or placebo for either TT or sprint intervals. Cr-pyruvate has been proposed as a more bioavailable form of Cr than monohydrate. However, the dose used in this study appeared to be too low to achieve the expected ergogenic effect of Cr over 7 days. Authors warned that higher doses of Cr-pyruvate (e.g., 20 g/day as in most Cr loading regimens) would be prohibitively expensive as well as highly acidic, thereby risking GI distress.
Kilduff et al. 2004	Endurance-trained cyclists (21 M) Experimental-placebo design	7 days at 20 g/day + 140 g/day carbohydrate	Cycling at 63% $\dot{V}O_2$max to exhaustion in the heat (30°C)	No overall but yes in responders to Cr loading	Cr increased intracellular water and reduced cardiovascular and thermoregulatory responses to exercise. No overall difference in time to exhaustion in Cr group from pre- to postsupplementation. However, subpopulation of Cr group determined to be "responders" with substantial uptake of Cr into muscle on the basis of lower urinary Cr excretion. In these participants, time to exhaustion increased as a result of supplementation (mean = 51.7 ± 7.4 vs. 47.3 ± 4.9 min, $p < .05$). Cr-induced hyperhydration was suggested to result in more efficient thermoregulatory response to exercise in the heat.

		Acute supplementation protocol			Few studies on trained athletes and performance changes, especially in cycling. No evidence of benefits from acute supplementation protocols
Carnitine					
Stuessi et al 2005	Well-trained participants (12 M) Crossover design	2 g 2 hr before first trial	2 × cycling at anaerobic threshold to exhaustion with 3 hr recovery	No	Increased plasma levels of carnitine are believed to have a vasodilatory effect, which was hypothesized to enhance recovery from prolonged high-intensity exercise. However, no difference in exercise times of either cycling task in carnitine or placebo trial (~21 min). No differences in substrate utilization or blood lactate levels. Therefore, carnitine not seen to have any effect on a single bout of prolonged high-intensity cycling or ability to recover over 3 hr.
Carnitine		Chronic supplementation protocol			**Studies of chronic carnitine intake generally fail to show increase in muscle carnitine levels following supplementation; therefore it is hard to imagine changes in metabolic function (e.g., enhanced fatty acid transport into mitochondria or acetyl carnitine "sink").**
Broad et al. 2005	Endurance-trained cyclists 15 M Crossover design (2-6 week washout)	28 days at 2 g/day	90 min cycling at 63% $\dot{V}O_2$max + 20 km TT (undertaken before and after supplementation periods)	No	Treatment trial produced an enhancement of TT performance at end of supplementation period compared with baseline trial. No difference in TT performance pre and post placebo trial. No difference in substrate utilization resulting from carnitine supplementation. Question over adequacy of washout period because plasma carnitine levels were still elevated in some participants undertaking carnitine supplementation in second trial.
Bovine colostrum		Chronic supplementation protocol			**Potential value presently undetermined since overall literature is unclear. No mechanisms identified to explain any potential benefits. Expense of supplement in moderate to large doses ($US40 per week) warrants additional supportive research before it can be recommended. The emergence of evidence that low dose colostrum might provide benefits to some athletes is of greater interest.**
Coombes et al. 2002	Trained cyclists (28 M) High dose colostrum = 10; low dose colostrum = 9; placebo = 9 Experimental–placebo design	8 weeks at 60 g/day colostrum or 20 g/day colostrum or placebo (40 g/day whey protein) 1.5 hr/day cycling	Tests at baseline and 8 weeks on separate days: • 2 × $\dot{V}O_2$max cycling tests separated by 20 min • 2 hr cycling at 65% $\dot{V}O_2$max + ~12 min TT	No Yes	No difference between groups or between weeks for performance of either $\dot{V}O_2$max test. Greater improvement in TT following 2 hr submaximal ride at week 8 in both colostrum groups (improvements = 4%, 19%, 16%, $p < .05$ for placebo, low-dose colostrum, and high-dose colostrum, respectively).

(continued)

Table 4.f *(continued)*

Publication	Participants	Supplement protocol	Exercise protocol	Enhanced performance	Comments
(Shing et al. 2006)	Highly-trained cyclists (29 M) Colostrum = 14; placebo = 15 Experimental–placebo design	8 weeks at 10 g/day colostrum or placebo (10 g/day whey protein) 5 weeks normal training + 5 d HIT + return to normal training	Tests at baseline, then at 5 weeks (normal training), 7 weeks (post HIT) and 8 weeks (return to normal training): • $\dot{V}O_2$max cycling test • Time to fatigue at 110% ventilatory threshold • 40 km TT	Normal training – no Immediately after HIT - yes	The results of the study were interpreted using inferences about the magnitude of change rather than statistical significance. The effect of colostrum on 40 km TT training after 5 week of normal training was unclear. After 5 d of HIT which induced fatigue, there was a likely benefit (~2% enhancement) to TT performance with colostrum treatment compared with placebo. However, this difference disappeared when normal training was resumed. Differences between groups in time to fatigue in short-term high-intensity protocol were unclear throughout the study.
β-Hydroxy β-methylbutyrate		**Chronic supplementation protocol**			**Potential value presently undetermined. HMB is usually studied in resistance athletes. Further study is needed over longer time periods with endurance athletes to test effect on muscle damage and recovery.**
Vukovich and Dreifort 2001	Trained cyclists (8 M) Crossover design (2-week washout)	2 weeks at 3 g/day HMB or leucine or placebo Cycling training	Tests pre and post each 2-week supplementation: cycling $\dot{V}O_2$peak	Yes	Significant increase in $\dot{V}O_2$peak following HMB supplementation but not other supplementation periods.
Zone (40:40:30) bars during ultra-endurance racing		**Acute supplementation protocol**			**No evidence that Zone bars used as race fuel are associated with enhanced performance, and there is evidence that carbohydrate replacement during exercise is of greater benefit.**
Rauch et al. 1999	Highly trained ultra-endurance cyclists (6 M) Crossover design	Hourly feeding schedule: 1.5 Zone bars + 700 ml of water or 1 g/kg BM CHO with 700 ml of water	5.5 hr cycling at 55% $\dot{V}O_2$max (~200 W) then TT (400 kJ, ~30 min)	No—in fact performance deterioration	Zone bars were associated with greater fat oxidation during prolonged exercise (~ 280 g of fat vs. 203 g). However, performance was impaired compared with energy-matched intake of carbohydrate during race. TT performance correlated with ability to sustain high rates of carbohydrate use.
Medium-chain triglyceride oils		**Acute supplementation protocol**			**Hypothesized role of MCT as an additional fuel source for ultra-endurance events doesn't appear to occur at the doses that are tolerated. Preexercise CHO meal may reduce potential for increased fat oxidation.**

Study	Participants/Design	Protocol	Performance enhanced	Results
Van Zyl et al. 1996	Trained cyclists (6 M) Crossover design	2 L of 4.3% MCT or 10% CHO or 10% CHO + 4.3% MCT Total intake of MCT = 86 g	2 hr cycling at 60% $\dot{V}O_2$max + 40 km TT (~70 min)	Yes	MCT + CHO enhanced TT performance times (65.1 min) compared with CHO (66.8 min) and MCT (72.1 min). Increase in FFA and glycogen sparing with MCT + CHO.
Jeukendrup et al. 1998	Well-trained cyclists and triathletes (9 M) Crossover design	20 ml/kg 10% CHO or 5% MCT or 10% CHO + 5% MCT or placebo Total intake of MCT = 86 g	2 hr cycling at 60% $\dot{V}O_2$max + TT (~15 min)	No	No difference between CHO, CHO + MCT, or placebo (~14 min). MCT alone impaired performance (17.3 min). MCT + CHO showed slightly higher fat oxidation than CHO alone. No glycogen sparing.
Goedecke, Elmer-English, et al. 1999	Well-trained cyclists (9 M) Crossover design	1.6 L of 10% CHO or 10% CHO + 1.7% MCT or 10% CHO + 3.4% MCT Total intake of MCT = 26 or 52 g	2 hr cycling at 63% $\dot{V}O_2$max + 40 km TT (~70 min)	No	No differences in TT performance. 2 participants experienced GI distress with higher MCT intake. Higher FFA with MCT but no change in CHO oxidation.
Angus et al. 2000	Well-trained cyclists and triathletes (8 M) Crossover design	1 L/hr of 6% CHO + 4% MCT (vs. 6% CHO or placebo) Total intake of MCT = 42 g/hr or ~120 g	100 km cycling TT (~3 hr)	No	CHO enhanced performance over placebo, but addition of MCT did not provide further benefits. 4 participants experienced GI problems with MCT. No differences in fat oxidation or plasma FFA between MCT and CHO + MCT. Suppression of fat oxidation may be attributable to high exercise intensity or pretrial CHO meal causing high insulin concentrations.
Vistisen et al. 2003	Well-trained cyclists (7 M) Crossover design	2.4 g/kg CHO or 2.4 g/kg CHO + 1.5 g/kg MCT/LCFA mixture over 4 hr Total intake of MCT mixture = 93-128 g over 4 hr	3 hr cycling at 55% $\dot{V}O_2$max + 800 kJ TT (~50 min)	No	No difference in TT performance between CHO and CHO + MCT mixture (50.8 ± 3.6 vs. 50.0 ± 1.8 min, NS). Significantly lower RER (greater fat use) during first hour of ride, but not significantly different thereafter, indicating only minor differences in substrate utilization as a result of the treatment. No major GI side effects during trial, but problems experienced next day with CHO + MCT mixture trial
Goedecke et al. 2005	Endurance-trained cyclists (8 M) Crossover design	1 hr before exercise: 75 g CHO or 32 g MCT During exercise: 600 mL/hr of 10% CHO or 10% CHO + 4.2% MCT Total intake: 148 g over 6 hr	4.5 hr cycling at 50% PPO (including 75 kJ sprint every hour) + 200 kJ TT (~15 min)	No—in fact impaired	No difference in substrate utilization (RER) during submaximal exercise. Half the participants experienced GI side effects with MCT. Hourly sprint times and TT performance compromised in MCT trial (TT mean = 12:36 ± 1:06 vs. 14:30 ± 0:58 min, $p < .05$).

Table 4.f (continued)

Publication	Participants	Supplement protocol	Exercise protocol	Enhanced performance	Comments
Coenzyme Q10		**Chronic supplementation protocol**			**No evidence that coenzyme Q10 increases antioxidant function in mitochondrial membrane or electron transport chain function. In fact, some studies show increased oxidative damage and impaired adaptation to high-intensity exercise program with CoQ10. Studies on untrained participants undertaking high-intensity training included to show potential for negative effects.**
Braun et al. 1991	Trained cyclists (10 M) Experimental–placebo design	8 weeks at 100 mg/day Training continued during period	Incremental cycling test to exhaustion pre and post supplementation period.	No	Performance increased equally in both groups after training period. Coenzyme Q10 had no effect on cycling performance or any measured parameters. Malondialdehyde concentrations in blood (marker of oxidative stress) reduced in both groups after training.
Snider et al. 1992	Highly trained triathletes (11 M) Crossover design	4 weeks at 3×100 mg/day (as part of "Coenzyme Athlete Performance System (CAPS)" supplement with vitamin E, inosine, cytochrome c) Normal training	Cycling and running 90 min on treadmill at 70% $\dot{V}O_2$max + cycling at 70% $\dot{V}O_2$max to exhaustion	No	No difference in time to exhaustion between trials. No differences in blood metabolites or RPE.
Laaksonen et al. 1995	Trained marathon runners and triathletes (11 M) Crossover design 4-week washout	6 weeks at 120 mg/day Normal training	60 min cycling at 60% $\dot{V}O_2$max + incremental cycling test to exhaustion	No—in fact, performance deterioration	No change in muscle coenzyme Q10 concentrations, despite increase in serum coenzyme Q10 with supplementation. No change in plasma malondialdehyde in either group. Negative effect on incremental cycling performance (placebo had greater endurance).
Weston et al. 1997	Trained cyclists and triathletes (18 M) Experimental–placebo design	28 days at 1 mg·kg^{-1}·day^{-1} Normal training undertaken	Incremental cycling test to exhaustion undertaken during pre and post periods	No	Coenzyme Q10 did not enhance any performance parameters.
Nielsen et al. 1999	Well-trained triathletes (7 M) Crossover design	6 weeks at 100 mg/day (+ vitamins E + C)	Incremental cycling $\dot{V}O_2$max test to exhaustion	No	No effect on maximal oxygen uptake or muscle energy metabolism (determined by NMRS).
Malm et al. 1996	Healthy participants (15 M) Experimental–placebo design	20 days at 120 mg/day Days 2-9: usual activity Days 11-15: 2/day anaerobic training Days 16-20: recovery	Anaerobic cycling tests undertaken at day 1, 11, 15, and 20	No—in fact, failure to adapt to training	Improvement in work capacity after 15 and 20 days of training with placebo group, but no improvement in coenzyme Q10 group. Increased CK levels with coenzyme Q10 group after test set on day 11 and during training block; no increase in CK with placebo group. Suggests increased cellular muscle damage with high-intensity training and coenzyme Q10.

Study	Participants/Design	Supplementation protocol	Test protocol	Performance benefit?	Results
Malm et al. 1997	Healthy participants (18 M) Experimental–placebo design	22 days at 120 mg/day Days 2-9: usual activity Days 11-14: 2/day anaerobic training Days 15-22: recovery	Anaerobic test (days 1, 11, 15, and 20) 30 s Wingate cycle + 5 min recovery + 10 × 10 s sprints Aerobic tests (pretrial and day 18 or 20) Cycling $\dot{V}O_2$max Running $\dot{V}O_2$max	No—in fact, failure to adapt to training No No	Placebo and Q10 group both improved performance of repeated sprint test after training; however, only placebo group maintained this improvement during recovery to day 20. Placebo group achieved higher average power and greater improvement in latter intervals during anaerobic training sessions. No change in running or cycling $\dot{V}O_2$max in either group over time or in oxygen use during submaximal cycling.
Branched-chain amino acids during exercise		**Acute supplementation protocol**			**No evidence that BCAA consumed during exercise have beneficial role above that of carbohydrate intake on central fatigue.**
Madsen et al. 1996	Well-trained cyclists (9 M) Crossover design	3.5 L at 5% glucose or 5% glucose + 18 g BCAA	100 km cycling TT	No	No performance differences between trials. Plasma BCAA and ammonia levels higher with BCAA trial.
Blomstrand et al. 1997	Trained cyclists (7 M) Crossover design	90 mg/kg (~6.5 g)	60 min cycling at 70% $\dot{V}O_2$max + 20 min TT Stroop CWT after ride	No Yes	No differences in work done in TT. However, RPE lower in BCAA trial during steady-state phase. Index of cognitive function (Stroop CWT) improved after exercise on BCAA trial.
Protein added to carbohydrate sports drinks during exercise		**Acute supplementation protocol**			**The support for claims that performance is enhanced by the addition of protein (~2%) to sports drinks (6-8% carbohydrate) is unclear. The original hypothesis proposed that the presence of protein would increase the insulin response to carbohydrate feedings and spare muscle glycogen utilization during exercise. However, an enhanced insulin response has not been seen, and no performance benefits have been seen in studies which use a performance (time trial) rather than endurance (time to exhaustion) protocol and in which carbohydrate intake is at rates considered to be optimal (~ 1 g/min). The addition of protein to sports drinks may change the flavor characteristics of the drink. Although the case for protein intake during exercise has not been made, there is good support for the combined intake of protein and carbohydrate during recovery after exercise.**
Ivy et al. 2003	Trained cyclists (9M) Crossover design	600 mL per hr of 8% CHO drink or 8% CHO + 2% protein or flavored placebo	3 h cycling alternating between 45% and 75% $\dot{V}O_2$max + time to exhaustion at 85% $\dot{V}O_2$max	Yes	Carbohydrate sports drink increased time to exhaustion vs placebo (19.7 ± 4.6 vs 12.7 ± 3.1 min, P< 0.05), while the CHO + protein drink enhanced this effect (26.9 ± 4.5 min, p < .05). No obvious mechanism since there were no differences in plasma glucose and insulin concentrations between CHO and CHO+protein trials. Cyclists consumed 48 g/hr or 0.67 g/kg/h carbohydrate intake in CHO trial

(continued)

Table 4.f *(continued)*

Publication	Participants	Supplement protocol	Exercise protocol	Enhanced performance	Comments
Saunders et al. 2004	Trained cyclists (15 M) Crossover design	7.2 mL/kg per hour of 7% CHO drink or 7% CHO + 2% protein	Cycling at 75% $\dot{V}O_2$max to exhaustion	Yes	Cyclists rode 29% longer ($P < 0.05$) in the CHO+Protein trial (106.3 ± 45.2 min) than the CHO beverage (82.3 ± 32.6 min). CHO intake was ~ 37g/hr or 0.53 g/kg/hr in CHO trial.
Van Essen et al. 2006	Trained cyclists (15 M) Crossover design	1000 mL per hour of 6% CHO drink or 6% CHO + 2% protein or flavored placebo	80 km time trial on cycle ergometer	No	Time to complete the 80 km was 4.4% faster with CHO (135 ± 9 min) and CHO+protein (135 ± 9 min) than with placebo CHO (141 ± 10 min, P< 0.05). However no differences between CHO and CHO+protein. CHO intake was 60 g/hr or 0.8 g/kg/hr in CHO trial. Authors suggest that no additional benefit is achieved by adding protein to CHO supplementation that is already at rate of optimal oxidation.
Burke, Arkinstall et al. in press	Trained triathletes (15 M) Crossover design	10 ml/kg per hr of 8% CHO drink or 8% CHO + 2% protein or 10% CHO drink (energy match for CHO+protein)	2.5 h cycling at 70% $\dot{V}O_2$max + time trial (7 kJ/kg)	No	No detectable differences in TT performance between trials (26.79 ± 2.36, 26.97 ± 2.40 and 26.71 ± 2.00 min for 8%CHO, 8%CHO+protein and 10%CHO, NS). Plasma glucose concentrations were higher with 10% CHO, but no differences in plasma insulin between trials. CHO intake was 57 g/hr or 0.8 g/kg/hr in 8% CHO trial.
Tyrosine during exercise		**Acute supplementation protocol**			**No evidence that tyrosine consumed during exercise has beneficial role above that of carbohydrate intake on central fatigue and performance.**
Chinevere et al. 2002	Well-trained cyclists (9 M) Crossover design	25 mg/kg tyrosine every 30 min beginning 1 hr before exercise, with or without CHO	90 min cycling at 70% $\dot{V}O_2$max + ~ 30 min TT	No	TT performance was enhanced with CHO (27.1 min) and CHO + tyrosine (26.1 min) trials compared with placebo (34.4 min) and tyrosine alone (32.6 min; $p < .05$). Therefore, tyrosine does not enhance performance despite increasing tyrosine–tryptophan ratio in blood and presumably changing amino acid uptake into brain.
Arginine aspartate		**Chronic supplementation protocol**			**Arginine aspartate has been promoted to enhance performance attributable to claimed effects of aspartate on metabolism during exercise and the claimed effects of arginine on secretion of hormones including growth hormone. The limited literature does not support the efficacy of this supplement.**
Abel et al. 2005	Endurance-trained participants (30 M) Experimental–placebo trial	28 days at high dose (5.7 g arginine + 8.7 g aspartate) or low dose (2.8 g arginine + 2.2 g arginine)	Cycling $\dot{V}O_2$max test pre and post supplementation	No	No difference between changes in $\dot{V}O_2$max and metabolic or hormonal parameters between placebo and various doses of supplement.
Inosine		**Chronic supplementation protocol**			**No evidence of increased production of ATP or performance enhancements. In fact, in one study inosine supplementation decreased endurance.**

Study	Subjects	Supplementation protocol	Exercise protocol	Ergogenic	Outcome
Snider et al. 1992	Highly-trained triathletes (11 M) Crossover design	4 weeks at 3 × 100 mg/day (+ vitamin E, coenzyme Q10, cytochrome c) Normal training	Cycling and running 90 min on treadmill at 70% $\dot{V}O_2$max + cycling at 70% $\dot{V}O_2$max to exhaustion	No	No difference in time to exhaustion between trials. No differences in blood metabolites or RPE.
Starling et al. 1996	Well-trained cyclists (10 M) Crossover design	5 days at 5,000 mg/day Normal training	Wingate bike test, 30 min self-paced cycle, supramaximal sprint to fatigue	No—in fact, performance deterioration	No difference in Wingate performance or 30 min cycle. Negative effect on time to fatigue. Increase in plasma uric acid concentration.
McNaughton, Dalton, and Tarr, 1999	Well-trained cyclists (7 M) Crossover design	5 or 10 days at 10,000 mg/day Normal training	5 × 6 s, 30 s, and 20 min TT	No	No improvements in sprint times or TT performance. Increase in plasma uric acid concentrations.
Antioxidant vitamins (C, E)		**Chronic supplementation protocol**			**No evidence of performance enhancement attributable to antioxidant supplementation. Further long-term studies are required in highly trained athletes. However, there is also possibility that chronic antioxidant supplementation causes negative effects by acting as pro-oxidant or by reducing valuable oxidative processes involved in training adaptations**
Nielsen et al. 1999	Well-trained triathletes (7 M) Crossover design	6 weeks at 270 mg/day vitamin E + 600 mg/d vitamin C (+ coenzyme Q10)	Incremental cycling test to exhaustion	No	No effect on maximal oxygen uptake or muscle energy metabolism (determined by NMRS).
CAPS		**Chronic supplementation protocol**			**No evidence of ergogenic benefits when manufacturer's recommended dose is consumed.**
Snider et al. 1992	Highly trained triathletes (11 M) Crossover design	4 weeks at 3 doses/day (each contains 100 mg of coenzyme Q10, 200 IU of vitamin E, 100 mg of inosine, 500 mg of cytochrome c) Normal training	Cycling and running 90 min on treadmill at 70% $\dot{V}O_2$max + cycling at 70% $\dot{V}O_2$max to exhaustion	No	No difference in time to exhaustion between trials. No differences in blood metabolites or RPE.

(continued)

Table 4.f (continued)

Publication	Participants	Supplement protocol	Exercise protocol	Enhanced performance	Comments
Pyruvate		**Chronic supplementation protocol**			**No evidence of ergogenic benefits when manufacturer's recommended dose of 3-6 g/day is consumed.**
Morrison et al. 2000	Well-trained cyclists (7 M) Crossover design	7 days at 7 g/day	Cycling at ~75% $\dot{V}O_2$max to exhaustion	No	No difference in time to exhaustion between groups (placebo ~91 min vs. pyruvate ~88 min).
van Schuylenbergh et al. 2003	Well-trained cyclists or triathletes (14 M) Experimental–placebo design	7 days at 7 g/day Cr-pyruvate (~3 g/day pyruvate)	1 hr self-paced cycling TT followed by 5 × 10 s intervals with 2 min rest	No for TT No for intervals	No difference between pre- and postsupplementation trials in either Cr-pyruvate group or placebo for either TT or sprint intervals. Manufacturer claims that ergogenic dose of pyruvate is 3-6 g/day.
Earnest et al. 2004	Endurance-trained cyclists (17 M) Experimental–placebo design	2 weeks at undisclosed amount pyruvate in Optygen supplement (+1 g/day cordyceps sinensis + 300 mg of *Rhodiola rosea*, 200 μg of chromium, + undisclosed amounts of phosphate, ribose, adenosine)	Incremental cycling time to exhaustion to assess peak power output, $\dot{V}O_2$peak	No	No change in cycling endurance or aerobic capacity in either group over time.
Tricarboxylic acid cycle intermediates		**Chronic supplementation protocol**			**No evidence of ergogenic benefits when manufacturer's recommended dose is provided.**
Brown et al. 2004	Endurance-trained cyclists (7 M) Crossover design	3 weeks of commercial supplement providing 40 g/day tricarboxylic acid cycle intermediates and other nutrients (amino acids, vitamins) vs. 40 g of CHO placebo	2 × cycling to exhaustion at 75% $\dot{V}O_2$max with 30 min recovery	No	No change in time to exhaustion in first cycling bout or subsequent endurance after 30 min recovery.

Microhydrin (silica-hydride)

Microhydrin is claimed to contain silica-hydride and therefore provide hydride ions to act as a reducing agent or buffer or antioxidant during exercise. Doses used in available studies exceed manufacturer's recommendation but mimic use among cyclists. Only study measuring exercise capacity failed to find evidence of alteration in metabolism or cycling performance.

Study	Subjects/design	Acute supplementation protocol		Exercise test	Results/comments
Glazier et al. 2004	Endurance-trained cyclists (7 M) Crossover design	9.6 g of Microhydrin over 48 hr (3.6 g at 24 hr pretrial and 6 g at 3 hr pretrial)	No	2 hr cycling at 70% $\dot{V}O_2$max with 5 × 2 min bursts at 85% $\dot{V}O_2$max + 7 kJ/kg TT	Infrared spectroscopy of supplement failed to find the presence of the claimed "ergogenically active" silica-hydride bonds in the product. There was no difference in blood parameters (e.g., lactate), substrate oxidation, or time performance between Microhydrin and placebo trials. Average power output in TT was ~221 W and 288 W for Microhydrin and placebo trials respectively, NS.

Oxygenated water

Oxygenated water products are claimed to increase blood oxygenation and enhance hydration levels, leading to enhanced athletic performance. Scientific proof of these claims is lacking, and the hypotheses underpinning of the proposed benefits seem physiologically unlikely.

Study	Subjects/design	Chronic supplementation protocols		Exercise test	Results/comments
Wing-Gaia et al. 2005	Recreational cyclists (9 M)	3 days at 35 ml/kg purified oxygenated water	No	Cycling TT at 600 kJ (~1 hr) under hypoxic conditions (~4,600 m)	Differences between TT performances were small (76.4 vs. 76.3 min for oxygenated water vs. control). No difference in aerobic intensity, rate of perceived exertion, or lactate concentrations during TT. No differences in urine specific gravity pre and post trial between trials.

Herbals: cordyceps sinensis

No evidence of ergogenic benefits when manufacturer's recommended dose is consumed.

Study	Subjects/design	Chronic supplementation protocol		Exercise test	Results/comments
Parcell et al. 2004	Well-trained cyclists (22 M) Experimental–placebo design	5 weeks at 3.15 g/day cordyceps sinensis (Cordy-Max Cs-4) Normal training	No No	Cycling at $\dot{V}O_2$peak TT lasting ~ 1 hr	No change in aerobic capacity ($\dot{V}O_2$peak) over time in either group. No change in time to complete cycling time trial over time or between groups.
Earnest et al. 2004	Endurance-trained cyclists (17 M) Experimental–placebo design	2 weeks at 1 g/day cordyceps sinensis (+300 mg of rhodiola rosea, 200 µg of chromium, and 800 mg mix of pyruvate, phosphate, ribose, and adenosine—individual amounts undisclosed) = Optygen	No	Incremental cycling time to exhaustion to assess peak power output, $\dot{V}O_2$peak	No change in cycling endurance or aerobic capacity in either group over time.

(continued)

Table 4.f (continued)

Publication	Participants	Supplement protocol	Exercise protocol	Enhanced performance	Comments
Herbals: rhodiola rosea		**Acute supplementation protocol**			**Preliminary evidence to show benefits to endurance in healthy volunteers following acute use, perhaps attributable to central nervous system effect. No effects seen in other tests of performance. This outcome needs to be replicated in further studies**
de Bock et al. 2004	Active participants (24 M) Crossover design	200 mg of rhodiola rosea taken 1 hr pretest	Battery of tests: • Incremental cycling to fatigue • Isokinetic knee torque • Speed of limb movement • Reaction time • Sustained attention	Yes No No No No	Compared with placebo, supplementation with rhodiola rosea product increased time to exhaustion in cycling protocol. No effect seen on muscle strength or measures of reaction time and responsiveness to stimuli.
Herbals: rhodiola rosea		**Chronic supplementation protocol**			**No effect on endurance seen with chronic use. Further studies are needed.**
de Bock et al. 2004	Active participants (23 M) Experimental–placebo design	4 weeks at 200 mg of rhodiola rosea	Battery of tests: • Incremental cycling to fatigue • Isokinetic knee torque • Speed of limb movement • Reaction time • Sustained attention	No No No No No	Neither treatment nor placebo group showed any changes in response to test battery. Previously seen benefits of acute intake of rhodiola rosea on exercise capacity not apparent after chronic supplementation
Earnest et al. 2004	Endurance-trained cyclists (17 M)	2 weeks at 300 mg of rhodiola rosea (+1 g/day cordyceps sinensis, 200 µg of chromium, and 800 mg mix of pyruvate, phosphate, ribose, and adenosine—individual amounts undisclosed) = Optygen	Incremental cycling time to exhaustion to assess peak power output, $\dot{V}O_2$peak	No	No change in cycling endurance or aerobic capacity in either group over time.

M = male; F = female; TT = time trial; RPE = rating of perceived exertion; CHO = carbohydrate; ATP = adenosine triphosphate; $\dot{V}O_2$max = maximal O_2 uptake; BM = body mass; Cr = creatine; HMB = b-hydroxy b-methylbutyrate; MCT = medium-chain triglyceride; LCFA = long chain fatty acids\bb\; FFA = free fatty acids; NS = not significant; RER = respiratory exchange rate; GI = gastrointestinal; PPO = Peak Power Output\; NMRS = nuclear magnetic resonance scanning; CK = creatine kinase; BCAA = branched-chain amino acids; CWT = Color Word Test; HIT = High intensity training.

Table 4.g   Longitudinal Studies Comparing High Carbohydrate Intakes (HCHO) and Moderate Carbohydrate Intakes (MCHO) on Training Adaptation and Performance of Athletes Undertaking Intensive Training

Publication	Athletes	Duration of study (days)	CHO intake ($g \cdot kg^{-1} \cdot day^{-1}$)	Effect on muscle glycogen	Performance protocol	Performance advantage with HCHO
Costill, Flynn, et al. 1988	Well-trained (collegiate) swimmers (12 M)	10 Participants self-selected into 2 dietary groups (8 HCHO and 4 MCHO)	8.2 vs. 5.3	Declined in MCHO Maintained in HCHO	Training: doubling of usual 1.5 hr/day training program. Performance battery: power (swim bench); 2×25-yard freestyle swim with 2-3 min recovery interval; $\dot{V}O_2$max in pool; swimming efficiency at submaximal pace	No for final performance. No difference in 25-yard swim, swim power, $\dot{V}O_2$max over trial and between groups. However, stroke efficiency reduced in MCHO. Yes for training performance. MCHO group reported "chronic fatigue" during training program.
Lamb et al. 1990	Well-trained (collegiate) swimmers (14 M)	9 Crossover design	12.1 vs. 6.5	NA	$2 \times$ daily training sessions: intervals over variety of distances + 1,500 m and 3,000 m timed for afternoon sessions during last 5 days	No. No difference in mean swimming times over range of distances between diets.
Kirwan et al. 1988	Well-trained runners (10 M)	5 Crossover design	8.0 vs. 3.9	Declined in both groups but greater reduction in MCHO	Training increased by 150% for 5 days. Economy tested on treadmill at 2 speeds on days 4 and 6. Overnight fasted	Yes. Reduction in running economy with MCHO.
Sherman et al. 1993	Trained runners (9 M + 9 M)	7 Experimental – placebo design	10 vs. 5	Declined in MCHO Maintained in HCHO	$2 \times$ time to exhaustion on a treadmill at 80% $\dot{V}O_2$max with 5 min recovery period. Trials undertaken at end of day after 1 hr training	No. No difference between groups on endurance during either run. Sum time = 613 ± 36 s and 560 ± 106 s for MCHO and HCHO respectively, NS.
Achten et al. 2004	Well-trained runners (7 M)	4 + intensified training Crossover design	8.5 vs. 5.4	Decrease in muscle glycogen utilization during training sessions at 58% and 77% $\dot{V}O_2$max during MCHO trial compared with HCHO	Preload + 8 km treadmill TT on days 1, 5, 8, 11. 16 km road TT on days 6, 7, 9, 10. Overnight fasted	Yes. Intensified training lead to deterioration of 8 km TT by 61 s in HCHO and 155 s in MCHO, and deterioration in 16 km TT in MCHO only. HCHO reduced symptoms of overreaching during intensified training compared with MCHO but did not prevent it.

(continued)

Table 4.g (continued)

Publication	Athletes	Duration of study (days)	CHO intake (g·kg⁻¹·day⁻¹)	Effect on muscle glycogen	Performance protocol	Performance advantage with HCHO
Simonsen et al. 1991	Well-trained (collegiate) rowers (12 M, 10 F)	28 Experimental–placebo	10 vs. 5	MCHO allowed maintenance of muscle glycogen stores, whereas HCHO allowed an increase in stores	3 × 2,500 m rowing ergometer TT with 8 min recovery interval undertaken on days 1, 3, 5 of each week Trials undertaken at evening workout	Yes. Power output maintained during ergometer rowing TT with MCHO, leading to overall improvement of 1.6% after 4 weeks. Improvement in power output in HCHO over same period = 10.7%.
Sherman et al. 1993	Trained cyclists (9 M + 9 M)	7 Experimental–placebo	10 vs. 5	Declined in MCHO Maintained in HCHO	2 × time to exhaustion on cycle ergometer at 80% $\dot{V}O_2$max with 5 min recovery period Trials undertaken at end of day after 1 hr training	No. No difference between groups on endurance during either bout. Sum time = 550 ± 85 s and 613 ± 45 s for MCHO and HCHO respectively, NS.
Vogt et al. 2003	Well-trained duathletes (11 M)	35 Crossover design	6.9 vs. 3.6	Maintained on both diets	$\dot{V}O_2$max cycling TT undertaken after progressive submaximal preload; outdoor 21 km run (all undertaken on separate days) Trials undertaken after meal (composition of meal varied with dietary treatment)	No. No difference in aerobic capacity, cycling TT power, or half marathon run time between diets (e.g., 21 km run = 80 min 12 s ± 86 s and 80 min 24 s ± 82 s for HCHO and MCHO).

M = male; F = female; NA = not available; TT = time trial; $\dot{V}O_2$max = maximal oxygen uptake; CHO = carbohydrate; NS = not significant.

Table 4.h Effect of Up to 28 Days Adaptation to High-Fat (HFAT) on Endurance and Ultra-Endurance Performance of Trained Participants

Publication	Athletes	Fat adaptation protocol	Performance protocol	Performance advantage with HFAT
Phinney et al. 1983	Well-trained cyclists (5 M) Crossover design with order effect (control diet first)	28 days CHO (57% CHO) then 28 days HFAT (fat = 85% E, CHO = <20 g/day)	Cycling time to fatigue at 80% $\dot{V}O_2$max Overnight-fasted + no CHO intake during exercise	No. No difference in time to fatigue between trials (151 vs. 147 min for HFAT and CHO. Group data skewed by 1 participant who increased time to fatigue by 156% on HFAT trial. Study design includes order effect.
O'Keeffe et al. 1989	Moderately trained cyclists (7 F) Crossover design	7 days HFAT (fat = 59% E, CHO =1.2 g/kg BM) CHO (CHO = 6.4 g/kg BM)	Cycling time to fatigue at 80% $\dot{V}O_2$max 3-4 hr after meal, no CHO intake during exercise	No—in fact, performance deteriorated with HFAT. Time to fatigue reduced by 47% on HFAT trial.
Lambert et al. 1994	Well-trained cyclists (5 M) Crossover design	14 days HFAT (fat = 67% E, CHO = 17% E[a]) CHO (CHO = 74% E[a])	Cycling time to fatigue at 60% $\dot{V}O_2$max (preceded by Wingate test and time to fatigue at 90% $\dot{V}O_2$max) Overnight-fasted + no CHO intake during exercise	Yes. Time to fatigue increased by 87% on HFAT trial. No significant differences in performance of preceding high intensity cycle tests.
Goedecke, Christie, et al. 1999	Well-trained cyclists (2 × 8 M) Parallel group design	15 days HFAT (fat = 69%E, CHO = 2.2 g/kg BM) CHO (CHO = 5.5 g/kg BM)	150 min cycling at 70% $\dot{V}O_2$max + ~60 min TT (time to complete 40 km) MCT intake 1.5 hr before event (~14 g); MCT (0.3 g·kg⁻¹·hr⁻¹) and CHO (0.8 g·kg⁻¹·hr⁻¹) during exercise Performance measured t = 0, 5, 10, and 15 days	No. TT performance increased over time in both groups as a result of training protocol. Significant improvements seen in both groups by Day 10, but no difference in mean improvement between groups. Important finding of study: adaptations achieved after only 5 days of high-fat diet.
Rowlands and Hopkins 2002	Well-trained cyclists (7 M) Crossover design	14 days HFAT (fat = 66% E, CHO = ~2.4 g/kg) High CHO (CHO = ~ 8.6 g/kg, 70% CHO)	5 hr cycling including 15 min TT + incremental test + 100 km TT HFAT = high-fat preevent meal HCHO = high CHO preevent meal Both: 0.8 g·kg⁻¹·hr⁻¹ CHO during ride	Yes—submaximal intensity exercise. No—higher-intensity exercise. Relative to baseline: HCHO showed small NS decreases in performance of both 15 min TT and 100 km TT. HFAT showed larger but NS decrease in performance of 15 min TT but small NS improvement in 100 km TT.

M = male; F = female; $\dot{V}O_2$max = maximal oxygen uptake; CHO = carbohydrate; TT = time-trial; BM = body mass; NS = not significant; E = energy.

[a]g/kg intakes unavailable.

Table 4.i Effect of Adaptation (5-10 days) to High-Fat, Low-Carbohydrate (CHO) Diet (Fat-adapt) Followed by CHO Restoration in Trained Participants

Publication	Participant characteristics	Fat adaptation protocol	CHO restoration	Performance protocol	Performance advantage with fat-adapt + CHO restoration
Burke et al. 2000	Well-trained cyclists and triathletes (8 M) Crossover design	5 days intensive supervised training + Fat-adapt (fat = 68% E; CHO = 18% E, 2.5 g/kg BM) or Control (CHO = 74% E, 9.6 g/kg BM CHO)	1 day rest + high CHO (CHO = 75% E, 10 g/kg BM)	120 min cycling at 70% V̇O₂max + ~30 min TT (time to complete 7 J/kg BM) Fasted + no CHO intake during exercise	Perhaps for individuals. 2 participants performed badly on control trial, probably because of hypoglycemia. Plasma glucose better maintained on Fat-adapt trial. TT not significantly different between trials: 30.73 ± 1.12 vs. 34.17 ± 2.62 min for Fat-adapt and control trial. However, mean difference in TT = 8% enhancement with Fat-adapt trial (p = .21, NS) (95% CI = −6% to 21%).
Burke et al. 2002	Well-trained M cyclists and triathletes (8 M) Crossover design	5 days intensive supervised training Fat-adapt (fat = 68% E; CHO = 18% E, 2.5 g/kg BM) or Control (CHO = 70% E, 9.3 g/kg BM CHO)	1 day rest + high CHO (CHO = 75% E, 10 g/kg BM)	120 min cycling at 70% V̇O₂max + ~30 min TT (time to complete 7 J/kg BM) CHO intake 2 hr before exercise (2 g/kg BM) and during exercise (0.8 g·kg⁻¹·hr⁻¹)	No. Plasma glucose maintained in both trials attributable to CHO intake during exercise. Difference in TT between trials was trivial: Fat-adapt = 25.53 ± 0.67 min; control = 25.45 ± 0.96 min (p = .86, NS). Mean difference in TT = 0.7% impairment with Fat-adapt trial (95% CI = −1.7% to 0.4%).
Carey et al. 2001	Highly-trained ultra-endurance cyclists and triathletes (7 M) Crossover design	6 days intensive supervised training Fat-adapt (fat = 69% E CHO = 16% E, 2.5 g/kg BM) or Control (CHO = 75% E, 11 g/kg BM)	1 day rest + high CHO (CHO = 75% E, 11 g/kg BM)	240 min cycling at 65% V̇O₂max + 60 min TT (distance in 1 hr) CHO intake before exercise (3 g/kg BM) and during exercise (1.3 g·kg⁻¹·hr⁻¹)	No or perhaps for individuals. TT performance NS between trials: 44.25 ± 0.9 vs. 42.1 ± 1.2 km for Fat-adapt and control trial. However, mean difference in TT performance = 4% enhancement with Fat-adapt (p = .11, NS) (95% CI = −3% to 11%).
Lambert et al. 2001	Trained cyclists and triathletes (5 M) Crossover design	10 days usual training + Fat-adapt (fat = 65% E, CHO = 15% E, 1.6 g/kg BM) or Control (CHO = 53% E, 5.8 g/kg BM)	3 days high CHO (CHO = 65% E, 7 g/kg BM) + 1 day rest	150 min cycling at 70% V̇O₂max+ 20 km (~30 min) TT MCT intake 1 hr before event (~14 g); MCT (0.3 g·kg⁻¹·hr⁻¹) and CHO (0.8 g·kg⁻¹·hr⁻¹) during exercise	Yes. Difference in TT performance = 4% enhancement with Fat-adapt: 29.35 ± 1.25 vs. 30.68 ± 1.55 min for Fat-adapt and control (p < .05).

Rowlands and Hopkins 2002	Well-trained cyclists (7 M) Crossover design	14 days HCHO (CHO = ~8.6 g/kg, 70% E) or 11.5 days Fat-adapt (~2.4 g/kg, 15% CHO; 66% fat)	2.5 days high CHO (6.8g/kg BM)	5 hr cycling protocol including 15 min TT + incremental test + 100 km TT HCHO = high-CHO preevent meal Both: 0.8 g·kg⁻¹·hr⁻¹ CHO during ride	Perhaps—submaximal intensity exercise. No—higher-intensity exercise. Relative to baseline testing: HCHO showed small NS decreases in performance of both 15 min TT and 100 km TT. Fat-adapt showed no change in 15 min TT but small NS enhancement of 100 km TT.
Havemann et al. 2006	Well-trained cyclists (8 M) Crossover design	6 days intensive training Fat-adapt (fat = 68% E, CHO = 17% E, 1.8 g/kg BM) or Control (CHO = 68% E, 7.5 g/kg BM)	1 day rest + High CHO (8-10 g/kg)	100 km cycling TT, including 4 × 4 km sprints 5 × 1 km sprints (10, 32, 52, 72, and 99 km) CHO consumed during ride	No, in fact, performance enhancement of 1 km sprints. Differences between 100 km TT performances not significant (156 min 54 s vs. 153 min 10 s for Fat-adapt vs. control. Trend to low power output during 4 km sprints with Fat-adapt. However, power during 1 km sprints (undertaken at >90% PPO) was significantly reduced in Fat-adapt trial. Confirms hypothesis that "glycogen impairment" as a result of fat adaptation limits performance of high intensity exercise.

M = male; TT = time trial; BM = body mass; MCT = medium-chain triglyceride; CHO = carbohydrate; NS = not significantly different; $\dot{V}O_2$max = maximal oxygen uptake; E = energy; CI = confidence interval; PPO = Peak Power Output\bb\. All values are mean ± SEM.

Table 5.a Studies of Carbohydrate (CHO) Intake Immediately Before or During High-Intensity Exercise ~1 hr Duration

Publication	Participants	Supplement protocol	Exercise protocol	Enhanced endurance/ performance	Comments
			HOT ENVIRONMENT		
Below et al. 1995	Well-trained cyclists (8 M) Crossover design with CHO ± fluid replacement	~1.1 g/kg CHO Treatments: 1,330 ml of 6% CHO or 200 ml of 40% CHO drink vs. fluid only Intake: ad libitum intake during trial	Cycling 50 min at 80% $\dot{V}O_2$max + ~10 min TT	Yes	Overall, CHO was associated with 6.3% enhancement of TT performance compared with no CHO replacement, $p < .05$. No differences in physiological parameters between CHO and no CHO trials.
Carter et al. 2003	Trained cyclists (8 M) Crossover design	~1 g/kg CHO Treatments: 6% CHO drink vs. placebo. Intake: 8 ml/kg immediately before trial + 3 ml/kg every 15 min	Cycling 73% $\dot{V}O_2$max to exhaustion	Yes	Time to exhaustion was increased by 13.5% with CHO (60.6 ±11.1 min) compared with flavored placebo (50.8 ± 7.5 min), $p < .05$. No difference between rate of rectal temperature rise, although trend to higher temperature at exhaustion with CHO. Blood glucose maintained in both trials but slightly higher with CHO.
Millard-Stafford et al. 1997	Well-trained runners (10 M) Crossover design with 2 different types of CHO drink	~0.7-1.0 g/kg: Treatments: 6% or 8% CHO drinks vs. placebo Intake: 1 L before run, ad libitum during run	Running 15 km treadmill run: 13.4 km at steady state and then 1.6 km TT	Yes	Both CHO drinks enhanced TT performance (6% CHO: 344 s for 1.6 km TT; 8% CHO: 341 s) compared with flavored placebo (358 s), $p < .05$.
			COOL OR MODERATE ENVIRONMENT OR ENVIRONMENT NOT STATED		
Neufer et al. 1987	Well-trained cyclists (10 M) Crossover design with solid and liquid CHO	~0.6 g CHO Treatments: solid CHO, CHO drink vs. placebo Intake: immediately before exercise	Cycling 45 min at 77% $\dot{V}O_2$max and then TT	Yes	Greater work done with solid and liquid forms of CHO (~175 kNm) compared with placebo (159 kNm), $p < .05$. No glycogen sparing with CHO intake.
Anantaraman et al. 1995)	Trained participants (5 M) Crossover design with pre-CHO and pre+during CHO	~0.5 or 2 g/kg CHO Treatments: 10% CHO drink vs. placebo Intake: 300 ml immediately before or 300 ml before and 300 ml every 15 min	Cycling 60 min protocol starting at 90% $\dot{V}O_2$max and declining as necessary	Yes	Workload maintained in all trials until 40-60 min, where decrease off in power with placebo trial. Total work done during trial was higher in both pre-CHO trial (619 ± 234 kJ) and pre+during CHO trial (599 ± 235 kJ) compared with placebo (560 ± 198 kJ), $p < .05$.

Study	Subjects/Design	CHO dose/Treatments	Exercise	Ergogenic benefit	Findings
Jeukendrup et al. 1997	Well-trained cyclists (19 M + F) Crossover design	1.1 g/kg CHO Treatments: 8% CHO drink vs. placebo Intake: 14 ml/kg consumed in equal portions immediately before and each 25% of TT	Cycling TT to complete work expected to last about ~1 hr	Yes	TT performance with CHO (58.74 ± 0.52 min; mean power = 297 W) was enhanced compared with performance with a flavored placebo (60.15 ± 0.65 min, mean power = 291 W), $p < .001$.
Kovacs et al. 1998	Well-trained cyclists (15 M) Crossover design	~1 g/kg CHO Treatments: 7% CHO drink vs. placebo Intake: 14 ml/kg immediately before and 3 ml/kg at ~20 and 40 min of TT.	Cycling TT lasting ~1 hr	No	Similar times to complete TT in CHO trial (62.5 ± 1.3 min) and placebo (61.5 ± 1.1 min), NS.
Nikolopoulos et al. 2004	Well-trained cyclists (8 M) Crossover design	~1 g/kg CHO Treatments: 6.4% CHO drink vs. placebo Intake: 14 ml/kg consumed as 8 ml/kg immediately before and 2 ml/kg at 15 min intervals	Cycling Time to fatigue at 85% $\dot{V}O_2$max	Probably	Strong trend for increase in endurance: 13% increase in time to exhaustion with CHO (58:54 ± 8:48 min) compared with flavored placebo (51:18 ± 5:54 min), NS. Surface EMG same for first 30 min in each trial; after 45 min and at fatigue, EMG lower in CHO trial. Suggests neural mechanism for CHO effect.
Desbrow et al. 2004	Well-trained cyclists and triathletes (9 M) Crossover design	0.8 g/kg Treatments: 6% CHO drink vs. placebo Intake: 14 ml/kg consumed as 8 ml/kg immediately before and 2 ml/kg at ~25%, 50%, 75% of TT	Cycling TT lasting ~1 hr	No	No difference in TT performance between CHO (62:34 ± 6:44 [min:s]) and placebo trials (62:40 ± 5:35). No differences in post-TT blood glucose concentrations between trials.
Van Nieuwenhoven et al. 2005	Trained to well-trained runners (90 M + 8 F) Crossover design	~0.6 g/kg Treatments: 7% CHO drink vs. water Intake: 600 ml consumed in equal portions before and at 4.5, 9, and 13.5 km of race	Running 18 km road race	No	No differences in performance of whole group between water (78:03 ± 8:30 [min:s]) and carbohydrate trials (78:23 ± 8:47) or for 10 fastest runners (63:50 vs. 63:54 for water and carbohydrate, respectively).
Burke et al. 2005	Highly trained distance runners (18M) Crossover design	1.1 g/kg Treatments: CHO gel vs. placebo Intake: dose split between immediately before and at 7 km and 14 km	Running Half-marathon (field study)	No	Differences in half-marathon time trivial: 73:56 (min:s) vs. 73:35 for placebo and CHO (difference = 0.3%, NS).

M = male; F = female; TT = time trial; $\dot{V}O_2$max = maximal oxygen uptake; NS = not significant; EMG = electromyogram.

Adapted from Burke et al. 2005.

Table 5.b **Reported Dietary Intakes of Male Middle- and Long-Distance Runners: Training (Mean Daily Intake ± SD)**

Publication	Running population	Survey method	Age (years)	BM (kg)	ENERGY MJ	ENERGY kJ/kg	CHO g	CHO g/kg	CHO %E	PROTEIN g	PROTEIN g/kg	PROTEIN %E	FAT g	FAT %E
Berry et al. 1949	International group of Olympians: • Middle distance (n = 6)	Duplicate food collection and chemical analysis (4 days)	25	73	15.92	218	468	6.4	50	148	2.1	15	146	34
	• Long distance (n = 2)		33	65	14.21	218	344	5.3	41	200	3.1	22	134	35
Saltin 1978	Scandinavian cross-country runners		—	—	14.87	—	408	—	46	130	—	14	—	—
Clement and Asmundson 1982	Canadian collegiate distance runners (n = 35)	7-day food diary (household measures)	22	—	12.62 ± 2.84	—	374 ± 86	—	50	119 ± 25	—	16	115 ± 33	34
Bilanin et al. 1989	U.S. runners (n = 8)	3-day food diary (household measures)	29	68	13.02 ± 3.56	200 ± 57	424	6.3	52 ± 10	117	1.7	15 ± 8	118	34 ± 11
Grandjean 1989	U.S. national-level and collegiate distance runners (n = 10)	3-day food diary (household measures)			12.68 ± 2.4	—	372	—	49 ± 9	135	—	17 ± 4	116	34 ± 8
Van Erp-Baart et al. 1989a	Dutch international-level runners (n = 56)	2 × 4- to 7-day food diary (household measures)	30	69	13.28	193	~417	~6.1	~50	~116	~1.7	~14	~122	~34
Heinemann and Zerbes 1989	German national team distance runners (n = 10)	3-day semi-weighed food diary	19-25	61	22.14	326	733	12.0	53	180	2.0	13	209	35
Couzy et al. 1990	French national- and international-level middle-distance runners (n = 6)	2 × 7-day weighed food diary	22	64	11.9	190	352	5.5	47	126	2.0	17	54	36
Moses and Manore 1991	U.S. elite distance runners (n = 17)	3 × 3-day food diary (household measures)	26	66	13.11	201	401	6.1	48	117	1.8	15	118	34
Burke et al. 1991	Australian national-level marathon runners (n = 19)	7-day food diary (household measures)	30	64	14.9 ± 2.8	230 ± 40	487 ± 111	7.6	52 ± 5	128 ± 22	2.0 ± 0.4	14.5 ± 2	128 ± 27	32 ± 7

Reference	Subjects	Method												
Ludbrook and Clark 1992	Australian well-trained distance runners (n = 12)	7-day weighed food diary	38	69	14.58 ± 2.65	211	482 ± 131	7.0	54	112 ± 20	1.6	13 ± 2	120 ± 37	30 ± 8
Robertson et al. 1992	Scots well-trained distance runners (n = 6)	7-day weighed food diary	32	58	13.8	238	449	7.7	52	109	1.9	13	146	39
Coetzer et al. 1993	South African distance runners	Food frequency question-naire												
	• Elite black (n = 11)			56	13.00 ± 5.49	260 ± 63	432	7.8	56	118	2.1	14.5 ± 3	105	30 ± 6
	• Elite white (n = 9)			70	14.34 ± 4.75	207 ± 75	437	6.2	51	154	2.2	18 ± 2	118	31 ± 8
Grandjean and Ruud 1994	U.S. Olympic team (n = 11)				13.05	189	420	6.1	53	124	1.8	16	106	29
Tanaka et al. 1995	U.S. collegiate cross-country runners (n = 14)	4-day food diary (house-hold measures)	19	64	15.17 ± 3.45	238 ± 55	504 ± 136	7.9	55 ± 6	128 ± 32	2.0	14 ± 3	115 ± 27	29 ± 5
Schena et al. 1995	Italian national-level runners (n = 35)	7-day food diary (house-hold measures)	27	62.7	14.03 ± 0.94	230	502 ± 36	8.0	60	90 ± 12	1.4	18	85 ± 6	22
Niekamp and Baer 1995	U.S. collegiate cross-country runners (n = 12)	2 × 4-day food diary (household measures)	20	66	13.58 ± 2.46	206	497 ± 134	7.5	61	104 ± 28	1.6	13	92 ± 29	26
Sugiura et al. 1999	Japanese national team distance runners (n = 8)	3-day food diary (house-hold measures)	25	60	14.32 ± 2.11	229 ± 18	382 ± 19	7.1 ± 0.8	52 ± 5	139 ± 37	2.3 ± 0.5	15 ± 2	131 ± 25	32 ± 3
Sugiura et al. 1999	Japanese national team middle-distance runners (n = 4)	3-day food diary (house-hold measures)	24	63	14.32 ± 2.11	229 ± 18	383 ± 19	6.2 ± 0.7	49 ± 7	131 ± 33	2.1 ± 0.4	15 ± 2	131 ± 40	36 ± 5
Onywera et al. 2004	Kenyan elite middle- and long-distance runners (n = 10)	7-day weighed food diary	22	56	12.5 ± 1.2	212	607 ± 57	10.4	76	75 ± 12	1.3	10	46 ± 14	13
Fudge et al. 2006	Kenyan elite middle- and long-distance runners (n = 10)	7-day weighed food diary	22	56	13.2 ± 1.3	236	549	9.8	67 ± 8	123	2.2	15 ± 4	61	17 ± 4

Table 5.c Reported Dietary Intakes of Female Middle- and Long-Distance Runners: Training (Mean Daily Intake ± SD)

Publication	Running population	Survey method	Age (years)	BM (kg)	ENERGY		CHO			PROTEIN			FAT	
					MJ	kJ/kg	g	g/kg	%E	g	g/kg	%E	g	%E
Dale and Goldberg 1982	Club-level marathon runners (n = 19)	4-day food diary (household measures)	29	53	9.59	182	248	4.7	44	80	1.5	16	98	40
Clement and Asmundson 1982	Canadian collegiate distance runners (n = 17)	7-day weighed food diary	22	—	8.47 ± 2.2	—	252 ± 56	—	50	74 ± 24	—	14	87 ± 31	38
Deuster et al. 1986	U.S. national-level marathon runners (n = 51)	3-day food diary (household measures)	29	52	10.02 ± 3.1	193	323 ± 109	6.2	55	81 ± 4	1.6	13.5	89 ± 6	33
Van Erp-Baart et al. 1989a	Dutch international-level distance runners (n = 18)	2 × 4- to 7-day food diary (household measures)	31	52	8.75	168	~301	~5.8	~50	~82	~1.6	~15	~68	~29
Haymes and Spillman 1989	U.S. collegiate distance runners (n = 11)	3-day food diary (household measures)	21	53	7.62 ± 2.8	144	268	5.0	56 ± 10	67 ± 28	1.3	15	137	30 ± 7
Nutter 1991	U.S. collegiate cross-country runners (n = 6)	7-day food diary (household measures)	19	53	6.96 ± 2.4	135 ± 49	247	4.8	57 ± 8	66	1.3	16 ± 7	50	27 ± 8
Ludbrook and Clark 1992	Australian well-trained distance runners (n = 11)	7-day weighed food diary	33	51	8.85 ± 2.1	174	299 ± 58	5.9	57	73 ± 16	1.4	14 ± 3	63 ± 28	26 ± 7
Schulz et al. 1992	U.S. national- and international-level distance runners (n = 9)	6-day food diary (household measures)	26	52	9.17	176	333	6.4	59	73	—	13	66	27
Baer and Taper 1992	U.S. high school runners (n = 7)	2 × 7-day food diary (household measure)	15	51	6.90 ± 2.1	135	206 ± 65	4.0	50	56 ± 14	1.1	14	66 ± 19	36

Edwards et al. 1993	U.S. collegiate cross-country runners (n = 9)	7-day food diary		55	8.53 ± 1.2	158 ± 37	—	—	—	—	—	—	—	—
Grandjean and Ruud 1994	U.S. Olympic team (n = 9)				9.0	176	275	5.4	50	82	1.6	15	74	30
Beidleman et al. 1995	U.S. trained distance runners (n = 10)	3-day weighed (?) food diary	22	54	8.16 ± 1.6	152 ± 37	296 ± 68	5.5	60 ± 8	70 ± 17	1.4 ± 0.3	14 ± 2	58 ± 22	26 ± 8
Tanaka et al. 1995	U.S. collegiate cross-country runners (n = 10)	4-day food diary (household measures)	20	55	8.31 ± 1.84	152 ± 33	331 ± 70	6.1 ± 1.3	67 ± 2	64 ± 15	1.2	13 ± 2	51 ± 18	23 ± 5
Wiita and Stombaugh 1996	U.S. state-level high school distance runners (n = 22)	3-day food diary (household measures). Longitudinal	17 20	50 53	8.99 6.88	175 130	283 253	5.5 4.7	53 60	81 57	1.6 1.1	15 14	76 48	32 26
Sugiura et al. 1999	Japanese national team distance runners (n = 7)	3-day food diary (household measures)	24	47	11.37 ± 1.48	244 ± 37	337 ± 59	7.2 ± 1.4	51 ± 5	109 ± 18	2.4 ± 0.5	16 ± 2	98 ± 15	33 ± 4
Sugiura et al. 1999	Japanese national team middle-distance runners (n = 4)	3-day food diary (household measures)	24	63	14.32 ± 2.11	229 ± 18	383 ± 19	6.2 ± 0.7	49 ± 7	111 ± 23	2.3 ± 0.4	16 ± 1	106 ± 33	34 ± 5

BM = body mass; CHO = carbohydrate; E = energy.

Table 5.d Relevant Studies of Supplements With Likely Benefit to Middle- and Long-Distance Running Performance

Publication	Participants	Supplement protocol	Exercise protocol	Enhanced performance	Comments
Caffeine		Acute supplementation protocol			**Strong evidence of enhancement of endurance and performance of prolonged moderate- and high-intensity running with caffeine. More sport-specific studies are needed to define caffeine intake protocols that may benefit middle- and long-distance events, including timing and dose of caffeine.**
Sasaki et al. 1987	Well-trained runners (5M) Crossover study	Caffeine before and during run (total = 420 mg = ~7.2 mg/kg) With and without sugar intake	Treadmill running at 80% $\dot{V}O_2$max for 45 min and then to exhaustion	Yes	Caffeine and caffeine + sucrose trials significantly increased time to exhaustion compared with placebo.
Graham and Spriet 1991	Well-trained runners (7 M) Crossover design undertaken with cycling and running protocols	9 mg/kg at 60 min pre-race	Treadmill running at 85% $\dot{V}O_2$max to exhaustion	Yes	Caffeine enhanced mean time to exhaustion by ~45%, from ~49 min to ~71 min (individual response = 5-87% enhancement). One nonresponder noted in group, and confirmed when same participants repeated test on cycle. Some urinary caffeine levels above 12 µg/ml.
French et al. 1991	Recreational runners (6 M)	10 mg/kg taken immediately before run	Treadmill running at 75% $\dot{V}O_2$max for 45 min and then incremental to exhaustion	Yes	Caffeine enhanced distance run to exhaustion compared with control trial ($p < .05$).
Wiles et al. 1992	Well-trained runners (18 M) Crossover study	3 g of coffee (150-200 mg of caffeine) at 60 min pre-race	1,500 m race on treadmill	Yes	Mean 1,500 time improved by ~4.2 s ($p < .05$) with caffeine compared with placebo.
Wiles et al. 1992	Well-trained runners (10 M) Crossover study	3 g of coffee (150-200 mg of caffeine) at 60 min pre-race	1,500 m race: 1,100 m at constant speed + 1 min "final burst" at self-selected speed	Yes	Caffeine enhanced speed of 1 min final burst by ~0.6 km/hr, equivalent to 10 m ($p < .05$).
Graham and Spriet 1995	Well-trained runners (8 M) Crossover design	3, 6, and 9 mg/kg at 60 min pre-race	Treadmill running at 85% $\dot{V}O_2$max to exhaustion	Yes for 3 mg/kg and 6 mg/kg	Time to exhaustion increased at 3 and 6 mg/kg doses compared with placebo ($p < .05$). Highest dose of caffeine had the greatest effect on epinephrine and metabolites yet had the least effect on performance.
Cohen et al. 1996	Trained runners (5 M + 2 F) Crossover study with different caffeine doses	5 and 9 mg/kg taken pre-race	Half-marathon (field study) in hot conditions	No	No effects on RPE or performance at either dose compared with placebo.

Reference	Subjects/design	Supplementation protocol	Event/test	Ergogenic?	Findings
Graham et al. 1998	Well-trained runners (7 M) Crossover design	4.5 mg/kg caffeine in capsule or added to decaf coffee or caffeinated coffee at 60 min pre-race	Treadmill running at 85% $\dot{V}O_2$max to exhaustion	Yes	Increase in time to exhaustion in caffeine capsule trial only. No enhancement of performance with coffee or caffeine taken with coffee trials. Other components of coffee antagonize the responses to caffeine.
Doherty et al. 2002	Trained runners (14 M) Crossover design	5 mg/kg taken 60 min before test. Participants had previously undertaken creatine loading protocol	Treadmill running at 125% $\dot{V}O_2$max to exhaustion	Yes	Total $\dot{V}O_2$ and time to exhaustion increased in caffeine trial compared with placebo (222 vs. 198 s, $p < .05$).
Van Nieuwenhoven et al. 2005	Trained to well-trained runners (90 M + 8 F) Crossover design	~1.3 mg/kg in 7% CHO sport drink vs. CHO sport drink alone and water. 600 ml consumed in equal portions before and at 4.5, 9, and 13.5 km of race	Running 18 km road race	No	No differences in performance of whole group between caffeinated sport drink (78:03 ± 8:42 [min:s]), sport drink (78:23 ± 8:47), or water (78:03 ± 8:30) or for 10 fastest runners (63:41, 63:54 vs. 63:50 for caffeine sport drink, sport drink, and water, respectively).
Bridge and Jones 2006	Distance runners (8 M) Crossover design with 3 trials (caffeine, placebo, and control)	3 mg/kg taken 60 min prerace	8 km race on track	Yes	Relative to the mean time of the control and placebo trials, caffeine supplementation resulted in a 23.8 s or 1.2% improvement in run time ($P < .05$) with individual results ranging from 10 to 61 s improvement. HR was significantly higher in caffeine trial, with trend to lower RPE despite faster running speed.
Bicarbonate or citrate		Acute supplementation protocol			**Some evidence of enhancement of middle distance, and even longer events with acute bicarbonate or citrate loading prior to run. Further event-specific studies are required to confirm benefits.**
Wilkes et al. 1983	Collegiate middle-distance runners (6 M) Crossover study	300 mg/kg sodium bicarbonate at 2.5 hr pre-race	800 m race	Yes	Improved running time with bicarbonate (2:02.9 [min:s]) vs. placebo (2:05.1) and control (2:05.8), $p < .05$. Elevated postexercise values for pH, lactate, and blood bicarbonate.
Tiryaki and Atterbom 1995	Collegiate runners (11 F) + untrained controls (4 F) Crossover study	300 mg/kg sodium citrate or sodium bicarbonate at 2.5 hr pre-race	600 m race	No	No performance effect despite significant changes to acid-base status.
Bird et al. 1995	Trained middle-distance runners (n = 12)	300 mg/kg sodium bicarbonate at 90 min pre-exercise	1,500 m	Yes	Performance in bicarbonate trial improved compared with placebo trial (253.9 vs. 256.8 s, $p < .05$).
Potteiger et al. 1996	Well-trained runners (7 M) Crossover study	300 mg/kg sodium bicarbonate or 500 mg/kg sodium citrate at 2 hr pre-race	30 min run on treadmill at LT plus time to exhaustion at 110% LT	No	Both citrate and bicarbonate supplementation increased blood pH during steady-state run. No significant differences in run to exhaustion: 287 s, 172.8 s, 222.3 s for bicarbonate, citrate, and placebo, respectively.

(continued)

Table 5.d (continued)

Publication	Participants	Supplement protocol	Exercise protocol	Enhanced performance	Comments
Shave et al. 2001	Highly trained competitive triathletes and pentathletes (7 M, 2 F) Crossover study	500 mg/kg sodium citrate at 1.5 hr pre-race	3,000 m race	Yes	Performance time significantly faster ($p < .05$) for citrate trial (610.9 s) compared with placebo trial (621.6 s). High risk of gastrointestinal distress.
Oopik et al. 2003	Well-trained collegiate distance runners (17 M) Crossover study	500 mg/kg sodium citrate at 2 hr pre-race	5,000 m treadmill run	Yes	Performance significantly faster ($p < .05$) for citrate trial (1,153 s) compared with placebo trial (1,183 s). High risk of gastrointestinal distress. Blood lactate concentration higher after race with citrate trial.
Oopik et al. 2004	Trained runners (10 M) Crossover study	500 mg/kg sodium citrate at 2 hr pre-race at 3 hr pre-race	5,000 m race in indoor stadium	No	No difference in 5 km running time or speed between trials was observed in this competitive setting.
Montfoort et al. 2004	Competitive distance runners (15 M) Crossover study	300 mg/kg sodium bicarbonate or 525 mg/kg sodium citrate or 400 mg/kg sodium lactate at 90-180 min pre-race	Treadmill run to exhaustion at speed designed to last 1-2 min	Yes, bicarb Possibly, citrate Possibly, lactate	Analysis estimated likelihood of treatments increasing endurance compared with chloride placebo by at least 0.5% (considered to be the smallest worthwhile improvement). Bicarbonate produced 2.7% enhancement of endurance (96% chance of improvement); lactate enhanced endurance by 1.7% (83% chance), and citrate enhanced endurance by 0.5% (50% chance). Overall, authors concluded that bicarbonate is most effective and citrate is possibly not as effective. No difference in gastrointestinal symptoms.
Bicarbonate and citrate		**Chronic supplementation protocol for training**			**There is new evidence that repeated use of bicarbonate loading before interval training sessions may enhance training adaptations and improve performance of sustained high-intensity exercise, at least in moderately trained individuals. It may also assist the athlete to train harder. Further research is needed to confirm these findings, especially for highly trained athletes.**
Edge at al. 2006	Moderately trained (16 F) Experimental-placebo design	8 wks at 400 mg/kg sodium bicarbonate in a split dose 90 min and 30 min before interval training Periodized interval training undertaken 3 d/wk: 2 min intervals with 1 min recovery, with 6 to 12 intervals completed at 140-170% of intensity at lactate threshold Both groups completed the same training load	0 and 8 wks (cycle): • $\dot{V}O_2$peak • lactate threshold • time to exhaustion at 100% pre-trial $\dot{V}O_2$peak	Yes	Both groups increased their $\dot{V}O_2$peak by similar amounts as a result of the 8 wk interval training. Both groups also increased their muscle-buffering capacity. This increase in muscle-buffering capacity was related to pre-training capacity rather than the treatment (subjects with lower pre-training muscle-buffering capacity achieved greater increases as a result of training). Although both groups showed an increase in lactate threshold and time to exhaustion at $\dot{V}O_2$peak, the improvements were greater in the bicarbonate group. The authors speculated that training intensity rather than accumulation of H^+ ions is responsible for increasing muscle buffering capacity. Furthermore, inducing alkalosis during exercise may enhance muscle adaptations by reducing the damage to mitochondria or protein synthesis.

M = male; F = female; LT = lactate threshold; $\dot{V}O_2$max = maximal oxygen uptake; RPE = rating of perceived exertion.

Table 5.e Relevant Studies of Supplements With Undetermined or Unlikely Benefit to Middle- and Long-Distance Runners

Study	Participants	Supplement protocol	Exercise protocol	Enhanced performance	Comments
Glycerol hyperhydration		**Acute supplementation protocol**			**The literature suggests that potential benefits may occur in prolonged events in the heat, where glycerol hyperhydration is used to increase total body water and provide a substantial reduction in the fluid deficit that is accrued. However, most studies have been undertaken with a cycling protocol and don't take into account the increase in BM that occurs with retention of ~600 ml of additional fluid. Further running-specific studies are needed to determine benefit. Should be undertaken only under scientific supervision because of potential for side effects.**
Latzka et al. 1998	Heat-acclimatized participants (8 M) Crossover design	1.2 g/kg lean BM + 29 ml/kg water, 1 hr pre-exercise (compared with water hyperhydration or control)	Treadmill running at 55% V̇O₂max until exhaustion or high rectal temperature Hot environment (35°C) without further fluid intake	Yes (better than control but equal to water hyperhydration)	Both hyperhydration trials increased body fluid by ~1,400 ml. Time to exhaustion longer in both trials compared with control. Performance changes not explained by differences in sweat losses, cardiac output, or temperature control. Some gastrointestinal and headache symptoms with glycerol.
Creatine		**Acute supplementation protocol**			**Most studies suggest that acute creatine supplementation does not benefit the performance of prolonged running and may even be detrimental to performance because of the accompanying increase in BM (~0.6 kg). Chronic supplementation may be of some benefit to the training adaptations achieved by the interval training programs undertaken by middle-distance runners, although weight gain concerns must be addressed.**
Viru et al. 1994	Trained middle-distance runners (10 M) Experimental–placebo design	6 days at 30 g/day creatine or placebo	Interval set: 4 × 300 m with 4 min rest plus 4 × 1,000 m with 3 min rest	Yes	Creatine increased BM by 1.8 kg. Compared with presupplementation trial, creatine group experienced a reduction in running time in the final 300 and 1,000 m runs of each interval set, an improvement in total running time for each set, and an enhancement of the best run of each set. Placebo group achieved only occasional enhancement of these parameters in postsupplementation trial.
Balsom et al. 1993	Trained runners (17 M) Experimental–placebo design	6 days at 20 g/day creatine or placebo	6 km cross-country run	No, in fact, impaired performance	Slower time to complete cross-country run after creatine supplementation (23.79 vs. 23.36 min), potentially attributable to increase in BM (~0.9 kg) with creatine loading. No difference in run times in placebo group (23.76 vs. 23.92 min).

(continued)

Table 5.e *(continued)*

Study	Participants	Supplement protocol	Exercise protocol	Enhanced performance	Comments
Terrillion et al. 1997	Well-trained runners (12 M) Experimental–placebo design	5 days at 20 g/day creatine or placebo	2×700 m run	No	No significant difference in postsupplementation performance of either 700 m run in creatine or placebo group compared with baseline.
Bovine colostrum		**Chronic supplementation protocol**			**Potential value undetermined. No mechanisms identified to explain any potential benefits. Expense of supplement ($US40 per week) warrants additional supportive research before it can be recommended.**
Buckley et al. 2002	Active males (30 M; colostrum = 17 M; placebo = 13 M) Experimental–placebo design	8 weeks at 60 g/day colostrum or placebo (60 g/day whey protein) Running program 3 × week at 45 min	Tests at baseline, 4 weeks, and 8 weeks: $2 \times \dot{V}O_2$max tests separated by 20 min	No, at 4 weeks Yes, at 8 weeks	Training improved peak running speed in both runs in both groups at week 8. No differences between groups in either run at week 4 although trend to lower peak speed in second run with colostrum group. At week 8, no difference in peak speed in first run but greater speed in second run in colostrum group ($p < .05$), suggesting better recovery between runs.
Carnitine		**Acute or chronic supplementation protocol**			**Few studies on trained athletes and performance changes, especially in running. Studies of chronic carnitine intake fail to show increase in muscle carnitine levels following supplementation; therefore, hard to imagine changes in metabolic function (e.g., enhanced fatty acid transport into mitochondria or acetyl carnitine "sink").**
Colombani et al. 1996	Endurance-trained athletes (7 M) Crossover design	2 g at 2 hr before run and at 20 km mark	Marathon run + submaximal performance test day after marathon	No	No change in exercise metabolism or marathon running time. No change in recovery and submaximal test performance on following day.
Marconi et al. 1985	National class walkers (6 M) Crossover design	4 g/day for 2 weeks	Submaximal run + treadmill $\dot{V}O_2$max + supramaximal jumps	Yes?	Increase in $\dot{V}O_2$max by 6%. However, no effects on oxygen utilization and RER at submaximal loads or change in lactate accumulation with jumps. Results appear inconsistent.
Coenzyme Q10		**Chronic supplementation protocol**			**No evidence that coenzyme Q10 increases antioxidant function in mitochondrial membrane or electron transport chain function. In fact, some cycling studies show increased oxidative damage and impaired adaptation to high-intensity exercise program when untrained participants take CoQ10 in conjunction with training. Need for more running-specific studies.**
Kaikkonen et al. 1998	Moderately trained runners (37 M) Experimental–placebo design	3 weeks at 90 mg/day (+ vitamin E) or placebo	Marathon (field test)	Not measured	No change in indexes of oxidative or muscle damage following marathon run.

Study	Participants / Design	Supplementation protocol	Performance measure	Ergogenic?	Findings
Ginseng—Eleutherococcus senticosus		Chronic supplementation protocol			**Limited data on runners. No clear evidence of any type of benefits of any type of ginseng (Panax or Eleutherococcus senticosus) on recovery or performance.**
Dowling et al. 1996	Highly trained runners (26 M + 4 F) Experimental–placebo design	6 weeks at 60 drops/day (maximum recommended dose) of Russian ginseng (Eleutherococcus senticosus) or placebo	10 min treadmill run test at • 10 km race pace • $\dot{V}O_2$max test on treadmill	No	No change in treadmill max test between groups. No change in metabolic characteristics at race pace or RPE. Low statistical power may prevent small changes from being detected.
Inosine		Chronic supplementation protocol			**Limited data on runners. No evidence of increased production of ATP or performance enhancements. In fact, inosine supplementation decreased maximal run performance. Data in cyclists also show evidence of performance impairment with inosine.**
Williams et al. 1990	Highly trained runners (9 M + F) Crossover design	2 days at 6,000 mg/day for 2 days (maximum recommended dose)	• Competitive 3-mile treadmill run • Maximal treadmill run	No / No, in fact performance impairment with inosine	No effect of inosine on 3 mile run time, $\dot{V}O_2$peak, or other variables. Negative effect on maximal run time to exhaustion in inosine trial compared with placebo ($p < .05$).
Cytochrome c		Chronic and acute supplementation protocol			**No evidence of benefits to performance**
Faria et al. 2002	Trained endurance runners (18 M + 1 F) Crossover design	6 days at 800 mg/day cytochrome c or placebo + 800 mg at 1 hr before trial	13 min submaximal treadmill run + 3 mile treadmill run at controlled intensities followed by $\dot{V}O_2$max test	No	No difference in oxygen utilization, HR, or RPE during submaximal or 3-mile runs. No difference in $\dot{V}O_2$max between trials.
Branched-chain amino acids		Acute supplementation protocol			**Limited data on runners, and existing studies have been criticized for contrived findings. More studies are needed to support claims of benefits related to reduction of "central fatigue." Needs also to be compared with intake of CHO, which can reduce both central and peripheral fatigue.**
Blomstrand et al. 1991	Cross-country runners (25 M) + marathon runners (193 M) Experimental–placebo design	16 g (marathon) or 7.5 g (cross-country) compared with placebo	Marathon or 30 km cross-country race • Run time • Stroop CWT given after cross-country run to measure cognitive function	Yes / Yes	Marathon study: participants divided (arbitrarily) into a slower and faster group. Authors claim that slower group ran faster with BCAA than placebo. This outcome has been criticized on statistical grounds. Cross-country study: CWT performance improved in BCAA trial after cross-country run.

(continued)

Table 5.e (continued)

Study	Participants	Supplement protocol	Exercise protocol	Enhanced performance	Comments
Hassmen et al. 1994	Cross-country runners (Study 1: 23 M) (Study 2: 29 M) Experimental–placebo design	Total amount BCAA = 5.3 g, served as 5 × 150 ml 7% CHO drink with BCAA vs. CHO alone throughout race	Cognitive performance (Stroop CWT) before and after 30 km cross-country race	No for running performance; Yes for cognitive performance	Difference in running time between groups not significant. Participants receiving BCAAs scored higher in various parts of the CWT after the race than pre-race, while there were no differences in scores over race in placebo group. Performance of more complex parts maintained in BCAA group but reduced in placebo group over race. Changes in mood not substantial in either group
L-tryptophan		Acute supplementation protocol			**No evidence of benefits to performance**
Stensrund et al. 1992	Well-trained runners (49 M) Experimental–placebo design	1.2 g of tryptophan during 24 hr period before second trial	Treadmill run at 100% $\dot{V}O_2$max until exhaustion before and after supplementation	No	No difference in improvements in run time to exhaustion from first to second trial between tryptophan and placebo group.
Magnesium		Chronic supplementation protocol			**Although magnesium is lost in sweat and is added to sport drinks produced in some countries, there is no evidence that runners or other athletes benefit from specific magnesium supplementation.**
Terblanche et al. 1992	Marathon runners (n = 20) Experimental–placebo design	365 mg/day magnesium or placebo for 4 weeks before and 6 weeks after a marathon	42 km marathon	No	No effect of supplementation on blood or muscle magnesium concentrations. No effects on marathon running performance, extent of muscle damage, or recovery of muscle function after the marathon.
Access sport nutrition bar (containing adenosine agonists)		Acute supplementation protocol			**No evidence of benefits to performance**
Oliver and Tremblay 2002	Trained runners (n = 12) Crossover design	1 Access bar or muesli bar or placebo drink, 15 min before trial	Treadmill run to complete set amount of work (~55 min)	No	No difference in time to complete running time trial between any of the treatments.
Medium-chain triglyceride (MCT)		Chronic supplementation protocol			**No change in metabolism or substrate utilization following chronic supplementation with this alternative source of dietary fat.**
Misell et al. 2001	Trained endurance runners (12 M) Crossover design	2 weeks at 60 g/day MCT oil (or long-chain fatty acid oil placebo)	• $\dot{V}O_2$max • 30 min at 85% $\dot{V}O_2$max for 30 min and then 75% $\dot{V}O_2$max to exhaustion	No; No	No difference in maximal aerobic capacity test or endurance time in following test.

M = male; F = female; BM = body mass; ATP = adenosine triphosphate; HR = heart rate; RPE = rating of perceived exertion; CHO = carbohydrate; $\dot{V}O_2$max = maximal oxygen uptake; RER = respiratory exchange rate; BCAA = branched-chain amino acid; CWT = Color Word Test; MCT = medium-chain triglyceride.

Table 6.a Reported Dietary Intakes of Male Swimmers: Training (Mean Daily Intake ± SD)

Publication	Swimming population	Survey method	Age (yr)	BM (kg)	Energy		CHO			Protein			Fat	
					MJ	kJ/kg	g	g/kg	%E	g	g/kg	%E	g	%E
Saltin 1978	Scandinavian swimmers				~15.70	—	~480	—	51	~118	—	12	~157	37
Van Handel et al. 1984	U.S. national-level swimmers (n = 13)	3-day food diary (household measures)	22	80	18.18 ± 4.18	227	531	6.6	49 ± 10	184	2.3	17 ± 2	164	34 ± 8
Barr 1989	Canadian national-level swimmers (n = 10)	3-day food diary (household measures)	16	72	14.79 ± 3.2	209 ± 46	456 ± 126	6.3	51 ± 5	143 ± 35	2.0 ± 0.4	16 ± 3	134 ± 27	34 ± 3
Van Erp-Baart et al. 1989a	Dutch international swimmers (n = 20)	4- to 7-day food diary (household measures)	18	73	16.11	221	~486	~6.7	~48	~161	~2.2	~16	~157	~36
Chen et al. 1989	Chinese elite swimmers (n = 3)	3- to 5-day weighed food diary	22	74	24.82 ± 3.3	334 ± 46	484 ± 228	6.5 ± 3.1	33 ± 7	320 ± 50	4.3 ± 0.7	22 ± 3	315 ± 39	48 ± 6
Grandjean 1989	U.S. national-level and collegiate swimmers (n = 15)	3-day food diary (household measures)			16.80 ± 2.62	—	513	—	51 ± 7	147	—	14 ± 2	159	35 ± 6
Berning et al. 1991	U.S. national-level swimmers (n = 22)	5-day food diary (household measures)	16	77	21.83 ± 2.97	282	600 ± 99	7.7	46	166 ± 23	2.1	13	248 ± 46	43
Barr and Costill 1992	U.S. collegiate swimmers		19											
	• Prestudy (n = 24)	2-day food diary (household measures)		75	15.3 ± 3.9	204	501 ± 141	6.7	55	121 ± 28	1.6	13	134 ± 42	32
	• ↑ training (n = 11)			72	17.7 ± 3.0	246	600 ± 126	8.3	57	136 ± 30	1.9	12	150 ± 33	31
	• Maintained training (n = 13)			79	13.5 ± 3	170	474 ± 144	6.0	59	112 ± 28	1.4	13	105 ± 25	29
Roberts and Smith 1992	Canadian international-level swimmers (n = 9)	5 × 2-day food diary (household measures)	23	76	19.16	252	718	9.6	60	179	2.4	15	124	24
Paschoal and Amancio 2004	Brazilian international-level (n = 8)	4-day food diary (household measures)	19	71	15.9	224 ± 43	504	7.1 ± 1.5	53	163	2.3 ± 0.5	17		30

BM = body mass; CHO = carbohydrate; E = energy.

Table 6.b   Reported Dietary Intakes of Female Swimmers: Training (Mean Daily Intake ± SD)

Publication	Swimming population	Survey method	Age (years)	BM (kg)	Energy MJ	Energy kJ/kg	CHO g	CHO g/kg	CHO %E	Protein g	Protein g/kg	Protein %E	Fat g	Fat %E
Smith et al. 1982	U.S. collegiate swimmers (n = 9)	4 × 4-day food record (household measures)	19	64	10.31 ± 2.23	161	315	4.9	49 ± 8	99	1.5	16 ± 3	99	36 ± 6
Short and Short 1983	U.S. collegiate swimmers (n = 20)	3-day food diary (household measures)			~12.98	—	~333	—	~42	~119	—	~15	~149	~42
Van Handel et al. 1984	U.S. national-level swimmers (n = 14)	3-day food diary (household measures)	17	62	9.64 ± 3.5	155	305	4.9	53 ± 6	92	1.3	16 ± 3	77	30 ± 7
Barr 1989	Canadian national-level swimmers (n = 10)	3-day food diary (household measures)	16	62	8.64 ± 2	140	284 ± 85	4.6	54 ± 7	89 ± 19	1.5 ± 0.3	17 ± 3	69 ± 15	30 ± 4
Tilgner and Schiller 1989	U.S. collegiate swimmers (n = 19)	2 × 3-day food diary (household measures)	19	63	10.42 ± 2.3	163	337 ± 84	5.3	54	79 ± 18	1.3	13	91 ± 22	33
Vallieres et al. 1989	Canadian collegiate swimmers (n = 6)	2 × 3-day food diary (household measures)	22	62	10.33	165	333 ± 91	5.4	55	90 ± 27	1.5	15	94 ± 38	33
Chen et al. 1989	Chinese elite swimmers (n = 3)	3- to 5-day weighed food diary	20	65	19.21 ± 0.72	297 ± 12	405 ± 58	6.2 ± 0.9	35 ± 5	230 ± 18	3.5 ± 0.3	26 ± 2	248 ± 14	49 ± 3
Risser et al. 1990	U.S. collegiate swimmers (n = 10)	3 × 24 hr recall	18	65	7.93 ± 2.65	122	258 ± 83	4.0	52	70 ± 23	1.1	14	67 ± 30	31
Barr 1991	U.S. collegiate swimmers (n = 14)	3-day food diary (household measures)	20	63	9.59 ± 1.95	152	324 ± 66	5.1	56	73 ± 18	1.2	13	82 ± 20	32
Berning et al. 1991	U.S. national-level swimmers (n = 21)	5-day food diary (household measures)	15	58	14.93 ± 2.8	256	428 ± 110	7.4	48	107 ± 21	1.8	12	164 ± 32	41

Reference	Subjects	Method												
Trappe et al. 1997	U.S. international-level swimmers (n = 5)	2-day food diary	19	65	13.1 ± 2.2	201	524	8.1	68	90	1.4	11	74	21
Almeras et al. 1997	Canadian national and international level (n = 6)	Monthly 3-day food diary (household measures) over 13 months	17	60	~10.5	~175	~370	~6.2	~60	~105	~1.8	~16	~68	~24
Ousley-Pahnke et al. 2001	U.S. collegiate swimmers during taper (n = 15)	4-day food diary (household measures)	20	66	9.53 ± 2.79	144	362 ± 109	5.5	63 ± 5	80 ± 25	1.2	14 ± 3	60 ± 24	23 ± 5
Gropper et al. 2003	U.S. collegiate swimmers (n = 5)	3-day food diary (household measures)	19	65	10.1									
Petersen et al. 2006	U.S. collegiate swimmers and divers (n = 18 swimmers and 6 divers) 16-week training period	2 x 3 day food diary (household measures) • Beginning of season • End of season	20	65	10.06 ± 3.62 9.86 ± 3.21	155 156	365 ± 108 381 ± 116	5.6 6.0	62 ± 7 65 ± 7	79 ± 29 83 ± 28	1.2 1.3	13 ± 2 14 ± 2	54 53	24 ± 6 22 ± 6

BM = body mass; CHO = carbohydrate; E = energy.

Table 6.c Reported Dietary Intakes of Rowers: Training (Mean Daily Intake ± SD)

Publication	Rowing population	Survey method	Age (years)	BM (kg)	Energy		CHO			Protein			Fat	
					MJ	kJ/kg	g	g/kg	%E	g	g/kg	%E	g	%E
MALES														
De Wijn et al. 1979	Dutch Olympic team rowers (n = 8)	7-day food diary (household measures)		87	17.31 ± 2.11	199	467	5.4	43	139	1.6	13	192	43
Short and Short 1983	U.S. collegiate rowers (n = 27)	1- to 3-day food diary (household measures)		85	16.99	200	456	5.4	44	183	2.2	17	168	37
Van Erp-Baart et al. 1989a	Dutch international-level rowers (n = 18)	2 × 4- to 7-day food diary (household measures)	22	77	14.59	189	~472	~6.1	~52	~118	~1.5	~13	~138	~35
Heinemann and Zerbes 1989	German national-level rowers (n = 3)	3-day food diary (household measures)	18-23	88	~25.2	286	~770	~8.8	52	~205	2.3	13	238	35
FEMALES														
Short and Short 1983	U.S. collegiate rowers (n = 24)	3-day food diary (household measures)		68	9.78	144	272	4.0	46	96	1.8	16	96	36
Van Erp-Baart et al. 1989a	Dutch international-level rowers (n = 8)	2 × 4- to 7-day food diary (household measures)	23	70	12.98	186	~374	~5.4	~46	~114	~1.6	~14	~140	~40
Steen et al. 1995	U.S. collegiate rowers (n = 16)	5-day food diary (household measures)	21	69	11.05 ± 1.8	160	337 ± 68	4.9	51	88 ± 15	1.3	13	104 ± 25	36

BM = body mass; CHO = carbohydrate; E = energy.

Table 6.d Available Data on Fluid Losses and Voluntary Fluid Intakes During Swimming and Rowing Workouts

Publication	Athlete	Session	Environmental conditions	Sweat rates	Voluntary fluid intake	Hydration change (%BM)
SWIMMERS						
Cox et al. 2002	Highly trained, internationally competitive swimmers (21 M + 20 F)	Interval training sessions in indoor pool, mean = 4 km (n = 295 observations)	31°C, 63% rh Water = 29°C	123 ml/km[a] ~365 ml/hr	127 ml/km ~365 ml/hr	0 (−1.7% to 1.7%)
		All male training sessions (n = 155 observations)		138 ml/km ~415 ml/hr	155 ml/kg ~465 ml/hr	+0.11% (−1.7% to 1.4%)
		All female training sessions (n = 140 observations)		107 ml/km	95 ml/km	−0.14% (−1.7% to +1%)
		Aerobic focused sessions (n = 81 observations)		92 ml/km	109 ml/km	
		Anaerobic threshold sessions (n = 23 observations)		167 ml/km	117 ml/km	
Soler et al. 2003	Competitive swimmers (9 M)	Interval training session in outdoor pool, 9 km, 180 min	30°C Water = 27°C	~600 ml/hr (1.8 ± 0.5 L total)	100 ml over 180 min	−2.5%
Lemon et al. 1989	Well-trained male swimmers			450 ml/hr		
Cade et al. 1991	Highly trained internationally competitive swimmers (20 M)	Interval training sessions over 3 weeks, each 2 hr		1,620 ml/hr		
	Highly trained swimmers (20 F)	Interval training sessions over 3 weeks, each 2 hr		1,440 ml/hr		
ROWERS						
Jurimae et al. 2000	Well-trained rowers (n = 12 M)	On-water session: 23 km, 137 min				−1.7%
Burke 1995	Highly trained rowers (M)	On-water sessions undertaken over 1 week (90-120 min per session)	10°C	1165 ml/hr (430-2,000)	582 ml/hr (215-1,265)	−0.6% (0-2.3%)

Table 6.d (continued)

Publication	Athlete	Session	Environmental conditions	Sweat rates	Voluntary fluid intake	Hydration change (%BM)
		SWIMMERS				
	Highly trained rowers (M)	On-water sessions undertaken over 1 week (90-120 min per session)	10°C	780 ml/hr (360-1,550)	405 ml/hr (145-660)	−0.5% (0-2%)
	Highly trained rowers (M)	On-water sessions undertaken over 1 week (90-120 min per session)	32°C	1,390 ml/hr (740-2,335)	780 ml/hr (290-1,390)	−1.2% (0-1.8%)

F = female, M = male, BM = body mass, rh = relative humidity.

[a]Estimates of changes in fluid balance were expressed in terms of the volume of training (km) undertaken in the session to account for the variable times between interval sets and between warm-up and cool-down of individual swimmers. Conversion to an estimate per hour was achieved by using mean value for the duration of the group session.

Table 6.e   Relevant Studies of Supplements With Likely Benefit to Swimming and Rowing Performance

Study	Participants	Supplement protocol	Exercise protocol	Enhanced performance	Comments
Caffeine		**Acute supplementation protocol**			**More sport-specific studies are needed, using highly trained athletes, to define the range of events and caffeine intake protocols in which benefits are achieved. There may be some merit in finding the lowest caffeine dose at which performance benefits are seen.**
Collomp et al. 1992	Trained swimmers (14 M + F) and recreational swimmers (7 M + F) Crossover design	250 mg (~4 mg/kg) taken 60 min prerace	2 × 100 m sprints	Yes in trained participants No in recreational participants	Authors suggest that specific training is required for caffeine to improve anaerobic capacity. However, another explanation is that trained swimmers are more reliable in performance, and this, in combination with the greater sample size in the current study, provided a greater opportunity to detect small changes in performance
MacIntosh and Wright 1995	Well-trained swimmers (11 M + F) Crossover design	6 mg/kg taken 60 min prerace	1,500 m freestyle race	Yes	23 s improvement in swimming time with caffeine ($p < .05$). Caffeine affected substrate and electrolyte balance.
Bruce et al. 2000	Well-trained rowers (8 M) Crossover design	6 mg/kg or 9 g/kg taken 60 min prerace	2,000 m ergometer row	Yes for both doses	Caffeine enhanced performance by mean of 1.3% and 1% for 6 mg/kg and 9 mg/kg doses, respectively, compared with placebo treatment ($p < .05$). Some participants had urinary caffeine concentrations above 12 ng/ml with higher caffeine dose. Effect presumed to be attributable to central nervous system effect, because "metabolic theory" of muscle glycogen sparing does not apply to this mode of exercise. However, participants were unable to identify caffeine trials, suggesting that effect is subtle.
Anderson et al. 2000	Well-trained rowers (8 F) Crossover design	6 mg/kg or 9 g/kg taken 60 min prerace	2,000 m ergometer row	Yes for both doses	Caffeine enhanced performance by mean of 0.7% and 1.3% for 6 mg/kg and 9 mg/kg doses, respectively, compared with placebo treatment ($p < .05$). Performance improvement achieve primarily by enhancing the first 500 m of row.
Burke, Anderson, and Pyne in press	Highly trained competitive swimmers (7 M + 8 F) Crossover design	2 mg/kg taken 60 min prerace	100 m race (best stroke)	No	No difference in reaction time, 50 m split, or 100 m race time between trials; however, rating of perceived exertion was lower in the caffeine trial (16.6 vs. 17.1, $p = .01$). Self-reports of sleeping patterns following the trial found that caffeine supplementation was associated with an increase in the time taken to fall asleep and a reduction in the quality of sleep.

(continued)

Table 6.e *(continued)*

Study	Participants	Supplement protocol	Exercise protocol	Enhanced performance	Comments
Bicarbonate or citrate		**Acute supplementation protocol**			**Few studies are available using highly elite or well-trained partici- pants and sport-specific studies. More studies are needed to define the range of swimming events that might benefit from bicarbonate or citrate loading and protocols that can be used in rowing and swimming from heats to finals.**
Gao et al. 1988	Well-trained col- legiate swimmers (10 M) Crossover design	250 mg/kg bicarbonate, sodium chloride placebo or control, 1 hr prerace	5 × 100 yd interval swim set with ~2 min rest between sprints (training simulation)	Yes	Faster times in 4th and 5th swim with bicarbonate trials ($p < .05$). Supplementation also associated with higher post-race blood lactate concentrations.
Pierce et al. 1992	Well-trained col- legiate swimmers (7 M) Crossover design	200 mg/kg bicarbonate, sodium chloride placebo, or control, 1 hr prerace	100 freestyle swim and 2 × 200 yd swims in preferred stroke, with recovery interval of 20 min between each race (simulation of competi- tion program)	No	No difference in swim times between trials.
McNaugh- ton and Cedaro 1991	Highly trained rowers (5M) Crossover design	300 mg/kg bicarbonate prerace	6 min maximal effort on rowing ergometer	Yes	Increased work and distance rowed (1,861 m vs. 1,813 m) with bicarbonate ($p < .05$). Increased lactate levels.
Mero et al. 2004	National-level swim- mers (8 M + 8 F) Crossover design, 30 day washout	300 mg/kg bicarbonate or gelatin placebo, 2 hr prerace (6 days at 20 g/day creatine also taken before bicarb trial)	2 × 100 m swims with 10 m passive recovery	Perhaps	Faster time for second swim with creatine/bicarb trial than with placebo: 1 s reduction in performance from first swim in placebo compared with 0.1 s drop-off in supplement trial ($p < .05$). Although study shows favorable outcome of supplement mixture, it is unable to indicate individual effect of bicarbonate.
Bicarbonate and citrate		**Chronic supplementation protocol for training**			**There is new evidence that repeated use of bicarbonate loading before interval training sessions may enhance training adaptations and improve performance of sustained high-intensity exercise, at least in moderately trained individuals. It may also assist the athlete to train harder. Further research is needed to confirm these findings, especially for highly trained atheletes.**

406

Study	Subjects and design	Supplementation protocol	Protocol/tests	Relevance to racing	Comments
Edge at al. 2006	Moderately trained (16 F) Experimental-placebo design	8 wks at 400 mg/kg sodium bicarbonate in a split dose 90 min and 30 min before interval training Periodized interval training undertaken 3 d/wk: 2 min intervals with 1 min recovery, with 6 to 12 intervals completed at 140-170% of intensity at lactate threshold Both groups completed the same training load	0 and 8 wks (cycle): • $\dot{V}O_2$peak • lactate threshold • time to exhaustion at 100% pre-trial $\dot{V}O_2$peak	Yes	Both groups increased their $\dot{V}O_2$peak by similar amounts as a result of the 8 wk interval training. Both groups also increased their muscle buffering capacity. This increase in muscle buffering capacity was related to pre-training capacity rather than the treatment (subjects with lower pre-training muscle buffering capacity achieved greater increases as a result of training). Although both groups showed an increase in lactate threshold and time to exhaustion at $\dot{V}O_2$peak, the improvements were greater in the bicarbonate group. The authors speculated that training intensity rather than accumulation of H^+ ions is responsible for increasing muscle buffering capacity. Furthermore, inducing alkalosis during exercise may enhance muscle adaptations by reducing the damage to mitochondria or protein synthesis.

Creatine

Acute (loading) supplementation protocol with relevance to racing

Any improvements in performance of single sprint swim appear to be too small to detect with conventional studies. May be useful for longer events and for rowing and kayaking races. More sport-specific studies are needed using highly trained athletes.

Study	Subjects and design	Supplementation protocol	Protocol/tests	Relevance to racing	Comments
Burke, Pyne, et al. 1996	Highly trained internationally competitive swimmers (32, M + F) Experimental-placebo design	5 days at 20 g/day creatine or placebo	Tests undertaken at baseline and after loading: • Swim races • 25 m • 50 m • 100 m • 10 s maximal test on cycle ergometer	No No No No	No significant differences between group means for sprint swim times or for 10 s cycle ergometer performance.
Mujika et al. 1996	Highly trained internationally competitive swimmers (32, M + F) Experimental-placebo design	5 days at 20 g/day creatine or placebo	Tests undertaken at baseline and after loading: • Swim races • 25 m • 50 m • 100 m	No No No	No significant performance changes in either group. Significant increase in BM in creatine group.
Grindstaff et al. 1997	Adolescent trained swimmers (18, M + F) Experimental-placebo design	9 days at 20 g/day creatine or placebo	Tests undertaken at baseline and after loading: • 3 × 100 m swim races • 3 × 20 s arm ergometer tests	Yes Perhaps	Improved performance after supplementation in creatine group for first and second swim races, and a trend to better cumulative swim time, compared with post-supplementation swim performance in the placebo group. A trend to greater increase work in the creatine group in post-supplementation arm ergometer tests, especially for the first test.

(continued)

Table 6.e (continued)

Study	Participants	Supplement protocol	Exercise protocol	Enhanced performance	Comments
Peyrebrune et al. 1998	Highly trained competitive swimmers (14 M) Experimental–placebo design	5 days at 9 g/day creatine or placebo	Tests undertaken at baseline and after loading; • 1 × 50 yd maximal swim	No	No difference in performance of single sprint.
McNaughton et al. 1998	Highly trained competitive surf ski and white-water kayak paddlers (16 M) Experimental–placebo trial	5 days at 20 g/day creatine or placebo	Tests undertaken at baseline and after loading; • 90 s, 150 s, and 300 s kayak ergometer tests	Yes	Significant increase in BM with creatine. Participants completed significantly more work in all tests.
Rossiter et al. 1996	Club-level rowers (38, M + F) Experimental–placebo design	5 days at 0.25 g/kg BM per day creatine or placebo	Tests undertaken at baseline and after loading; • 1,000 m ergometer row	Perhaps	Trend to improved 100 m rowing performance by ~1% ($p = .088$) in creatine group but no change in placebo group.
Lawrence et al. 1997	Trained rowers (M + F) Experimental–placebo design	5 days at 0.6 g/kg BM/day creatine or placebo	Tests undertaken at baseline and after loading; • 2,500 m ergometer row	Yes	Creatine supplemented group improved ergometer performance by 3.4 s ($p < .05$). Speculation that enhancement of early stage of row resulted from enhanced ATP resynthesis from CrP system, whereas later improvements may have been attributable to enhanced buffering of hydrogen ions produced by anaerobic glycolysis.
Syrotuik et al. 2001	Well-trained collegiate rowers (12 M + 10 F) Experimental–placebo design	5 days at 0.3 g/kg BM/day creatine or placebo	Tests undertaken at baseline and after loading; • 2,000 m ergometer row	No	No difference in performances after creatine or placebo supplementation. Creatine group gained 0.7 kg BM.
Chwalbinska-Moneta 2003	Highly trained elite rowers (n = 16 M) Experimental–placebo design	5 days at 20 g/day creatine or placebo	Tests undertaken at baseline and after loading; • Rowing to exhaustion at 7 W/kg	Yes	Increase in rowing time to exhaustion by 12.1 s in creatine group ($p <.05$) but only by 2.4 s (NS) in placebo group. Incremental test protocol on rowing ergometer also showed a beneficial shift in relationship between blood lactate and work intensity in creatine group following treatment.
Mendes et al. 2004	Highly trained competitive swimmers (12 M + 6 F) Experimental–placebo design	8 days at 20 g/day creatine or placebo (each 5 g dose taken with 20 g carbohydrate)	Tests undertaken at baseline and after loading; • 50 m maximal swim • 100 m maximal swim	No No	Study undertaken during period of high volume training. Creatine supplementation associated with weight gain of ~1.3 kg, while no change was seen in placebo group. No difference in performance of 50 m and 100 m swims between groups or over time

Reference	Subjects/Design	Supplementation	Tests		Results/Comments
Anomasiri et al. 2004	Trained swimmers (38M) Experimental–placebo design	5 days at 10 g/day creatine or placebo	Tests undertaken at baseline and after loading: • 400 m maximal swim • 30 s Wingate cycle test	Perhaps Perhaps	Creatine supplementation associated with weight gain of ~0.7 kg, while smaller change was seen in placebo group. Both groups achieved faster 400 m swim time after supplementation (p < .05) but enhancement with creatine group was numerically greater. In addition, the creatine group recorded a faster time over the last 50 m of this swim (p < .05). Both groups increased their anaerobic capacity (mean power) on Wingate test, but creatine group also improved their fatigue index (p < .05) following supplementation.
Creatine		**Acute supplementation protocol with relevance to interval training**			**Main benefit of creatine loading appears to be in enhancing response to repeated high-intensity efforts with short recovery—e.g., interval and resistance training.**
Peyrebrune et al. 1998	Highly trained competitive swimmers (14 M) Experimental–placebo design	5 days at 9 g/day creatine or placebo	Tests undertaken at baseline and after loading: • 8 × 50 yd maximal swims	Yes	Reduced total sprint time for 8 × 50 yd swims in creatine group resulting from a smaller percentage decline in performance times over interval set.
Theodorou et al. 1999	Highly trained competitive swimmers (22, M + F) Pre- and posttest in all swimmers (order effect)	4 days at 25 g/day creatine or placebo	Tests undertaken at baseline and after loading: • Intervals swimming sets (5-10 repeats on 1 or 2 min depending on swimmer's usual event)	Yes	Improvement of 1.5% in mean swim time in interval set. Significant increase in BM after creatine supplementation. Order effect dismissed by failure to improve further with longer-term study.
Syrotuik et al. 2001	Well-trained collegiate rowers (12 M + 10 F) Experimental–placebo design	5 days at 0.3 g/kg BM/day creatine or placebo	Tests undertaken at baseline and after loading: • Repeated power interval (6 × 250 m) • Strength tests: 3 sets × 10 RM with 2 min recovery	No No	No difference in performances after creatine or placebo supplementation. Creatine group gained 0.7 kg BM.
Mero et al. 2004	National-level swimmers (8 M + 8 F) Crossover design 30-day washout	6 days at 20 g/day creatine or placebo (acute bicarbonate loading also undertaken on morning of creatine trial)	2 × 100 m swims with 10 m passive recovery	Yes (?)	Faster time for second swim with creatine and bicarb trial than with placebo: 1 s reduction in performance from first swim in placebo compared with 0.1 s drop-off in supplement trial (p < .05). Study unable to indicate individual effect of creatine.

(continued)

Table 6.e (continued)

Study	Participants	Supplement protocol	Exercise protocol	Enhanced performance	Comments
Mendes et al. 2004	Highly trained competitive swimmers (12 M + 6 F) Experimental–placebo design	8 days at 20 g/day creatine or placebo (each 5 g dose taken with 20 g carbohydrate)	Tests undertaken at baseline and after loading: • 3 × (3 × 50 m) swims with 30 s rest between intervals and 150 s rest between sets	No	Study undertaken during period of high-volume training. Creatine supplementation associated with weight gain of ~1.3 kg, while no change was seen in placebo group. No difference in performance of 50 m and 100 m swims between groups or over time.
Creatine		**Chronic supplementation protocol for enhanced training adaptations and long-term performance enhancement**			**More studies are needed with highly trained athletes to show clear benefits from enhanced training being translated into superior competition performance.**
Thompson et al. 1996	Well-trained collegiate swimmers (10 F) Experimental–placebo design	6 weeks at 2 g/day creatine or placebo (slow loading dose)	Tests undertaken at baseline and after 6 weeks: • Resistance calf exercise to fatigue • 100 m and 400 m swim	No	No differential effect on calf exercise duration or swim time between groups after 6 weeks of training and supplementation protocol.
Leenders et al. 1999	Well-trained collegiate swimmers (32, M + F) Experimental–placebo design	6 days at 20 g/day (loading) + 8 days at 10 g/day (maintenance) creatine or placebo	Tests undertaken at baseline and after 14 days: • 6 × 50 m swims • 10 × 25 yd swims	Yes for M No for F	14 days of creatine supplementation was associated with improvement in mean overall swimming velocity in M swimmers in the 6 × 50 m intervals set (p = .02). Body composition not changed with creatine supplementation.
Theodorou et al. 1999	Highly trained competitive swimmers (22, M + F) Pre- and posttest in all swimmers (order effect)	8 weeks at 5 g/day creatine or placebo (maintenance dose following initial loading dose)	Tests undertaken at baseline and after 8 weeks: • Interval session according to usual stroke/event	No	No difference between groups or across time in mean interval swim times after 8 weeks of supplementation and training.
Dawson et al. 2002	Adolescent trained swimmers (10 M + 10 F) Experimental–placebo design	5 days at 20 g/day creatine or placebo (loading) + 22 days at 5 g/day (maintenance)	Tests undertaken at baseline and after 28 days: • 50 m, 100 m hand-timed swims with long recovery interval • 2 × swim bench test for 30 s with long recovery interval	No Yes	No significant improvement in swimming performance for creatine or placebo group after 4 weeks of supplementation and training. Swim bench test showed 7.5% increase in anaerobic work during both 30 s trials in creatine group after 4 weeks (p <.05) but not in placebo group. No change in BM over period in either group.

Reference / Design	Supplementation protocol	Tests	Benefit	Findings
Selsby et al. 2003	Well-trained collegiate swimmers (8 M + 7 F) Experimental–placebo design	5 days at 0.3 g/kg BM/day (loading) + 9 days at 2.2 g/day (maintenance dose) creatine or placebo	Tests undertaken at baseline and after 14 days: • 50 yd and 100 yd swim	Yes	Improvement in creatine group: 2% improvement for the 100 yd swim ($p < .01$) and 1% improvement for 50 yd swim (NS). No improvement seen in the placebo group.
Syrotuik et al. 2001	Well-trained collegiate rowers (12 M + 10 F) Experimental–placebo design	22 days at 0.03 g/kg BM/day creatine or placebo (maintenance dose) taken after loading phase	Tests undertaken at baseline and after 22 days: • 2,000 m rowing ergometer • Repeated power interval (6 × 250 m) • Strength tests: 3 sets × 10 RM with 2 min recovery • $\dot{V}O_2$max	No No No No	No difference between groups in the training volume undertaken during 4 weeks; therefore, creatine supplement does not allow a greater training stimulus. Training caused an enhancement of 2,000 m rowing performance and repeated power intervals in both groups; no additional effect of creatine.
Theodorou et al. 2005	Highly trained, competitive swimmers (6 M + 4 W) Experimental–placebo design	4 days at 25 g/day creatine (5 split doses each day) with or without 100 g CHO with each dose Squad swimming training	Tests undertaken: 2 × baseline + postcreatine + further 2 weeks + 4 weeks Strength tests: 3 sets • 10 × 50 m intervals on 60 s cycle (n = 8) or • 8 × 100 m intervals on 120 m cycle	Not directly tested	Weight gain of 0.6 kg in creatine only group and 1.0 kg in creatine + CHO group. All swimmers increased swim velocity with creatine loading and continued to improve swimming up to 4 weeks postsupplementation. Authors recognized small sample size and lack of placebo group for creatine; study only tested the additional effect of adding CHO to creatine intake rather than creatine per se. CHO group showed greater weight increase (CHO loading or increase in energy balance with additional 8 MJ/day intake?) and increased risk of gastrointestinal discomfort.
Peyrebrune et al. 2005	Highly trained, competitive swimmers Experimental–placebo design	Both groups: 5 days at 20 g/day (acute loading) at baseline and precompetition after 22-27 weeks Intermediate period: 22-27 weeks at 3 g/day or placebo Squad swimming training	Tests undertaken at baseline, 1 week, and ~27 weeks • 8 × 50 yd intervals Tests undertaken at end of ~27 weeks • Competition performance compared with previous personal best time	Not directly tested Perhaps	Interval swimming improved by acute supplementation in both groups (no control group). This study directly compared the effect of maintenance following acute loading on long-term performance. Competition times in best event improved by ~1.9% vs. 0.86% (short-course swimming for creatine and placebo group) and ~0.14% vs. −0.49% (long-course swimming). No significant differences between groups; however, practical significance curves showed a 90% probability of any improvement with creatine maintenance, 64% of this improvement being >1% and 26% of this improvement being >2%. Therefore, performance enhancement may be worthwhile in real world.

M = male; F = female; BM = body mass; RM = maximal repetition; CrP = creatine phosphate; ATP = adenosine triphosphate; NS = not significant.

Table 6.f Relevant Studies of Supplements With Undetermined or Unlikely Benefit to Swimmers and Rowers

Study	Participants	Supplement protocol	Exercise protocol	Enhanced performance	Comments
Bovine colostrum		Chronic supplementation protocol			**Potential value presently undetermined. No mechanisms identified to explain any potential benefits. Expense of supplement in moderate to large doses ($US40 per week) warrants additional supportive research before it can be recommended. Emerging evidence that benefits might be seen at lower doses is also of interest.**
Brinkworth et al. 2002	Highly trained competitive rowers (13 F) (colostrum = 6; placebo = 7) Experimental–placebo design	9 weeks at 60 g/day of colostrum or placebo (whey protein) 18 hr/week rowing + 3/week resistance training	Tests at baseline and 9 weeks: 2 × incremental rowing tests with 15 min recovery interval (each = 3 × 4 min submaximal workloads + 4 min maximal effort)	No	Rowing performance increased by week 9 in both groups. No difference between groups at week 9 for either maximal rowing performance. Higher value for index of blood buffering capacity at week 9 in colostrum group.
Branched-chain amino acids (e.g., leucine)		Chronic supplementation protocol			**Inconclusive work on effect of supplementation with BCAA or individual amino acids such as leucine. The positive results from studies need to be compared with the intake of protein per se.**
Crowe et al. 2005	Outrigger canoeists (19 F, 3 M) Experimental–placebo design	6 weeks at 45 mg·kg^{-1}·day^{-1} leucine ~8 hr/week outrigger training + cross-training	Tests at baseline and 6 weeks: • Rowing at 70-75% $\dot{V}O_2$max to exhaustion • 10 s upper-body power test (arm cranking)	Yes Yes	Both groups increased total work done in upper-body test with no difference between groups; leucine group showed greater increase in peak power ($p < .05$). Significant increase in rowing time to exhaustion in leucine group over 6 weeks; not seen in placebo group. Effect could not be attributed to "central fatigue" mechanism along with BCAA supplementation hypothesis.
β-Hydroxy β-methylbutyrate		Chronic supplementation protocol			**Potential value in reducing muscle damage and enhancing recovery from resistance training is presently undetermined. The overall literature involving resistance training is equivocal. Some studies suggest that benefits are limited to novice trainers or to the initial response to an increase in training load. Further studies are required in highly trained athletes to support any benefits.**
Slater et al. 2001	Highly trained competitive rowers (and water polo players) (27 M) Experimental–placebo design	6 weeks at 3 g/day conventional or time-release HMB or placebo Resistance training 3/week + sport-related training Nutritional advice + carbohydrate and protein supplement	Tests at baseline, 3 weeks, and 6 weeks for 3 RM: • Bench press • Leg press • Chin-ups	No No No	All groups increased strength and lean BM (assessed by DEXA), in response to training and dietary intervention, with no differences in response between groups. No differences between groups of urinary 3-methyl histidine or plasma creatine kinase concentrations, crude markers of muscle breakdown and damage

Supplement / Study	Subjects & Design	Protocol	Tests	Ergogenic?	Findings
Carnitine		Chronic supplementation protocol			**Few studies on trained athletes and performance changes, especially in swimming or rowing. Studies of chronic carnitine intake fail to show increase in muscle carnitine levels following supplementation; therefore, hard to imagine changes in metabolic function (e.g., fatty acid transport into mitochondria or acetyl carnitine "sink").**
Trappe et al. 1994	Highly trained collegiate swimmers (20 M) Experimental–placebo design	7 days at 4 g/day HMB or placebo	Tests at baseline and at 7 days: • 5 × 100 yd swims	No	No difference in performance times between trials or between groups.
Ribose		Chronic supplementation protocol			**Literature fails to show consistent benefits to performance of high-intensity exercise following ribose supplementation. Expense of ribose (~US$40/week) warrants additional supportive research before it can be recommended.**
Dunne et al. 2006	Collegiate rowers, including novice and experienced rowers (n = 31 F) Experimental–placebo design	10 weeks at 20 g per day (split dose before and after training) 5-6 days/week at rowing, resistance training and running	Tests at 0 and 8 weeks: • 2,000 m ergometer test	No	Placebo group, receiving low-dose dextrose pre- and posttraining, had larger enhancement of 2,000 m rowing ergometer tests than ribose group (15.2 vs. 5.2 s, $p = .03$).
Pyruvate		Chronic supplementation protocol			**No evidence that pyruvate supplementation enhances performance of sustained high-intensity exercise.**
Ebersole et al. 2000	Well-trained collegiate rowers (9 M + 9 F) Experimental–placebo design	14 days at 8.1 g/day pyruvate or placebo	Tests at baseline and at 14 days: 3 bouts of cycling to exhaustion at workload allowing 4-6 min of work (2 on one day and 3rd on following day): • Critical power calculated from relationship between work limit and time limit	No	No difference in critical power between groups and over time.

(continued)

Table 6.f (continued)

Study	Participants	Supplement protocol	Exercise protocol	Enhanced performance	Comments
Magnesium-aspartate		**Protocol**			**No evidence that exercise causes magnesium deficiency or that magnesium supplementation enhances performance.**
Ruddel et al. 1990	Adolescent trained swimmers (14 M + 10 F) Experimental–placebo design	3 months at 20 mmol/day magnesium aspartate or placebo	Tests at baseline and at 3 months: • 100 m, 400 m swim • Bike ergometer tests: PWC170 and $\dot{V}O_2$max	No	Magnesium supplementation led to increase in magnesium concentration in serum but not red blood cells. No change in any performance parameter between groups. Some reports of gastrointestinal disturbances (diarrhea) in supplemented group.
Vitamin E		**Chronic supplementation protocol**			**No evidence that vitamin E supplementation enhances performance.**
Sharman et al. 1971	Adolescent trained swimmers (26 M) Experimental–placebo design	6 weeks at 400 mg/day α-tocopherol or placebo	Tests at baseline and at 6 weeks: • 1 mile run • 400 m swim • Pull-ups, press-ups, sit-ups • Cardiorespiratory function tests	No	Training effects on performance and functional measures but no differences between response of treatment and placebo group.
Sharman et al. 1976	Adolescent trained swimmers (27, M + F) Experimental–placebo design	6 weeks at 400 mg/day α-tocopherol or placebo	Tests at baseline and 6 weeks: • 400 m swim • Pull-ups, press-ups, sit-ups • Cardiorespiratory function tests	No	Training effects on performance and functional measures but no differences between response of treatment and placebo group.
Lawrence, Bower, et al. 1975	Adolescent trained swimmers (48, M + F) Experimental–placebo design	6 months at 900 IU/day α-tocopherol or placebo	Tests at baseline at 1, 2, 5, and 6 months 10 or 5 × 100 yd swim with 10 s rest interval	No	Training improved times in both groups to similar extent. No difference in postswim lactate concentrations.

Reference	Subjects/Design	Supplementation protocol	Tests	Sig.	Findings
Talbot and Jamieson 1977	Adolescent and adult well-trained swimmers (25 F + 20 M) Partial crossover design	5 weeks at 400 IU/day or 1,600 IU/day α-tocopherol or placebo	Tests at baseline and after 5 and 10 weeks: • 100 m, 400 m swim	No	No difference in performance between treatments; 64% of swimmers who had previously been taking vitamin E voluntarily ceased treatment after study because of findings that there was no performance change with or without treatment.
Vitamin B$_6$ (pyridoxine)		Chronic supplementation protocol			**No evidence that vitamin B$_6$ supplementation enhances performance.**
Lawrence, Smith, et al. 1975	Adolescent trained swimmers (32 M + 15 F) Experimental–placebo design	6 months at 17 mg/day pyridoxine Cl or placebo	Tests at baseline and at 1, 2, 5, and 6 months • 10 or 5 yd × 100 yd swim with 10 s rest interval	No	Training improved times in both groups to similar extent. Postswim lactate concentrations higher in pyridoxine group.
Bee pollen		Chronic supplementation protocol			**No evidence that bee pollen supplementation enhances performance.**
Maughan and Evans 1982	Adolescent trained swimmers (16 M + 4 F) Experimental–placebo design	6 weeks at 2-4/day Pollitabs (bee pollen + vitamin B, C, E in undeclared amounts) or placebo	Tests at baseline and at 6 weeks: • Handgrip strength • Quadriceps isometric strength and endurance • $\dot{V}O_2$max • Vital capacity and forced expiratory volume	No	Some small training induced changes over the 6-week period; however, no differences in response of pollen and placebo group. Pollen group had fewer missed days of training than placebo group because of upper respiratory tract infections (4 vs. 27 days) but this finding was not able to be statistically evaluated.
Velvet antler		Chronic supplementation protocol			**Velvet antler from various deer and elk species has been promoted in Asian medicine, and more recently to athletes, with claims of enhanced recovery and performance and stimulation of gonadal hormones. There is little evidence to support these claims.**
Syrotuik et al. 2005	Collegiate rowers (25 M + 21 F) Experimental–placebo design	10 weeks at 560 g/day elk velvet antler Training at 3/week strength and 3/week endurance sessions	Tests at baseline and 5 and 10 weeks • 2,000 m ergometer rowing • 1RM leg press • 1RM bench press	No No No	Both groups of males and female rowers improved rowing performance and strength and reduced body fat with training, but these was no difference between the deer velvet and placebo groups. There were also no differences in resting or exercise-stimulated concentrations of testosterone, cortisol, and growth hormone as a result of supplementation.

BCAA = branched-chain amino acid; HMB = β-hydroxy β-methylbutyrate; RM = repetition maximum; DEXA = duel energy X-ray absorptiometry; RM = repetition maximum; PWC170 = Physical Work Capacity at heartrate 170.

Table 6.g Situations in Sports With Varying Goals for Recovery

Moderate to severe dehydration requiring aggressive rehydration	Moderate to severe muscle glycogen depletion requiring aggressive refueling	Desire for gain of muscle size and strength (hypertrophy)	Need for general protein recovery and adaptation	Energy requirements	Examples in sport
+	+	+	+	High	Australian football games and training sessions; rugby union and league games and training sessions; rowing training sessions
+	+	+	+	Restricted	Training sessions and games for Australian rules and rugby players requiring loss of body fat; training sessions for rowers requiring loss of body fat (e.g., lightweight and females)
-	+	+	+	High	Swimming and water polo workouts; prolonged resistance workouts in air-conditioned gym
-	+	+	+	Restricted	Workouts for swimmers and water polo players undertaking loss of body fat (especially females)
+	-	+	+	High	Workouts for sprinters or male gymnasts in hot weather
+	-	+	+	Restricted	Workouts for freestyle skiers requiring high power-to-weight ratio and loss of body fat
-	-	+	+	High	Workouts for male gymnasts in air-conditioned gym
+	+	-	+	High	Workouts or races for endurance athletes (e.g., cyclists, distance runners, triathletes)
+	+	-	+	Restricted	Workouts for female endurance athletes (cyclists, distance runners, triathletes) especially during loss of body fat or lightweight rowers during "weight-making" periods
-	+	-	+	High	Middle and distance swim race for males
-	+	-	+	Restricted	Middle and distance race for females in taper
+	-	-	+	High	Workouts or races in motor sports
+	-	-	+	Restricted	Skilled-based training sessions (e.g., archery) in a hot environment
-	-	-	+	Restricted	Skill-based training sessions (e.g., archery, female gymnastics) in a cool environment

+ = presence of this factor; − = absence of this factor

Table 6.h Guidelines for Postexercise Recovery, Adapted From the Australian Institute of Sport Guidelines, Prepared by the Department of Sports Nutrition

A. Recovery from key training or competition sessions based on endurance or "quality" work	• Effective refueling begins only after a substantial amount of carbohydrate has been consumed. When there is less than 8 hr between workouts or events that deplete glycogen stores, maximize effective recovery time by eating a high-carbohydrate meal or snack within 30 min of completing each session. Be organized to have suitable food and drinks available—at the exercise venue if necessary.
	• Consume foods and drinks providing 1 g of carbohydrate per kg BM immediately after exercise, and repeat after an hour or until normal meal patterns are resumed (see sections A–E). Recovery snacks and meals should contribute toward a daily carbohydrate total of 7-12 g per kg BM. Total carbohydrate intake should be individualized to your exercise program and energy budget. Seek expert advice from a sports dietitian, especially if you are trying to restrict total energy intake.
	• Consuming protein within recovery snacks and meals may enhance the synthesis of new proteins underpinning adaptations to the workout as well as help to meet any increase in protein requirements related to exercise. The intake of a protein source providing 3-6 g of essential amino acids (~10-20 g of protein from a high-quality source) has a substantial effect on net protein synthesis. Most meals within a well-chosen diet will meet this target. Examples of snacks that provide a good source of carbohydrate and protein include breakfast cereal and milk, flavored milk drinks, and specially formulated sport bars and liquid meal supplements (see section E).
	• Compact forms of carbohydrate are valuable when fuel needs are high and intake is limited by a suppressed appetite or gastric discomfort. Examples include low-fiber versions of carbohydrate-rich foods, sugar-rich foods and drinks, and special sport supplements such as sport bars.
	• Carbohydrate-containing fluids are appealing when one is fatigued or dehydrated. These include sport drinks, soft drinks and juices, commercial liquid meal supplements, milk shakes, and fruit smoothies.
	• Low glycemic index carbohydrate foods such as lentils and legumes may be less suitable for speedy glycogen recovery and should not be the principal carbohydrate source in recovery meals. This is generally not a problem because typical Western diets are based on carbohydrate-rich foods of moderate and high glycemic index.
	• A pattern of small, frequent meals may achieve high carbohydrate intakes without the discomfort of overeating. However, you should organize a routine of meals and snacks to suit individual preferences, timetable, appetite, and comfort. In long-term recovery (24 hr), as long as enough carbohydrate is consumed, it doesn't appear to matter how intake is spaced throughout the day. An increased frequency of intake of carbohydrate (e.g., snacks every 30-60 min) may be useful during the first hours of recovery.
	• When stomach comfort or total energy requirements limit total food intake, don't consume high-fat foods and excessive amounts of protein at the expense of carbohydrate choices.
	• Choose nutritious carbohydrate foods and drinks that contain other nutrients, such as vitamins and minerals. These nutrients are important in the overall diet but may also assist other postexercise recovery processes. Future research may show that intake early after exercise could enhance other activities of repair and rebuilding, as well as the immune system.
	• Avoid excessive intake of alcohol during the recovery from exercise. Alcohol may directly impair refueling and recovery processes, but its main effect is indirect. If you are intoxicated, you are unlikely to follow sound nutritional practices and are more likely to undertake risky behavior with a high risk of accidents.
	• Drink fluids to restore fluid balance. When your total fluid deficit (sweat losses minus fluid intake during the workout) exceeds 2% of body mass, implement a special hydration plan (see Section D:"Special comments for the dehydrated athlete").

(continued)

Table 6.h (continued)

B. Recovery from key resistance training workouts	**Guidelines for preexercise recovery strategies** • Consume a source of amino acids before the session—the intake of 3-6 g essential amino acids (~10-20 g of a high-quality protein) enhances protein recovery after the workout. Protein-rich foods should be consumed 30-60 min before the session to allow for digestion to take place. Consume carbohydrate at the same time to enhance the protein response; an intake >1 g per kg BM will provide a substantial "top up" of fuel stores and avoid the risk of rebound hypoglycemia in susceptible athletes. It may not always be practical to consume foods before a heavy workout; nutrient-rich drinks such as liquid meal supplements, fruit smoothies, or sport bars provide a more compact alternative (see Section E for ideas). **Guidelines for postexercise recovery strategies** • Consume a source of amino acids within the hour after the session—the intake of 3-6 g amino acids (~10-20 g of a high-quality protein) enhances protein recovery after the workout. Carbohydrate consumed at the same time may enhance the protein response and promotes rapid recovery of muscle glycogen stores (see section E for protein–carbohydrate recovery snacks and light meals that can be consumed until normal meal patterns are resumed). • When strength training sessions are prolonged, or undertaken in conjunction with an aerobic exercise session, add refueling strategies to recovery plans (see Section A: Recovery from an endurance workout). • Avoid the intake of excessive amounts of alcohol during the hours following a strength workout, because alcohol may impair protein synthesis. A sensible approach to alcohol intake is beneficial for all aspects of postexercise recovery. • Ensure that your daily diet provides adequate energy and protein intake to meet goals for gain of muscle mass. Daily maximum protein needs are likely to be ~1.5-2.0 g per kg BM. Intakes greater than this are not likely to confer any additional benefits for muscle gain.
C. Special comments for the athlete with an energy-restricted diet	• Pre- or postexercise recovery snacks should not contribute additional energy to a restricted energy budget. Rather, when rapid recovery is desirable, change the timing of your existing meal schedule to allow for immediate intake after exercise sessions. One option is to reschedule training sessions or meals to eat an existing meal as soon as possible after the workout. Where this is not practical, take a small snack from within your usual meal plan to consume immediately after training or as a preresistance training snack and then consume the remainder of the meal at the usual time (e.g. save the fruit and flavored yogurt usually consumed as dessert for a recovery snack). • Make up recovery snacks from foods and drinks that can also contribute to overall nutrient intake goals. Nutrient-rich choices (e.g., fruit, flavored milk drinks and dairy foods, sandwiches with meat and salad fillings) are more valuable than lower-nutrient choices (e.g., confectionery, soft drink, bread with jam or honey). • Make meals and snacks filling by choosing foods with a high-fiber content (e.g., fresh fruit rather than juice), high volume and low energy density (e.g., salad fillings added to sandwiches), or low glycemic index (e.g., rolled oat cereals rather than cornflakes). The addition of protein to meals and snacks (e.g., yoghurt with fruit, meat or cheese in a sandwich) also improves satiety. Follow guidelines for low-fat eating. • Recognize that an energy-restricted budget may not cover the guidelines for optimal intakes of some macronutrients (e.g., carbohydrate for optimal daily glycogen synthesis). See a sports dietitian for advice to balance the priority of recovery needs and physique goals and to organize meal plans that optimize nutrient intake within your energy budget. You may need to periodize your nutritional goals—that is, restrict energy during periods suitable for loss of body fat while liberalizing energy and carbohydrate intake to promote better fueling and recovery for key sessions or competition.

D. Special comments for the dehydrated athlete	• A fluid deficit needs to be corrected because it will impair the outcomes of subsequent exercise sessions. However, moderate to severe fluid deficits can also affect recovery, because the increased risk of gastrointestinal upset and discomfort can limit your ability to consume substantial amounts of nutrients. Attack hydration needs as an immediate priority. You may need to consume dilute fluids before moving on to more complex drinks and foods.
	• Do not rely on thirst or opportunity to dictate fluid needs. A "hit and miss" approach may be acceptable when fluid deficits are 1 L or less, but when fluid losses are greater, a fluid plan is required.
	• Monitor changes in body mass over the session to evaluate the success of drinking strategies during exercise and the residual fluid deficit that must now be replaced (1 kg = ~1 L of fluid). Because fluid losses will continue during the recovery period via urine losses and ongoing sweating, you will need to consume additional fluid to counter this. Typically, you will need to drink a volume equal to ~125-150% of the postexercise fluid deficit over the next 2-4 hr to fully restore fluid balance.
	• Ensure an adequate supply of palatable drinks. This may be difficult when you are at a remote competition venue or traveling in a country where bottled water must be consumed.
	• Encourage fluid intake by making flavored fluids available. Because most people prefer sweet-tasting drinks, these drinks are likely to increase voluntary intake of such fluids. Keep drinks at a refreshing temperature to encourage greater intake. Cool drinks (10-15°C) are preferred in most situations. Ice-cold fluids (0-5°C) may seem ideal when the conditions are hot; however, such cold fluid is often challenging to drink quickly or in large volumes.
	• Choose fluids that can meet a range of recovery goals simultaneously (e.g., sport drinks provide carbohydrate and fluid, whereas liquid meals provide carbohydrate, protein, fluid, and micronutrients).
	• When the fluid deficit is moderate to large (e.g., >2 L), minimize urine losses and maximize the retention of fluids by actively replacing the sodium lost in sweat. A high-sodium beverage such as an oral hydration solution (50-90 mmol or 2-5 g of salt per liter) or salt added to postexercise meals and consumed with substantial volumes of fluid will replace both fluid and sodium. Dietary strategies that minimize urine losses during the rehydration period not only enhance the speed of regaining fluid balance but also help the athlete to achieve better-quality rest or sleep without frequent disturbances related to having to get up to urinate.
	• Be aware that "urine checks" over the first hours of rehydration can provide false readings. Athletes are often educated that the production of "copious amounts of clear urine" is a sign of good hydration status. Urine color and measurements of urinary specific gravity or osmolality provide a reliable indicator of hydration status over the long term (e.g., morning urine samples). However, during the period of fluid replacement immediately following dehydration, mismatch of fluid and sodium replacement can mean that large amounts of dilute urine are produced despite the continuing existence of substantial fluid deficits.
	• Value fluids that are well liked. Caffeine-containing fluids (e.g., cola drinks, tea, coffee, and energy drinks) are generally not considered to be ideal rehydration beverages because caffeine may increase urine losses. However, the diuretic effect of caffeine is overstated in habitual caffeine drinkers. Consider that the greater voluntary consumption of favorite beverages such as cola drinks may lead to better hydration status even if these drinks are associated with a slightly greater urine production.
	• Avoid excessive alcohol intake. Alcohol also causes an increase in urine losses, and drinks containing significant amounts of alcohol (4% or more of volume) are not considered ideal rehydration beverages. Nevertheless, remember that the main effect of alcohol on recovery is indirect. If you are intoxicated, you are unlikely to follow sound nutritional practices and are more likely to undertake high-risk behavior.
	• Where possible, avoid postexercise activities that exacerbate sweat losses—for example, long exposure to hot spas, saunas, or sun.

(continued)

Table 6.h (continued)

E. Putting it together—ideas for recovery snacks	Use this guide to consume snacks or light meals providing at least 1 g of carbohydrate per kg of BM. This will ensure speedy recovery of glycogen stores (postexercise recovery) or allow you to "top up" fuel stores before a workout (preexercise snack). In the case of postexercise recovery, this strategy should be repeated after 1-2 hr or until normal eating patterns have been resumed. The intake of protein (10-20 g) in conjunction with carbohydrate snacks will help to meet goals for enhanced net protein synthesis.

Carbohydrate-rich snacks (50 g CHO servings) providing at least 10 g of protein:

- 250-350 ml of liquid meal supplement
- 250-350 ml of milk shake or fruit smoothie
- 500 ml of flavored low-fat milk
- Many sport bars (check labels for protein and carbohydrate content)
- 60 g (1.5-2 cups) of breakfast cereal with 1/2 cup of milk
- 1 round of sandwiches including cheese, meat, or chicken filling, and 1 large piece of fruit or 300 ml of sport drink
- 1 cup of fruit salad with 200 g of fruit-flavored yogurt or custard
- 200 g of fruit-flavored yoghurt or 300 ml of flavored milk and 30-35 g cereal bar
- 2 crumpets or English muffins with thick spread of peanut butter or 2 slices of cheese
- 200 g (cup or small tin) of baked beans on 2 slices of toast
- 250 g (large) baked potato with cottage cheese or grated cheese filling
- 150 g thick crust pizza with meat, chicken, or seafood topping

50 g carbohydrate snacks:

- 800-1,000 ml of sport drink
- 800 ml of cordial
- 500 ml of fruit juice, soft drink, or flavored mineral water
- 60-70 g packet of jelly beans or jube sweets
- 2 sport gels
- 3 medium pieces of fruit or 2 bananas
- 1 round of thickly spread jam or honey
- 2 large (35 g) or 3 small (25 g) cereal bars
- 1 large chocolate bar (70-80 g)
- 3 thick rice cakes with jam or honey
- 2 crumpets or English muffins with vegemite
- 1 cup of thick vegetable soup with large bread roll
- Jaffle or toasted sandwich with banana filling
- 100 g (1 medium or 2 small) American muffin, fruit bun, or scone
- 250 g (1 cup) of creamed rice
- 250 g (large) baked potato with salsa filling
- 100 g pancakes (1-2 large) + 30 g of syrup

BM = body mass; CHO = carbohydrate.

Table 7.a Reported Dietary Intakes of Sprint and Jump Athletes: Training (Mean Daily Intake ± SD)

Publication	Sprint population	Survey method	Age (year)	BM (kg)	ENERGY		CHO			PROTEIN			FAT	
					MJ	kJ/kg	g	g/kg	%E	g	g/kg	%E	g	%E
MALES														
Short and Short 1983	U.S. collegiate track athletes (n = 10)	3-day food diary (household measures)			17.3		526		49	144		14	161	36
Short and Short 1983	U.S. collegiate track-and-field athletes (n = 7)	3-day food diary (household measures)			14.82		489		55	116		28	107	13
Sugiura et al. 1999	Japanese national team sprinters (n = 10)	3-day food diary (household measures)	22	67	11.09 ± 1.52	167 ± 33	340 ± 57	5.1 ± 1.0	54 ± 4	102 ± 20	1.5 ± 0.4	15 ± 2	90 ± 16	30 ± 3
Sugiura et al. 1999	Japanese national team jumpers (n = 4)	3-day food diary (household measures)	26	69	11.97 ± 1.16	174 ± 25	359 ± 51	5.2 ± 1.0	54 ± 5	104 ± 13	1.5 ± 0.1	15 ± 3	99 ± 15	31 ± 3
FEMALE														
Haymes and Spillman 1989	U.S. collegiate sprinters (n = 12)	3-day food diary (household measures)	20	55	8.43 ± 3.16	153	237	4.3	45 ± 12	80 ± 18	1.5	16	87	39 ± 9
Sugiura et al. 1999	Japanese national team sprinters (n = 11)	3-day food diary (household measures)	20	52	10.0 ± 2.2	192 ± 46	305 ± 79	5.8 ± 1.6	53 ± 5	89 ± 25	1.7 ± 0.5	15 ± 2	86 ± 17	33 ± 4
Sugiura et al. 1999	Japanese national team jumpers (n = 4)	3-day food diary (household measures)	21	54	8.28 ± 2.21	152 ± 37	244 ± 60	4.5 ± 1.0	51 ± 3	82 ± 33	1.5 ± 0.6	16 ± 2	72 ± 17	33 ± 2
Mullins et al. 2001	U.S. national-level heptathletes (n = 19)	4-day food diary (household measures)	26	67	9.90 ± 3.8	151 ± 67	339 ± 124	5.2 ± 2.2	57	95 ± 39	1.4 ± 0.6	16	71 ± 46	27

BM = body mass; CHO = carbohydrate; E = energy.

421

Table 7.b   Relevant Studies of Supplements With Likely Benefit to Sprint and Jump Performance

Study	Participants	Supplement protocol	Exercise protocol	Enhanced performance	Comments
Creatine		**Acute supplementation protocol with relevance to racing (i.e., single sprint)**			**Although there is some evidence that creatine supplementation can enhance the performance of a single sprint race, it is generally considered that these improvements are small and hard to detect with conventional studies. More sport-specific studies are needed using highly trained athletes.**
Bosco et al. 1997	Well-trained runners and jumpers (14 M) Experimental–placebo design	5 days at 20 g/day creatine Standardized training: 6/week at 2-3 hr/days	Treadmill sprint to exhaustion ~1 min	Yes	13% increase in time to exhaustion in creatine group following supplementation compared with baseline trial (67 vs. 59 s, $p < .05$), whereas no change seen in placebo group. Increase in postrun blood lactate after creatine supplementation ($p < .05$).
Skare et al. 2001	Competitive sprinters (18 M) Experimental–placebo design	5 days at 20 g/day creatine	100 m running sprint	Yes	Creatine supplementation was associated with a weight gain of 0.6 kg, but also an increase in running velocity in 100 m sprint after supplementation (sprint time = 11.59 vs. 11.68 s, post- vs. presupplementation, $p < .05$). No detectable changes in placebo group.
Creatine		**Acute supplementation with relevance to interval training**			**Main benefit of creatine loading appears to be in enhancing response to repeated high-intensity efforts with short recovery (e.g., interval and resistance training).**
Harris et al. 1993	Trained middle-distance runners (10 M) Experimental–placebo design	6 days at 30 g/day creatine	4 × 300 m running with 4 min recovery	Yes	Creatine trial associated with greater reduction in running time in the final 300 m run in set (0.7 s) than placebo trial (0.3 s).
Redondo et al. 1996	Team athletes and sprinters (18, M + F) Experimental–placebo design	7 days at 25 g/day creatine	3 × 60 m running sprints	No	No difference between baseline and postsupplementation testing for either group in overall sprinting velocity or velocity through 3 testing zones within the 60 m sprint.
Bosco et al. 1997	Well-trained runners and jumpers (14 M) Experimental–placebo design	5 days at 20 g/day creatine Standardized training: 6/week at 2-3 hr/day	45 s continuous jumping	Yes	Average jumping height in jumping trial increased by 7% ($p < .05$) after supplementation in creatine group, with major changes occurring during first 2 × 15 s periods. No change in placebo group.

Reference	Subjects/Design	Supplementation	Protocol	Ergogenic effect	Results
Schedel, Terrier, et al. 2000	Interval-trained participants (judoka and tennis players) (7 M) Crossover study with order effect: placebo followed by creatine	7 days at 20 g/day creatine	4 × 80 m running sprints with 5 min recovery	Yes	Increase in BM of 0.8 kg with creatine trial ($p < .05$). Creatine trial also showed increase in average running speed for all sprints by 1.4% ($p < .05$), principally resulting from 1.5% increase in stride frequency. Major changes seen in 4th sprint in each series.
Skare et al. 2001	Competitive sprinters (18 M) Experimental–placebo design	5 days at 20 g/day creatine,	6 × 60 m sprints	Yes	Increase in running velocity after supplementation for creatine group for overall 6 × 60 m sprints (45.12 vs. 45.63 min). Improvement in 5 of 6 sprints. Increase in blood lactate levels postsupplementation. No changes in placebo group.
Finn et al. 2001	Trained triathletes (16 M) Experimental–placebo design	5 days at 20 g/day creatine	4 × 20 s cycling sprints with 20 s recovery	No	Trend for improvement in performance of 1 s peak power, 5 s peak power, and fatigue index for first sprint after creatine supplementation. No improvement in mean power for first sprint or other sprints.
Ziegenfuss et al. 2002	Collegiate sprint-trained athletes (team sports, wrestling, track) (10 M + 10 F) Experimental–placebo design	3 days at 0.35 g/kg LBM/day creatine	6 × 10 s cycle sprints with 60 s recovery	Yes	Increase in BM of 0.9 kg in creatine group ($p < .05$). MRI of thighs showed a 6% increase in thigh volume in 5 of 6 creatine participants ($p = .05$). Creatine group showed increase in total work in final sprint compared with baseline and increase in peak power during sprints 2-6. Effect was greater in female athletes.
Havenitidis et al. 2003	Sprint-trained athletes (28 M) Unusual design: control + experimental groups. Order effect with baseline, placebo then experimental and control trials	4 days at 10 g/day, 25 g/day, or 34 g/day creatine	3 × 30 s cycle sprints with 6 min recovery	No for 10 g/day dose Yes for 25 and 34 g/day dose	Increase in BM of 0.4 kg with creatine. No change in power characteristics of Wingate cycling test across trials in control group. No difference in mean power across 3 sprints in low-dose creatine (0.7% increase, NS). Improvements in mean power with 25 and 34 g/day creatine were 11.8% and 11.1% ($p < .05$).
Delecluse et al. 2003	Highly trained sprinters (5 M + 4 F) Crossover design with 7 weeks washout	7 days at 0.35 g·kg^{-1}·day^{-1} creatine	• 2 × 40 m running sprints with 5 min recovery • 6 × 40 m sprints with 30 s recovery	No No	Difference in BM of ~0.7 kg between end of creatine and supplement trials. Trend to better performance in 40 m sprint in creatine trial (~0.05 s) but differences not significant. No difference in running velocity over 40 m between trials. 6 × 40 m intervals associated with high degree of fatigue in both trials.

(continued)

Table 7.b (continued)

Study	Participants	Supplement protocol	Exercise protocol	Enhanced performance	Comments
Javierre et al. 2004	Well-trained runners (19 M)	5 days at 20 g/day creatine	• 6 × 60 m running sprints with 2 min recovery	No	Both groups showed fatigue over successive sprints (increase in running time) and improved performance of sprints in postsupplementation trial. No differences between groups. However, creatine group showed reduction in ventilation and $\dot{V}O_2$ during postexercise period, suggesting enhanced recovery.
			• Countermovement jump	No	
			• Static jump	No	
Creatine		**Chronic supplementation protocol for training adaptations**			**More studies are needed with highly trained athletes to show clear benefits from enhanced training being translated into superior competition performance.**
Kirksey et al. 1999	Track-and-field athletes (36, M + F) Experimental–placebo design	6 weeks at 0.3 mg/kg creatine Supervised preseason resistance training program	Tests at 0, 8 weeks: • 5 × 10 s cycling sprints with 50 s recovery	Yes	Greater increase in average, peak, and initial rate of production of power, and work done in cycling sprints in creatine group, compared with placebo group ($p < .05$). Greater increase also in countermovement jump power ($p < .05$). Results attributed to a greater (2.5 kg) increase in LBM.
			• Countermovement jump	Yes	
Lehmkuhl et al. 2003	Collegiate track-and-field athletes (19, M + F) Experimental–placebo design	7 days at 0.3 g/kg BM/day + 7 weeks at 0.03 g/kg BM creatine Supervised event-specific resistance training program—no difference in training volume between groups	Tests at 0 and 8 weeks: • 5 × 5 s cycling sprints with 50 s recovery	Yes	Greater increase in BM and LBM with creatine group than placebo over 8 weeks. No differences in improvement in jumps over period, and no differences in peak power or average power for the 5 cycle sprints. However, greater increase in initial rate of power production in cycle sprints ($p < .05$).
			• Static jump	No	
			• Countermovement jump	No	
Caffeine		**Acute supplementation protocol with relevance to racing**			**Sport-specific studies are needed with highly trained sprinters or jumpers to ascertain the potential benefits of caffeine as a training and competition aid.**
Williams et al. 1988	Untrained participants (9 M) Crossover design	7 mg/kg caffeine	15 s cycling sprint	No	Caffeine failed to increase maximal power output or alter rate or magnitude of fatigue.
Collomp et al. 1991	Untrained participants (6, M + F) Crossover design	5 mg/kg caffeine at 60 min pretrial	30 s cycling sprint	No	No difference in maximal anaerobic capacity or power and power decrease between trials. Blood lactate concentrations higher with caffeine trial.
Doherty 1998	Well-trained athletes (9 M) Crossover design	5 mg/kg caffeine at 60 min pretrial	Running to exhaustion at 125% $\dot{V}O_2$max	Yes	Caffeine increased time to exhaustion and maximal accumulated oxygen deficit compared with placebo trial ($p < .05$). No difference in blood lactate concentrations between trials.

Study	Participants/Design	Supplementation protocol	Exercise protocol	Ergogenic	Results/Comments
Bell et al. 2001	Untrained participants: 1. 16 M, 2. 8 M, Crossover design	5 mg/kg caffeine at 90 min pretrial	• 30 s cycling sprint • Cycling to exhaustion at 125% $\dot{V}O_2$max	No Yes	Caffeine increased time to exhaustion and maximal accumulated oxygen deficit compared with placebo trial ($p < .05$). Increased blood lactate concentrations with caffeine trial.
Doherty et al. 2002	Trained athletes (14 M), Crossover design	5 mg/kg caffeine at 60 min pretrial (following creatine loading)	Running to exhaustion at 125% $\dot{V}O_2$max	Yes	Caffeine increased time to exhaustion but no difference in maximal accumulated oxygen deficit.
Wiles et al. 2006	Cyclists (9 M), Crossover design	5 mg/kg caffeine at 60 min pre-trial	Cycling: 1 km TT on lab ergometer	Yes	Cycling performance was significantly improved in caffeine trial, but no difference between the placebo trial and control trial. Improvements were 2.3 s decrease in time (3.1%), and increases of 1.6 km/h in speed, 18 W in mean power (3.6%) and 76W peak power (8.8%)
Caffeine		**Acute supplementation protocol with relevance to interval training**			**Sport-specific studies are needed with highly trained sprinters or jumpers to ascertain the potential benefits of caffeine as a training and competition aid.**
Anselme et al. 1992	Untrained participants (14, M + F), Crossover design	250 mg (~4 mg/kg) caffeine at 30 min pretrial	Repeated 6 s cycling sprints, force and velocity test	Yes	Increased pedaling frequency and W_{max} in caffeine trial compared with placebo ($p < .05$) Caffeine elevated blood lactate.
Greer et al. 1998	Recreationally active participants (9 M), Crossover design	6 mg/kg caffeine at 60 min pretrial	4 × 30 s cycling sprints	No	No difference in overall peak or average power outputs between trials. No difference in blood lactate levels but increase in ammonia in caffeine trial.
Vanakoski et al. 1998	Trained athletes (7 M), Crossover design	7 mg/kg caffeine at 70 min pretrial	3 × 1 min cycling sprints	No	No difference in maximal cycling speed, maintenance of speed, or total work output between trials. No difference in blood lactate levels between trials.
Paton et al. 2001	Team athletes (16 M), Crossover design	6 mg/kg caffeine at 60 min pretrial	10 × 20 m sprints on interval of 10 s	No	Negligible difference between caffeine and placebo trials for time to complete 10 sprints and decay in performance over 10 sprints.
Bicarbonate or citrate		**Acute supplementation protocol with relevance to racing**			**More studies are needed to define the range of track events that might benefit from bicarbonate or citrate loading and the protocols that can be used for multievent competitions (e.g., heats and finals). In these situations it may be prudent to use a chronic loading protocol or repeated protocols of acute loading, manipulated to take the effect of a preceding dose into account.**
Goldfinch et al. 1988	Trained runners (6 M), Crossover study	400 mg/kg sodium bicarbonate or placebo or control, at 60 min pretrial	400 m run	Yes	Improved running time with bicarbonate (56.94 s vs. 58.63 and 58.46 s for bicarbonate, placebo, and control trials, respectively, $p < .05$). Elevated postexercise values for pH and base excess.

(continued)

Table 7.b (continued)

Study	Participants	Supplement protocol	Exercise protocol	Enhanced performance	Comments
McNaughton, Backx, et al. 1999	Active participants (8 M) Crossover study with order effect: baseline testing then bicarbonate, then control trial 1 month later	5 days at 0.5 g·kg⁻¹·day⁻¹ bicarbonate	60 s supramaximal cycling	Yes	Chronic intake of bicarbonate over a period of days increased blood pH. Work done in bicarbonate trial was greater than that achieved in baseline testing and control trial (24.1 vs. 21.1 and 21.1 MJ, $p < .05$).
Bicarbonate and citrate		Chronic supplementation protocol for training			**There is new evidence that repeated use of bicarbonate loading before interval training sessions may enhance training adaptations and improve performance of sustained high-intensity exercise, at least in moderately trained individuals. It may also assist the athlete to train harder. Further research is needed to confirm these findings, especially for highly trained athletes.**
Edge at al. 2006	Moderately trained (16 F) Experimental–placebo design	8 wks at 400 mg/kg sodium bicarbonate in a split dose 90 min and 30 min before interval training Periodized interval training undertaken 3 d/wk: 2 min intervals with 1 min recovery, with 6 to 12 intervals completed at 140-170% of intensity at lactate threshold Both groups completed the same training load	0 and 8 wks (cycle): • V̇O₂peak • lactate threshold • time to exhaustion at 100% pre-trial V̇O₂peak	Yes	Both groups increased their V̇O₂peak by similar amounts as a result of the 8 wk interval training. Both groups also increased their muscle buffering capacity. This increase in muscle buffering capacity was related to pre-training capacity rather than the treatment (subjects with lower pre-training muscle buffering capacity achieved greater increases as a result of training). Although both groups showed an increase in lactate threshold and time to exhaustion at V̇O₂peak, the improvements were greater in the bicarbonate group. The authors speculated that training intensity rather than accumulation of H+ ions is responsible for increasing muscle buffering capacity. Furthermore, inducing alkalosis during exercise may enhance muscle adaptations by reducing the damage to mitochondria or protein synthesis.

M = male; F = female; BM = body mass; LBM = lean body mass; W$_{max}$ = maximal work; MRI = magnetic resonance imaging; NS = not significant.

Table 7.c Relevant Studies of Supplements With Undetermined or Unlikely Benefit to Sprinters and Jumpers

Study	Participants	Supplement protocol	Exercise protocol	Enhanced performance	Comments
Bovine colostrum		**Chronic supplementation protocol**			Potential value presently undetermined. No mechanisms identified to explain any potential benefits. Expense of supplement in moderate and large doses ($US40 per week) warrants additional supportive research before it can be recommended. Emerging evidence that benefits might be seen at lower doses is also of interest.
Mero et al. 1997	Elite sprinters and jumpers (9 M) Crossover design with 13-day washout	8 days at 25 ml/day colostrum or 125 ml/day placebo (milk whey) 6 sessions speed and resistance training	Tests at day 6 of each program: • Countermovement jump	No	No difference in jump performance. Serum IGF increased over time with colostrum supplementation (although still within physiological ranges) compared with placebo. No change in serum or saliva immunoglobulins between treatments.
Buckley et al. 2003	Active participants (51 M) Experimental–placebo design	8 weeks at 60 g/day bovine colostrum or placebo (whey protein) 3 weeks resistance and plyometrics training	Tests at baseline and 4 and 8 weeks: • 3 × 10 s cycling sprints with 2 min recovery • 3 × vertical jumps with 2 min recovery	Yes at 8 weeks only Yes at 8 weeks only	No differences in performance measures at baseline. At week 4, no differences in peak cycling power, anaerobic work capacity, or peak vertical jump power. At week 8, peak vertical jump power and peak cycle power higher in colostrum group, but no differences in anaerobic work capacity. No changes in IGF-1 in either group.
ATP supplements		**Acute supplementation protocol**			**Some animal studies show that supplementation with ATP produces increase in blood and cell ATP levels, with changes in physiological function. However, in humans, oral presentation of ATP is likely to be challenged by denaturation in the gut, poor absorption because of the high molecular weight, and poor transport to the muscle cell. Recent development of "enterically coated" ATP supplements has allowed some of these challenges to be addressed. However, there needs to be clear evidence that acute or chronic intake of such supplements increases blood and cellular levels of ATP or alters physiological function. Data to support these outcomes are lacking.**
Jordan et al. 2004	Strength-training athletes (27 M) Experimental–placebo design	On day 7: 150 mg or 225 mg enterically coated ATP 75 min pretrial	Baseline and 7 days: • 2 × 30 s cycling Wingate test, separated by 5 min	No	No difference between baseline and day 7 results for either group for total work, peak power, or mean power in Wingate tests. No difference in posttest lactate accumulation. No change in blood ATP levels, 60 min after ingestion of supplements.

(continued)

Table 7.c *(continued)*

Study	Participants	Supplement protocol	Exercise protocol	Enhanced performance	Comments
ATP supplements		**Chronic supplementation protocol**			**There is no evidence that chronic supplementation with ATP enhances performance. See comments above.**
Jordan et al. 2004	Strength-training athletes (27 M) Experimental–placebo design	From day 7 to 21 14 days at 150 mg or 225 mg enterically coated ATP	Tests at baseline, 21 days (after 14 days of supplementation) • 2 × 30 s cycling Wingate test, separated by 5 min	No	No difference between baseline and day 21 results for either group for total work, peak power, or mean power in Wingate tests. No difference in posttest lactate accumulation. No change in blood ATP levels, 60 min after ingestion of supplements.
Inosine		**Chronic supplementation protocol**			**No evidence of increased production of ATP or performance enhancements with inosine. In fact, inosine supplementation has been shown to impair some performance protocols in runners and cyclists.**
Starling et al. 1996	Competitive cyclists (10 M) Crossover design	5 days at 5,000 mg/day inosine	Tests at 1 and 6 days • 30 s cycling Wingate test • Supramaximal cycling sprint to exhaustion	No No, in fact, impairment	No difference in peak power, end power, or fatigue index during 30 s cycling between inosine and placebo trials. Placebo trial associated with better supramaximal cycling sprint outcome (109.7 vs. 99.7 s). Uric acid higher following inosine supplementation.
McNaughton, Dalton, and Tarr et al. 1999	Trained participants (7 M) Crossover design	5 and 10 days at 10,000 mg/day inosine	Tests at 0, 6, and 11 days • 5 × 6 s cycling sprints • 30 s cycling sprint	No No	No changes in performance in either test after 5 and 10 days of inosine supplementation compared with placebo. Increase blood uric acid concentration with inosine supplementation.
Ribose supplementation		**Acute supplementation protocol**			**Literature fails to show benefits to performance of repeated high-intensity bouts of exercise with ribose supplementation. Expense of ribose (~US$40/week) warrants additional supportive research before it can be recommended.**
Kerksick et al. 2005	Collegiate cyclists (n = 12 M) Crossover design 1 week washout	2 × (3 g of ribose + 150 µg of folate), before and during repeated sprint protocol	Cycling protocol • 5 × 30 s cycling sprints with 30 s recovery	No	Peak power and total work decreased significantly across sprints in both trials. Ribose supplementation did not alter performance or metabolism during repeated sprints.
Ribose supplementation		**Chronic supplementation protocol**			**Literature fails to show benefits to performance of repeated high-intensity bouts of exercise with chronic ribose supplementation. Expense of ribose (~US$40/week) warrants additional supportive research before it can be recommended.**

Op 't Eijnde et al. 2001	Athletes in sports involving sprint and resistance activities (19 M) Experimental–placebo design	6 days at 16 g/day ribose Training program of 2/day × 1 bout of 15 × 12 knee extensions with 15 s recovery	Test protocol: 2 bouts: 15 × 12 knee extensions with 15 s recovery 60 min between bouts	No	Test protocol undertaken on PM of day 6, with rest during AM. 6-day training protocol increased power output profiles of contraction series and overall mean power output achieved in postsupplementation testing compared with pretesting by ~10%. No difference between groups. Biopsy sampling of participants undertaking similar exercise protocol in a separate study showed that the sprint protocol decreased muscle ATP concentrations by ~20–25% with little restoration of ATP over next 24 hr with either ribose or placebo supplementation.
Kreider, Melton, Greenwood, et al. 2003	Resistance-trained athletes (19 M) Experimental–placebo design	5 days at 10 g/day ribose	Tests at 0, 6 days • 2 × 30 s cycling sprints with 3 min recovery	No	Test protocol achieved a decrease in power output across 30 s of sprinting and a lower work output in sprint 2 compared with sprint 1. No difference between pre- and postsupplementation values for peak power, average power, fatigue index, or time to peak power for either group. Ribose group showed a higher total work for second sprint during postsupplementation trial than placebo group, as a result of deterioration in placebo group. No difference in blood lactate and ammonia profiles between groups
Berardi and Ziegenfuss 2003	Active formerly competitive athletes (8 M) Crossover design with 5-day washout	3 days at total 32 g of ribose (day 1: 8 g; day 2: 8 + 8 g; day 3: 8 g)	Test protocol undertaken day 1 (AM and PM) and day 3 (PM) • 6 × 10 s cycling sprints with 60 s recovery	No	Comparison of sprints on day 3 of each protocol showed that ribose trial showed a marginal but inconsistent increase in peak power and mean power across sprints. Increase was significantly greater for sprint 2 but not other sprints. Authors concluded that because treatment dose was already in excess of manufacturers' recommendations, ribose is not a cost-effective supplement.
Hellsten et al. 2004	Active participants (8 M) Crossover design with 5-day washout	3 days at 3 × 200 mg/kg ribose or placebo following 7 days of 2/day sprint training (15 × 10 all-out sprints)	Tests after 72 hr: 15 × 10 s sprints with 50 s recovery	No	Immediately after the last training session, muscle ATP was ~25% lower in both trials and remained lower at 5 and 24 hr of supplementation. After 72 hr, muscle ATP had returned to pretraining in ribose trial but was still lower in placebo trial. However, mean and peak power outputs during the test performed at 72 hr were similar in both trials. Therefore, even though the availability of ribose in the muscle may be a limiting factor for the rate of resynthesis of ATP, it appears that the reduction in muscle ATP observed after intense training does not appear to be limiting for high-intensity exercise performance.
Glutamine	**Chronic supplementation protocol**				
Lehmkuhl et al. 2003	Collegiate track-and-field athletes (19, M + F) Experimental–placebo design	8 weeks at 4 g/day glutamine in addition to creatine (i.e., creatine vs. glutamine + creatine) Supervised event-specific resistance training program—no difference in training volume between groups	Tests at 0 and 8 weeks: • 5 × 5 s cycling sprints with 50 s recovery • Static jump • Countermovement jump	Yes No No	**No evidence of enhancement of response to training with low to moderate dose glutamine supplementation.** Creatine supplementation in conjunction with training was associated with an increase in cycling power and increase in lean body mass. However, the addition of glutamine did not further enhance these gains.

M = male; F = female; IGF = insulin-like growth factor; ATP = adenosine triphosphate.

Table 8.a Reported Dietary Intakes of Male Team Athletes—Field Games: Training (Mean Daily Intake ± SD)

Publication	Team population	Survey method	Age (years)	BM (kg)	ENERGY		CHO			PROTEIN			FAT	
					MJ	KJ/kg	g	g/kg	%E	g	g/kg	%E	g	%E
Short and Short 1983	U.S. collegiate American football players	3-day food diary (household measures)												
	• Offensive team (n = 33)			96	20.38	212	550	5.7	44	201	2.0	16	208	38
	• Defensive team (n = 23)			94	20.25	215	528	5.6	43	191	2.0	16	218	41
Hickson, Johnson, et al. 1987	U.S. collegiate American football players (n = 11)	3-day semiweighed food diary (recorded by observer)	20	108	15.02 ± 3.0	139	329 ± 86	3.0	39	190 ± 40	1.8	22	158 ± 48	39
Hickson, Duke, et al. 1987	U.S. high school American football players (n = 88)	24 hr dietary recall	15-18	76	14.06 ± 6.65	200 ± 87	366 ± 170	4.8	42					
Grandjean 1989	U.S. national-level and collegiate American football players (n = 55)	3-day food diary (household measures)			16.25 ± 2.8		428		46	152		16	167	38
Millard-Stafford et al. 1989	U.S. collegiate American football players (n = 35)	3-day food diary (household measures)	20	99	15.87 ± 3.75	160	443	4.5	45	157	1.6 ± 0.6	17 ±	130	35 ± 5
Cole et al. 2005	U.S. collegiate American football players (n = 28)	2 × 3-day food diary (household measures)	19-23	110	13.78 ± 0.39	125	392 ± 15	3.6	53	169 ± 5	1.5	22	103	23
Jacobs, Westlin, et al. 1982	Swedish professional soccer players (n = 15)	7-day food diary (household measures)	24	74	20.7 ± 4.71	282	596 ± 127	8.1	47 ± 3	170 ± 27	2.3	13.5 ± 1.5	217 ± 36	29 ± 8
Short and Short 1983	U.S. collegiate soccer players (n = 8)	3-day food diary (household measures)			12.39		320		43	113		16	135	41

Hickson, Johnson, et al. 1987	U.S. collegiate soccer players: • Conditioning on campus (n = 17)	3-day food diary (household measures)	20	72	18.7	260	596	8.3	52			14		34
	• Season on campus (n = 8)				15.92 ± 2.69	221	487 ± 107	6.8	52 ± 11			16		32 ± 9
	• Season off campus (n = 9)				12.79 ± 4.89	178	306 ± 118	4.2	42 ± 15			16		42 ± 18
Van Erp-Baart et al. 1989a	Dutch international-level soccer players (n = 20)	4- to 7-day food diary (household measures)	20	74	14.3	192	420	5.6	47	111	1.5	13	134	35
Caldarone et al. 1990	Italian professional soccer players (n = 33)	7-day dietary recall (household measures)	26	76	12.81 ± 2.37	169	449	5.9	56					
Bangsbo et al. 1992	Danish professional soccer players (n = 7)	10-day food diary (household measures)	23	77	15.7	204	426	5.5	46	144	1.9	16	152	38
Schena et al. 1995	Italian national-level soccer players (n = 16)	7-day food diary (household measures)	25	74	13.44 ± 1.48	180	454 ± 32	6.1	57	86 ± 16	1.2	19	90 ± 14	24
Zuliani et al. 1996	Italian professional soccer players (n = 25)	4-day food diary (household measures)	25	71	15.26 ± 1.81	213	532	7.4	56					
Maughan 1997	Scottish professional soccer players—two clubs (n = 51)	7-day weighed food diary	23	80	11.0 ± 2.6	137	354 ± 95	4.4	51 ± 8	103 ± 26	1.3	16 ± 2	93 ± 33	31 ± 5
			26	75	12.8 ± 2.2	171	397 ± 94	5.3	48 ± 4	108 ± 20	1.4	14 ± 2	118 ± 24	35 ± 4
Rico-Sanz et al. 1998	Puerto Rico Olympic team soccer players (n = 8)	12-day food diary (household measures)	17	63	16.52 ± 4.48	260 ± 50	526 ± 62	8.3	53 ± 6	143 ± 23	2.3	14 ± 2	142 ± 17	32 ± 4
Ebine et al. 2002	Japanese professional soccer players (n = 7)	7-day food diary (household measures)	22	70	13.0 ± 2.4	186	—	—	—	—	—	—	—	—
Reeves and Collins 2003	English professional soccer players (n = 21)	7-day food diary (household measures)	20	74	12.83 ± 0.8	173	437 ± 40	5.9	57 ± 4	115 ± 2	1.6	15 ± 2	94 ± 1	27 ± 3

(continued)

Table 8.a *(continued)*

Publication	Team population	Survey method	Age (years)	BM (kg)	ENERGY MJ	ENERGY KJ/kg	CHO g	CHO g/kg	CHO %E	PROTEIN g	PROTEIN g/kg	PROTEIN %E	FAT g	FAT %E
Wray et al. 1994	Professional Australian football players (n = 15)				13.6		410 ± 123	4.7 ± 1.4	48	138 ± 35	1.6 ± 0.4		116 ± 45	31
Graham and Jackson 1998	Professional Australian football players (n = 10)				14.0		489 ± 89	5.9 ± 1.2	57	148 ± 30	1.8 ± 0.2	19	88 ± 32	24
Schokman et al. 1999	Professional Australian football players (n = 40)	4-day food diary (household measures)	23	86	13.2 ± 2.5	154 ± 28	415 ± 110	4.8 ± 1.3	52 ± 9	139 ± 27	1.6 ± 0.3	18 ± 3	104 ± 35	29 ± 8
Lundy et al. 2006	Australian professional rugby league players (n = 34)	4-day food diary (household measures)	~25	~93	17.71 ± 3.69	192 ± 39	563 ± 146	6 ± 1	51 ± 6	184 ± 42	2.0 ± 0.5	18 ± 3	120 ± 35	25 ± 5
Van Erp-Baart et al. 1989a	Dutch international-level field hockey players (n = 8)	4- to 7-day food diary (household measures)	27	75	13.58	181	365	4.9	43	105	1.4	12	132	36
Grandjean and Ruud 1994	U.S. Olympic field hockey players (n = 8)				15.57	181	343	4.2	39	156	1.9	18	155	39
Short and Short 1983	U.S. collegiate lacrosse players: • Season (n =10) • Season (n = 10)	3-day food diary (household measures)			17.46 15.52		542 398		46 43	140 154		14 17	145 130	
Reeves and Collins 2003	Gaelic football players: • County players (n = 12) • Club players (n = 13)	7-day food diary (household measures)	25 24	83 81	12.53 ± 1.0 12.16 ± 1.4	151 ± 11 150 ± 16	432 ± 23 360 ± 30		52 ± 5 49 ± 6	120 ± 14 105 ± 13		16 ± 2 14 ± 2	86 ± 1 96 ± 2	26 ± 4 30 ± 6
Grandjean 1989	U.S. national-level and collegiate baseball players (n = 11)	3-day food diary (household measures)			19.45 ± 3.74	—	523	—	45 ± 11	219	—	18 ± 7	195	37 ± 8

BM = body mass; CHO = carbohydrate; E = energy.

Table 8.b Reported Dietary Intakes of Female Team Athletes—Field Games: Training (Mean Daily Intake ± SD)

Publication	Team population	Survey method	Age (years)	BM (kg)	ENERGY		CHO			PROTEIN			FAT	
					MJ	KJ/kg	g	g/kg	%E	g	g/kg	%E	g	%E
Short and Short 1983	U.S. collegiate lacrosse players (n = 7)	3-day food diary (household measures)			9.32		257		50	89		16	95	35
Van Erp-Baart et al. 1989a	Dutch international-level field hockey players (n = 9)	4- to 7-day food diary (household measures)	24	62	9.0	145	264	4.3	47	62	1.0	11	85	35
Tilgner and Schiller 1989	U.S. collegiate field hockey players (n = 8)	2 × 3-day food diaries (household measures)	19	60	8.18 ± 1.57	136	228 ± 44	3.8	47	76 ± 18	1.3	16	84 ± 17	39
Nutter 1991	U.S. collegiate field hockey players (n = 9): • Season • Postseason	7-day food diary (household measures)	19	64	6.35 ± 1.7 / 5.99 ± 1.7	100 ± 26 / 94 ± 24	213 / 192	3.4 / 3.0	54 ± 8 / 54 ± 8	57 / 57	0.9 / 0.9	15 ± 4 / 16 ± 4	45 / 47	27 ± 9 / 30 ± 7
Clark et al. 2003	U.S. collegiate soccer players (n = 13): • Season • Postseason	3-day food diary (household measures)	20	62	9.61 ± 1.3 / 7.83 ± 2.2	155 / 126	320 ± 70 / 263 ± 71	5.2 ± 1.1 / 4.3 ± 1.2	55 ± 8 / 57 ± 7	87 ± 19 / 59 ± 17	1.4 ± 0.3 / 1.0 ± 0.3	15 ± 3 / 13 ± 2	75 ± 13 / 66 ± 29	29 ± 6 / 31 ± 7
Gropper et al. 2003	U.S. collegiate soccer players (n = 15)	3-day food diary (household measures)	19	59	8.46 ± 2.5	143				71 ± 29	1.3	14		
Martin et al. 2006	England national soccer players (n = 16)	7-day food diary (household measures)	25	61	7.98 ± 1.53	130	252	4.1 ± 1	54 ± 7	74	1.2 ± 0.3	17 ± 2	55	29 ± 7
Gropper et al. 2003	U.S. collegiate softball players (n = 6)	3-day food diary (household measures)	20	66	7.65 ± 2.9	116				64 ± 30	1.0	14		

BM = body mass; CHO = carbohydrate; E = energy.

Table. 8.c Available Data on Voluntary Fluid Intakes and Sweat Losses During Training and Competition in Field-Based Team Sports (mean ± SD, or range)

Publication	Participants	Temperature (°C)	Humidity (%)	SWEAT LOSS		FLUID INTAKE		
				Total (ml)	Rate (ml/hr)	Total (ml)	Rate (ml/hr)	Hypohydration (% BM)
AMERICAN FOOTBALL—TRAINING								
Stofan et al. 2003	Professional football players (NFL) (16 M)	1 2 - 3 1 WBGT		1,300-5,200		300-5,000		1.2 ± 1.0
Stofan et al. 2005	Collegiate football players • Crampers (5 M) • Noncrampers (5 M)			4,000±1,200 3,500 ± 1,600	1,600 1,400	2,600 ± 800 2,800 ± 700	1,040 1,120	1.3 ± 0.9 0.7 ± 1.2
Godek, Godek, et al. 2005	Collegiate football players (10 M; 36 observations)	~30	40-70	~4,800	2,140 ± 530	~3200	1,425 ± 480	~1.8
Godek, Bartolozzi, et al. 2005	Collegiate football players (10 M; multiple observations) • Tepid water • Cold water	~23	40-70		~2,000			1.8 1.3
AMERICAN FOOTBALL—MATCH								
Hoffman et al. 2002	Collegiate football players (23 M)	10						1.0
AUSTRALIAN FOOTBALL—MATCH								
Pyke and Hahn 1980	Semiprofessional players: • (8 M) • (6 M)	27 38	52 25	3,190 3,630	1,800 2,100	740 1,500	410 870	3.0 2.7
Pohl et al. 1981	Semiprofessional players (23 M)	12-15	55-88	1,430		190		1.8 (0.6-3.4)
RUGBY LEAGUE—TRAINING								
Meir and Murphy 1998	Professional players (23 M, 4 sessions)	20-25						0.7

Meir et al. 1990	Professional players (11 M, forwards) (11 M, backs)	20-24	67-73			2.4 ± 0.9 1.5 ± 0.7
Walsh et al., 1995, cited in Meir and Murphy 1998	Professional players (6 games played by same team)	Winter		1,965	852	1.2 ± ~0.6
Jennings et al. 1998	Professional players (28 M, 16 games)	23	73			1.1
Meir et al. 1990	Professional players (22 M) • Forwards • Backs	24	70			2.4 ± 0.89 1.5 ± 0.66
Meir and Murphy 1998	Professional players (23 M, 3 matches)	22-27	75-90			1.9 ± 1
Meir et al. 2003	Professional players (25 M, 10 matches) • All matches (n = 165) • Backs • Forwards • Day matches • Night matches	12 17 10	83 83 83			0.92 ± 0.82 0.85 ± 0.90 0.99 ± 0.72 1.47 ± 0.11 0.65 ± 0.26

Cohen et al. 1981	Professional players (15 M) • 8 M, forwards • 7 M, backs	24-25	30-32	2,100 2,560 1,570	150	2.5 2.9 2.1
Goodman et al. 1985	Well-trained amateurs • 15 M • 14 M • 13 M	18-20 21-23 20-22	18-20 78-85 74-82	2,160 1,740 2,250	751	1.6 1.4 1.5

(continued)

Table. 8.c *(continued)*

Publication	Participants	Temperature (°C)	Humidity (%)	SWEAT LOSS		FLUID INTAKE		Hypohydration (% BM)
				Total (ml)	Rate (ml/hr)	Total (ml)	Rate (ml/hr)	
RUGBY UNION—MATCH								
Meir and Halliday 2005	International players • Game 1 (22 M) • Game 2 (22 M) • Game 3 (20 M) • Game 4 (20 M)	19 20 18 16	20 30 49 56					0.76 ± 0.78 0.69 ± 0.92 1.25 ± 0.93 1.28 + 1.17 Across games 14 players > 2% BM loss and 2 players > 3% BM loss
SOCCER—TRAINING								
Broad et al. 1996	Junior elite players • 80 M, summer • 46 M, winter	25 9	41 61	1,555 ± 510 1,095 ± 425	985 ± 320 745 ± 260	670 ± 425 435 ± 350	430 ± 310 310 ± 255	1.2 ± 0.7 0.8 ± 0.5
Broad et al. 1996	International players (30 W, summer)	30	35	1,160 ± 430	815 ± 245	570 ± 290	395 ± 155	0.9 ± 0.5
Shirreffs et al. 2005	Elite professional players (26 M)	32	20	2,193 ± 365	1,462	972 ± 335	648	1.59 ± 0.6
Maughan et al. 2004	Elite professional players (24 M)	24-29	46-64	2,033 ± 413	1,355	971 ± 303	647	1.4 ± 0.5
Maughan, unpublished observations, cited in Maughan et al. 2005	Elite professional players (20 M)	28	56	2,221 (1,515-2,895)	1,481	1,401 (721-2,278)	934	1.15 (−0.24-2.3)
Maughan, unpublished observations, cited in Maughan et al. 2005	Elite professional players (24 M)	25	60	1,827 (884-3,100)	1218	834 (243-2,057)	556	1.22 (−0.24-2.6)
Maughan et al. 2005	Elite professional players (16 M)	5	81	1,690 ± 450	1,130 ± 300	413 ± 215	282	1.62 ± 0.55

							BM
SOCCER—MATCHES								
Mustafa and Mahmoud 1979	International-level players (8 M)	33 26 13	40 78 7	2,089 ± 637 2,546 ± 750 846 ± 162		657 ± 328 242 ± 930 0		1.4 kg 2.3 kg 0.8 kg
Leatt 1986	Collegiate players (7 M)	19	55	2,000		1,000		1.0 kg
Kirkendall 1993	Collegiate players			1,310		1,135		0.5
Zeederberg et al. 1996	Junior elite players (22 M)	13-15	63-69	1,700	1,133	700 (controlled)	467	1.0 ± 0.2 kg
Broad et al. 1996	International-level players (10 F, summer)	26	78	1,505 ± 435	760 ± 220	810 ± 310	410 ± 155	1.2 ± 0.9
Broad et al. 1996	Junior elite players • 46 M, summer • 13 M, winter	25 10	41 56	1,935 ± 620 1,585 ± 585	1,210 ± 330 1,025 ± 265	825 ± 525 530 ± 235	515 ± 335 360 ± 195	1.4 ± 0.9 1.4 ± 0.7
CRICKET—MATCHES								
Gore et al. 1993	National-level players (7 M) • Batsmen • Bowlers	23	65		540 470 710		430	0.3
	National-level players (7 M) • Batsmen • Bowlers	33	22		700 600 690		510	1.2
	National-level bowlers (3 M)	33	30		1,370		525	4.3
CRICKET—TRAINING								
Burke et al. 2006 unpublished observations	International-level players (11 M)	29	50	3,004 ± 1,014	1,202 ± 406	2,172 ± 482	870 ± 193	1.0 ± 0.7

BM = body mass; M = male; F = female; WBGT = wet bulb globe temperature.

Table 8.d Studies of Supplements With Likely Benefit to Field-Based Team Sports

Publication	Participants	Supplement protocol	Exercise protocol	Enhanced performance	Comments
Caffeine		**Acute (loading) supplementation protocol with relevance to movement patterns during matches**			**General literature suggests that intake of small to moderate doses of caffeine before or during matches may enhance performance by reducing perception of fatigue. This theory has not been tested in situations simulating team sports; the only study involving team athletes focused on performance of a brief period of high-intensity sprints.**
Paton et al. 2001	Team athletes (16 M) Crossover design	6 mg/kg caffeine taken 60 min pretest	10 × 20 m sprints on interval of 10 s	No	Negligible difference between caffeine and placebo trials for time to complete 10 sprints and decay in performance over 10 sprints.
Stuart et al. 2006	Rugby union players (9 M) Crossover design	6 mg/kg caffeine taken 70 min pretest	2 × 40 min circuits (simulated rugby union protocol) involving repetitions of • 20 m sprint speed — Possible • 30 m sprint speed — Very likely • Offensive sprint — Likely • Defensive sprint — Likely • Drive 1 power — Likely • Drive 2 power — No—harm possible • Tackle speed — Likely • Passing ability — Likely		Study involved probability statistics rather than testing of null hypothesis. Interpretation included change in fatigue with caffeine compared with placebo trial. Mean improvements of 0.5-3% in performance of sprint tasks, with greater improvement in second half. Suggests caffeine effect achieved by reduction in fatigue. 10% improvement in ability to pass ball accurately—because of enhancement of arousal or attention.
Schneiker et al. 2006	Team athletes (10M) Crossover design	6 mg/kg caffeine taken 60 min pretest	2 × 36 min min cycle protocol, each involving • 18 × 4 s sprint with 2 min recovery	Yes	Total work during sprints in first half was 8.5% greater in caffeine trial than placebo, and work in second half was 7.6% greater in caffeine trial (both p < .05). Mean peak power score achieved during sprints in first and second halves were 7% and 6.6% greater in caffeine trial than placebo (both p < .05).
Creatine		**Acute (loading) supplementation protocol with relevance to movement patterns during matches**			**Reasonable evidence that creatine loading is associated with enhanced ability to undertake repeated brief sprints with short recovery intervals as found in movement patterns of field-based team sports.**
Mujika et al. 2000	National-level soccer players (17 M) Experimental–placebo trial	6 days @ 20 g/day creatine or placebo	Soccer-specific exercise protocol completed before and after supplementation: • Included series of countermovement jumps, 6 × 15 m sprints, and intermittent endurance test (40 × 15 s sprints)	Yes	Gain of 0.6 g BM in creatine group. Significant improvement in average time and sum of times for the 6 × 15 m sprints in posttest for creatine group, with improvements evident over the first 5 m. Decline in countermovement jumps seen in placebo group at the end of the protocol prevented in creatine group. No difference in intermittent endurance test between groups. No difference in blood lactate concentrations between groups in postsupplementation trial despite better sprint performance in creatine group; lower ammonia concentrations. Suggests creatine supplementation reduced adenine nucleotide degradation and reduced reliance on anaerobic glycolysis.

Study	Subjects	Supplementation	Exercise protocol	Performance enhancement	Results
Preen et al. 2001	Active participant (14 M) Experimental–placebo trial	5 days @ 20 g/day creatine or placebo	Intermittent exercise protocol completed before and after supplementation: • 80 min intermittent cycling protocol: 10 sets of 5-6 × 6 s maximal bike sprints with various rest intervals (24, 54, or 84 s)	Yes	Creatine supplementation increased resting muscle content of creatine and creatine phosphate. Gain of BM of 0.9 kg in creatine group. Compared with first trial, creatine group increased total work done over 80 min as well as work done and peak power during each set of sprints, especially sprints with longer recovery intervals. Performance enhancements seen throughout the 80 min of protocol. Blood lactate concentrations peaked after set 4; no difference between treatments. No change in muscle glycogen utilization. No performances changes seen in posttesting with placebo group.
Cox et al. 2002	International-level soccer players (12 F) Experimental–placebo trial	6 days @ 20 g/day creatine or placebo	Soccer-specific exercise protocol (60 min) competed before and after supplementation: • Included blocks of 20 m sprints, agility tests, and ball-shooting skills	Yes	Gain of 0.8 kg BM with creatine supplementation. Compared with pretest, creatine group enhanced a substantial number of individual 20 m sprints and agility tests during middle section of protocol. Despite not reaching statistical significance because of low statistical power, mean enhancement of 20 m time = 1.7% and 30 cm, and agility test = 2.7% and 70 cm, meaningful in a game. No alteration of shooting skill. Blood lactate reduced in creatine trial during first half of protocol, suggesting that early benefits to phosphagen system that reduced glycolysis were replaced by growing dependence on aerobic system in late phase of protocol. No changes seen with posttest on placebo trial.
Ziegenfuss et al. 2002	Collegiate athletes including basketball, field hockey, ice hockey, softball players (10 M, 10 F) Experimental–placebo design	3 days @ 0.35 g/kg LBM or placebo	Before and after supplementation: • 6 × 10 s cycling sprints with 60 s recovery	Yes	Gain of BM of 0.9 kg in creatine group. Creatine supplementation significantly increased peak power during sprints 2-6. Increase in mid-thigh muscle volume in creatine group (assessed by magnetic resonance imaging).
Biwer et al. 2003	Collegiate soccer players (8 F + 7 M) Crossover design, 4 weeks washout	5 days @ 0.3 g/kg creatine or placebo	Intermittent exercise protocol completed before and after supplementation • 20 min treadmill run with repeated 1 min hill sprint (incline, maintain and decline) + 2 min rest, followed by incremental hill run to fatigue	No	Significant increase in BM with creatine supplementation in males (~1.2 kg) but not females (0.4 kg). No difference between posttest and pretest results for RPE during hill sprints or time to fatigue for either creatine or placebo trials. Suggestion that length of hill sprint may not reflect movement patterns of soccer or activity stressing phosphagen system.

(continued)

Table 8.d *(continued)*

Publication	Participants	Supplement protocol	Exercise protocol	Enhanced performance	Comments
Ayoama et al. 2003	Collegiate softball players (26 F) Experimental–placebo design	7 days of heavy exercise then 7 days @ 20 g/day + 14 days @ 3 g/day creatine or 20 g/day creatine in second week only or placebo	Testing at baseline and 1, 2, 3, and 4 weeks: • 2 × maximal knee extensions • 30 repeated knee extensions	No Yes	Loading with creatine did not benefit maximal static strength but enhanced mean strength and endurance of repeated contractions. Benefits lost after a week when creatine supplementation ceased.
Ostojic 2004	Junior elite soccer players (20 M) Experimental–placebo design	7 days @ 30 g/day creatine or placebo	Testing at baseline and after 7 days: • Dribble test • Sprint-power test • Countermovement jump • Endurance shuttle run	 Yes Yes Yes No	Significant improvement in postsupplementation performance of dribble test (10.2 vs. 13 s, $p < .05$), sprint-power test (2.2 vs. 2.7 s, $p < .05$), and jumping ability (55 vs. 49 cm, $p < .05$) in creatine group. No change in shuttle run score. Performances in placebo group unchanged by supplementation.
Ahmun et al. 2005	Highly trained rugby union players (14 M) Crossover design, 4 week washout	5 days @ 20 g/day creatine or placebo	Testing at baseline and after 6-7 days • 10 × 6 s cycling Wingate test • 10 × 40 m running tests	Perhaps No	~5% increase in peak power production and minimum power production in cycling test, compared with no change in placebo group. Although not statistically significant because of high participant variability, authors stated that the difference would be useful in real life.
Creatine		Chronic supplementation protocol to enhance resistance training outcomes in team sport players			Literature provides reasonable support for creatine supplementation as an aid to increase outcomes from resistance training. More sports-specific work is needed to investigate if this transfers into better performance in game.
Noonan et al. 1998	Collegiate American football players (39 M) Experimental–placebo design	8 weeks @ 100 mg·kg $BM^{-1}·day^{-1}$ or 300 mg·kg $BM^{-1}·day^{-1}$ creatine or placebo Resistance training 4/week	Testing at baseline, 8 weeks • 1RM bench press • 40 yd sprint • Vertical jump	 Yes Yes No	6% increase in 1RM bench press in 300 mg/kg BM creatine group ($p < .05$). No change in placebo group or 100 mg/kg group. 40 yd sprint enhanced in 100 mg/kg group ($p < .05$) but not other groups; no difference in vertical jump in any group postsupplementation.
Kreider et al. 1998	Collegiate American football players (25 M) Experimental–placebo design	28 days @ 16 g/day creatine or placebo Resistance training 5/week, conditioning 3/week	Testing at baseline, 4 weeks: 4-8RM lifting volume • Bench press • Power clean • Squat	 Yes No No	Greater increase in BM and LBM (assessed by DEXA) in creatine group ($p < .05$). Greater increase in lifting volume in bench press ($p < .05$) but not other lifts in creatine group.

Study	Population / Design	Protocol	Testing measures	Significant	Results
Pearson et al. 1999	Collegiate American football players (16 M) Experimental–placebo design	10 weeks @ 5 g/day creatine or placebo Off-season resistance training 4/week	Testing at baseline, 10 weeks: • 1RM bench press • 1RM power clean • 1RM squat	Yes Yes Yes	Creatine group increased 1 RM lifts by 3-11% ($p < .05$). BM increase of 1.5 kg in creatine group ($p < .05$). No changes in placebo group. Lack of training effect in control group explained by preexisting training status of participants and reduction in energy intake during intense training program attributable to lifestyle interruptions.
Stone et al. 1999	Collegiate American football players (42 M) Experimental–placebo design	5 weeks @ 0.22 g/kg creatine or 0.13 g/kg creatine+ 0.09 g/kg pyruvate or placebo Resistance training 3/week, football practice 2/week	Testing at baseline, 5 weeks: • 1RM bench press • 1RM squat • Vertical jump	Yes No Yes	Compared with placebo, creatine groups increased BM, LBM (assessed by densitometry), bench press, and vertical jump ($p < .05$).
Stout et al. 1999	Collegiate American football players (24 M) Experimental–placebo design	Creatine (5 days @ 20 g/day then 7 weeks @ 10 g/day), creatine + CHO (33 g CHO taken with creatine dose) or CHO alone Resistance training 4/week and running 2/week	Testing at baseline, 8 weeks: • 1RM bench press • 100 m sprint • Vertical jump	No for creatine alone Yes for creatine + CHO	Improvements in LBM, vertical jump, 100 yd sprint, and bench press in creatine and CHO group compared with CHO alone ($p < .05$). With creatine alone, improvements in bench press and LBM ($p < .05$) but other changes only as trends. CHO supplementation with creatine thought to increase muscle creatine uptake.
Brenner et al. 2000	Collegiate lacrosse players (16 F) Experimental–placebo design	7 days @ 20 g/day + 25 days @ 2 g/day for 25 days Resistance training	Testing at baseline, 5 weeks: • 1RM bench press • 1RM leg extension • Muscular endurance test (5 sets × 30 repetitions)	Yes No No	Increase in leg extension in both groups following training. Greater increase in bench press in creatine group than placebo group (17% vs. 3%, $p < .05$).
Larsen-Meyer et al. 2000	Collegiate soccer players (14 F) Experimental–placebo design	13 weeks creatine protocol or placebo Resistance training	Testing at baseline, 13 weeks: • 1RM bench press • 1RM squat	No No	Both groups increased strength in bench press and squat over off-season resistance training program. No significant difference between groups.
Bemben et al. 2001	Collegiate American football players (17 M) Experimental–placebo design	5 weeks @ 20 g/day then 8 weeks @ 5 g/day or placebo or control Resistance training 4/week	Testing at baseline, 9 weeks: • 1RM bench press • 1RM power clean • 1RM squat • Wingate cycling test	Yes No Yes Yes	Increase in bench press and squat in creatine group greater than in placebo group. Significant increase in BM and LBM in creatine group compared with other groups. Increase in BM and LBM and TBW (assessed by densitometry) in creatine group but unchanged in other groups. Increase in anaerobic power and capacity in Wingate test with creatine group compared with placebo or control groups.

(continued)

Table 8.d *(continued)*

Publication	Participants	Supplement protocol	Exercise protocol	Enhanced performance	Comments
Wilder et al. 2002	Collegiate American football players (25 M) Experimental–placebo design	6 days @ 20 g/day then 9 weeks @ 3 g/day creatine or 10 weeks @ 5 g/day or placebo Resistance 4/week and agility training 4/week	Testing at baseline and at 5 and 10 weeks: • 1RM back squat	No	Both groups increased 1RM strength and LBM (assessed by densitometry) over the 10-week training program. No difference between groups.
Creatine		Chronic supplementation protocol to enhance interval or other intermittent training			Some evidence, but not consistent findings, that creatine supplementation enhances training outcomes leading to better performance at the end of training block. More sport-specific research needed.
Kreider et al. 1998	Collegiate American football players (28 M) Experimental–placebo design	28 days @ 16 g/day creatine or placebo Resistance training 5/week, conditioning 3/week	Testing at baseline, 4 weeks: • 12 × 6 s cycling sprints with 30 s recovery	Yes	Mean improvement in work achieved in first 5 sprints of repeated cycling protocol in creatine group ($p < .05$) but dissipated after this.
Stone et al. 1999	Collegiate American football players (42 M) Experimental–placebo design	5 weeks @ 0.22 g/kg creatine or 0.13 g/kg creatine+ 0.09 g/kg pyruvate or placebo Resistance training 3/week, football practice 2/week	Testing at baseline, 5 weeks: • 15 × 5 s cycling sprint with 1 min recovery	No	No change in performance of repeated sprints with either creatine group compared with placebo.
O'Connor and Crowe 2003	Elite rugby league players (27 M) Experimental–placebo design	6 weeks @ 3 g/day creatine (+HMB) or control Resistance training 3/week, conditioning work 4/week, and speed work 1/week during preseason	Testing at baseline, 6 weeks: • Multistage fitness test (aerobic capacity) • 60 s cycling sprint (anaerobic capacity)	No No	No difference in aerobic power between creatine group and control at end of trial. Parameters of anaerobic capacity (peak power, total work) increased with training, but no difference between groups at posttrial testing.

TBW = total body water; LBM = lean body mass; BM = body mass; M = male; F = female; CHO = carbohydrate; RPE = rating of perceived exertion; RM = repetition maximum; DEXA = dual-energy X-ray absorptiometry; HMB = β-hydroxy β-methylbutyrate.

Table 8.e Studies of Supplements With Undetermined or Unlikely Benefits to Field-Based Team Sports

Publication	Participants	Supplement protocol	Exercise protocol	Enhanced performance	Comments
Bicarbonate		**Acute supplementation protocol**			**Although 2 studies provide support for beneficial effects of bicarbonate loading on the performance of an intermittent high-intensity protocol suggested to represent team sports, further sport-specific research is needed, particularly in elite athletes. In general, time-motion studies of most team sports do not report high lactate levels and pH changes to limit performance.**
Price et al. 2003	Active participants (8 M) Crossover study	300 mg/kg bicarbonate @ 60 min preexercise	Intermittent cycling protocol of 30 min involving 10 × repetition of 90 s @ 40%, 60s @ 60%, and 14 s @ 90% $\dot{V}O_2$max	Yes	Significant main effect with greater PPO achieved in 14 s sprints across protocol in bicarbonate trial, whereas placebo trial showed gradual decline in PPO across time. Blood lactate levels elevated to 10-12 mmol/L by 10 min and remained elevated across rest of protocol. Such values are higher than is generally reported in team sports; thus movement patterns may not reflect true workloads or physiological limitations of team sports.
Bishop and Claudius 2005	Team sports players (7 F) Crossover study	2 × 200 mg/kg bicarbonate @ 90 min and 20 min preexercise	Intermittent cycling protocol of 2 × 36 min • "Halves" • Repeated 2 min blocks (all-out 4 s sprint, 100 s active recovery at 35% $\dot{V}O_2$peak, and 20 s of rest)	Yes	Bicarbonate supplementation failed to produce any effect on performance in first half but caused trend toward improved total work in the second half ($p = .08$). In particular, participants completed significantly more work in 7 of 18 4 s sprints in the second half in the bicarbonate trial.
Bicarbonate and citrate		**Chronic supplementation protocol for training**			**There is new evidence that repeated use of bicarbonate loading before interval training sessions may enhance training adaptations and improve performance of sustained high-intensity exercise, at least in moderately trained individuals. It may also assist the athlete to train harder. Further research is needed to confirm these findings, especially for highly trained athletes.**
Edge at al. 2006	Moderately trained (16 F) Experimental-placebo design	8 wks at 400 mg/kg sodium bicarbonate in a split dose 90 min and 30 min before interval training Periodized interval training undertaken 3 d/wk: 2 min intervals with 1 min recovery, with 6 to 12 intervals completed at 140-170% of intensity at lactate threshold Both groups completed the same training load	0 and 8 wks (cycle): • $\dot{V}O_2$peak • lactate threshold • time to exhaustion at 100% pre-trial $\dot{V}O_2$peak	Yes	Both groups increased their $\dot{V}O_2$peak by similar amounts as a result of the 8 wk interval training. Both groups also increased their muscle buffering capacity. This increase in muscle buffering capacity was related to pre-training capacity rather than the treatment (subjects with lower pre-training muscle buffering capacity achieved greater increases as a result of training). Although both groups showed an increase in lactate threshold and time to exhaustion at $\dot{V}O_2$peak, the improvements were greater in the bicarbonate group. The authors speculated that training intensity rather than accumulation of H^+ ions is responsible for increasing muscle buffering capacity. Furthermore, inducing alkalosis during exercise may enhance muscle adaptations by reducing the damage to mitochondria or protein synthesis.

(continued)

Table 8.e *(continued)*

Publication	Participants	Supplement protocol	Exercise protocol	Enhanced performance	Comments
Bovine colostrum		**Chronic supplementation protocol**			**Potential value presently undetermined in overall literature. No mechanisms identified to explain any potential benefits. Expense of moderate and large doses of supplement ($US40 per week) warrants additional supportive research before it can be recommended. Interest in emerging evidence that low doses might provide benefits is of interest.**
Hofman et al. 2002	Elite hockey players (17 F + 18 M) Experimental–placebo design	8 weeks @ 60 g/day of colostrum or placebo (whey protein) 3/week training + game 1/week	Tests at baseline and 8 weeks: • 5 × 10 m sprint • Vertical jump • Shuttle run • "Suicide" agility test	Yes No No No	No improvements in shuttle run, jump, or agility run over 8 weeks in either group. Significant improvement in sprint performance for both groups with larger improvement in colostrum group (0.64 s vs. 0.33 s, $p < .05$). Similar increases in LBM in both groups.
β-hydroxy β-methylbutyrate (HMB)		**Chronic supplementation protocol**			**Potential value in reducing muscle damage and enhancing recovery from resistance training is presently undetermined. Present literature is equivocal. Some studies suggest that benefits are limited to novice trainers or to initial response to an increase in training load. Further studies are required in highly trained athletes to support any benefits.**
O'Connor and Crowe 2003	Elite rugby league players (27 M) Experimental–placebo design	6 weeks @ 3 g/day HMB or (3 g/day HMB + creatine) or control Resistance training 3/week, conditioning work 4/week, and speed work 1/week during preseason	Testing at baseline, 6 weeks: • Multistage fitness test (aerobic capacity) • 60 s cycling sprint (anaerobic capacity)	No No	No difference in aerobic power in either HMB group compared with control group at posttrial testing. Parameters of anaerobic capacity (peak power, total work) improved with training but there was no difference between control group and HMB groups at end of trial.
Ransone et al. 2003	Collegiate American football players (35 M) Crossover design	4 weeks @ 3 g/day HMB or placebo Sport-specific training (20 hr/week) including resistance training (4/week)	Tests at baseline, 4 weeks: 1RM for • Bench press • Power cleans • Squats	No No No	No significant changes in muscle strength over time in either trial. No change in BM or body fat (assessed via anthropometry).

Reference	Subjects/Design	Supplementation protocol	Tests		Results
Hoffman et al. 2004	Collegiate American football players (26 M) Experimental–placebo design	3 g/day HMB for 10 days Sport-related training	Tests at baseline and at 10 days • Anaerobic power test	No	No difference in anaerobic power seen between groups. Plasma concentrations of cortisol decreased and creatine kinase increased over the 10 days of training in both groups.
Chromium or chromium picolinate		**Acute supplementation protocol**			**No enhancement of insulin action with either acute or chronic supplementation. No effect on body composition or strength changes in response to resistance training.**
Davis et al. 2000	Active participants (8 M) Crossover design Conditions not stated; presumably moderate	400 µg of chromium preexercise + 15 ml/kg 6% carbohydrate–electrolyte drink before and during exercise, or carbohydrate drink alone or placebo drink	5 × 15 min intermittent shuttle running + intermittent run to fatigue	No	Carbohydrate increased time to fatigue in last shuttle run compared with placebo trial. However, no further improvement with carbohydrate + chromium (11.2 vs. 11.1 min).
Chromium or chromium picolinate		**Chronic supplementation protocol**			**No enhancement of insulin action with chronic supplementation. No effect on body composition or strength changes in response to resistance training.**
Clancy et al. 1994	Collegiate football players (36 M) Experimental–placebo design	9 weeks @ 200 µg/day 9 weeks of resistance and conditioning training	Testing at baseline, 5 and 10 weeks: • Isometric and concentric strength of knee and elbow measured by dynamometer	No	No enhancement of LBM, body fat (assessed by densitometry), or girths in chromium group above placebo group. No changes in strength measurements in either group. Urinary chromium losses increased in chromium supplementation group.
Pyruvate		**Chronic supplementation protocol**			**No evidence of benefits to metabolism or training outcomes**
Stone et al. 1999	Collegiate American football players (42 M) Experimental–placebo design	5 weeks @ 0.22 g/kg creatine or 0.13 g/kg creatine+ 0.09 g/kg pyruvate or placebo Resistance training 3/week, football practice 2/week	Testing at baseline, 5 weeks: • 1RM bench press • 1RM squat • Vertical jump • 15 × 5 s cycling sprint with 1 min recovery	No No No No	Compared with creatine alone, creatine–pyruvate did not further increase enhancements seen over 5 weeks of training, suggesting that pyruvate is ineffective.

(continued)

Table 8.e *(continued)*

Publication	Participants	Supplement protocol	Exercise protocol	Enhanced performance	Comments
Ginseng		**Chronic supplementation protocol**			**Literature does not show any consistent benefits to performance following ginseng supplementation. Ginseng supplements have variable amounts of active ingredients**
Ziemba et al. 1999	Trained soccer players (15 M) Experimental–placebo design	6 weeks @ 350 mg/day Panax ginseng	• Incremental cycling test to exhaustion • Reaction time measured at each stage (time to respond to lights)	No Yes	No change in lactate threshold or $\dot{V}O_2$max. However, enhanced reaction time at rest and at submaximal workloads.
Branched-chain amino acids (BCAA)		**Acute supplementation protocol**			**Literature does not show any consistent benefits to motor or mental performance following BCAA supplementation.**
Blomstrand et al. 1991	National-level soccer players (6 F) Crossover design	6% carbohydrate drink + 7.5 g BCAA or carbohydrate alone	Soccer match: Stroop Color Word Test given before and after match	Yes	Stroop Color Word Test score enhanced after game with carbohydrate + BCAA compared with carbohydrate alone.
Davis et al. 1999	Active participants (3 M + 5 F) Crossover design	6% carbohydrate drink 1 hr pre + during exercise + 7 g BCAA in 1 hr preexercise drink or carbohydrate drink alone or placebo	5 × 15 min intermittent shuttle running + intermittent run to fatigue	No	Time to fatigue in last test with CHO trial compared with placebo trial, but no extra advantage with BCAA (9.66 vs. 9.00 min, $p < .05$).

LBM = lean body mass; BM = body mass; M = male; F= female; PPO = Peak Power Output; RM = repetition maximum; CHO = carbohydrate..

Table 9.a Reported Dietary Intakes of Male Team Athletes—Court and Indoor Games: Training (Mean Daily Intake ± SD)

Publication	Team population	Survey method	Age (years)	BM (kg)	ENERGY		CHO			PROTEIN			FAT	
					MJ	KJ/kg	g	g/kg	%E	g	g/kg	%E	g	%E
Berry et al. 1949	Mexican basketball player at 1948 Olympic Games (n = 1)	4-day duplicate meal collection, chemical assay	26	82	12.85	156	397	4.8	52	134	1.6	18	104	30
Short and Short 1983	U.S. collegiate basketball players • Season (n = 8) • Season (n = 13)	3-day food diary (household measures)			16.26 23.31		421 584		43 42	152 212		16 15	169 254	39 41
Nowak et al. 1988	U.S. collegiate basketball players (n = 16)	3-day food diary (household measures)	19	83	14.87 ± 4.51	179	437 ± 158	5.3	47	159 ± 70			139 ± 48	
Grandjean 1989	U.S. national-level and collegiate basketball players (n = 11)	3-day food diary (household measures)			17.04 ± 3.2	—	448	—	44 ± 7	160	—	15 ± 2	189	41 ± 6
Schroder et al. 2000	Professional basketball players (n = 16)	24 hr recall	23	96	~17.9		~380		~45	~211		~19	~211	~36
Van Erp-Baart et al. 1989a	Dutch international-level water polo players (n = 30)	4- to 7-day food diary (household measures)	24	86	16.59	194	~467	~5.5	~45	~162	~1.9	~17	~166	~37
Schena et al. 1995	Italian national-level ice hockey players (n = 20)	7-day food diary (household measures)	24	73	14.25 ± 1.12	190	456 ± 38	6.5	53	112 ± 53	1.5	23	96 ± 11	24

BM = body mass; CHO = carbohydrate; E = energy.

Table 9.b Reported Dietary Intakes of Female Team Athletes—Court and Indoor Games: Training (Mean Daily Intake ± SD)

Publication	Team population	Survey method	Age (years)	BM (kg)	ENERGY		CHO			PROTEIN			FAT	
					MJ	KJ/kg	g	g/kg	%E	g	g/kg	%E	g	%E
Short and Short 1983	U.S. collegiate basketball players (n = 9)	3-day food diary (household measures)		71	13.6	192	379	5.3	46	108	1.5	14	145	40
Hickson et al. 1986	U.S. collegiate basketball players (n = 13)	3 × 24 hr dietary recall	19	68	8.38 ± 2.3	126 ± 121	—	—	—	—	—	—	—	—
Nowak et al. 1988	U.S. collegiate basketball players (n = 10)	3-day food diary (household measures)	19	72	7.23 ± 2.4	100	229 ± 95	3.2	51	68 ± 28			63 ± 19	
Risser et al. 1990	U.S. collegiate basketball players (n = 9)	3 × 24 hr dietary recall	20	70	7.52 ± 3.64	109	227 ± 104	3.3	48	69 ± 37	1.0	15	52 ± 26	26
Short and Short 1983	U.S. collegiate volleyball players • Season (n = 11) • Season (n = 7)	3-day food diary (household measures)			10.27 7.61		314 244		49 53	103 61		16 13	95 69	34 34
Van Erp-Baart et al. 1989a	Dutch international-level volleyball players (n = 9)	4- to 7-day food diary (household measures)	23	66	9.24	140	263	4.0	46	73	1.1	13	92	37
Risser et al. 1990	U.S. collegiate volleyball players (n = 12)	3 × 24 hr dietary recall	20	66	6.73 ± 2.4	102	216 ± 69	3.3	51	70 ± 31	1.1	17	54 ± 27	30
Papadopoulou et al. 2002	Greek junior national volleyball players (n = 16)	3-day food diary (household measures)	17	66	8.45 ± 4.1	128	228 ± 97	3.5 ± 1.4	45 ± 13	67 ± 25	1.0 ± 0.4	15 ± 5	98 ± 67	41 ± 11
Van Erp-Baart et al. 1989a	Dutch international-level handball players (n = 8)	4- to 7-day food diary (household measures)	22	63	8.97	142	251	4.0	45	76	1.2	14	101	42
Ersoy 1995	Turkish handball players (n = 10)	3-day food diary (household measures)	22	62	7.30	118	229	3.7	53	51	0.8	12	68	35

BM = body mass; CHO = carbohydrate; E = energy.

Table 9.c Available Data on Voluntary Fluid Intakes and Sweat Losses During Training and Competition in Court and Indoor Sports (Mean ± SD)

Publication	Participants	Temperature (°C)	Humidity (%)	SWEAT LOSS Total (ml)	SWEAT LOSS Rate (ml/hr)	FLUID INTAKE Total (ml)	FLUID INTAKE Rate (ml/hr)	Dehydration (= % change in BM^)
BASKETBALL—TRAINING								
Broad et al. 1996	Junior elite players • 36 M[a], summer • 36 M, winter	27[b](27)[c] 20 (10)	34 (30) 24 (43)	2,300 ± 830 2,145 ± 535	1,370 ± 235 1,040 ± 170	1,380 ± 640 1,015 ± 425	795 ± 235 490 ± 175	1.0 ± 0.5 1.2 ± 0.4
Broad et al. 1996	Junior elite players • 69 F, summer • 39 F, winter	25 (24) 17 (12)	43 (24) 56 (77)	1,240 ± 225 1,320 ± 360	680 ± 140 685 ± 115	760 ± 310 655 ± 365	410 ± 160 330 ± 155	0.7 ± 0.4 1.0 ± 0.4
Burke et al. 2006b unpublished data	Elite international players (16 M)	12	59	2058 ± 601	895 ± 261	1086 ± 597	472 ± 260	1.3 ± 0.5 (2 players > 2% loss)
BASKETBALL—MATCH PLAY								
Broad et al. 1996	Junior elite players • 44 M, summer • 38 M, winter	23 (22) 19 (9)	41 (22) 36 (61)	2,310 ± 600 2,200 ± 610	1,600 ± 370 1,585 ± 360	151 5 ± 640 1,260 ± 625	1,080 ± 615 915 ± 460	0.9 ± 0.7 1.0 ± 0.6
Broad et al. 1996	Junior elite players • 32 F, summer • 24 F, winter	26 (25) 17 (10)	60 (58) 58 (60)	1,420 ± 385 1,320 ± 400	915 ± 255 975 ± 255	930 ± 265 810 ± 245	600 ± 170 600 ± 165	0.7 ± 0.5 0.7 ± 0.5
NETBALL—TRAINING								
Broad et al. 1996	Junior elite players • 39 F, summer • 39 F, winter	28[b](28)[c] 19 (8)	36 (34) 30 (58)	1,300 ± 290 915 ± 320	725 ± 140 715 ± 265	785 ± 355 620 ± 285	440 ± 190 500 ± 275	0.7 ± 0.5 0.4 ± 0.5

(continued)

Table 9.c *(continued)*

Publication	Participants	Temperature (°C)	Humidity (%)	SWEAT LOSS Total (ml)	SWEAT LOSS Rate (ml/hr)	FLUID INTAKE Total (ml)	FLUID INTAKE Rate (ml/hr)	Dehydration (= % change in BM^)
NETBALL—MATCH PLAY
Broad et al. 1996	Junior elite players • 16 F, summer • 16 F, winter	22 (20) 14 (16	66 (72) 43 (45)	1,295 ± 435 1,065 ± 210	980 ± 255 880 ± 185	695 ± 300 820 ± 360	520 ± 190 660 ± 250	0.9 ± 0.5 0.3 ± 0.6
WATER POLO—TRAINING
Cox, Broad, et al. 2002	International level (81 M)	27^d		455 ± 60	285 ± 60	230 ± 60	140 ± 55	0.3 ± 0.1
WATER POLO—MATCH PLAY
Cox, Broad, et al. 2002	International level (33 M)	27^d		595 ± 95	785 ± 90	285 ± 90	380 ± 85	0.4 ± 0.1

BM = body mass.

^{a}Figures refer to numbers of observations in males (M) and females (F); ^{b}court temperature, ^{c}outside temperature, ^{d}pool temperature. ^The weight change occurring over the session is presumed to represent a body fluid deficit, and has not been corrected for change in BM that occurs in very prolonged events due to factors other than fluid loss (e.g., metabolic fuel losses).

Table 9.d Studies of Supplements With Likely Benefit to Court-Based and Indoor Team Sports

Publication	Participants	Supplement protocol	Exercise protocol	Enhanced performance	Comments
Acute (loading) supplementation protocol with relevance to movement patterns during matches					**Reasonable evidence that creatine loading is associated with enhanced ability to undertake repeated brief sprints with short recovery intervals as found in movement patterns of court and indoor team sports. —More sport-specific research needed.**
Aaserud et al. 1998	Well-trained handball players (14 M) Experimental–placebo design	5 days @ 15 g/day + 9 days @ 2 g/day creatine or placebo	Tests at baseline, after 5 days (large dose) and 14 days (low dose) • 8 × 40 m running sprint with 25 s recovery	Yes	Run time on last 3 sprints reduced after 5 days of high-dose creatine ($p < .05$). No change seen in placebo group. Similar increase in blood lactate concentration with sprint set in both groups.
Jones et al. 1999	High-level ice hockey players (16 M) Experimental–placebo design	5 days @ 20 g/day + 10 weeks @ 5 g/day creatine or placebo	Tests at baseline, after 10 days and 10 weeks • Cycle tests 5 × 15 s with 15 s recovery • 6 × 80 m skate sprints on 30 s time cycle	Yes Yes	No changes seen in placebo group. Average mean and peak power outputs in cycling test increase in creatine group after 10 days ($p < .05$). Mean on-ice sprint performance also enhanced at 10 days.
Ziegenfuss et al. 2002	Collegiate athletes including basketball, field hockey, ice-hockey, softball players (10 M, 10 F) Experimental–placebo design	3 days @ 0.35 g/kg LBM creatine or placebo	Tests at baseline and 3 days • 6 × 10 s cycling sprints with 60 s recovery	Yes	Gain of BM of 0.9 kg in creatine group. Creatine supplementation significantly increased peak power during sprints 2-6. Increase in mid-thigh muscle volume in creatine group (assessed by magnetic resonance imaging).
Izquierdo et al. 2002	Well-trained handball players (19 M) Experimental–placebo design	5 days @ 20 g/day creatine or placebo	Tests at baseline and 5 days • Repeated sprint running test (15 m) • Discontinuous incremental running test (endurance test) • 1RM bench press • Repetition bench press • 1RM half squat • Repetition half squat • Countermovement jump	Yes—first 5 m No No Yes Yes Yes Yes	Increase of 0.6 kg BM in creatine group ($p < .05$) but not placebo group. Increase in maximal strength in lower-body test, and greater improvement in total repetitions performed to fatigue in lower-body strength tests compared with upper body in creatine group. Improved performance in the first 5 m of 15 m sprint runs and attenuated decline in jumping ability over testing protocol with creatine group compared with placebo. No change in endurance test in either group.

(continued)

Table 9.d *(continued)*

Publication	Participants	Supplement protocol	Exercise protocol	Enhanced performance	Comments
Chronic supplementation to enhance training outcomes					There is reasonable evidence that chronic creatine supplementation can provide a training aid, improving game practice, interval training or resistance training. More sport-specific research is needed to see if this transfers into better outcomes in a game
Aaserud et al. 1998	Well-trained handball players (14 M) Experimental–placebo design	5 days @ 15 g/day + 9 day @ 2 g/day creatine or placebo	Tests at baseline, after 5 days (large dose) and 14 days (low dose) • 8 × 40 m running sprint with 25 s recovery	Yes	See preceding details in acute supplementation information. Performance enhancements maintained but not further improved after 9 days.
Jones et al. 1999	High-level ice hockey players (16 M) Experimental–placebo design	5 days @ 20 g/day + 10 weeks @ 5 g/day	Tests at baseline, after 10 days and 10 weeks • Cycle tests 5 × 15 s with 15 s recovery • 6 × 80 m skate sprints on 30 s time cycle	Yes Yes	See details in acute supplementation information. Performance enhancements for mean peak power and on-ice skate performance maintained but not further improved after 10 weeks.

M = male; F = female, BM = body mass; LBM = lean body mass; RM = repetition maximum.

Table 9.e Studies of Hydration or Carbohydrate (CHO) Intake and Performance of Prolonged Intermittent High-Intensity Exercise

Publication	Participants	Fluid or CHO intake protocol	Exercise protocol	Enhanced performance	Comments
			FLUID		
Hoffman et al. 1995	Junior competitive basketball players (10 M) Crossover design 21°C, 64% rh	No fluid or fluid intake throughout game to replace sweat losses. No fluid achieved hypohydration of ~1% at half time, ~1.9% at end of game	Warm-up plus 2 × 20 min game simulations. Jump testing protocol undertaken at warm-up, halftime, and postgame • Vertical squat • Countermovement jump • 30 s vertical jump	Perhaps	No significant change in vertical jump or countermovement jump between trials or across game. Trend to improvement in performance of 30 s vertical jump test from pregame to postgame, with anaerobic power being 19% higher in fluid trial at postgame testing compared with no-fluid trial. Authors claim that this may be of practical importance despite failing to reach statistical significance.
McGregor et al. 1999	Semiprofessional soccer players (9 M) Crossover design 13-15°C, 57% rh	No fluid or 15 ml/kg artificially flavored water consumed before and throughout 90 min protocol. Overall difference in fluid status = 1.4% vs. 2.4% hypohydration	90 min intermittent high-intensity shuttle running (LIST) • Performance of 15 m sprints monitored throughout LIST	Yes	No difference over time or between trials for mean sprint time for first 5 × 15 min blocks. In last 15 min, mean sprint time was longer in no-fluid trial than fluid trial ($p < .05$). Higher ratings of perceived exertion and serum cortisol during last 30 min of LIST of no-fluid trial. Mean heart rate higher in no-fluid trial.
Devlin et al. 2001	Competitive medium to fast cricket bowlers (7 M) Crossover design Bowling test undertaken in moderate environment (16°C)	Artificially flavored ice cubes (placebo) or intake of fluid before (600 ml) and during (250 ml per break) intermittent exercise to replace 80% of fluid losses: Overall difference in fluid status = 0.5% vs. 2.8% hypohydration	1 hr intermittent exercise in the heat. Testing pregame • Shuttle run	Yes	Number of shuttles run in pretest shuttle protocol similar for both trials (~92). However, in posttest protocol, placebo associated with lower number of shuttles completed (76 vs. 82, $p < .05$).
Magal et al. 2003	Competitive tennis players (11 M) Crossover design (glycerol vs. water hyperhydration) Hot environment: ~31°C, 75% rh	Hyperhydration (22 ml/kg fluid) with or without glycerol during 150 min prior to protocol. During protocol, 10 ml/kg of 8% CHO–electrolyte drink consumed during protocol with overall during-game hypohydration of 2.7% BM. Rehydration over 90 min postprotocol with 11 ml/kg fluid with and without glycerol	Exercise protocol = 75 min match play. Performance testing: • 5 and 10 m sprint tests • Agility test undertaken preexercise, postexercise, and postrehydration	Yes (?) No (?)	Performance of 5 and 10 m sprints reduced in both trials after exercise, with authors claiming this was attributable to 2.7% hypohydration. No change in performance of agility test. No difference between trials, although glycerol trial associated with better maintenance of plasma volume. Performance restored after rehydration period. There is an order effect in this study, and performance changes may result from the the effect of the exercise protocol and subsequent rest as well as hypohydration.

(continued)

Table 9.e *(continued)*

Publication	Participants	Fluid or CHO intake protocol	Exercise protocol	Enhanced performance	Comments
			FLUID		
Kobayashi et al. 2004	Collegiate table tennis players (8M) Crossover design with some order effect (moderate trial first then hot trials in counterbalanced order) Moderate environment = 17°C, 50% Hot environment = 30°C, 70%	Moderate environment trial with no fluid intake (loss of 0.34 L/h over 101 min); 2 trials in hot environment with no fluid replacement (loss of 1.47 kg = 2.4% BM), or ad lib replacement with sports drink (subjects consumed 1.94L)		Yes, in hot conditions	Although study is targeted as an investigation of dehydration, fluid trial involved a sports drink, thereby introducing carbohydrate intake as an additional factor in performance changes. No fluid intake in hot conditions resulted in an elevated rectal temperature compared to moderate conditions and hot conditions with fluid intake. Anaerobic power decreased by 14% in Hot/no fluid trial compared with 2% decrement in Moderate/no fluid and Hot/fluid trials (p <.05). Performance scores increased across first 4 bouts in all trials, then decreased in Hot/no fluid trial compared with other trials. Average scores across the trials showed significantly lower performance for Hot/no fluid trial (436) compared to Moderate/no fluid (484) and Hot/fluid (469).

Dougherty et al. 2006	Skilled adolescent basketball players (15 M)
	Crossover design
	Presumably moderate environment following 2 hr exposure to hot environment and moderate exercise to incur a fluid deficit of ~ 2% BM
		Prior to protocol, participants prepared by drinking artificially flavored water (Placebo trial) or limiting fluid intake to achieve fluid deficit of 2% (Dehydration trial). Fluid intake continued during basketball protocol to maintain these differences	Basketball simulation protocol = 4 × 12 min quarters with 10 min half-time break:
			Drills included
			• Sprint tests:
			  -Suicides
			  -10 court widths
			• Lateral movement tests:
			  -Zigzags
			  -20 lane slides
			• 10 vertical jumps
			• Defensive drills
				Yes
				
				Yes
				
				No
				No
					Compared with Placebo (euhydration) trial, the performance of each of the sprints and suicides was impaired in Dehydration trial. Average sprinting times for both drills was 42 ± 5 vs 39 ± 4 s for Dehydration and Placebo respectively (p <.05). Lateral movement drills, individually and combined, were impaired in Dehydration trial compared to Placebo trial (average lateral movement times were 37 ± 4 vs 34 ± 4 s for Dehydration and Placebo respectively; p <.05). There was no difference between trials in time to complete vertical jumps or defensive drills.

			CARBOHYDRATE		
Muckle 1973	Competitive male soccer team. n = 40 matches: 20 = CHO, 20 = control Crossover design Outdoors—presumably moderate conditions	105-110 g of CHO (glucose and mineral syrup) given 30 min prematch	40 matches over season: • Movement analysis of one player per match chosen at random	Yes	Individual analysis showed enhanced number of ball contacts over last 15 min of CHO match compared with control matches.

Study	Supplement	Exercise protocol	Ergogenic?	Results
Burke and Ekblom 1982 Active tennis players (5 M + 5 F) Crossover design Indoor court 23-25°C	5 trials: • Control (no exercise) • Sauna induced dehydration by 2.4% BM • Exercise + no fluid • Exercise + ad lib water throughout (505 ml) • Exercise + ad lib CHO–electrolyte drink (736 ml + 55 g CHO)	Exercise protocol = 2 hr of tennis Tests undertaken pre- and post-2 hr of tennis or rest: • Sargent jump	Yes	Plasma glucose maintained at higher levels with CHO trial. Sargent jump increased posttrial with CHO and maintained on water trial. Trend to reduction in Sargent jump with dehydration and control.
Kirkendall et al. 1988 Collegiate soccer players (10 M) Crossover design Outdoors—presumably moderate conditions	125 g of CHO (glucose polymer syrup) or placebo consumed before and during match	Match play • Movement analysis of players undertaken for 3 × 5 min of each half and extrapolated to 90 min	Yes	CHO match showed 25% greater distance covered in 2nd half than placebo match ($p < .05$). In addition, greater distance covered at "strategic intensities" of cruise and sprint.
Simard et al. 1988 Collegiate ice hockey players (7 M) Crossover design Presumably cool-moderate environment or ice rink	120 g glucose in lemon drink over 3 hr pregame and during real ice hockey game or placebo drink	2 × ice hockey games (3 × 20 min period) • Movement analysis of players Muscle biopsies taken pre- and postgame	Yes	Carbohydrate trial associated with 5% greater playing time and 10% greater distance skated than control trial. Blood glucose concentrations higher at end of CHO trial. After normalizing for distance skated, CHO trial associated with reduction in glycogen utilization ($p < .05$).
Criswell et al. 1991 High-school football players (44 M) Experimental–placebo design Hot outdoor environment: 28°C, 66% rh	6 × 170 ml of 7% CHO–electrolyte fluid or placebo consumed at 10 min intervals during scrimmage (71 g of CHO)	Simulated field-play: 50-play scrimmage. Tests undertake pre- and post-session • 8 × 40 yd sprints (40 s recovery)	No	Compared with presession testing, both CHO and placebo group reduced peak and mean velocity for the 8 × 40 yd sprints at the end of the scrimmage session. No differences between groups in terms of performance decay. Plasma glucose concentrations higher in CHO group at end of scrimmage session.
Mitchell et al. 1992 Competitive tennis players (10 M + 2 F) Crossover design	11.4 ml·kg^{-1}·hr^{-1} placebo or 7.5% CHO drink, consumed as 200 ml per 15 min (800 ml/hr fluid + 60 g/hr CHO = 2.5 g/kg CHO)	3 hr match play. Tests undertaken pre- and postplay • 10 ball shuttle run (183 m)	No	Blood glucose concentrations maintained in both trials over 3 hr of match practice. 2-3% decline in time to complete shuttle run from pre- to postplay tests, but no difference between trials.
Nicholas et al. 1995 Trained games players (9 M) Crossover design Lab conditions kept <20°C	15 ml/kg 7% CHO-electrolyte drink or placebo, consumed before and throughout 90 min protocol to provide 1.1 g/kg CHO	75 min intermittent high-intensity shuttle running followed by • Intermittent run to exhaustion	Yes	Time to exhaustion in intermittent run was 33% longer in CHO trial than placebo (8.9 min vs. 6.7 min, $p < .05$). Blood glucose concentrations maintained within normal range for both trials but tended to be higher in CHO trial.

(continued)

Table 9.e (continued)

Publication	Participants	Fluid or CHO intake protocol	Exercise protocol	Enhanced performance	Comments
			FLUID		
Ferrauti et al. 1997	Competitive tennis players (8 M + 8 F) Crossover design Hot outdoor environment: 28°C, 42% rh	100 ml (women) and 150 ml (men) of 7.6% CHO–electrolyte drink or placebo consumed every 15 min to provide a total of 2.8 L of fluid and 243 g of CHO (men) and 2.0 L of fluid and 182 g of CHO (women) over 4 hr	4 hr tennis singles play (with 30 min break after 150 min). Tests of speed undertaken at end of 4 hr: • 6 × 15 min sprint with 30 min rest	Yes	Better running time for tennis sprint test with CHO than placebo. Blood glucose concentration greater in CHO trial than placebo from 90-180 min. In both studies, decline in blood glucose concentration when play resumed after 30 min break.
Nassis et al. 1998	Active participants (8 M + 1 F) Crossover design Presumably moderate laboratory conditions	13 ml/kg 7% CHO–electrolyte drink or placebo spread throughout protocol (0.9 g/kg CHO)	Intermittent treadmill running protocol (15 s sprints, 10 s rest) with speed of sprint increasing over protocol, until >100 min to fatigue: 90% $\dot{V}O_2$max	No	Performance times not different between trials (112.5 vs. 110 min for placebo and CHO, NS). Blood glucose concentration higher only at 40 min with CHO trial, and no difference in rates of CHO oxidation between trials.
Vergauwen et al. 1998	Well-trained tennis players (13 M) Crossover design Conditions not stated; presumably moderate	CHO–electrolyte or placebo to provide total of 0.7 g·kg^{-1}·hr^{-1} CHO and 800 ml/hr fluid	Tests undertaken pre- and post-2 hr match play • 70 m shuttle run	Yes	Compared with prematch test, time to complete postmatch shuttle run increased in placebo trial by ~2.5% ($p < .05$). No deterioration in shuttle run seen in CHO trial
Davis et al. 1999	Active participants (3 M + 5 F) Crossover design Conditions not stated; presumably moderate	15 ml/kg 6% CHO–electrolyte or placebo drink before and during exercise (0.9 g/kg CHO)	5 × 15 min intermittent shuttle running followed by • Intermittent run to fatigue	Yes	Heart rate lower with CHO trial from 30 min onward. Blood glucose higher for first 45 min with CHO trial. Time to fatigue in last test 52% longer with CHO trial (9.66 vs. 6.36 min, $p < .05$).
Davis et al. 2000	Active participants (8 M) Crossover design Conditions not stated; presumably moderate	15 ml/kg 6% CHO–electrolyte or placebo drink before and during exercise (0.9 g/kg CHO)	5 × 15 min intermittent shuttle running followed by • Intermittent run to fatigue	Yes	Heart rate lower with CHO trial. Blood glucose higher for first 45 min with CHO trial. Time to fatigue in last test 32% longer with CHO trial (11.2 vs. 8.5 min, $p < .05$).
Welsh et al. 2002	Collegiate basketball and soccer players (5 F + 5 M) Crossover design Presumably moderate lab conditions	6% CHO–electrolyte drink (quarters) and 18% CHO drink (halftime) or placebo drinks to provide total of 22 ml/kg fluid and 1.9 g/kg CHO (127 g CHO)	Warm-up + 60 min "game" of intermittent high-intensity running and jumping protocol (4 × 15 min quarters with 20 min halftime break) followed by • Shuttle run to fatigue	Yes	Mean "time to fatigue" in shuttle run at end of 60 min "game" protocol was 37% longer with CHO trial than placebo (3.58 vs. 2.61 min, $p < .05$). Mean time for 20 min sprints was better maintained in 4th quarter with CHO than placebo, leading to 14% enhancement of speed. No differences in 30 s vertical jump between trials. Plasma glucose concentrations maintained at higher levels throughout CHO trial than placebo.

Study	Participants / Design	CHO intervention	Protocol	Significant	Findings
Kipp et al. 2003	Collegiate soccer players (15 F) Crossover design Presumably moderate lab conditions	900 ml of 7% CHO–2% protein–electrolyte drink (63 g CHO) or sweetened placebo	75 min practice session including warm-up, skills, and 40 m scrimmaging followed by • 4 × 280 sprints (agility + straight sprinting)	Yes	Mean time for the 4 sprints completed after practice session showed 4% faster time for the last sprint with CHO trial than placebo trial (91.5 vs. 95.5 s, $p < .05$).
Morris et al. 2003	Collegiate rugby or soccer players (9 M) Crossover design 30°C	27 ml/kg of 6.5% CHO–electrolyte drink or placebo or flavored water, before and throughout the protocol to provide 1.8 g/kg CHO	5 × 15 min intermittent high-intensity protocol (modified LIST) followed by • Intermittent run to exhaustion	No	Sprint performance reduced over duration of the protocol. Time to exhaustion protocol showed order effect with 3rd trial being longer than first trial (effect of acclimation?). Hard to interpret other results in light of this effect. Trend for CHO trial to reduce endurance and higher rectal temperatures compared with flavored water trial. Reduced gastric emptying. Blood glucose concentrations higher with CHO trial, suggesting that CHO availability not a limiting factor for endurance in the heat.
Winnick et al. 2005	Participants in team sports (10 M + 10 F) Crossover design Presumably moderate lab conditions:	22 ml/kg 6% CHO–electrolyte drink or placebo or flavored water, before and throughout the protocol to provide 1.3 g/kg CHO (~41 g/hr)	4 × 15 min intermittent high-intensity protocol with tests throughout • 20 m sprints • 60 s jumping tests	Yes Yes	Mean times for the 20 m sprint declined over the test protocol in the placebo trial but were maintained in the CHO trial so that 4th quarter times were faster for CHO vs. placebo (0.1 s, $p < .01$). Similarly, average jump height was maintained in the CHO trial but declined over time in the placebo trial, so that 4th quarter performance was better in the 4th quarter in CHO trial. Therefore, physical performance was enhanced with CHO intake, because of the preservation of function that would otherwise decline in latter stages of protocol in placebo trial.
Dougherty et al. 2006	Skilled adolescent basketball players (15 M) Crossover design Presumably moderate environment following 2 hr exposure to hot environment and moderate exercise to incur a fluid deficit of ~2% BM	Prior to protocol, participants prepared by drinking artificially flavored water (Placebo trial) or 6% CHO–electrolyte drink to maintain hydration, and continued intakes of these fluids during basketball protocol to maintain hydration	Basketball simulation protocol = 4 × 12 min quarters with 10 min half-time break: Drills included • Sprint tests: -Suicides -10 court widths • Lateral movement tests: -Zigzags -20 lane slides • 10 vertical jumps • Defensive drills	Yes No No No	There were no differences between trials in time to complete vertical jumps or to complete defensive drills, although defensive drills were completed faster in CHO trial than in a third trial involving dehydration (see column above in section involving fluid). Sprint tests were completed faster in CHO trial compared to Placebo trial (38 ± 4 vs 39 ± 4 s for CHO and Placebo respectively ($p < .05$). Times for the lateral movement tests were similar between CHO and Placebo trials.

CHO = carbohydrate; M = male; BM = body mass; rh = relative humidity; LIST = Loughborough Intermittent Shuttle Test; NS = not significant.

Table 9.f Studies of Hydration or Carbohydrate (CHO) Intake and Cognitive and Skill Performance

Publication	Participants	Fluid or CHO intake protocol	Exercise protocol	Enhanced performance	Comments
			FLUID		
Hoffman et al. 1995	Junior competitive basketball players (10 M) Crossover design 21°C, 64% rh	No fluid or fluid intake throughout game to replace sweat losses. No fluid achieved hypohydration of ~1% at halftime, ~1.9% at end of game	Warm-up plus 2 × 20 min game simulations with testing of jumps following warm-up, halftime, and postgame. Skill tests throughout game: • Success of free throws and field goals	Perhaps	No significant change in percentage of successful free throws between trials or between halves of simulated game. Although differences between fluid and no-fluid trial did not reach statistical significance, no-fluid trial showed an 8% decrease in percentage of successful field goals in second half compared with first half, whereas fluid trial showed 1.6% improvement in percentage success. Authors noted that this difference is likely to be of practical significance.
McGregor et al. 1999	Semiprofessional soccer players (9 M) Crossover design 13-15°C, 57% rh	15 ml/kg artificially flavored water or no fluid, consumed before and throughout 90 min protocol. Overall difference in fluid status = 1.4% vs. 2.4% hypohydration	90 min intermittent high-intensity shuttle running (LIST) Tests undertaken pre- and post-LIST • Soccer skill test (dribble test) • Mental concentration test (number recognition)	Yes No	Performance of skill and mental concentration tests were identical in pre-LIST testing. Mental concentration maintained in both trials, but performance of dribble test deteriorated by 5% in no-fluid trial (130 vs. 136 s, p < .05).
Devlin et al. 2001	Competitive medium–fast cricket bowlers (7 M) Bowling test undertaken in moderate environment (16°C)	Intake of fluid before (600 ml) and during (250 ml per break) intermittent exercise to replace 80% of fluid losses: Overall difference in fluid status = 0.5% vs. 2.8% hypohydration	1 hr intermittent exercise in the heat. Tests undertaken pre- and post: • Bowling test for 36 deliveries (line, length, and speed)	Yes	Hypohydration trial was associated with a reduction in posttest scores for line (16% reduction) and length (15% reduction) of accuracy of bowling (p < .05) compared with fluid trial. No impairment of the bowling velocity with hypohydration trial.

Study	Participants & design	Intervention	Exercise/skills protocol	Effect	Results
Magal et al. 2003	Competitive tennis players (11 M) Crossover design (glycerol vs. water hyperhydration) Hot environment: ~31°C, 75% rh	Hyperhydration (22 ml/kg fluid) with or without glycerol during 150 min prior to protocol. During protocol, 10 ml/kg 8% CHO–electrolyte drink consumed during protocol with overall hypohydration of 2.7% BM. Rehydration over 90 min postprotocol with 11 ml/kg fluid with or without glycerol	Exercise protocol = 75 min match play. Skills tests undertaken preexercise, postexercise, and postrehydration • Ground strokes test • Serve test	No	No change in performance of ground strokes or serve tests over time (with changes in hydration status) or between trials. Authors claim that participants achieve relatively high percentile scores throughout, and the test may not have been sufficiently sensitive to detect real changes in skill performance.
Dougherty et al. 2006	Skilled adolescent basketball players (15 M) Crossover design Presumably moderate environment following 2 hr exposure to hot environment and moderate exercise to incur a fluid deficit of ~ 2% BM	Prior to protocol, participants prepared by drinking artificially flavored water (Placebo trial) or limiting fluid intake to achieve fluid deficit of 2% (Dehydration trial). Fluid intake continued during basketball protocol to maintain these differences	Basketball simulation protocol = 4 × 12 min quarters with 10 min half-time break: Skills included in drills: Shooting percentage from • Around the World shooting • 3-point shooting • Free throw shooting	Yes	Combined shooting percentage over the protocol was reduced in Dehydration trial (45 ± 9%, p < .05) compared to Placebo (euhydration) trial, (53 ± 11%). There was no difference in shooting percentage for short-range layups between trials.

CARBOHYDRATE

Study	Participants & design	Intervention	Exercise/skills protocol	Effect	Results
Muckle 1973	Competitive male soccer players n = 40 matches: 20 = control 20 = CHO Outdoors—presumably moderate conditions	105-110 g of CHO (glucose and mineral syrup) given 30 min prematch	40 matches over season: • Team performance = goals scored vs. goals conceded • One player chosen at random per match for movement analysis	Yes	During matches with CHO, team scored more goals in second half and conceded fewer goals than in control matches. Further analysis showed that goal scoring fell by 20-50% in last 30 min of control matches compared with CHO matches. Individual analysis showed enhanced number of ball contacts over last 15 min of CHO match compared with glucose control.
Burke and Ekblom 1982	Active tennis players (5 M + 5 F) Crossover design Indoor court 23-25°C	5 trials: • Control (no exercise) • Sauna-induced dehydration by 2.4% BM • Exercise + no fluid • Exercise + ad lib water throughout (505 ml) • Exercise + ad lib CHO–electrolyte drink (736 ml + 55 g CHO)	Exercise protocol = 2 hr tennis. Skills tests undertaken pre- and post-2 hr of tennis or rest: • 100 ball accuracy test	Yes	Plasma glucose maintained at higher levels with CHO trial. Accuracy test scores maintained from pre- to post-trial with CHO and control (no exercise) but reduced with water, no fluid, and dehydration trials.

(continued)

459

Table 9.f *(continued)*

Publication	Participants	Fluid or CHO intake protocol	Exercise protocol	Enhanced performance	Comments
			CARBOHYDRATE		

Mitchell et al. 1992	Competitive tennis players (10 M + 2 F) Crossover design	11.4 ml·kg⁻¹·hr⁻¹ placebo or 7.5% CHO drink, consumed as 200 ml per 15 min (800 ml/hr fluid + 60 g/hr CHO = 2.5 g/kg CHO)	3 hr match play. Tests undertaken pre- and postplay
			• 10 serves
			• Skill monitoring over 3 hr play:
			  • Serve percentage
			  • Unforced errors
				No	Blood glucose concentrations maintained in both trials over 3 hr of match practice. No difference in serve velocity from pre- to postplay testing or between trials. Increase in first serve percentage over 3 hr of match play, but no difference between trials. No change or differences between trials for second serve or unforced errors.

Zeederberg et al. 1996	Junior elite soccer players (22 M—2 teams) Crossover design Cool outdoor environment: 13-15°C, 63-69% rh	5 ml/kg 7% CHO–electrolyte drink or placebo consumed before and at halftime of match to provide total 10 ml/kg fluid and 0.7 g/kg CHO	2 matches played 7 days apart: each team divided into two for treatment or placebo: Match analysis undertaken by video and scored by trained personnel regarding
			  • Number and success of tackling
			  • Controlling
			  • Passing
			  • Dribbling
			  • Heading
			  • Shooting
				No	Blood glucose concentrations maintained over the duration of the match at similar levels (~5 mmol/L) in both trials. No significant difference in the total number or number of successful executions of each of the soccer motor skills between trials.

Ferrauti et al. 1997	Competitive tennis players (8 M + 8 F) Crossover design Hot outdoor environment: 28°C, 42% rh	100 ml (women) and 150 ml (men) of 7.6% CHO–electrolyte drink or placebo consumed every 15 min to provide a total of 2.8 L of fluid and 243 g CHO (men) and 2.0 L and 182 g of CHO (women) over 4 hr	4 hr tennis singles play (with 30 min break after 150 min). Tests of skill undertaken at end of 4 hr • Hitting accuracy with standardized ball machine test	No	No difference in hitting accuracy on standardized ball machine test between trials.
Vergauwen et al. 1998	Well-trained tennis players (13 M) Crossover design Conditions not stated; presumably moderate	CHO–electrolyte or placebo to provide total of 0.7 g·kg⁻¹·hr⁻¹ CHO and 800 ml/hr fluid	2 hr match play. Prep and postplay • Leuven Tennis Performance Test—4 games × 10 rallies played on court	Yes	In placebo trial, postmatch testing revealed reduction in stroke quality for first service and for defensive rallies. CHO trial attenuated the reduction in stroke precision with smaller increase in error rate and nonreached balls.

Study	Subjects/design	Protocol	Fluid/CHO provision	Skill	Findings
Graydon et al. 1998	Club standard squash players (8 M) Crossover design Conditions not stated; presumably moderate	Protocol simulating 3 squash games with 90 s rest period between (total = 79 rallies) Test undertaken after warm-up and after game 3: • Accuracy with 20 balls from feeder	CHO drink containing glucose polymer or placebo. Total amount N/A; but consumed 50% after warm-up and 25% after game 1 and game 2	Yes	Significant trial effect; accuracy scores maintained from pregame to postgame on CHO trial (62.6-59.1) but showed 19% decline in placebo trial (60.6-47.6, $p < .01$). RPE scores showed an increase in fatigue between all games in placebo trial, but a smaller overall increase in perception of effort in CHO trial.
Ostojic and Mazic 2002	Professional soccer players (22 M) Experimental–placebo design 25°C, 57% rh	90 min on-field soccer simulation: first half = game play + second half = soccer-specific skill tests • Precision rate • Power • Coordination • Dribble	7% CHO–electrolyte drink or placebo to provide total 15 ml/kg fluid and 1.1 g/kg CHO before and throughout 90 min	Yes	Blood glucose concentrations higher at the end of the first and second half in CHO group compared with placebo. CHO group performed significantly better in precision and dribble skill tests than placebo group. No difference in coordination tests and power tests between groups. Ratings of perceived effort higher in placebo group at the end of the second half.
Welsh et al. 2002	Collegiate basketball and soccer players (5 F + 5 M) Crossover design Presumably moderate laboratory conditions:	Warm-up + 60 min "game" of intermittent high-intensity running and jumping protocol (4 × 15 min quarters with 20 min half-time break) followed by shuttle run to fatigue. • Motor skills test (hopping skills) throughout • POMS • Stroop Color Word Test	6% CHO–electrolyte drink (quarters) and 18% CHO drink (halftime) or placebo drinks to provide total of 22 ml/kg fluid and 1.9 g/kg CHO (127 g CHO)	Yes	Better maintenance of speed and agility of motor skills (hopping test) in 4th quarter of "game" protocol with CHO treatment than placebo trial, although differences disappeared when test was undertaken at end of shuttle run to fatigue following "game." Stroop Color Word Test improved with exercise but no significant differences between trials. No differences between treatments for POMS apart from lower fatigue score at end of shuttle run to fatigue in CHO trial.
Kipp et al. 2003	Collegiate soccer players (15 F) Crossover design Presumably moderate laboratory conditions:	75 min practice session including warm-up, skills, and 40 m scrimmaging Skill test throughout play: • Touches of ball during scrimmaging	900 ml of 7% CHO–2% protein–electrolyte drink (63 g CHO) or sweetened placebo. Drink consumed as 6 × 150 ml throughout exercise	Yes	Players demonstrated more touches of the ball during scrimmaging with CHO trial than with placebo.
Wallis and Galloway 2003	Well-trained squash players (10 M) Crossover design Presumably moderate laboratory conditions:	20 min moderate-intensity treadmill running + 9 min on-court high-intensity "ghosting." Skill test undertaken before and after play: • 120 shot boast and drive test: scores given according to line and length of ball	666 ml of 6% CHO–electrolyte drink (40 g CHO) or sweetened placebo. Drink consumed as 2 × 333 ml pre- and during exercise	Yes	No difference in scoring for preexercise skill test between trials (141 vs. 140). Postexercise skill test was higher in CHO trial than placebo trial (110 vs. 94, $p < .05$). Change in skill was the result of a lower number of "zero" scores caused by better positioning of player on court relative to the ball.

(continued)

Table 9.f *(continued)*

Publication	Participants	Fluid or CHO intake protocol	Exercise protocol	Enhanced performance	Comments
			CARBOHYDRATE		
Winnick et al. 2005	Participants in team sports (10 M + 10 F) Crossover design Presumably moderate lab conditions	22 ml/kg 6% CHO–electrolyte drink or placebo or flavored water, before and throughout the protocol to provide 1.3 g/kg CHO (~41 g/hr)	4 × 15 min intermittent high-intensity protocol with tests before, halftime, and after • Motor skills test • Force sensation • Target jumping • Stroop Word Color Test • POMS	Yes Yes No No Perhaps	Stroop tests increased in both trials over the protocol, and differences were not significant between trials. Fatigue and vigor scores on POMS declined over the protocol. The trend to a better mood state with CHO trial did not reach statistical significance. Performance of motor skills test, corrected for errors was greater in CHO trial in 3rd and 4th quarters, as a result of increased number of errors in placebo trial in second half of game. Force sensation in wrist was significantly lower in CHO trial at posttrial testing compared with placebo. Therefore, performance of CNS function was enhanced with CHO, because of the preservation of skills that would otherwise decline in latter stages of protocol in placebo trial.
Dougherty et al. 2006	Skilled adolescent basketball players (15 M) Crossover design Presumably moderate environment following 2 hr exposure to hot environment and moderate exercise to incur a fluid deficit of ~2% BM	Prior to protocol, participants prepared by drinking artificially flavored water (Placebo trial) or 6% CHO–electrolyte drink to maintain hydration, and continued intakes of these fluids during basketball protocol to maintain hydration	Basketball simulation protocol = 4 × 12 min quarters with 10 min halftime break: Skills included in drills: Shooting percentage from • Around the World shooting • 3-point shooting • Free throw shooting	Yes	Combined shooting percentage over the protocol was greater with Carbohydrate trial (60 ± 8%, p < .05) compared to Placebo trial, (53 ± 11%). There was no difference in shooting percentage for short-range layups between trials.
Bottoms et al. 2006	1st division/national squash players (16M). Crossover design Presumably moderate lab conditions	1000 of 6% CHO–electrolyte drink (60 g CHO) or sweetened placebo throughout protocol	20 min shuttle run + 9 min on court high-intensity "ghosting". Skill test undertaken before and after protocol: • Reaction time • Wrist maximal voluntary conttraction • 120 shot bost and drive skill test scores given axccordfing to line and length of ball	Yes No Perhaps	CHO trial associated with higher blood glucose concentrations although hypoglycaemia did not occur with placebo trial. Auditory reaction time increased from pre- to post-exercise protocol in both trials, but increase in visual reaction time only occurred in CHO trial. There was a trend to better squash skill at the end of the CHO trial compared with placebo, especially due to fewer balls going outside the scoring zone. This difference was significant with backhand shots—a weaker skill in these subjects.

CHO = carbohydrate; M = male; BM = body mass; POMS = Profile of Mood States test; rh = relative humidity; LIST = Loughborough Intermittent Shuttle Test; RPE = rating of perceived exertion; N/A = not applicable; CNS = central nervous system.

Table 10.a Reported Dietary Intakes of Female Racket Sport Athletes: Training (Mean Daily Intake ± SD)

Publication	Participants	Survey method	Age (years)	BM (kg)	ENERGY		CHO			PROTEIN			FAT	
					mJ	KJ/kg	g	g/kg	%E	g	g/kg	%E	g	%E
Nutter 1991	U.S. collegiate tennis players (n = 4)	3-day food diary (household measures)												
		• Season	19	53	6.96 ± 2.2	130 ± 31	213	4.0	49 ± 3	71	1.3	17 ± 3	61	33 ± 4
		• Postseason			6.14 ± 2.4	113 ± 33	202	3.8	55 ± 4	64	1.2	17 ± 3	46	28 ± 3
Grandjean and Ruud 1994	U.S. Olympic team tennis players (n = 9)				8.57	147	279	4.8	54	80	1.4	15	68	29
Gropper et al. 2003	U.S. collegiate tennis players (n = 7)	3-day food diary (household measures)	20	63	7.62 ± 3.85	121				53 ± 17	0.8	12		

BM = body mass; CHO = carbohydrate; E = energy.

Table 10.b Available Data on Voluntary Fluid Intakes and Sweat Losses During Training and Competition in Racket Sports (Mean ± SD)

Publication	Participants	Temperature (°C)	Humidity (%)	SWEAT LOSS Total (ml)	SWEAT LOSS Rate (ml/hr)	FLUID INTAKE Total (ml)	FLUID INTAKE Rate (ml/hr)	Dehydration (= % change in BM^)
TENNIS—TRAINING								
Bergeron et al. 2006	Skilled adolescent players (9M + 5F)	WBGT = 30						
	• Water trial			2,291 ±708	1,145	1,736 ±543	868	0.9 ± 0.6
	• Carbohydrate–electrolyte trial			2,172 ±577	1,086	1,897 ±645	948	0.5 ± 0.7
TENNIS—MATCH PLAY								
Bergeron et al. 1995	Collegiate players							
	• 12 M	32	54	2,700 ±800	1,800	1,700 ±500	1,122	1.3 ± 0.8
	• 8 F			1,700 ±600	1,133	1,300 ±600	867	0.7 ± 0.5
Bergeron 1996	Cramp-prone nationally ranked junior player (1 M)	32	62	4,500	2,500	3,300	1,800	1.4
McCarthy et al. 1998	Junior regionally competitive players (14 M + 6 F)	28	43	2,389	1,707	1,089 ±427	780	2.3 ± 0.9
Bergeron 2003	Competitive cramp-prone players (17 M)	29-36	35-64		2,600 ±400		1,600 ±400	
SQUASH—MATCH PLAY								
Noakes et al. 1982	Competitive squash players			2,000	1,333			
van Rensburg et al. 1982	Club-level and nationally ranked squash players (23 M)			2,040 ±480	1,805	420 ± 300	370	2.2
Hansen 1995	Club-level squash players (6 M, 63 observations)	>24[a] 19-23[a] <19*						2.2 1.8 1.3
Brown and Winter 1998	International-level squash players (3 M, 8 matches)	25	64	2,110±1,020	2,370 ±450	830 ± 400	976	2,110±1,020 kg

BM = body mass; M = males; F = females; WBGT = wet bulb globe temperature.

[a]Temperature index equal to mean of dry bulb and wet bulb measures. ^The weight change occurring over the session is presumed to represent a body fluid deficit, and has not been corrected for change in BM that occurs in very prolonged events due to factors other than fluid loss (e.g., metabolic fuel losses).

Table 10.c Studies of Supplements With Likely Benefit to Racket Sports

Publication	Participants	Supplement protocol	Exercise protocol	Enhanced performance	Comments
Creatine		**Acute (loading) supplementation protocol with relevance to movement patterns during matches**			**Good evidence that creatine loading is associated with enhanced ability to undertake repeated brief sprints with short recovery intervals as found in movement patterns of racket sports. More sport-specific research is needed to test the possible benefits to match play.**
Romer et al. 2001	Squash players (9 M) Crossover design with 4-week washout	5 days @ 0.3 g/kg creatine	On-court "ghosting" session involving 10 sets of 2 repetitions of simulated play with 30 s recovery	Yes	Creatine treatment enhanced mean set sprint time by 3.2% above that seen in placebo trial ($p < .05$). Sets 2-10 completed in significantly shorter time following creatine supplementation.
Op 't Eijnde et al. 2001	Well-trained tennis players (8 M) Crossover design with 5-week washout	5 days @ 20 g/day creatine	Tests undertaken pre and post 2 hr match play • Skills test (Leuven Tennis Performance Test) measuring stroke quality • 70 m shuttle run.	No No	No effect of creatine supplementation on shuttle run speed or on stroke quality (velocity or precision of serves, baseline strokes, or volleys). Authors suggest that tennis play may not totally deplete phosphocreatine stores to create opportunity for benefits from acute creatine supplementation. Does not rule out potential for benefits of chronic supplementation on training or long-term outcomes.
Pluim et al. 2006	Competitive tennis players (36M) Experimental–placebo design	6 days @ 0.3 g/kg/d creatine	• Service test • Ground stroke test (60 forehand and 60 backhand shots) • $3 \times 5 \times 20$ m sprints (30 s recovery) • Leg press and bench press strength	No No No No	Body mass increase of 1.4 kg in creatine group. There were no differeences in performance tests between groups at presupplementation testing or for absolute changes in performance over the supplementation period. Performance was measured as speed of service or gound strokes, total sprint time, or specific muscle strength. No measurements of shot accuracy were recorded.
Creatine		**Chronic supplementation protocol with relevance to training practices and tournament/circuit play**			**Possibility as training aid (match practice or interval training, resistance training) and competition aid. More sport-specific research is needed to test this.**
Pluim et al. 2006	Competitive tennis players (24M) Experimental–placebo design	28 days @ 0.3 g/kg/d creatine	• Service test • Ground stroke test • Sprint test • Strength test (see above)	No No No No	There were a large number of drop outs (12) from the study following the acute loading phase. No differences in absolute changes in performance measures between creatine and placebo group after 4 w training. Needs to be studied in players who undertake strength training.

(continued)

Table 10.c (continued)

Publication	Participants	Supplement protocol	Exercise protocol	Enhanced performance	Comments
Caffeine					May enhance performance of prolonged exercise (e.g., matches) where fatigue would otherwise occur. To date this theory is not adequately tested in racket sports on the basis of 2 studies. More studies are needed in situations specific to racket sports to better test the potential of caffeine supplementation.
Ferrauti et al. 1997	Competitive tennis players (8 M + 8 F) Crossover design Hot outdoor environment: 28°C, 42% rh	Placebo, CHO, or caffeine consumed before and throughout 4 hr of tennis play (364 mg of caffeine for males, 260 mg for females—4-4.5 mg/kg)	4 hr tennis singles play (with 30 min break after 150 min). Tests of skill and speed undertaken at end of 4 hr: • 6 × 15 min sprint with 30 min rest • Hitting accuracy and success during games	No Yes for females No for males	No effect of caffeine supplementation on tennis-specific running speed; caffeine trial not different than placebo trial. No effect on hitting accuracy and success of games played during 4 hr with male participants. However, female players had greater success during tennis play on caffeine trial than placebo.
Vergauwen et al. 1998	Well-trained tennis players (13 M) Crossover design Conditions not stated; presumably moderate	Placebo, CHO, or CHO + caffeine (5 mg/kg 1 hr pretest + 0.75 mg·kg⁻¹·hr⁻¹) over 2 hr	Tests undertaken pre and post 2 hr match play • Skills test (Leuven Tennis Performance Test) measuring stroke quality • 70 m shuttle run	No No	CHO trial resulted in maintenance of stroke quality and shuttle run speed, whereas placebo trial resulted in deterioration of these aspects of performance. Caffeine added to CHO did not further enhance posttrial performance. Authors suggest that caffeine dose was too high. However, perhaps effect could only be expected if addressing situation of fatigue, which did not occur because of CHO intake.
Strecker et al. 2006	Collegiate tennis players (10M) Crossover design Summer outside conditions, WBGT = 30° for both trials	Placebo or 3 mg/kg caffeine consumed with 1 L carbonated soft drink, 90 min pre-test 1.2 L water consumed during protocol	Skill test performed pre-, 30 min, 60 min and post-90 min of simulated tennis play against a ball machine, 15 ground strokes in all 4 directions (60 shots total): • forehand cross-court • forehand up the line • backhand cross-court • backhand up the line	 Yes Yes No No	Caffeine trial showed better performance of both forehand shots across the 90 min of simulated tennis play. There was no difference in skill in backhand shots between trials.

M = male; F = female; CHO = carbohydrate; rh = relative humidity; WBGT = wet bulb globe temperature.

Table 11.a Reported Dietary Intakes of Male Strength and Power Athletes: Training (Mean Daily Intake ± SD)

Publication	Team population	Survey method	Age (years)	BM (kg)	ENERGY		CHO			PROTEIN			FAT	
					MJ	KJ/kg	g	g/kg	%E	g	g/kg	%E	g	%E
Saltin 1978	Scandinavian shot put throwers	(not available)			~18.0	—	~452	—	~42	~145	—	~13	~170	~35
Ward et al. 1976	U.S. national-level discus throwers (n = 16)	24 hr dietary recall	26	111	19.5 ± 5.0	176	446 ± 153	4.0	37	237 ± 68	2.1	21	203 ± 79	39
Chen et al. 1989	Chinese elite throwers (n = 6)	3- to 5-day weighed food diary	25	109	22.38 ± 2.9	205 ± 25	450 ± 52	4.1 ± 0.5	34 ± 1	265 ± 44	2.4 ± 0.4	20 ± 3	277 ± 97	47 ± 16
Faber et al. 1990	South African national-level throwers (n = 20)	7-day food diary (household measures)	22	99	14.61 ± 3.27	152 ± 36	358	3.6	41 ± 7	163	1.6 ± 1	19 ± 4	162	41 ± 5
Sugiura et al. 1999	Japanese national team throwers (n = 2)	3-day food diary (household measures)	31	104	15.01 ± 2.79	144 ± 20	429 ± 81	4.1 ± 0.6	55 ± 7	134 ± 2	1.3 ± 0.1	15 ± 3	119 ± 8	30 ± 4
Chen et al. 1989	Chinese elite weightlifters (n = 10)	3- to 5-day weighed food diary	21	80	19.21 ± 2.52	238 ± 25	431 ± 96	5.4 ± 1.2	38 ± 8	257 ± 47	3.2 ± 0.6	22 ± 4	205 ± 33	40 ± 7
Van Erp-Baart et al. 1989a	Dutch international-level weightlifters (n = 7)	4- to 7-day food diary (household measures)	27	76	12.76	167	320	4.2	40	97	1.3	13	134	39
Grandjean 1989	U.S. national-level and collegiate weightlifters (n = 28)	3-day food diary (household measures)			15.2 ± 3.9	—	392	—	43 ± 8	161	—	18 ± 4	160	39 ± 6
Heinemann and Zerbes 1989	German national team weightlifters (n = 15)	3-day semiweighed food diary	15-19	95	~31.35	~330	~764	~8.0	39	~295	~3.3	16	~380	45
Burke et al. 1991	Australian national-level weightlifters (n = 19)	7-day food diary (household measures)	22	84	15.2 ± 5.0	190 ± 60	373 ± 94	4.8	42 ± 5	156 ± 42	1.9 ± 0.6	18 ± 5	155 ± 62	38 ± 4

(continued)

Table 11.a (continued)

Publication	Team population	Survey method	Age (years)	BM (kg)	ENERGY		CHO			PROTEIN			FAT	
					MJ	KJ/kg	g	g/kg	%E	g	g/kg	%E	g	%E
Faber et al. 1986	South African competitive bodybuilders (n = 76)	7-day food diary (household measures)	27	82	15.01 ± 4.22	183	320 ± 132	3.9	36	200 ± 79	2.4	21	157 ± 50	39
Tarnopolsky et al. 1988	Canadian elite bodybuilders (n = 6)	7-day food diary (household measures)	24	80	20.07 ± 0.2	251	592	7.4 ± 0.5	49	216	2.7 ± .04	19	168	32
Van Erp-Baart et al. 1989a	Dutch international-level bodybuilders (n = 8)	4- to 7-day food diary (household measures)	30	87	13.71	157	424	4.9	50	201	2.5	25	118	32
Kleiner et al. 1989	U.S. competitive bodybuilders (n = 35)	2 × 3-day food diary (household measures)	28	88	24.1 ± 10.5	270	637 ± 259	7.2	44	324 ± 163	3.7	22	214 ± 109	34
Heyward et al. 1989	U.S. competitive bodybuilders (n = 7) • Training (non-competition) • Competition	3-day food diary (household measures)	28	91 86	15.04 ± 4.86 9.8 ± 1.1	165 114	457 ± 148 365 ± 76	5.0 4.2	52 ± 11 63 ± 10	215 ± 59 163 ± 59	2.4 1.9	25 ± 6 28 ± 9	110 ± 71 32 ± 18	26 ± 12 13 ± 8
Baldo-Enzi et al. 1990	Italian bodybuilders • Steroid users (n = 14) • Nonusers (n = 17)	4-day food diary (household measures)	27 25	82 78	11.27 ± 11.58 13.69 ± 13.77	137 176	331 436	4.0 5.6	47 ± 52 51 ± 23	218 171	2.7 2.2	31 ± 28 20 ± 10	67 107	22 ± 20 29 ± 12
Bazzarre et al. 1990	U.S. competitive bodybuilders (n = 19)	7-day food diary (household measures)	28	80	8.5 ± 4.4	106	243 ± 121	3.0	46	169 ± 94	2.1	34	40 ± 51	17
Steen 1991	U.S. bodybuilder (n = 1) • Off-season • Weight reduction • Precontest	5- to 6-day food diary (weighed + household measures)	25	86 81 76	17.61 12.68 8.13	206 155 105	747 491 145	8.7 6.1 1.9	72 65 30	238 219 310	2.8 2.7 4.0	23 29 64	24 20 13	5 6 6

Keith et al. 1996	U.S. state and regional bodybuilders (n = 14)	3-day food diary (household measures)	26	93	18.68 ± 5.88	201	544 ± 193	5.8	48	252 ± 109	2.7	23	151 ± 93	29
Zuliani et al. 1996	Italian well-trained bodybuilders (n = 20)	4-day food diary (household measures)	25	77	15.4 ± 4.34	200	531	6.9	55 ± 5	163	2.1	18 ± 4	121	29 ± 7

BM = body mass; CHO = carbohydrate; E = energy.

Table 11.b Reported Dietary Intakes of Female Strength and Power Athletes: Training (Mean Daily Intake ± SD)

Publication	Team population	Survey method	Age (years)	BM (kg)	ENERGY		CHO			PROTEIN			FAT	
					MJ	KJ/kg	g	g/kg	%E	g	g/kg	%E	g	%E
Chen et al. 1989	Chinese elite throwers (n = 6)	3- to 5-day weighed food diary	21	84	18.58 ± 3.1	222 ± 38	386 ± 57	4.6 ± 0.7	35 ± 5	208 ± 28	2.5 ± 0.3	19 ± 3	230 ± 14	47 ± 21
Faber et al. 1990	South African national throwers (n = 10)	7-day food diary (household measures)	22	88	9.28 ± 2.0	112 ± 28	257	3.0	46 ± 8	93	1.1 ± 0.3	17 ± 2	95	38 ± 6
Sugiura et al. 1999	Japanese national team throwers (n = 8)	3-day food diary (household measures)	25	67	10.94 ± 2.36	167 ± 39	336 ± 58	5.1 ± 1.1	54 ± 3	93 ± 23	1.4 ± 0.4	14 ± 1	94 ± 24	32 ± 3
Van Erp-Baart et al. 1989a	Dutch international-level bodybuilders (n = 4)	4- to 7-day food diary (household measures)	25	56	6.16	110	196	3.5	51	112	2.0	16	47	28
Heyward et al. 1989	U.S. competitive bodybuilders (n = 12) • Training (noncompetition) • Competition	3-day food diaries (household measures)	29	58 52	6.85 ± 2.3 6.10 ± 2.7	120 117	208 ± 60 261 ± 112	3.6 5.0	53 ± 11 72 ± 11	102 ± 30 77 ± 57	1.8 1.5	26 ± 4 21 ± 6	42 ± 30 15 ± 7	21 ± 9 10 ± 3
Lamar-Hildebrand et al. 1989	U.S. competitive bodybuilders (n = 6)	3-day food record (household measures) • Training • Competition	18-30	59 53	5.25 9.35	88 176	196 359	3.3 6.8	60 65	76 57	1.3 1.1	23 10	21 49	15 19
Bazzarre et al. 1990	U.S. competitive bodybuilders (n = 8)	7-day food diary (household measures)	28	57	9.49 ± 11.2	166	332 ± 525	5.8	49 ± 18	162 ± 93	2.8	37 ± 16	33 ± 41	13 ± 9

BM = body mass; CHO = carbohydrate; E = energy.

Table 11.c Studies of Chronic Creatine Supplementation With Likely Benefit to Resistance Training in Strength and Power Sports

Publication	Participants	Supplement protocol	Exercise protocol	Enhanced performance	Comments
Earnest et al. 1995	Resistance-trained participants (8 M)	4 weeks of creatine (dose not provided) or placebo Habitual resistance training continued	Tests at baseline, 4 weeks: • 1RM bench press • Repetition 70% RM bench press to fatigue	Yes Yes	Creatine group increased 1 RM lift by 6% ($p < .05$) and repetitions by 26% ($p < .05$). No changes in placebo group. Increase in BM in creatine group.
Volek et al. 1997	Resistance-trained participants (14 M) Experimental–placebo design	1 weeks @ 25 g/day creatine or placebo Habitual resistance training continued	Tests at baseline, 4 weeks: • 10RM bench press: 5 sets of repetitions to fatigue • Jump squat: 5 sets @ 30% 1RM	Yes Yes	Creatine group increased bench press repetitions by 30% and increased power in jump squats ($p < .05$) No changes in placebo group. Increase in BM of 1.4 kg in creatine group.
Kelly and Jenkins 1998	Competitive powerlifters (18 M) Experimental–placebo design	5 days @ 20 g/day + 21 days @ 5 g/day creatine or placebo Habitual precompetition training continued	Tests at baseline, 26 days: • 3RM bench press • Repetition 85% RM bench press to fatigue	Yes Yes	Creatine group increased 3RM lift by 8% ($p < .05$) and repetitions by 39% ($p < .05$), significantly greater than increases in placebo group.
Volek et al. 1999	Resistance-trained participants (19 M) Experimental–placebo design	1 week @ 25g/day + 11 weeks @ 5 g/day creatine or placebo Resistance training program with preparation, hypertrophy, strength and peaking phases	Tests at baseline, 12 weeks: • 1RM bench press • 1RM squat • Repetition 80% RM bench press to fatigue	Yes Yes No	Greater increases in type I, IIa, and IIb muscle fiber cross-sectional areas and increase in BM and FFM with creatine group. Both groups increased 1RM lifts for bench press and squat, with gains being greater in creatine group ($p < .05$). No enhancement of repetition bench press in either group.
Peeters et al. 1999	Resistance-trained participants (35 M) Experimental–placebo design	3 days @ 20 g/day + 39 days @ 10 g/day creatine or placebo Periodized resistance training program	Tests at baseline, 6 weeks: • 1RM bench press • 1RM leg press • Repetition 8RM-10RM curl	Yes No No	Increases in bench press, leg press, and repetition curls in both groups, with only the 10% gain in bench press being greater in creatine group than placebo group ($p < .05$).
Becque et al. 2000	Resistance-trained participants (23 M) Experimental–placebo design	5 days @ 20 g/day + 5 weeks @ 2 g/day creatine or placebo 2/week resistance training for preacher curls	Tests at baseline, 6 weeks: • 1RM preacher curl	Yes	Increases in 1RM preacher curl in both groups with the 28% gain in creatine group being greater than placebo group ($p < .05$). 2 kg increase in BM with creatine group including increase in LBM ($p < .05$). No change in placebo group.
Syrotuik et al. 2000	Resistance-trained participants (21 M) Experimental–placebo design	5 days @ 0.3 g·kg⁻¹·day⁻¹ creatine (acute) or 5 d @ 0.3 g·kg⁻¹·day⁻¹ + 32 days @ 0.03 g·kg⁻¹·day⁻¹ creatine (acute or maintenance) or placebo 8-week resistance training program, including 3 weeks pretrial phase	Tests at baseline, 5 days, 37 days: • 1RM bench press • 1RM leg press • Repetition 80% RM bench press to fatigue • Repetition 80% RM leg press to fatigue	No No No No	All groups significantly increased strength performance measures after 37 days. No statistically significant differences between groups, although trend for improvements to be larger in creatine groups. Note that training volume was controlled and standardized for all groups, so that opportunity for creatine to allow better or greater training was removed.

(continued)

471

Table 11.c *(continued)*

Publication	Participants	Supplement protocol	Exercise protocol	Enhanced performance	Comments
Stevenson and Dudley 2001	Resistance-trained participants (23 M) Experimental–placebo design	7 days @ 20 g/day creatine or placebo Habitual resistance training continued	Testing at baseline, 7 days: • 1RM leg extensions • Repetition 12RM-15RM leg extensions	No No	Enhancement of leg extensions and repetitions in both groups.
Jowko et al. 2001	Untrained participants (40 M) Experimental–placebo design	7 days @ 20 g/day + 14 days @ 10 g/day creatine or placebo Resistance training	Tests at baseline and 3 weeks: • IRM for 6 separate lifts (bench press, power clean biceps curl, behind the neck press, squat, triceps extension)	Yes for accumulative strength	Creatine caused greater increase in LBM and accumulative strength than placebo group. Accumulative effect of Cr and HMB supplementation summarized in table 11.d.
Burke, Chilibeck, et al. 2001	Resistance-trained participants (36 M) Experimental–placebo design	7 weeks @ 0.1 g·kg^{-1}·day^{-1} creatine or placebo Habitual resistance training continued	Testing at baseline, 6 weeks: • 1RM bench press • 1RM squat	Yes No	Increase in bench press in both groups, but 17-20% increase in creatine group greater than in placebo ($p < .05$). Greater increase in lean body mass in creatine group ($p < .05$). Increases in squat strength equal in both groups.
Kilduff et al. 2002	Resistance-trained participants (32 M) Experimental–placebo design	5 days @ 20 g/day creatine or placebo Resistance training	Testing at baseline, 6 days: • Bench press 5 × 1RM	Yes	Creatine group divided into responders and nonresponders according to increase in muscle creatine content. Responders showed increase in BM of 1.2 kg ($p < .05$) and bench press ($p < .05$). No change in nonresponders and placebo group.
Falk et al. 2003	Resistance-trained participants (28 M) Experimental–placebo design	8 weeks @ 5 g/day creatine (+ ribose + glutamine) or placebo 8 weeks resistance training 4/week	Testing at baseline, 8 weeks: • 1RM bench press • Repetitions 80% RM bench press to fatigue	No No	Both groups increased LBM, muscle strength, and muscle endurance over the 8 weeks, but no differences between groups.
Volek et al. 2004	Resistance-trained participants (17 M) Experimental–placebo design	6 weeks @ 0.3 g·kg^{-1}·day^{-1} creatine or placebo 5/week resistance training including 4 weeks "overreaching" + 2 weeks taper	Testing at baseline, 8 weeks: • 1RM bench press • 1RM squat	Yes initially Yes initially	Squat and bench press were reduced during the initial weeks of heavy training in placebo but not creatine group ($p < .05$). Greater increase in BM and LBM with creatine at 6 weeks ($p < .05$). Trend for greater improvement in squat at 6 weeks. Authors conclude that creatine helps to maintain muscular performance during initial phase of high-volume "overreaching" program that otherwise results in performance decrements.

LBM = lean body mass; BM = body mass; M = male; F = female; RM = repetition maximum; FFM = fat-free mass; Cr = creatine; HMB = β-hydroxy β-methylbutyrate.

Table 11.d Studies of Supplements With Undetermined or Unlikely Benefits to Resistance Training in Power and Strength Sports

Publication	Participants	Supplement protocol	Exercise protocol	Enhanced performance	Comments
Bovine colostrum		**Chronic supplementation protocol**			**Potential value presently undetermined in overall literature. No mechanisms identified to explain any potential benefits. Expense of moderate to large doses of supplement ($US40 per week) warrants additional supportive research before it can be recommended. Information about benefits from lower doses is particularly valuable.**
Antonio et al. 2001	Active participants (14 M + 8F) Experimental–placebo design	8 weeks @ 20 g/day colostrum or placebo (whey protein) 3/week aerobic and resistance training	Tests at baseline and 8 weeks: • 1RM bench press • Maximal repetitions to exhaustion	No No	No enhancement of strength outcomes with colostrum. Colostrum group experienced significant increase in lean BM (1.5 kg), whereas placebo group showed increase in BM (2 kg) possibly from fat mass. Body composition assessed by DEXA.
Buckley et al. 2003	Active participants (51 M) Experimental–placebo design	8 weeks @ 60 g/day colostrum or placebo (whey protein) 3/week plyometrics and resistance training	Tests at baseline, 4 and 8 weeks: • 1RM bench press • 1RM chin-up • 1RM parallel dip • 1RM biceps curl • 1RM leg press • 1RM knee extension • 1RM knee flexion • 1RM calf raise	No No No No No No No No	No differences between groups in the improvement in strength for any of the protocols at 4 or 8 weeks. No change in plasma IGF-1 in either group
Brinkworth et al. 2004	Active participants (34 M) Experimental–placebo design	8 weeks @ 60 g/day colostrum or placebo (whey protein) 4/week one-arm resistance training	Tests at baseline and 8 weeks: • 1RM biceps curl	No	Increase in biceps curl 1RM in trained arm but no difference between placebo and colostrum group. Increase in circumference and MRI determined cross-sectional area of trained arm of colostrum group compared with placebo group ($p < .05$), principally because of an increase in subcutaneous fat and skin.

(continued)

Table 11.d (continued)

Publication	Participants	Supplement protocol	Exercise protocol	Enhanced performance	Comments
β-Hydroxy β-methylbutyrate (HMB)		Chronic supplementation protocol			**Potential value in reducing muscle damage and enhancing recovery from resistance training is presently undetermined. The results of the present literature are equivocal. Some studies suggest that benefits are limited to novice trainers or to the initial response following an increase in training load. Further studies are required in highly trained athletes to support any benefits. Although a meta-analysis has reported that the overall effect of HMB on resistance training is significant, this study has been criticized—see chapter 3.**
Nissen et al. 1996	Untrained participants (41 M) Experimental–placebo design	3 weeks @ 1.5 or 3 g/day HMB or placebo Groups subdivided into moderate or high protein (117 or 175 g/day) Resistance training 3/week	Tests at baseline and 3 weeks: • Weight lifted in training session	Yes	HMB associated with decrease in urinary 3-MH (measure of protein breakdown) and plasma CK (measure of muscle damage). Trend to increased gain in lean BM with HMB. Dose-responsive increase in weight lifted during training session with HMB compared with placebo.
Nissen et al. 1996	Resistance-trained participants (28 M) Experimental–placebo design	7 weeks @ 3 g/day HMB or placebo Resistance training 2-3 hr/day	Tests at baseline and 7 weeks: • Bench press • Squat • Clean	Yes No No	Control group was stronger at baseline in upper body strength; gains made by HMB group simply caused groups to be equal in upper- and lower-body strength at end of study. Greater increase in LBM during early part of study in HMB group was absent by 7 weeks. Effects of HMB diminish over time. Diet not controlled.
Kreider et al. 1999	Resistance-trained participants (40 M) Experimental–placebo design	4 weeks @ 3 or 6 g/day HMB or placebo Resistance training 7 hr/week	Tests at baseline and 4 weeks: • 1RM bench press • 1RM leg press	No No	No difference in improvements in strength between groups or changes in lean BM or body fat levels. No differences between plasma concentrations of CK and LDH (another marker of muscle damage).
Gallagher et al. 2000	Untrained participants (37 M) Experimental–placebo design	8 weeks @ 3 or 6 g/day HMB or placebo Resistance training 3/week	Tests at baseline and 8 weeks: • 1RM strength for 10 separate lifts (bench press, arm curl, arm extensions, shoulder press, lat pull-down, abdominal crunch, hip sled, leg curl, leg extension, calf raise)	No for all lifts	No differences in strength gains between treatments. 3 g/day HMB supplementation increased LBM and decreased the increase in plasma CK compared with placebo. Larger HMB dose not associated with increase in LBM.

Study	Participants/Design	Supplementation protocol	Tests	Benefit	Findings
Panton et al. 2000	Participants with various training status (39 M + 36 F) Experimental–placebo design	4 weeks @ 3 g/day HMB or placebo Resistance training 3/week	Tests at baseline and 4 weeks: • 1RM bench press • 1RM leg press and extension	Yes No	No sex differences, allowing data to be pooled. HMB group showed greater increase in upper-body strength than placebo group, but changes in leg strength were similar between HMB and placebo ($p < .01$). No differences in strength gains according to prior training status. Trend to increase in LBM and decrease in fat mass, and reduction in plasma CK in HMB group compared with placebo.
Jowko et al. 2001	Untrained participants (40 M) Experimental–placebo design	3 weeks @ 3 g/day HMB, creatine (20 g/day for 7 days + 10 g/day for 14 days), HMB-creatine, or placebo Resistance training	Tests at baseline and 3 weeks: • 1RM for 6 separate lifts (bench press, power clean biceps curl, behind the neck press, squat, triceps extension)	Yes for accumulative strength	Creatine caused greater increase in LBM and accumulative strength than placebo group. Greater increase in accumulative strength and trend to greater increase in LBM with HMB than placebo. Effects of Cr and HMB were additive. HMB reduced plasma CK levels and urea, suggesting nitrogen sparing.
Chromium or chromium picolinate		Chronic supplementation protocol			**Literature involving untrained participants fails to support enhancement of strength gains or loss of body fat with chronic supplementation and resistance training—also tested in weight division and team sport athletes without evidence of benefits.**
Hasten et al. 1992	Untrained participants (59 M) Experimental–placebo design	12 weeks @ 200 µg/day chromium picolinate 12-week resistance training program	Tests at baseline, 12 weeks: • 1RM bench press • 1RM squat	No No	No differences in strength changes attributable to chromium picolinate. Greater increase in BM in females with chromium but no difference with males. No difference with loss of body fat.
Lukaski et al. 1996	Untrained participants (36 M) Experimental–placebo design	8 weeks @ 3.4 µmol/day (~200 µg/day) chromium picolinate or chloride 8-week resistance training program	Tests at baseline, 8 weeks: • 1RM bench press • 1RM leg press • 1RM lat pull-down • 1RM leg curl	No No No No	No beneficial effects on lean BM, body fat, or strength above training effect. No difference between chromium preparations. Resistance training caused reduction in iron status that was exacerbated (decreased transferrin status) with chromium picolinate.
Hallmark et al. 1996	Untrained participants (16 M) Experimental–placebo design	12 weeks @ 200 µg/day 12-week resistance training program	Tests at baseline, 12 weeks: • 1RM leg press • 1RM leg extension • 1RM chest press • 1RM lat pull-down • 1RM seated rows • 1RM overhead press	No No No No No No	No differences in body composition with training in either supplement or placebo group. Strength increased in both groups, independent of supplement.

(continued)

Table 11.d (continued)

Publication	Participants	Supplement protocol	Exercise protocol	Enhanced performance	Comments
Walker et al. 1998	Collegiate wrestlers (20 M) Experimental–placebo design	14 weeks @ 200 µg/day	Tests at baseline, 14 weeks: • 1RM power clean • 1RM bench press • Lower-body endurance • Lower-body power • Upper-body endurance • Upper-body power	No No No No No No	Chromium picolinate supplementation coupled with a typical preseason training program does not enhance body composition or performance variables beyond improvements seen with training alone.
Amino acid supplementation		**Chronic supplementation protocol**			**Literature does not show any consistent benefits to hormonal environment or strength gains following oral supplementation with various amino acids.**
Elam et al. 1989	Untrained participants (22 M) Experimental–placebo design	5 weeks @ 1 g ornithine + 1 g arginine for 5 days/week 5-week resistance training program	Tests only at end of 5 weeks: Total strength (1RM for bench press, squat, deadlift, hip press, and incline press)	Yes claimed by authors, but data can't support such conclusion	At end of 5 weeks, treatment group had higher LMB and significantly greater in total strength (total of 1RM for 5 lifts) than placebo group. However, no pretrial testing undertaken to show that groups were equally matched at commencement of trial. No dietary control. No outcomes can be concluded from this poorly designed trial.
Gater et al. 1992a	Physically active participants (37M) Experimental–placebo design	10 weeks @ • Rest + placebo • RT + placebo • Rest + 66 mg/kg LBM/day each of arginine + lysine • RT + 66 mg/kg LBM/day each of arginine + lysine • RT + liquid meal (energy) supplement	Tests at baseline, 10 weeks: • 1RM bench press • 1RM squat • 1RM deadlift	No No No	No change in strength in any lift or total strength with arginine and lysine and rest, compared with rest and placebo. All resistance-trained groups showed increase in strength in each of the lifts, but no difference between groups in strength gains. All resistance-trained groups showed greater increases in LBM ($p < .05$) compared with rest groups. However, increase in LBM was greatest in resistance-trained group receiving energy supplement than other groups (placebo and lysine and arginine). No difference in strength or LBM gains between lysine and arginine and respective placebo groups. No change in resting levels of IGF-1 over time between groups, suggesting no stimulation of human growth hormone release.
Glutamine supplementation		**Acute supplementation protocol**			**No evidence that high-dose glutamine consumed before high-intensity work bout can enhance performance via increase in extracellular pH and additional buffering capacity.**
Antonio et al. 2002	Resistance-trained participants (6 M) Crossover design	300 mg/kg consumed 1 hr preexercise	2 sets of • Repetitions at BM for bench press to fatigue • Repetitions at 2 × BM for leg press	No No	No difference in performance of repetitions between trials. Plasma lactate and pH not measured to test theory of enhanced buffering capacity.

Glutamine supplementation

No evidence that chronic glutamine supplementation reduces post-training protein breakdown, thus enhancing recovery.

Glutamine supplementation	Chronic supplementation protocol	Tests		Results
Candow et al. 2001	Resistance-trained participants (31 M) Experimental–placebo design	6 weeks @ 0.9 g/kg LBM/day glutamine or placebo Resistance training program	Tests at baseline, 6 weeks: • 1RM bench press • 1RM squat	No No	No improvement above placebo group for strength in bench press and squat. No difference in changes in LBM between groups. 3-MH (marker of muscle protein degradation) increased with training, but no difference between groups.
Falk et al. 2003	Resistance-trained participants (28 M) Experimental–placebo design	8 weeks @ 3 g/day glutamine (+ creatine + ribose) or placebo 8 weeks resistance training 4/week	Tests at baseline, 8 weeks: • 1RM bench press • Repetitions 80% RM bench press to fatigue	No No	Both groups increased LBM, muscle strength, and muscle endurance over the 8 weeks, but no differences between groups.

Ribose supplementation

Overall literature fails to show consistent benefits to performance of repeated high-intensity bouts of exercise with ribose supplementation. Expense of ribose (~US$40/week) warrants additional supportive research before it can be recommended.

Ribose supplementation	Chronic supplementation protocol	Tests		Results
Van Gammeren et al. 2002	Recreational bodybuilders (19 M) Experimental–placebo design	4 weeks @ 10 g/day ribose or placebo Resistance training	Tests at baseline, 4 weeks: • 1RM bench press • 10 sets to fatigue at BM bench press	Yes Yes	No difference in LBM assessed by DEXA over time or between groups. Increase in strength and strength endurance over 4 weeks in both groups. However, only ribose group reached statistical significance: Bench press 1RM: 20% vs. 12% improvement. Total work performed in 10 sets to fatigue: 3.2% vs. 1.7% improvement for ribose vs. placebo.
Falk et al. 2003	Resistance-trained participants (28 M) Experimental–placebo design	8 weeks @ 2 g/day ribose (+ creatine + glutamine) or placebo 8 weeks of resistance training 4/week	Tests at baseline, 8 weeks: • 1RM bench press • Repetitions 80% RM bench press to fatigue	No No	Both groups increased LBM, muscle strength, and muscle endurance over the 8 weeks, but no differences between groups.

(continued)

Table 11.d *(continued)*

Publication	Participants	Supplement protocol	Exercise protocol	Enhanced performance	Comments
ATP supplements		**Acute supplementation protocol**			Some animal studies show that supplementation with ATP produces increase in blood and cell ATP levels, with changes in physiological function. However, in humans, oral intake of ATP is likely to be challenged by denaturation in the gut, poor absorption attributable to the high molecular weight, and poor transport to the muscle cell. Recent development of "enterically coated" ATP supplements has allowed some of these challenges to be addressed. However, there needs to be clear evidence that acute or chronic intake of such supplements increases blood and cellular levels of ATP and alters physiological function. Data to support these outcomes are currently lacking.
Jordan et al. 2004	Strength-training athletes (27 M) Experimental–placebo design	On day 7: 150 mg or 225 mg enterically coated ATP 75 min pretrial	Baseline, and 7 days: • 1RM bench press • 3 × 70% RM bench press to fatigue	Perhaps	Group receiving higher dose ATP had significantly higher 1RM bench press, whereas no difference was seen with low-dose and placebo group. However, authors note that change was small and was within technical error of measurement. Overall changes with supplement (acute and chronic application) not consistent.
ATP supplements		**Chronic supplementation protocol**			**There is a lack of evidence that chronic intake of ATP will increase muscle ATP concentration and improve function.**
Jordan et al. 2004	Strength-training athletes (27 M) Experimental–placebo design	From day 7 to 21 14 days @ 150 mg or 225 mg enterically coated ATP	Tests at baseline, 21 days (after 14 days of supplementation) • 1RM bench press • 3 × 70% RM bench press to fatigue	Perhaps	Muscular endurance was increased in one set in posttesting of high-dose ATP group but not in other two sets or in other groups. No difference in muscular strength. Authors note that change was small and was within technical error of measurement. Overall changes with supplement (acute and chronic application) not consistent.
Tribulus terrestris		**Chronic supplementation protocol**			**There is no evidence to support the claims that tribulus terrestris increases plasma testosterone levels and enhances muscle hypertrophy.**
Antonio et al. 2000	Resistance-trained participants (15 M) Experimental–placebo design	8 weeks @ 3.2 mg·kg⁻¹·day⁻¹ *tribulus terrestris* or placebo Periodized resistance training 3/week	Tests at baseline, 8 weeks: • Repetitions at BM for bench press to fatigue • Repetitions at 2 × BM for leg press	No—in fact, p l a c e b o group better No	Both groups increased muscular endurance in leg press by ~30% (p < .05) with no difference between groups. However, only placebo group showed a significant enhancement of bench press repetitions (~30% vs. 3% in tribulus group). No change in body composition in either group or change in profile of mood states.

ZMA supplement	**Chronic supplementation protocol: 30 mg of zinc monomethionine aspartate, 450 mg of magnesium aspartate, 10.5 mg of vitamin B$_6$**			**ZMA was first formulated in conjunction with Victor Conte and the BALCO laboratory. One study undertaken by Conte reported beneficial outcomes in a group of strength-training athletes following use of this supplement. Other companies now make versions of this product. A second study failed to find any benefits to the training adaptations achieved by a resistance-trained population.**
Brilla and Conte 2000	Collegiate American football players (27 M) Experimental–placebo design	8 weeks of ZMA at night Resistance training program	Testing at baseline, 8 weeks: • Muscle strength by dynamometer in lower extremities	Yes	Supplement group increased blood concentrations of anabolic hormones (testosterone, IGF-1) and minerals (zinc and magnesium) whereas concentrations decreased in placebo group. Torque and power increased to a greater extent in the supplement group than placebo group.
Wilborn et al. 2004	Resistance-trained men (M) Experimental–placebo design	8 weeks of ZMA at night (plus additional herbal compounds) Resistance training program	Testing at baseline, 8 weeks: • 1RM bench press • 80% RM bench press to fatigue • 1RM bench press • 80% RM bench press to fatigue • 30 s Wingate cycling test	No No No No No	Supplementation group showed a small but significant increase in plasma zinc concentrations over the 8 weeks but no difference in magnesium concentrations. No differences between groups in terms of changes in testosterone or cortisone hormones, muscular strength and endurance, or anaerobic cycling capacity.
Myostatin inhibitors	**Chronic supplementation**			**Myostatin is a cytokine that acts as a growth differentiating factor. An increase in myostatin increases proteolysis and atrophy of type IIa and IIb muscle fibers. The binding or "knocking out" of myostatin is associated with an increase in lean body mass and strength. Supplements containing agents claimed to bind myostatin have been released with claims of increasing muscle size and function. There is currently no evidence to support the claims for these supplements.**
Willoughby 2004	Untrained participants (22 M) Experimental–placebo design	12 weeks @ 4/day myostim supplement (@300 mg of cystoseira canariensis extract) Resistance training program	Testing at baseline and 3, 6, 9, and 12 weeks • Upper-body relative strength • Lower-body relative strength	No No	Participants increased muscle strength, lean body mass and body mass, and serum myostatin with training. There were no differences between myostim and placebo groups. Analysis of the supplement confirmed the presence of cystoseira canariensis in the cited quantities and its ability to bind myostatin as well as another chemical FRLG that also inhibits myostatin. This may nullify the effect of the supplement on myostatin. However, the authors suggested that a longer duration of study or use with well-trained participants should be undertaken.

LBM = lean body mass; BM = body mass; M = male; F= female; DEXA = dual-energy X-ray absorptiometry; MRI = magnetic resonance imaging; RM = repetition maximum; IGF-1 = insulin-like growth factor 1; 3-MH = 3-methylhistidine; CK = creatine kinase; LDH = lactate dehydrogenase; ATP = adenosine triphosphate; RT = resistance training; FRLG = follistatin-like related gene

Table 13.a Reported Dietary Intakes of Male Gymnasts: Training (Mean Daily Intake ± SD)

Publication	Team population	Survey method	Age (years)	BM (kg)	ENERGY			CHO			PROTEIN			FAT	
					MJ	kJ/kg	g	g/kg	%E	g	g/kg	%E	g	%E
Short and Short 1983	U.S. collegiate gymnasts (n = 10)	3-day food diary (household measures)			8.74		231		44	78		15	90	39
Chen et al. 1989	Chinese elite gymnasts (n = 4)	3- to 5-day weighed food diary	21	59	13.84 ± 0.23	234 ± 38	357 ± 77	6.1 ± 1.3	43 ± 9	151 ± 28	2.6 ± 0.5	18 ± 3	141 ± 18	38 ± 5
Weimann et al. 2000	German junior elite gymnasts (n = 18)	3-day intake assessed by interview	13		8.85 ± 0.17		158 ± 63		47	74 ± 12		13	91 ± 17	36

BM = body mass; CHO = carbohydrate; E = energy.

Table 13.b Reported Dietary Intakes of Female Gymnasts: Training (Mean Daily Intake ± SD)

Publication	Team population	Survey method	Age (years)	BM (kg)	ENERGY		CHO			PROTEIN			FAT	
					MJ	kJ/kg	g	g/kg	%E	g	g/kg	%E	g	%E
Moffatt 1984	U.S. high school gymnasts (n = 13)	2 × 3-day food diary (household measures)	15	50	8.04 ± 2.82	159	222 ± 77	4.4	46 ± 4	74 ± 23	1.4	15 ± 2	82 ± 17	38 ± 5
Loosli et al. 1986	U.S. special school gymnasts (n = 97)	3-day food diary (household measures)	13	43	7.68	178	220	5.1	49	71	1.6	15	74	36
Hickson et al. 1986	U.S. collegiate gymnasts (n = 9)	3 × 24 hr dietary recall	19	58	7.67 ± 2.1	134 ± 150	—	—	—	—	—	—	—	—
Benardot et al. 1989	U.S. junior elite gymnasts (n = 22)	2-day food diary (household measures)	11-14	31	7.13 ± 1.76	230	227 ± 64	7.3	53 ± 6	67 ± 20	2.0	15 ± 2	62 ± 18	33 ± 5
Grandjean 1989	U.S. national-level and collegiate gymnasts (n = 10)	3-day food diary (household measures)		—	8.09 ± 1.66	—	237	—	49 ± 5	76	—	15 ± 2	79	36 ± 4
Reggiani et al. 1989	U.S. artistic gymnasts (n = 26)	6-day food diary (household measures)	12	38	6.49 ± 2.13	171	194	5.1	48 ± 7	62 ± 25	1.5	15 ± 3	62	36 ± 7
Chen et al. 1989	Chinese elite gymnasts (n = 5)	3- to 5-day weighed food diary	18	45	9.61 ± 1.4	213 ± 29	242 ± 49	5.4 ± 1.1	42 ± 9	94 ± 5	2.1 ± 0.6	16 ± 4	106 ± 14	42 ± 6
Van Erp-Baart et al. 1989a	Dutch international-level gymnasts (n = 11)	4- to 7-day food diary (household measures)	15	47	7.41	158	246	5.2	53	66	1.4	14	66	32
Benson et al. 1990	Swiss national gymnasts (n = 12)	7-day food diary (household measures)	12	35	6.45 ± 1.66	165 ± 56	205	5.9	53 ± 6	69	2.0	17 ± 3	55	31 ± 6
Kirchner et al. 1995	U.S. collegiate gymnasts (n = 26)	Food frequency questionnaire	20	54	5.77 ± 2.3	107	180 ± 60	3.3	52	53 ± 4	1.0	15.5	48 ± 6	31
Jonnalagadda et al. 1998	U.S. national artistic gymnasts (n = 29)	3-day food diary (household measures)	15 (12-19)	49	7.01 ± 2.27	143	283 ± 96	5.8	66	72 ± 23	1.5	17	32 ± 17	18
Weimann et al. 2000	German junior elite gymnasts (n = 22)	3-day intake assessed by interview	14	—	5.81 ± 0.21	—	195 ± 81	—	55	47 ± 18	—	13.5	49 ± 20	31
Gropper et al. 2003	U.S. collegiate gymnasts (n = 9)	3-day food diary (household measures)	19	57	7.18 ± 2.09	126	—	—	—	61 ± 12	1.1	14	—	—

BM = body mass; CHO = carbohydrate; E = energy.

Table 14.a Studies of Iron Depletion and Deficiency in Winter Sport Athletes Published After 1985

Publication	Team population	Gender	Sample size	Serum ferritin (µg/L)	Hb (g/dL)	Serum ferritin cutoff (µg/L)	Athletes with iron depletion or deficiency (%)	Athletes with anemia (%)
Haymes et al. 1986	U.S. national cross-country skiers	Females Males	10 9	32.8 56.1	14.3 16.3	<28/<12 <28	40/20 22	0 0
Clement et al. 1987	Olympic cross-country skiers	Females Males	14 23	44.5 ± 32.0 48.6 ± 28.1	13.8 ± 1.1 15.5 ± 0.9	<30	57 26	7 (<12 g/dL) 0
Clement et al. 1987	Olympic alpine skiers	Females Males	10 10	43.4 ± 23.1 47.8 ± 17.1	13.7 ± 1.1 14.9 ± 1.2	<30	20 20	20 20
Clement et al. 1987	Olympic speed skaters	Females	8	36.8 ± 20.7	13.7 ± 0.8	<30	50	0
Couzy et al. 1989	French national-level alpine ski racers	Females	20	20.8 ± 1.8 (transferrin saturation)	13.7 ± 0.1	<16% (transferrin saturation)	35	0
Ingjer et al. 1990	Norwegian cross-country skiers	Male	7		15.0 ± 0.9			
Roberts and Smith 1990	Canadian elite-level speed skaters	Males Females	6	94.0 ± 27.0 57.0 ± 14.0				
Fogelholm et al. 1992	Finnish international-level cross-country skiers	Females Males	7 8	29 66	14.0 14.8	<20	29-42 0	0 0
Schena et al. 1995	Italian international-level alpine skiers	Males	17	82.4 ± 12.2	16.4 ± 1.4	<20	0	0
Schena et al. 1995	Italian international-level cross-country skiers	Males	73	39.5 ± 2.7	15.4 ± 1.2	<20	19	0
Meyer et al. 1999	Swiss international-level alpine skiers	Females	10	34.5 ± 20.2	14.1 ± 0.9	<20	30	0

Hb = hemoglobin.

references

Aaserud, R., P. Gramvik, S.R. Olsen, and J. Jensen. 1998. Creatine supplementation delays onset of fatigue during repeated bouts of sprint running. *Scandinavian Journal of Medicine and Science in Sports* 8: 247-251.

Abel, T., B. Knechtle, C. Perret, P. Eser, P. von Arx, and H. Knecht. 2005. Influence of chronic supplementation of arginine aspartate in endurance athletes on performance and substrate metabolism. *International Journal of Sports Medicine,* 26: 344-349.

Abt, G., S. Zhou, and R. Weatherby. 1998. The effect of a high-carbohydrate diet on the skill performance of midfield soccer players after intermittent treadmill exercise. *Journal of Science and Medicine in Sport* 1: 203-212.

Abt, G., and S. Armstrong. 2002. How does he do it? *International Herald Tribune,* July 26: p. 18.

Achten, J., S.H. Halson, L. Moseley, M.P. Rayson, A. Casey, and A.E. Jeukendrup. 2004. Higher dietary carbohydrate content during intensified running training results in better maintenance of performance and mood state. *Journal of Applied Physiology* 96: 1331-1340.

Achten, J., and A.E. Jeukendrup. 2003. Effects of pre-exercise ingestion of carbohydrate on glycaemic and insulinaemic responses during subsequent exercise at differing intensities. *European Journal of Applied Physiology* 88: 466-471.

Ackland, T., B. Elliot, and J. Richards. 2003. Growth in body size affects rotational performance in women's gymnastics. *Sports Biomechanics* 2: 163-176.

Agostini, R. 2000. Alpine skiing. In *Women in Sport* (edited by B.L. Drinkwater), pp. 613-625. Oxford, UK: Blackwell Science.

Ahlborg, G., J. Bergstrom, and J. Brohult. 1967. Human muscle glycogen content and capacity for prolonged exercise after difference diets. *Foersvarsmedicin* 3: 85-99.

Ahmun, R.P., R.J. Tong, and P.N. Grimshaw. 2005. The effects of acute creatine supplementation on multiple sprint cycling and running performance in rugby players. *Journal of Strength and Conditioning Research* 19: 92-97.

Akermark, C., I. Jacobs, M. Rasmusson, and J. Karlsson. 1996. Diet and muscle glycogen concentration in relation to physical performance in Swedish elite ice hockey players. *International Journal of Sport Nutrition* 6: 272-284.

Alderman, B.L., D.M. Landers, J. Carlson, and J.R. Scott. 2004. Factors related to rapid weight loss practices among international-style wrestlers. *Medicine and Science in Sports and Exercise* 36: 249-252.

Allen, J.D., J. McLung, A.G. Nelson, and M. Welsch. 1998. Ginseng supplementation does not enhance healthy young adults' peak aerobic exercise performance. *Journal of the American College of Nutrition* 17: 462-466.

Almeras, N., S. Lemieux, C. Bouchard, and A. Tremblay. 1997. Fat gain in female swimmers. *Physiology and Behavior* 61: 811-817.

Almond, C.S.D., A.Y. Shin, E.B. Fortescue, R.C. Mannix, D. Wypij, B.A. Binstadt, C.N. Duncan, D.P. Olson, A.E. Salerno, J.W. New-

burger, and D.S. Greenes. 2005. Hyponatremia among runners in the Boston marathon. *New England Journal of Medicine* 352: 1550-1556.

American Academy of Pediatrics (Committee on Sports Medicine and Fitness). 2005. Use of performance-enhancing substances. *Pediatrics* 115: 1103-1106.

American College of Sports Medicine. 1975. Position statement of the American College of Sports Medicine: Prevention of heat injuries during distance running. *Medicine and Science in Sports and Exercise* 7: vii-ix.

American College of Sports Medicine. 1976. Position statement: Weight loss in wrestlers. *Medicine and Science in Sports* 8: xi-xiii.

American College of Sports Medicine. 1982. Position statement on the use of alcohol in sports. *Medicine and Science in Sports and Exercise* 14: ix-x.

American College of Sports Medicine. 1987. Position stand of the American College of Sports Medicine: The prevention of thermal injuries during distance running. *Medicine and Science in Sports and Exercise* 19: 529-533.

American College of Sports Medicine. 1996. Position stand: Exercise and fluid replacement. *Medicine and Science in Sports and Exercise* 28: i-vii.

American College of Sports Medicine. 2000. Roundtable: The physiological and health effects of oral creatine supplementation. *Medicine and Science in Sports and Exercise* 32: 706-717.

American College of Sports Medicine. 2007. Position stand: Exercise and fluid replacement. *Medicine and Science in Sports and Exercise.*

American College of Sports Medicine, American Dietetic Association and Dietitians of Canada. 2000. Nutrition and athletic performance. *Medicine and Science in Sports and Exercise* 32: 2130-2145.

American Dietetic Association. 1993. Position stand of the American Dietetic Association and the Canadian Dietetic Association: Nutrition for physical fitness and athletic performance for adults. *Journal of the American Dietetic Association* 93: 691-696.

American Medical Association. 1967. Wrestling and weight control. *Journal of the American Medical Association* 201: 541-543.

American Psychiatric Association. 1994. *Diagnostic and Statistical Manual of Mental Disorders* (4th ed.). Washington, D.C.: American Psychiatric Association.

Anantaraman, R., A.A. Carmines, G.A. Gaesser, and A. Weltman. 1995. Effects of carbohydrate supplementation on performance during 1 hour of high-intensity exercise. *International Journal of Sports Medicine* 16: 461-465.

Andersen, R.E., and D.L. Montgomery. 1988. Physiology of alpine skiing. *Sports Medicine* 6: 210-221.

Anderson, M.E., C.R. Bruce, S.F. Fraser, N.K. Stepto, R. Klein, W.G. Hopkins, and J.A. Hawley. 2000. Improved 2000-meter rowing performance in competitive oarswomen after caffeine ingestion. *International Journal of Sport Nutrition and Exercise Metabolism* 10: 436-447.

Anderson, M.J., J.D. Cotter, A.P. Garnham, D.J. Casley, and M.A. Febbraio. 2001. Effect of glycerol-induced hyperhydration on thermoregulation and metabolism in the heat. *International Journal of Sport Nutrition and Exercise Metabolism* 11: 315-333.

Andrews, J.L., D.A. Sedlock, M.G. Flynn, J.W. Navalta, and H. Ji. 2003. Carbohydrate loading and supplementation in endurance trained women runners. *Journal of Applied Physiology* 95: 584-590.

Angus, D.J., M. Hargreaves, J. Dancey, and M.A. Febbraio. 2000. Effect of carbohydrate or carbohydrate plus medium-chain triglyceride ingestion on cycling time trial performance. *Journal of Applied Physiology* 88: 113-119.

Anselme, F., K. Collomp, B. Mercier, S. Ahmaidi, and C. Prefaut. 1992. Caffeine increases maximal anaerobic power and blood lactate concentration. *European Journal of Applied Physiology* 65: 188-191.

Antonio, J., M.S. Sanders, D. Kalman, D. Woodgate, and C. Street. 2002. The effects of high-dose glutamine ingestion on weightlifting performance. *Journal of Strength and Conditioning Research* 16: 157-160.

Antonio, J., M.S. Sanders, and D. Van Gammeren. 2001. The effects of bovine colostrum supplementation on body composition and exercise performance in active men and women. *Nutrition* 17: 243-247.

Antonio, J., J. Uelmen, R. Rodriguez, and C. Earnest. 2000. The effects of tribulus terrestris on body composition and exercise performance in resistance-trained males. *International Journal of Sport Nutrition and Exercise Metabolism* 10: 208-215.

Archer, D.T., and S.M. Shirreffs. 2001. Effect of fluid ingestion rate on post-exercise rehydration in man. *Proceedings of the Nutrition Society* 60: 200A.

Ariel, G., and W. Saville. 1972. Anabolic steroids: The physiological effects of placebos. *Medicine and Science in Sports and Exercise* 4: 124-126.

Arkinstall, M.J., C.R. Bruce, V. Nikolopoulos, A.P. Garnham, and J.A. Hawley. 2001. Effect of carbohydrate ingestion on metabolism during running and cycling. *Journal of Applied Physiology* 91: 2125-2134.

Armstrong, L. 2000. *It's Not About the Bike: My Journey Back to Life.* Sydney, Australia: Allen & Unwin.

Armstrong, L. 2003. *'Every Second Counts.* Sydney, Australia: Bantam Books.

Armstrong, L.E. 2002. Caffeine, body fluid-electrolyte balance, and exercise performance. *International Journal of Sport Nutrition and Exercise Metabolism* 12: 189-206.

Ashenden, M.J., P.A. Fricker, R.K. Ryan, N.K. Morrison, G.P. Dobson, and A.G. Hahn. 1998. The haematological response to an iron injection amongst female athletes. *International Journal of Sports Medicine* 19: 474-478.

Ashenden, M.J., D.T. Martin, G.P. Dobson, C. Mackintosh, and A.G. Hahn. 1998. Serum ferritin and anemia in trained female athletes. *International Journal of Sport Nutrition* 8: 223-229.

Askew, E.W. 1995. Environmental and physical stress and nutrient requirements. *American Journal of Clinical Nutrition* 61: 631S-637S.

Askew, E.W. 2002. Work at high altitude and oxidative stress: Antioxidant nutrients. *Toxicology* 180: 107-119.

Asp, S., T. Rohde, and E.A. Richter. 1997. Impaired muscle glycogen resynthesis after a marathon is not caused by decreased muscle GLUT-4 content. *Journal of Applied Physiology* 83: 1482-1485.

Ayoama, R., E. Hiruma, and H. Sasaki. 2003. Effects of creatine loading on muscular strength and endurance of female softball players. *Journal of Sports Medicine and Physical Fitness* 43: 481-488.

Baer, J.T., and L.J. Taper. 1992. Amenorrheic and eumenorrheic adolescent runners: Dietary intake and exercise training status. *Journal of the American Dietetic Association* 92: 89-91.

Bahrke, M.S., and W.P. Morgan. 1994. Evaluation of the ergogenic properties of ginseng. *Sports Medicine* 18: 229-248.

Bahrke, M.S., and W.P. Morgan. 2000. Evaluation of the ergogenic properties of ginseng: An update. *Sports Medicine* 29: 113-133.

Bailes, J.E., R.C. Cantu, and A.L. Day. 2002. The neurosurgeon in sport: Awareness of the risks of heatstroke and dietary supplements. *Neurosurgery* 51: 283-286.

Baldo-Enzi, G., F. Giada, G. Zuliani, L. Baroni, E. Vitale, G. Enzi, P. Magnanini, and R. Fellin. 1990. Lipid and apoprotein modifications in body builders during and after self-administration of anabolic steroids. *Metabolism* 39: 203-208.

Bale, P., and J. Goodway. 1990. Performance variables associated with the competitive gymnast. *Sports Medicine* 10: 139-145.

Balik, J. 1993. Who killed Momo Benaziza? *Ironman* January: 10.

Balon, T.W., J.F. Horowitz, and K.M. Fitzsimmons. 1992. Effects of carbohydrate loading and weight-lifting on muscle girth. *International Journal of Sport Nutrition* 2: 328-334.

Balsom, P.D., G.C. Gaitanos, K. Soderlund, and B. Ekblom. 1999. High-intensity exercise and muscle glycogen availability in humans. *Acta Physiologica Scandinavica* 165: 337-345.

Balsom, P.D., S.D.R. Harridge, K. Soderlund, B. Sjodin, and B. Ekblom. 1993. Creatine supplementation per se does not enhance endurance exercise performance. *Acta Physiologica Scandinavica* 149: 521-523.

Balsom, P.D., K. Wood, P. Olsson, and B. Ekblom. 1999. Carbohydrate intake and multiple sprint sports: With special reference to football (soccer). *International Journal of Sports Medicine* 20: 48-52.

Bangsbo, J., L. Norregaard, and F. Thorsoe. 1992. The effect of carbohydrate diet on intermittent exercise performance. *International Journal of Sports Medicine* 13: 152-157.

Barr, S.I. 1987. Women, nutrition and exercise: A review of athletes' intakes and a discussion of energy balance in active women. *Progress in Food and Nutrition Science* 11: 307-361.

Barr, S.I. 1989. Energy and nutrient intakes of elite adolescent swimmers. *Journal of the Canadian Dietetic Association* 50: 20-24.

Barr, S.I. 1991. Relationship of eating attitudes to anthropometric variables and dietary intakes of female collegiate swimmers. *Journal of the American Dietetic Association* 91: 976-977.

Barr, S.I., and D.L. Costill. 1989. Water: Can the endurance athlete get too much of a good thing? *Journal of the American Dietetic Association* 89: 1629-1632.

Barr, S.I., and D.L. Costill. 1992. Effect of increased training volume on nutrient intake of male collegiate swimmers. *International Journal of Sports Medicine* 13: 47-51.

Barr, S.I., K.C. Janelle, and J.C. Prior. 1995. Energy intakes are higher during the luteal phase of ovulatory menstrual cycles. *American Journal of Clinical Nutrition* 61: 39-43.

Barr, S.I., and H.A. McKay. 1998. Nutrition, exercise, and bone status in youth. *International Journal of Sport Nutrition* 8: 124-142.

Barrow, G.W., and S. Saha. 1988. Menstrual irregularity and stress fractures in collegiate female long distance runners. *American Journal of Sports Medicine* 16: 209-216.

Bass, S., M. Bradney, G. Pearce, E. Hendrich, K. Inge, S. Stuckey, S.K. Lo, and E. Seeman. 2000. Short stature and delayed puberty in gymnasts: Influence of selection bias on leg length and the duration of training in trunk length. *Journal of Pediatrics* 136: 149-155.

Bass, S., G. Pearce, M. Bradney, E. Hendrich, P.D. Delmas, A. Harding, and E. Seeman. 1998. Exercise before puberty may confer residual benefits in bone density in adulthood: Studies in active prepubertal and retired female gymnasts. *Journal of Bone and Mineral Research* 13: 500-507.

Batterham, A.M., and W.G. Hopkins. 2006. Making meaningful inferences about magnitudes. *International Journal of Sports Physiology and Performance* 1: 50-57.

Baume, N., N. Mahler, M. Kamber, P. Mangin, and M. Saugy. 2006. Research of stimulants and anabolic steroids in dietary supplements. *Scandinavian Journal of Medicine and Science in Sports* 16: 41-48.

Baylis, A., D. Cameron-Smith, and L.M. Burke. 2001. Inadvertent doping through supplement use by athletes: Assessment and management of the risk in Australia. *International Journal of Sport Nutrition and Exercise Metabolism* 11: 365-383.

Bazzarre, T.L., S.M. Kleiner, and M.D. Litchford. 1990. Nutrient intake, body fat, and lipid profiles of competitive male and female bodybuilders. *Journal of the American College of Nutrition* 9: 136-142.

Beals, K.A. 2004. *Disordered Eating Among Athletes: A Comprehensive Guide for Health Professionals*. Champaign, IL: Human Kinetics.

Beals, K.A., and M.M. Manore. 1994. The prevalence and consequences of subclinical eating disorders in female athletes. *International Journal of Sport Nutrition* 4: 175-195.

Beals, K.A., and M.M. Manore. 2002. Disorders of the female athlete triad among collegiate athletes. *International Journal of Sport Nutrition and Exercise Metabolism* 12: 281-293.

Becque, M.D., J.D. Lochmann, and D.R. Melrose. 2000. Effects of oral creatine supplementation on muscular strength and body composition. *Medicine and Science in Sports and Exercise* 32: 654-658.

Beidleman, B.A., J.L. Puhl, and M.J. De Souza. 1995. Energy balance in female distance runners. *American Journal of Clinical Nutrition* 61: 303-311.

Bell, D.G., I. Jacobs, and K. Ellerington. 2001. Effect of caffeine and ephedrine ingestion on anaerobic exercise performance. *Medicine and Science in Sports and Exercise* 33: 1399-1403.

Bell, D.G., and T.M. McLellan. 2003. Effect of repeated caffeine ingestion on repeated exhaustive exercise endurance. *Medicine and Science in Sports and Exercise* 35: 1348-1354.

Below, P.R., R. Mora-Rodriguez, J. Gonzalez-Alonso, and E.F. Coyle. 1995. Fluid and carbohydrate ingestion independently improve performance during 1 h of intense exercise. *Medicine and Science in Sports and Exercise* 27: 200-210.

Bemben, D.A., T.D. Buchanan, M.G. Bemben, and A.W. Knehans. 2004. Influence of type of mechanical loading, menstrual status, and training season on bone density in young women athletes. *Journal of Strength and Conditioning Research* 18: 220-226.

Bemben, M.G., D.A. Bemben, D.D. Loftiss, and A.W. Knehans. 2001. Creatine supplementation during resistance training

in college football athletes. *Medicine and Science in Sports and Exercise* 33: 1667-1673.

Benardot, D. 1996. Working with young athletes: Views of a nutritionist on the sports medicine team. *International Journal of Sport Nutrition* 6: 110-120.

Benardot, D. 2000. Gymnastics. In *Nutrition in Sport* (edited by R.J. Maughan), pp. 588-608. Oxford, UK: Blackwell Science.

Benardot, D., and C. Czerwinski. 1991. Selected body composition and growth measures of junior elite gymnasts. *Journal of the American Dietetic Association* 91: 29-33.

Benardot, D., M. Schwarz, and D.W. Heller. 1989. Nutrient intake in young, highly competitive gymnasts. *Journal of the American Dietetic Association* 89: 401-403.

Benson, J.E., Y. Allemann, G.E. Theintz, and H. Howald. 1990. Eating problems and calorie intake levels in Swiss adolescent athletes. *International Journal of Sports Medicine* 11: 249-252.

Benson, R. 1991. Weight control among elite women swimmers. In *Eating Disorders Among Athletes: Theory, Issues, and Research* (edited by D. R. Black), pp. 97-109. Reston, VA: Association for the Advancement of Health Education; National Association for Girls and Women in Sport; Associations of the American Alliance for Health, Physical Education, Recreation and Dance.

Bent, S., T.N. Tiedt, M.C. Odden, and M.G. Shlipak. 2003. The relative safety of ephedra compared with other herbal products. *Annals of Internal Medicine* 138: 468-471.

Berardi, J.M., and T.N. Ziegenfuss. 2003. Effects of ribose supplementation on repeated sprint performance in men. *International Journal of Sport Nutrition and Exercise Metabolism* 17: 47-52.

Berg, H.E., and O. Eiken. 1999. Muscle control in elite alpine skiing. *Medicine and Science in Sports and Exercise* 31: 1065-1067.

Berg, H.E., O. Eiken, and P.A. Tesch. 1995. Involvement of eccentric muscle actions in giant slalom racing. *Medicine and Science in Sports and Exercise* 27: 1666-1670.

Bergeron, M. 1996. Heat cramps during tennis: A case report. *International Journal of Sport Nutrition* 6: 62-68.

Bergeron, M.F. 2003. Heat cramps: Fluid and electrolyte challenges during tennis in the heat. *Journal of Science and Medicine in Sport* 6: 19-27.

Bergeron, M.F., C.M. Maresh, L.E. Armstrong, J.F. Signorile, J.W. Castellani, R.W. Kenefick, K.E. LaGasse, and D.A. Riebe. 1995. Fluid-electrolyte balance associated with tennis match play in a hot environment. *International Journal of Sport Nutrition* 5: 180-193.

Bergeron, M.F., C.M. Maresh, W.J. Kraemer, A. Abraham, B. Conroy, and C. Gabaree. 1991. Tennis: A physiological profile during match play. *International Journal of Sports Medicine* 12: 474-479.

Bergh, U. 1987. The influence of body mass in cross-country skiing. *Medicine and Science in Sports and Exercise* 19: 324-331.

Berglund, B. 1992. High-altitude training. Aspects of haematological adaptation. *Sports Medicine* 14: 289-303.

Bergstrom, J., L. Hermansen, E. Hultman, and B. Saltin. 1967. Diet, muscle glycogen and physical performance. *Acta Physiologica Scandinavica* 71: 140-150.

Bergstrom, J., and E. Hultman. 1966. Muscle glycogen synthesis after exercise: An enhancing factor localized to the muscle cells in man. *Nature* 210: 309-310.

Berning, J.R., J.P. Troup, P.J. VanHandel, J. Daniels, and N. Daniels. 1991. The nutritional habits of young adolescent swimmers. *International Journal of Sport Nutrition* 1: 240-248.

Berry, W.T.C., J.B. Beveridge, E.R. Bransby, A.K. Chalmers, B.M. Needham, H.E. Magee, H.S. Townsend, and C.G. Daubney. 1949. The diet, haemoglobin values, and blood pressures of Olympic athletes. *British Medical Journal* 19: 300-304.

Best, C.H., and R.C. Partridge. 1930. Observations on Olympic athletes. *Proceedings of the Royal Society, London Series B*: 323-332.

Bijlsma, H., and G.J. van Ingen Schenau. 1999. Introduction. In *Handbook of Competitive Speed Skating* (edited by H. Gemser, J.J. de Koning, and G.J. van Ingen Schenau), pp. 1-11. Lausanne, Switzerland: International Skating Union.

Bilanin, J.E., M.S. Blanchard, and E. Russek-Cohen. 1989. Lower vertebral bone density in male long distance runners. *Medicine and Science in Sports and Exercise* 21: 66-70.

Biolo, G., K.D. Tipton, S. Klein, and R.R. Wolfe. 1997. An abundant supply of amino acids enhances the metabolic effect of exercise on muscle protein. *American Journal of Physiology Endocrinology and Metabolism* 273: E122-E129.

Biolo, G., B.D. Williams, R.Y. Fleming, and R.R. Wolfe. 1999. Insulin action on muscle protein kinetics and amino acid transport during recovery after resistance exercise. *Diabetes* 48: 949-957.

Bird, S.R., J. Wiles, and J. Robbins. 1995. The effect of sodium bicarbonate ingestion on 1500-m racing time. *Journal of Sports Sciences* 13: 399-403.

Bishop, D., and B. Claudius. 2005. Effects of induced metabolic alkalosis on prolonged intermittent-sprint performance. *Medicine and Science in Sports and Exercise* 37: 759-767.

Bishop, N.C., A.K. Blannin, P.J. Robson, N.P. Walsh, and M. Gleeson. 1999. The effects of carbohydrate supplementation on immune responses to a soccer-specific exercise protocol. *Journal of Sports Sciences* 17: 787-796.

Biwer, C.J., R.J. Jensen, W.D. Schmidt, and P.B. Watts. 2003. The effect of creatine on treadmill running with high-intensity intervals. *Journal of Strength and Conditioning Research* 17: 439-445.

Black, A.E., A.M. Prentice, G.R. Goldberg, S.A. Jebb, S.A. Bingham, M.B.E. Livingstone, and W.A. Coward. 1993. Measurements of total energy expenditure provide insights into the validity of dietary measurements of energy intake. *Journal of the American Dietetic Association* 93: 572-579.

Blom, C.S.B., D.L. Costill, and N.K. Vollestad. 1987. Exhaustive running: Inappropriate as a stimulus of muscle glycogen supercompensation. *Medicine and Science in Sports and Exercise* 19: 398-403.

Blomstrand, E., P. Hassmen, S. Ek, B. Ekblom, and E.A. Newsholme. 1997. Influence of ingesting a solution of branched-chain amino acids on perceived exertion during exercise. *Acta Physiologica Scandinavica* 159: 41-49.

Blomstrand, E., P. Hassmen, and E.A. Newsholme. 1991. Effect of branched-chain amino acid supplementation on mental performance. *Acta Physiologica Scandinavica* 143: 225-226.

Boardman, C. 2000. *The Complete Book of Cycling*. London, UK: Partridge.

Bohe, J., A. Low, R.R. Wolfe, M.J. Rennie, and R.R. Wolfe. 2003. Human muscle protein synthesis is modulated by extracellular, not intracellular amino acid availability: A dose-response study. *Journal of Physiology* 552: 315-324.

Boirie, Y., M. Dangin, P. Gachon, M.-P. Vasson, J.-L. Maubois, and B. Beaufrere. 1997. Slow and fast dietary proteins differently modulate postprandial protein accretion. *Proceedings of the National Academy of Science* 94: 14930-14935.

Borsheim, E., A. Aarsland, and R.R. Wolfe. 2004. Effect of an amino acid, protein, and carbohydrate mixture on net muscle protein balance after resistance exercise. *International Journal of Sport Nutrition and Exercise Metabolism* 14: 255-271.

Borsheim, E., M.G. Cree, K.D. Tipton, T.A. Elliott, A. Aarsland, and R.R. Wolfe. 2004. Effect of carbohydrate intake on net muscle protein synthesis during recovery from resistance exercise. *Journal of Applied Physiology* 96: 674-678.

Borsheim, E., K.D. Tipton, S.E. Wolf, and R.R. Wolfe. 2002. Essential amino acids and muscle protein recovery from resistance exercise. *American Journal of Physiology Endocrinology and Metabolism* 283: E648-E657.

Bosch, A.N., S.C. Dennis, and T.D. Noakes. 1994. Influence of carbohydrate ingestion on fuel substrate turnover and oxidation during prolonged exercise. *Journal of Applied Physiology* 76: 2364-2372.

Bosco, C., F. Cotelli, R. Bonomi, P. Mognoni, and G.S. Roi. 1994. Seasonal fluctuations of selected physiological characteristics of elite alpine skiers. *European Journal of Applied Physiology and Occupational Physiology* 69: 71-74.

Bosco, C., J. Tihanyi, J. Pucspk, I. Kovacs, A. Gabossy, R. Colli, G. Pulvirenti, C. Tranquilli, C. Foti, M. Viru, and A. Viru. 1997. Effect of oral creatine supplementation on jumping and running performance. *International Journal of Sports Medicine* 18: 369-372.

Bottoms, L.M., A.M. Hunter, and S.D.R. Galloway. 2006. Effects of carbohydrate ingestion on skill maintenance in squash players. *European Journal of Sport Science* 6(3): 187-196.

Bouchard, C., A. Tremblay, J.P. Despres, A. Nadeau, P.J. Lupien, G. Theriault, J. Dussault, S. Moorjani, S. Pinault, and G. Fournier. 1990. The response to long-term overfeeding in identical twins. *New England Journal of Medicine* 322: 1477-1482.

Braakhuis, A.J., K. Meredith, G.R. Cox, W.G. Hopkins, and L.M. Burke. 2003. Variability in estimation of self-reported dietary intake data from elite athletes resulting from coding by different sports dietitians. *International Journal of Sport Nutrition and Exercise Metabolism* 13: 152-165.

Branch, J.D. 2003. Effect of creatine supplementation on body composition and performance: A meta-analysis. *International Journal of Sport Nutrition and Exercise Metabolism* 13: 198-226.

Branth, S., L. Hambraeus, K. Westerterp, A. Andersson, R. Edsgren, M. Mustelin, and R. Nilsson. 1996. Energy turnover in a sailing crew during offshore racing around the world. *Medicine and Science in Sports and Exercise* 28: 1272-1276.

Braun, B., P.M. Clarkson, P.S. Freedson, and R.L. Kohl. 1991. Effects of coenzyme Q10 supplementation and exercise performance, VO2 max, and lipid perodixation in trained subjects. *International Journal of Sport Nutrition* 1: 353-365.

Brenner, M., J. Walberg-Rankin, and D. Sebolt. 2000. The effect of creatine supplementation during resistance training in women. *Journal of Strength and Conditioning Research* 14: 207-213.

Bridge, C.A., and M.A. Jones. 2006. The effect of caffeine ingestion on 8 km run performance in a field setting. *Journal of Sports Sciences* 24: 433-439.

Brigham, D.E., J.L. Beard, R.S. Krimmel, and W.L. Kenney. 1993. Changes in iron status during competitive season in female collegiate swimmers. *Nutrition* 9: 418-422.

Brilla, L.R., and V. Conte. 2000. Effects of a novel zinc-magnesium formulation on hormones and strength. *Journal of Exercise Physiology* [Online] 3: 26-36. Available http://faculty.css.edu/tboone2/asep/fldr/fldr.htm [accessed September 7, 2006].

Brinkworth, G.D., and J. D. Buckley. 2003. Concentrated bovine colostrum protein supplementation reduces the incidence of self-reported symptoms of upper respiratory track infection in adult males. *European Journal of Nutrition* 42: 228-232.

Brinkworth, G.D., J.D. Buckley, P.C. Bourdon, J.P. Gulbin, and A.Z. David. 2002. Oral bovine colostrum supplementation enhances buffer capacity but not rowing performance in elite female rowers. *International Journal of Sport Nutrition and Exercise Metabolism* 12: 349-363.

Brinkworth, G.D., J.D. Buckley, J.P. Slavotinek, and A.P. Kurmis. 2004. Effect of bovine colostrum supplementation on the composition of resistance trained and untrained limbs in healthy young men. *European Journal of Applied Physiology and Occupational Physiology* 91: 53-61.

Broad, E.M., L.M. Burke, G.R. Cox, P. Heeley, and M. Riley. 1996. Body weight changes and voluntary fluid intakes during training and competition sessions in team sports. *International Journal of Sport Nutrition* 6: 307-320.

Broad, E., R.J. Maughan, and S.D.R. Galloway. 2005. Effects of 4 weeks L-carnitine L-tartrate ingestion on substrate utilization during prolonged exercise. *International Journal of Sport Nutrition and Exercise Metabolism* 15: 665-679.

Brotherhood, J., B. Brozovic, and L.G.C. Pugh. 1975. Hematological status of middle- and long-distance runners. *Clinical Science and Molecular Medicine* 48: 139-145.

Brotherhood, J.R., and M. Swanson. 1979. Nutrient intakes and body weight changes of distance runners using the glycogen loading procedure. *Australian Journal of Sports Medicine* 11: 45-47.

Brouns, F., W.H.M. Saris, E. Beckers, H. Adlercreutz, G.J. Van Der Vusse, H.A. Keizer, H. Kuipers, P. Menheere, A.J.M. Wagenmakers, and F. Ten Hoor. 1989. Metabolic changes induced by sustained exhaustive cycling and diet manipulation. *International Journal of Sports Medicine* 10: S49-S62.

Brouns, F., W.H.M. Saris, and N.J. Rehrer. 1987. Abdominal complaints and gastrointestinal function during long-lasting exercise. *International Journal of Sports Medicine* 8: 175-189.

Brouns, F., W.H. Saris, and F. Ten Hoor. 1986. Nutrition as a factor in the prevention of injuries in recreational and competitive downhill skiing. Considerations based on the literature. *Journal of Sports Medicine and Physical Fitness* 26: 85-91.

Brown, A.C., and R.A. Herb. 1990. Dietary intake and body composition of Mike Pigg—1988 triathlete of the year. *Clinical Sports Medicine* 2: 129-137.

Brown, A.C., H.S.H. MacRae, and N.S. Turner. 2004. Tricarboxylic-acid-cycle intermediates and cycling endurance capacity. *International Journal of Sport Nutrition and Exercise Metabolism* 14: 720-729.

Brown, D., and E.M. Winter. 1998. Fluid loss during international standard match-play in squash. In *Science and Racquet Sports II* (edited by A. Lees, I. Maynard, M. Hughes, and T. Reilly), pp. 56-59. London: E & FN Spon.

Brownell, K.D., J. Rodin, and J.H. Wilmore. 1988. Eat, drink and be worried? *Runner's World* August 28: 28-34.

Brownell, K.D., J. Rodin, and J.H. Wilmore. 1992. *Eating, Body Weight and Performance in Athletes: Disorders of Modern Society.* Philadelphia, PA: Lea & Febiger.

Brownell, K.D., S.N. Steen, and J.H. Wilmore. 1987. Weight regulation practices in athletes: Analysis of metabolic and health effects. *Medicine and Science in Sports and Exercise* 19: 546-556.

Brownlie, T., V. Utermohlen, P.S. Hinton, and J.D. Haas. 2004. Tissue iron deficiency without anemia impairs adaptations in endurance capacity after aerobic training in previously untrained women. *American Journal of Clinical Nutrition* 79: 427-443.

Bruce, C.R., M.E. Anderson, S.F. Fraser, N.K. Stepto, R. Klein, W.G. Hopkins, and J.A. Hawley. 2000. Enhancement of 2000-m rowing performance after caffeine ingestion. *Medicine and Science in Sports and Exercise* 32: 1958-1963.

Brukner, P., and K. Bennell. 1997. Stress fractures in female athletes: Diagnosis, management and rehabilitation. *Sports Medicine* 24: 419-429.

Brukner, P., K. Bennell, and G. Matheson, 1999. *Stress Fractures.* Sydney, Australia: Blackwell Science.

Bucci, L.R., J.F. Hickson, I. Wolinsky, and J.M. Pivarnik. 1992. Ornithine supplementation and insulin release in bodybuilders. *International Journal of Sport Nutrition* 2: 287-291.

Buckley, J.D., M.J. Abbott, G.D. Brinkworth, and P.B.D. Whyte. 2002. Bovine colostrum supplementation during endurance running training improves recovery, but not performance. *Journal of Science and Medicine in Sport* 5: 65-79.

Buckley, J.D., G.D. Brinkworth, and M.J. Abbott. 2003. Effect of bovine colostrum on anaerobic exercise performance and plasma insulin-like growth factor. *Journal of Sports Sciences* 21: 577-588.

Burge, C.M., M.F. Carey, and W.R. Payne. 1993. Rowing performance, fluid balance, and metabolic function following dehydration and rehydration. *Medicine and Science in Sports and Exercise* 25: 1358-1364.

Burke, D.G., P.D. Chilibeck, K.S. Davison, D.G. Candow, J. Farthing, and T. Smith-Palmer. 2001. The effect of whey protein supplementation with and without creatine monohydrate combined with resistance training on lean tissue mass and muscle strength. *International Journal of Sport Nutrition and Exercise Metabolism* 11: 349-364.

Burke, D.G., P.D. Chilibeck, G. Parise, D.G. Candow, D. Mahoney, and M.A. Tarnopolsky. 2003. Effect of creatine and weight training on muscle creatine and performance in vegetarians. *Medicine and Science in Sports and Exercise* 35: 1946-1955.

Burke, E.R., and B. Ekblom. 1982. Influence of fluid ingestion and dehydration on precision and endurance performance in tennis. *Athletic Training* Winter: 275-277.

Burke, L. 1994. Sports amenorrhea, osteopenia, stress fractures and calcium. In *Clinical Sports Nutrition* (edited by L. Burke and V. Deakin), pp. 200-226. Sydney, Australia: McGraw-Hill.

Burke, L. 1995. *The Complete Guide to Food for Sports Performance.* Sydney, Australia: Allen and Unwin.

Burke, L.M. 2001a. An interview with Dr. Gary Green about supplements and doping problems from an NCAA perspective. *International Journal of Sport Nutrition and Exercise Metabolism* 11: 397-400.

Burke, L.M. 2001b. Energy needs of athletes. *Canadian Journal of Applied Physiology* 26: S202-S219.

Burke, L. 2006a. Preparation for competition. In *Clinical Sports Nutrition, 3rd ed.* (edited by L. Burke and V. Deakin), pp. 355-384. Sydney, Australia: McGraw-Hill.

Burke, L.M., M.E. Anderson, and D.B. Pyne. in press. Low levels of caffeine intake fail to enhance performance of swimming sprints by elite swimmers. *International Journal of Sport Nutrition Exercise Metabolism.*

Burke, L.M., D.J. Angus, G.R. Cox, N.K. Cummings, M.A. Febbraio, K. Gawthorn, J.A. Hawley, M. Minehan, D.T. Martin, and M. Hargreaves. 2000. Effect of fat adaptation and carbohydrate restoration on metabolism and performance during prolonged cycling. *Journal of Applied Physiology* 89: 2413-2421.

Burke, L.M., M. Arkinstall, L. Bell, and G.R. Cox. in press. Addition of amino acids to sports drink fails to enhance insulin concentration or cycling performance. *International Journal of Sport Nutrition Exercise Metabolism.*

Burke, L.M., L. Bell, G. Cox, R. Crawford, M. Minehan, and C. Wood. 2004. *Survival Around the World.* Sydney, Australia: Allen and Unwin.

Burke, L.M., A. Claassen, J.A. Hawley, and T.D. Noakes. 1998. Carbohydrate intake during prolonged cycling minimizes effect of glycemic index of preexercise meal. *Journal of Applied Physiology* 85: 2220-2226.

Burke, L.M., G.R. Collier, S.K. Beasley, P.G. Davis, P.A. Fricker, P. Heeley, K. Walder, and M. Hargreaves. 1995. Effect of coingestion of fat and protein with carbohydrate feedings on muscle glycogen storage. *Journal of Applied Physiology* 78: 2187-2192.

Burke, L.M., G.R. Collier, E.M. Broad, P.G. Davis, D.T. Martin, A.J. Sanigorski, and M. Hargreaves. 2003. Effect of alcohol intake on muscle glycogen storage after prolonged exercise. *Journal of Applied Physiology* 95: 983-990.

Burke, L.M., G.R. Collier, P.G. Davis, P.A. Fricker, A.J. Sanigorski, and M. Hargreaves. 1996. Muscle glycogen storage after prolonged exercise: Effect of the frequency of carbohydrate feedings. *American Journal of Clinical Nutrition* 64: 115-119.

Burke, L.M., G.R. Collier, and M. Hargreaves. 1993. Muscle glycogen storage after prolonged exercise: The effect of the glycemic index of carbohydrate feedings. *Journal of Applied Physiology* 75: 1019-1023.

Burke, L.M., M. Cort, G.R. Cox, R. Crawford, B. Desbrow, L. Farthing, M. Minehan, N. Shaw, and O. Warnes. 2006. Supplements and sports foods. In *Clinical Sports Nutrition, 3rd ed.* (edited by L. Burke and V. Deakin), pp. 485-579. Sydney, Australia: McGraw-Hill.

Burke, L.M., G.R. Cox, N.K. Cummings, and B. Desbrow. 2001. Guidelines for daily CHO intake: Do athletes achieve them? *Sports Medicine* 31: 267-299.

Burke, L.M., R.A. Gollan, and R.S.D. Read. 1986. Seasonal changes in body composition measurements in Australian rules footballers. *British Journal of Sports Medicine* 20: 69-71.

Burke, L.M., R.A. Gollan, and R.S.D. Read. 1991. Dietary intakes and food use of groups of elite Australian male athletes. *International Journal of Sport Nutrition* 1: 378-394.

Burke, L.M., and J.A. Hawley. 2002. Effects of short-term fat adaptation on metabolism and performance of prolonged exercise. *Medicine and Science in Sports and Exercise* 34: 1492-1498.

Burke, L.M., J.A. Hawley, D.J. Angus, G.R. Cox, S. Clark, N.K. Cummings, B. Desbrow, and M. Hargreaves. 2002. Adaptations to short-term high-fat diet persist during exercise despite high carbohydrate availability. *Medicine and Science in Sports and Exercise* 34: 83-91.

Burke, L.M., and B. Kiens. 2006. "Fat adaptation" for athletic performance—The nail in the coffin? *Journal of Applied Physiology* 100: 7-8.

Burke, L.M., B. Kiens, and J.L. Ivy. 2004. Carbohydrates and fat for training and recovery. *Journal of Sports Sciences* 22: 15-30.

Burke, L.M., A.B. Loucks, and N.P. Broad. 2006. Energy and carbohydrate for training and recovery. *Journal of Sports Sciences* 24: 675-685.

Burke, L.M., and R.J. Maughan 2000. Alcohol in sport. In *Nutrition in sport* (edited by R.J. Maughan), pp. 405-414. Oxford, UK: Blackwell Science.

Burke, L.M., D.B. Pyne, and R.D. Telford. 1996. Effect of oral creatine supplementation on single-effort sprint performance in elite swimmers. *International Journal of Sport Nutrition* 6: 222-233.

Burke, L.M., and R.S.D. Read. 1987a. A study of carbohydrate loading techniques used by marathon runners. *Canadian Journal of Sports Science* 12: 6-10.

Burke, L.M., and R.S.D. Read. 1987b. Diet patterns of elite Australian male triathletes. *The Physician and Sportsmedicine* 15: 140-155.

Burke, L.M., and R.S.D. Read 1988a. Food use and nutritional practices of elite Olympic weightlifters. In *Food habits in Australia* (edited by A.S. Truswell and M.L. Wahlqvist), pp. 112-121. Melbourne, Australia: Rene Gordon.

Burke, L.M., and R.S.D. Read. 1988b. A study of dietary patterns of elite Australian football players. *Canadian Journal of Sports Science* 13: 15-19.

Burke, L.M., C. Wood, D.B. Pyne, R.T. Telford, and P. Saunders. 2005. Effect of carbohydrate intake on half-marathon performance of well-trained runners. *International Journal of Sport Nutrition and Exercise Metabolism* 15: 573-589.

Burns, J., and L. Dugan. 1994. Working with the professional athletes in the rink: The evolution of a nutrition program for an NHL team. *International Journal of Sport Nutrition* 4: 132-134.

Bussau, V.A., T.J. Fairchild, A. Rao, P.D. Steele, and P.A. Fournier. 2002. Carbohydrate loading in human muscle: An improved 1 day protocol. *European Journal of Applied Physiology and Occupational Physiology* 87: 290-295.

Butterfield, G.E. 1987. Whole-body protein utilisation in humans. *Medicine and Science in Sports and Exercise* 19: S157-S165.

Cade, J.R., R.H. Reese, R.M. Privette, N.M. Hommen, J.L. Rogers, and M.J. Fregly. 1991. Dietary intervention and training in swimmers. *European Journal of Applied Physiology* 63: 210-215.

Caine, D., R. Lewis, P. O'Connor, W. Howe, and S. Bass. 2001. Does gymnastics training inhibit growth of females? *Clinical Journal of Sports Medicine* 11: 260-267.

Caldarone, G., C. Tranquilli, and M. Giampietro. 1990. Assessment of the nutritional state of top level football players. In *Sports Medicine Applied to Football* (edited by G. Santilli), pp. 133-141. Rome: Instituto Dietitian Scienza della Sport del Coni.

Caldwell, J.E., E. Ahonen, and U. Nousiainen. 1984. Differential effects of sauna-, diuretic-, and exercise-induced hypohydration. *Journal of Applied Physiology* 57: 1018-1023.

Campbell, W.W., J.L. Beard, L.J. Joseph, S.L. Davey, and W.J. Evans. 1997. Chromium picolinate supplementation and resistive training by older men: Effects on iron-status and hematologic indexes. *American Journal of Clinical Nutrition* 66: 944-949.

Candow, D.G., P.D. Chilibeck, D.G. Burke, K.S. Davison, and T. Smith-Palmer. 2001. Effect of glutamine supplementation combined with resistance training in young adults. *European Journal of Applied Physiology and Occupational Physiology* 86: 142-149.

Cann, C.E., M.C. Martin, H.K. Genant, and R.B. Jaffe. 1984. Decreased spinal mineral content in amenorrheic women. *Journal of the American Medical Association* 251: 626-629.

Carey, A.L., H.M. Staudacher, N.K. Cummings, N.K. Stepto, V. Nikolopoulos, L.M. Burke, and J.A. Hawley. 2001. Effects of fat adaptation and carbohydrate restoration on prolonged endurance exercise. *Journal of Applied Physiology* 91: 115-122.

Carrithers, J.A., D.L. Williamson, P.M. Gallagher, M.P. Godard, K.E. Schulze, and S.W. Trappe. 2000. Effects of postexercise carbohydrate-protein feedings on muscle glycogen restoration. *Journal of Applied Physiology* 88: 1976-1982.

Carter, J.E.L., and T.R. Ackland (eds.). 1994. *Kinanthropometry in Aquatic Sports: A Study of World Class Athletes.* Champaign, IL: Human Kinetics.

Carter, J.E., and C.V. Gisolfi. 1989. Fluid replacement during and after exercise in the heat. *Medicine and Science in Sports and Exercise* 21: 532-539.

Carter, J.M., A.E. Jeukendrup, and D.A. Jones. 2004. The effect of carbohydrate mouth-rinse on 1 h cycle time-trial performance. *Medicine and Science in Sports and Exercise* 36: 2107-2111.

Carter, J.M., A.E. Jeukendrup, C.H. Mann, and D.A. Jones. 2004. The effect of glucose infusion on glucose kinetics during a 1-h time trial. *Medicine and Science in Sports and Exercise* 36: 1543-1550.

Carter, J., A.E. Jeukendrup, T. Mundel, and D.A. Jones. 2003. Carbohydrate supplementation improves moderate and high-intensity exercise in the heat. *Pflugers Archives—European Journal of Physiology* 446: 211-219.

Casey, A., D. Constantin-Teodosiu, S. Howell, E. Hultman, and P.L. Greenhaff. 1996. Creatine ingestion favorably affects performance and muscle metabolism during maximal exercise in humans. *American Journal of Physiology Endocrinology and Metabolism* 271: E31-E37.

Casey, A., and P.L. Greenhaff. 2000. Does dietary creatine supplementation play a role in skeletal muscle metabolism and performance? *American Journal of Clinical Nutrition* 72: 607S-617S.

Catlin, D.H., B.Z. Leder, B. Ahrens, B. Starcevic, C.K. Hatton, G.A. Green, and J.S. Finkelstein. 2001. Trace contamination of over-the-counter androstenedione and positive urine test results for a nandrolone metabolite. *Journal of the American Medical Association* 284: 2618-2621.

Centers for Disease Control and Prevention. 1998. Hyperthermia and dehydration-related deaths associated with intentional rapid weight loss in three collegiate wrestlers—North Carolina, Wisconsin, and Michigan, November-December 1998. *Journal of the American Medical Association* 279: 824-825.

Cerretelli, P., and C. Marconi. 1990. L-carnitine supplementation in humans. The effects on physical performance. *International Journal of Sports Medicine* 11: 1-14.

Chandler, R.M., H.K. Byrne, J.G. Patterson, and J.L. Ivy. 1994. Dietary supplements affect the anabolic hormones after weight-training exercise. *Journal of Applied Physiology* 76: 839-845.

Chanutin, A. 1926. The fate of creatine when administered to man. *Journal of Biological Chemistry* 67: 29-37.

Charatan, F. 2003. Ephedra supplement may have contributed to sportsman's death. *British Medical Journal* 326: 464.

Chatard, J.-C., I. Mujika, C. Guy, and J.-R. Lacour. 1999. Anaemia and iron deficiency in athletes. *Sports Medicine* 27: 229-240.

Chen, J.D., J.F. Wang, K.J. Li, S.W. Wang, Y. Jiao, and X.Y. Hou. 1989. Nutritional problems and measures in elite and amateur athletes. *American Journal of Clinical Nutrition* 49: 1084-1089.

Cheuvront, S.N. 1999. The Zone diet and athletic performance. *Sports Medicine* 27: 213-228.

Cheuvront, S.N., E.M. Haymes, and M.N. Sawka. 2002. Comparison of sweat loss estimates for women during prolonged high-intensity running. *Medicine and Science in Sports and Exercise* 34: 1344-1350.

Chinevere, T.D., R.D. Sawyer, A.R. Creer, R.K. Conlee, and A.C. Parcell. 2002. Effects of L-tyrosine and carbohydrate ingestion on endurance exercise performance. *Journal of Applied Physiology* 93: 1590-1597.

Choma, C.W., G.A. Sforzo, and B.A. Keller. 1998. Impact of rapid weight loss on cognitive function in collegiate wrestlers. *Medicine and Science in Sports and Exercise* 30: 746-749.

Chong, S.K.F., and V.G.P. Oberholzer. 1988. Ginseng—Is there a clinical use in medicine? *Postgraduate Medicine* 65: 841-846.

Christensen, E.H., and O. Hansen. 1939. Arbeitsfahigkeit und Ehrnahrung. *Skandinavian Archives Physiology* 81:160-171.

Chryssanthopoulos, C., and C. Williams. 1997. Pre-exercise carbohydrate meal and endurance running capacity when car- bohydrates are ingested during exercise. *International Journal of Sports Medicine* 18: 543-548.

Chwalbinska-Moneta, J. 2003. Effect of creatine supplementation on aerobic performance and anaerobic capacity in elite rowers in the course of endurance training. *International Journal of Sport Nutrition and Exercise Metabolism* 13: 173-183.

Chynoweth, C. 2001. *Herald Sun* newspaper, Melbourne, Australia, October 20, p. 12.

Clancy, S.P., P.M. Clarkson, M.E. DeCheke, K. Nosaka, P.S. Freedson, J.J. Cunningham, and B. Valentine. 1994. Effects of chromium picolinate supplementation on body composition, strength, and urinary chromium loss in football players. *International Journal of Sport Nutrition* 4: 142-153.

Clark, M., D.B. Reed, S.F. Crouse, and R.B. Armstrong. 2003. Pre- and post-season dietary intake, body composition, and performance indices of NCAA Division I female soccer players. *International Journal of Sport Nutrition and Exercise Metabolism* 13: 303-319.

Clark, N., M. Nelson, and W. Evans. 1988. Nutrition education for elite female runners. *The Physician and Sportsmedicine* 16: 124-136.

Clark, V.R., W.G. Hopkins, J.A. Hawley, and L.M. Burke. 2000. Placebo effect of carbohydrate feedings during a 40-km cycling time trial. *Medicine and Science in Sports and Exercise* 32: 1642-1647.

Clarkson, P.M. 1992. Nutritional ergogenic aids: Carnitine. *International Journal of Sport Nutrition* 2: 185-190.

Clarkson, P.M. 1997. Effects of exercise on chromium levels. Is supplementation necessary? *Sports Medicine* 23: 341-349.

Clement, D.B., and R.C. Asmundson. 1982. Nutritional intake and hematological parameters in endurance runners. *The Physician and Sportsmedicine* 10: 37-43.

Clement, D.B., D.R. Lloyd-Smith, J.G. Macintyre, G.O. Matheson, R. Brock, and M. Dupont. 1987. Iron status in winter Olympic sports. *Journal of Sports Science* 5: 261-271.

Coetzer, P., T.D. Noakes, B. Sanders, M.I. Lambert, A.N. Bosch, T. Wiggins, and S.C. Dennis. 1993. Superior fatigue resistance of elite black South African distance runners. *Journal of Applied Physiology* 75: 1822-1827.

Coggan, A.R., and E.F. Coyle. 1987. Reversal of fatigue during prolonged exercise by carbohydrate infusion or ingestion. *Journal of Applied Physiology* 63: 2388-2395.

Cohen, B.S., A.G. Nelson, M.C. Prevost, G.D. Thompson, B.D. Marx, and G.S. Morris. 1996. Effects of caffeine ingestion on endurance racing in heat and humidity. *European Journal of Applied Physiology and Occupational Physiology* 73: 358-363.

Cohen, I., D. Mitchell, R. Seider, A. Kahn, and F. Phillips. 1981. The effect of water deficit on body temperature during rugby. *South African Medical Journal* 60: 11-14.

Cole, C.R., G.F. Salvaterra, J.E. Davis, M.E. Borja, L.M. Powell, E.C. Dubbs, and P.L. Bordi. 2005. Evaluation of dietary practices of National Collegiate Athletic Association Division I football players. *Journal of Strength and Conditioning Research* 19: 490-494.

Colgan, M. 1988. Inosine. *Muscle and Fitness* 49: 94-96, 204, 206, 210.

Collomp, K., S. Ahmaidi, M. Audran, J.L. Chanal, and C. Prefaut. 1991. Effects of caffeine ingestion on performance and anaerobic metabolism during the Wingate Test. *International Journal of Sports Medicine* 12: 439-443.

Collomp, K., S. Ahmaidi, J.C. Chatard, M. Audran, and C. Prefaut. 1992. Benefits of caffeine ingestion on sprint performance in trained and untrained swimmers. *European Journal of Applied Physiology* 64: 377-380.

Colombani, P., C. Wenk, I. Kunz, S. Krahenbuhl, M. Kuhnt, M. Arnold, P. Frey-Rindova, W. Frey, and W. Langhans. 1996. Effects of L-carnitine supplementation on physical performance and energy metabolism of endurance-trained athletes: A double-blind crossover field study. *European Journal of Applied Physiology* 73: 434-439.

Colson, S.N., F.B. Wyatt, D.L. Johnston, L.D. Autrey, Y.L. FitzGerald, and C.P. Earnest. 2005. Cordyceps sinensis- and Rhodiola rosea-based supplementation in male cyclists and its effect on muscle tissue oxygen saturation. *Journal of Strength and Conditioning Research* 19: 358-363.

Conlee, R.K., C.M. McGown, A.G. Fisher, G.P. Dalsky, and K.C. Robinson. 1982. Physiological effects of power volleyball. *The Physician and Sportsmedicine* 10: 93-97.

Constantini, N.W., A. Eliakim, L. Zigel, M. Yaaron, and B. Falk. 2000. Iron status of highly active adolescents: Evidence of depleted iron stores in gymnasts. *International Journal of Sport Nutrition and Exercise Metabolism* 10: 62-70.

Convertino, V.A., L.E. Armstrong, E.F. Coyle, G.W. Mack, M.N. Sawka, L.C. Senay, Jr., and W.M. Sherman. 1996. American College of Sports Medicine position stand. Exercise and fluid replacement. *Medicine and Science in Sports and Exercise* 28: i-vii.

Conway, K.J., R. Orr, and S.R. Stannard. 2003. Effect of a divided dose of endurance cycling performance, postexercise urinary caffeine concentration and plasma paraxanthine. *Journal of Applied Physiology* 94: 1557-1562.

Coombes, J.S., M. Conacher, S.K. Austen, and P.A. Marshall. 2002. Dose effects of oral bovine colostrum on physical work capacity in cyclists. *Medicine and Science in Sports and Exercise* 34: 1184-1188.

Coombes, J.S., and K.L. Hamilton. 2000. The effectiveness of commercially available sports drinks. *Sports Medicine* 29: 181-209.

Coombes, J.S., S.K. Powers, B. Rowell, K.L. Hamilton, S.L. Dodd, R.A. Shanely, C.K. Sen, and L. Packer. 2001. Effects of vitamin E and alpha-lipoic acid on skeletal muscle contractile properties. *Journal of Applied Physiology* 90: 1424-1430.

Costill, D.L., G.P. Dalsky, and W.J. Fink. 1978. Effects of caffeine ingestion on metabolism and exercise performance. *Medicine and Science in Sports and Exercise* 10: 155-158.

Costill, D.L., M.G. Flynn, J.P. Kirwan, J.A. Houmard, J.B. Mitchell, R.T. Thomas, and S.H. Park. 1988. Effects of repeated days of intensified training on muscle glycogen and swimming performance. *Medicine and Science in Sports and Exercise* 20: 249-254.

Costill, D.L., D. Hinrichs, W.J. Fink, and D. Hoopes. 1988. Muscle glycogen depletion during swimming interval training. *Journal of Swimming Research* 4: 15-18.

Costill, D.L., W.M. Sherman, W.J. Fink, C. Maresh, M. Witten, and J.M. Miller. 1981. The role of dietary carbohydrates in muscle glycogen resynthesis after strenuous running. *American Journal of Clinical Nutrition* 34: 1831-1836.

Coutts, A., P. Reaburn, K. Mummery, and M. Holmes. 2002. The effect of glycerol hyperhydration on Olympic distance triathlon performance in high ambient temperatures. *International Journal of Sport Nutrition and Exercise Metabolism* 12: 105-119.

Couzy, F., C.Y. Guezennec, and H. Legrand. 1989. Low transferrin saturation, hemoglobin and plasma zinc values in female alpine skiers. *Science and Sports* 4: 243-244.

Couzy, F., P. Lafargue, and C.Y. Guezennec. 1990. Zinc metabolism in the athlete: Influence of training, nutrition and other factors. *International Journal of Sports Medicine* 11: 263-266.

Cox, G.R., E.M. Broad, M.D. Riley, and L.M. Burke. 2002. Body mass changes and voluntary fluid intakes of elite level water polo players and swimmers. *Journal of Science and Medicine in Sport* 5: 183-193.

Cox, G.R., B. Desbrow, P.G. Montgomery, M.E. Anderson, C.R. Bruce, T.A. Macrides, D.T. Martin, A. Moquin, A. Roberts, J.A. Hawley, and L.M. Burke. 2002. Effect of different protocols of caffeine intake on metabolism and endurance performance. *Journal of Applied Physiology* 93: 990-999.

Cox, G.R., I. Mujika, D. Tumilty, and L.M. Burke. 2002. Acute creatine supplementation and performance during a field test simulating match play in elite female soccer players. *International Journal of Sport Nutrition and Exercise Metabolism* 12: 33-46.

Coyle, E.F. 1991. Timing and method of increased carbohydrate intake to cope with heavy training, competition and recovery. *Journal of Sports Sciences* 9: 29-52.

Coyle, E.F. 2004. Fluid and fuel intake during exercise. *Journal of Sports Sciences* 22: 39-55.

Coyle, E.F., A.R. Coggan, M.K. Hemmert, and J.L. Ivy. 1986. Muscle glycogen utilisation during prolonged strenuous exercise when fed carbohydrate. *Journal of Applied Physiology* 61: 165-172.

Coyle, E.F., A.R. Coggan, M.K. Hemmert, R.C. Lowe, and T.J. Walters. 1985. Substrate usage during prolonged exercise following a preexercise meal. *Journal of Applied Physiology* 59: 429-433.

Coyle, E.F., J.M. Hagberg, B.F. Hurley, W.H. Martin, A.A., Ehsani and J.O. Holloszy. 1983. Carbohydrate feeding during prolonged strenuous exercise can delay fatigue. *Journal of Applied Physiology* 55: 230-235.

Coyle, E.F., A.E. Jeukendrup, M.C. Oseto, B.J. Hodgkinson, and T.W. Zderic. 2001. Low-fat diet alters intramuscular substrates and reduces lipolysis and fat oxidation during exercise. *American Journal of Physiology Endocrinology and Metabolism* 280: E391-E398.

Coyle, E.F., and S.J. Montain. 1992. Carbohydrate and fluid ingestion during exercise: Are there trade-offs? *Medicine and Science in Sports and Exercise* 24: 671-678.

Creer, A., P. Gallagher, D. Slivka, B. Jemiolo, W. Fink, and S. Trappe. 2005. Influence of muscle glycogen availability on ERK1/2 and Akt signaling after resistance exercise in human skeletal muscle. *Journal of Applied Physiology* 99: 950-956.

Crespo, M., M. Reid, D. Miley, and F. Atienza. 2003. The relationship between professional tournament structure on the national level and success in men's professional tennis. *Journal of Science and Medicine in Sport* 6: 3-13.

Criswell, D., S. Powers, J. Lawler, J. Tew, S. Dodd, Y. Iryiboz, R. Tulley, and K. Wheeler. 1991. Influence of a carbohydrate-electrolyte beverage on performance and blood homeostasis during recovery from football. *International Journal of Sport Nutrition* 1: 178-191.

Crooks, C.V., C.R. Wall, M.L. Cross and K.J. Rutherfurd-Markwick. 2006. The effect of bovine colostrum supplementation on salivary IgA in distance runners. *International Journal of Sport Nutrition and Exercise Metabolism* 16: 47-64.

Crowe, M.J., D.M. O'Connor, and J.E. Lukins. 2003. The effects of β-hydroxy-β-methylbutyrate (HMB) and HMB/creatine supplementation on indices of health in highly trained athletes. *International Journal of Sport Nutrition and Exercise Metabolism* 13: 184-197.

Crowe, M.J., J.N. Weatherson, and B.F. Bowdon. 2005. Effects of dietary leucine supplementation on exercise performance. *European Journal of Applied Physiology* 97: 664-672.

Cui, J., M. Garle, P. Eneroth, and I. Bjorkhem. 1994. What do commercial ginseng preparations contain? *Lancet* 344: 134.

Cummings, N., R. Crawford, M. Cort, and F. Pelly. 2006. Providing meals for athletic groups. In *Clinical Sports Nutrition, 3rd ed.* (edited by L. Burke and V. Deakin), pp. 785-805. Sydney, Australia: McGraw-Hill.

Cunningham, J.J. 1980. A reanalysis of the factors influencing basal metabolic rate in normal adults. *American Journal of Clinical Nutrition* 33: 2372-2374.

Dabinett, J.A., K. Reid, and N. James. 2001. Educational strategies used in increasing fluid intake and enhancing hydration status in field hockey players preparing for competition in a hot and humid environment: A case study. *International Journal of Sport Nutrition and Exercise Metabolism* 11: 334-348.

Dale, E., and D.L. Goldberg. 1982. Implications of nutrition in athletes' menstrual cycle irregularities. *Canadian Journal of Applied Sports Science* 7: 74-78.

Dale, K.S., and D.M. Landers. 1999. Weight control in wrestling: Eating disorders or disordered eating? *Medicine and Science in Sports and Exercise* 31: 1382-1389.

Daly, R.M., P.A. Rich, R. Klein, and S. Bass. 1999. Effects of high-impact exercise on ultrasonic and biochemical indices of skeletal status: A prospective study in young male gymnasts. *Journal of Bone and Mineral Research* 14: 1222-1230.

Dangin, M., Y. Boirie, C. Garcia-Rodenas, P. Gachon, J. Fauquant, P. Callier, O. Ballevre, and B. Beaufrere. 2001. The digestion rate of protein is an independent regulating factor of postprandial protein retention. *American Journal of Physiology Endocrinology and Metabolism* 280: E340-E348.

Dangin, M., C. Guillet, C. Garcia-Rodenas, P. Gachon, C. Bouteloup-Demange, K. Reiffers-Magnani, J. Fauquant, O. Ballevre, and B. Beaufrere. 2003. The rate of protein digestion affects protein gain differently during aging in humans. *Journal of Physiology* 549(Pt. 2): 635-644.

Daries, H.N., T.D. Noakes, and S.C. Dennis. 2000. Effect of fluid intake volume on 2-h running performances in a 25°C environment. *Medicine and Science in Sports and Exercise* 32: 1783-1789.

Davis, J.M., R.S. Welsh, and N.A. Alderson. 2000. Effects of carbohydrate and chromium ingestion during intermittent high-intensity exercise to fatigue. *International Journal of Sport Nutrition and Exercise Metabolism* 10: 476-485.

Davis, J.M., R.S. Welsh, K.L. De Volve, and N.A. Alderson. 1999. Effects of branched-chain amino acids and carbohydrate on fatigue during intermittent, high-intensity running. *International Journal of Sports Medicine* 20: 309-314.

Dawson, B., C. Goodman, T. Blee, G. Claydon, P. Peeling, J. Beilby, and A. Prins. 2006. Iron supplementation: Oral tablets versus intramuscular injection. *International Journal of Sport Nutrition and Exercise Metabolism* 16: 180-186.

Dawson, B., T. Vladich, and B.A. Blanksby. 2002. Effects of 4 weeks of creatine supplementation in junior swimmers on freestyle sprint and swim bench performance. *Journal of Strength and Conditioning Research* 16: 485-490.

De Benedette, V. 1987. For jockeys, injuries are not a long shot. *The Physician and Sportsmedicine* 15: 237-245.

de Bock, K., B.O. Eijnde, M. Ramaekers, and P. Hespel. 2004. Acute rhodiola rosea intake can improve endurance exercise performance. *International Journal of Sport Nutrition and Exercise Metabolism* 14: 298-307.

de Boer, R.W., E. Vos, W. Hutter, G. de Groot, and G.J. van Ingen Schenau. 1987. Physiological and biomechanical comparison of roller skating and speed skating on ice. *European Journal of Applied Physiology and Occupational Physiology* 56: 562-569.

De Lorenzo, A., I. Bertini, N. Candeloro, R. Piccinelli, I. Innocente, and A. Brancati. 1999. A new predictive equation to calculate resting metabolic rate in athletes. *Journal of Sports Medicine and Physical Fitness* 39: 213-219.

De Wijn, J.F., J. Leusink, and G.B. Post. 1979. Diet, body composition and physical condition of champion rowers during periods of training and out of training. *Bibliotheca Nutritio Dieta* 27: 143-148.

De Wijn, J.F., and M. Van Erp-Baart. 1980. Foodpattern, body composition and physical condition of heavy weight competition-rowers. *Voeding* 41: 13-18.

Deakin, V. 2006. Iron depletion in athletes. In *Clinical Sports Nutrition, 3rd ed.* (edited by L. Burke and V. Deakin), pp. 174-199. Sydney, Australia: McGraw-Hill.

Decombaz, J., A. Bury, and C. Hager. 2003. HMB meta-analysis and the clustering of data sources [letter to the editor]. *Journal of Applied Physiology* 95: 2180-2182.

Degoutte, F., P. Jouanel, R.J. Begue, M. Colombier, G. Lac, J.M. Pequignot, and E. Filaire. 2006. Food restriction, performance, biochemical, psychological, and endocrine changes in judo athletes. *International Journal of Sports Medicine* 27: 9-18.

Delecluse, C., R. Diels, and M. Goris. 2003. Effect of creatine supplementation on intermittent sprint running performance in highly trained athletes. *Journal of Strength and Conditioning Research* 17: 446-454.

Dempsey, R.L., M.F. Mazzone, and L.N. Meurer. 2002. Does oral creatine supplementation improve strength? A meta-analysis. *Journal of Family Practice* 51: 945-951.

Dennehy, C.E., C. Tsourounis, and A.J. Horn. 2005. Dietary supplement-related adverse events reported to the California Poison Control System. *American Journal of Health-System Pharmacy* 62: 1476-1482.

Dennig, H., J.H. Talbot, H.T. Edwards, and B. Dill. 1931. Effects of acidosis and alkalosis upon the capacity for work. *Journal of Clinical Investigation* 9: 601-613.

Dennis, S.C., and T.D. Noakes. 1999. Advantages of a smaller bodymass in humans when distance-running in warm, humid conditions. *European Journal of Applied Physiology* 79: 280-284.

Depalma, M.T., W.M. Koszewski, J.G. Case, R.J. Barile, B.F. Depalma, and S.M. Oliaro. 1993. Weight control practices of lightweight football players. *Medicine and Science in Sports and Exercise* 25: 694-701.

Desbrow, B.D., M. Leveritt, R. Hughes, P. Scheelings, L. Jones. in press. Variation in caffeine content of commercial ground coffee. *Australia New Zealand Journal of Public Health.*

Desbrow, B., S. Anderson, J. Barrett, E. Rao, and M. Hargreaves. 2004. Carbohydrate-electrolyte feedings and 1 h time trial cycling performance. *International Journal of Sport Nutrition and Exercise Metabolism* 14: 541-549.

Deuster, P.A., S.B. Kyle, P.B. Moser, R.A. Vigersky, A. Singh, and E.B. Schoomaker. 1986. Nutritional intakes and status of highly trained amenorrheic and eumenorrheic women runners. *Fertility and Sterility* 46: 636-643.

Deutz, R.C., D. Benardot, D.T. Martin, and M.M. Cody. 2000. Relationship between energy deficits and body composition in elite female gymnasts and runners. *Medicine and Science in Sports and Exercise* 32: 659-668.

Devlin, J.T., and C. Williams. 1991. Foods nutrition and sports performance. Final consensus statement. *Journal of Sports Sciences* 9 (suppl): iii.

Devlin, L.H., S.F. Fraser, N.S. Barras, and J.A. Hawley. 2001. Moderate levels of hypohydration impairs bowling accuracy but not bowling velocity in skilled cricket players. *Journal of Science and Medicine in Sport* 4: 179-187.

Diehl, D.M., T.G. Lohman, S.C. Smith, and R. Kertzer. 1986. Effects of physical training and competition on the iron status of field hockey players. *International Journal of Sports Medicine* 7: 264-270.

DiGioacchino DeBate, R., H. Wethington, and R. Sargent. 2003. Sub-clinical eating disorder characteristics among male and female triathletes. *Eating and Weight Disorders* 7: 210-220.

Dill, D.B., H.T. Edwards, and J.H. Talbot. 1932. Alkalosis and the capacity for work. *Journal of Biological Chemistry* 97: 58-59.

Doherty, M. 1998. The effects of caffeine on the maximal accumulated oxygen deficit and short-term running performance. *International Journal of Sport Nutrition* 8: 95-104.

Doherty, M., P.M. Smith, R.C. Davison, and M.G. Hughes. 2002. Caffeine is ergogenic after supplementation of oral creatine monohydrate. *Medicine and Science in Sports and Exercise* 34: 1785-1792.

dopinginfo.de. 2000. Firmen- und Produktnamen von Nahrungsergänzungsmitteln, in denen verbotene anabol-androgene Steroide enthalten sind. http://www.dshs-koeln.de/biochemie/rubriken/07_info/020513.html [accessed September 7 2006].

Doscher, N. 1944. The effect of rapid weight loss upon the performance of wrestlers, boxers, and upon the physical proficiency of college students. *Research Quarterly* 15: 317-324.

Dougherty, K.A., L.B. Baker, M. Chow, and W.L. Kenney. 2006. 2% dehydration impairs and 6% carbohydrate drink improves boys basketball skills. *Medicine and Science in Sports and Exercise* 38: 1650-1658.

Douglas, P.D. 1989. Effect of competition and training on hematological status of women field hockey and soccer players. *Journal of Sports Medicine and Physical Fitness* 29: 179-183.

Dowling, E.A., D.R. Redondo, J.D. Branch, S. Jones, G. McNabb, and M.H. Williams. 1996. Effect of eleutherococcus senticosus on submaximal and maximal exercise performance. *Medicine and Science in Sports and Exercise* 28: 482-489.

Doyle, J.A., W.M. Sherman, and R.L. Strauss. 1993. Effects of eccentric and concentric exercise on muscle glycogen replenishment. *Journal of Applied Physiology* 74: 1848-1855.

Drinkwater, B.L., K. Nilson, C.H. Chesnut, W.J. Bremner, S. Shainholtz, and M.B. Southworth. 1984. Bone mineral content of amenorrheic and eumenorrheic athletes. *New England Journal of Medicine* 311: 277-281.

Drinkwater, B.L., K. Nilson, S. Ott, and C.H. Chesnut. 1986. Bone mineral density after resumption of menses in amenorrheic athletes. *Journal of the American Medical Association* 256: 380-382.

Dubnov, G., and N.W. Constantini. 2004. Prevalence of iron depletion and anemia in top-level basketball players. *International Journal of Sport Nutrition and Exercise Metabolism* 14: 30-37.

Dummer, G.M., L.W. Rosen, W.W. Heusner, P.J. Roberts, and J.E. Counsilman. 1987. Pathogenic weight-control behaviours of young competitive swimmers. *The Physician and Sportsmedicine* 15: 75-86.

Dunne, L., S. Worley, and M. Macknin. 2006. Ribose versus dextrose supplementation, association with rowing performance. *Clinical Journal of Sports Medicine* 16: 68-71.

Durnin, J.V.G.A. 1982. Muscle in sports medicine—Nutrition and muscular performance. *International Journal of Sports Medicine* 3: 52-57.

Duthrie, G., D.B. Pyne, and S. Hooper. 2003. Applied physiology and game analysis of rugby union. *Sports Medicine* 33: 973-1001.

Earnest, C.P., G.M. Morss, F. Wyatt, A.N. Jordan, S. Colson, T.S. Church, Y. Fitzgerald, L. Autrey, R. Jurca, and A. Lucia. 2004. Effects of a commercial herbal-based formula on exercise performance in cyclists. *Medicine and Science in Sports and Exercise* 36: 504-509.

Earnest, C.P., P.G. Snell, R. Rodriguez, A.L. Almada, and T.L. Mitchell. 1995. The effect of creatine monohydrate ingestion on anaerobic power indices, muscular strength and body composition. *Acta Physiologica Scandinavica* 153: 207-209.

Ebersole, K.T., J.R. Stout, J.M. Eckerson, T.J. Housh, T.K. Evetovich, and D.B. Smith. 2000. The effect of pyruvate supplementation on critical power. *Journal of Strength and Conditioning Research* 14: 132-134.

Ebert, T.E., D.T. Martin, N. Bullock, M.J. Quod, I. Mujika, L. Farthing, K. Fallon, L.M. Burke, and R.T. Withers. 2005. Effects of exercise-induced dehydration on thermoregulation and cycling hill-climbing performance [abstract]. *Medicine and Science in Sports and Exercise* 37 (5 suppl): S169.

Ebine, N., J.-Y. Feng, M. Homma, S. Saitoh, and P.J.H. Jones. 2000. Total energy expenditure of elite synchronized swimmers measured by the doubly labeled water method. *European Journal of Applied Physiology* 83: 1-6.

Ebine, N., H.H. Rafamantanantsoa, Y. Nayuki, K. Yamanaka, K. Tashima, T. Ono, S. Saitoh, and P.J.H. Jones. 2002. Measurement of total energy expenditure by the doubly labelled water method in professional soccer players. *Journal of Sports Sciences* 20: 391-397.

Edge, J., D. Bishop, and C. Goodman. 2006. Effects of chronic bicarbonate ingestion during interval training on changes to muscle buffering capacity and short-term endurance performance. *Journal of Applied Physiology* 101: 918-925.

Edwards, J.E., A.K. Lindeman, A.E. Mikesky, and J.M. Stager. 1993. Energy balance in highly trained female endurance runners. *Medicine and Science in Sports and Exercise* 25: 1398-1404.

Edwards, T.L., D.M. Santeusanio, and K.B. Wheeler. 1986. Endurance of cyclists given carbohydrate solutions during moderate-intensity rides. *Texas Medicine* 82: 29-31.

Eichner, E.R. 1995. Overtraining: consequences and prevention. *Journal of Sports Sciences* 13: S41-S48.

Eichner, E.R. 2000. Minerals: Iron. In *Nutrition in sport* (edited by R.J. Maughan), pp. 326-338. Oxford, UK: Blackwell Science.

Ekblom, B. 1986. Applied physiology of soccer. *Sports Medicine* 3: 50-60.

Ekblom, B., and U. Bergh. 2000. Cross-country skiing. In *Nutrition in Sport* (edited by R.J. Maughan), pp. 656-662. Oxford, UK: Blackwell Science.

Ekblom, B., and C. Williams. 1994. Final consensus statement: foods, nutrition and soccer performance. *Journal of Sports Sciences* 12: S3.

Ekelund, U., A. Yngve, K. Westerterp, and M. Sjostrom. 2002. Energy expenditure assessed by heart rate and doubly labeled water in young athletes. *Medicine and Science in Sports and Exercise* 34: 1360-1366.

Elam, R.P. 1988. Morphological changes in adult males from resistance exercise and amino acid supplementation. *Journal of Sports Medicine and Physical Fitness* 28: 35-39.

Elam, R.P., D.H. Hardin, R.A.L. Sutton, and L. Hagen. 1989. Effects of arginine and ornithine on strength, lean body mass and urinary hydroxyproline in adult males. *Journal of Sports Medicine and Physical Fitness* 29: 52-56.

Elliot, T.A., M.G. Cree, A.P. Sanford, R.R. Wolfe and K.D. Tipton. 2006. Milk ingestion stimulates net muscle protein synthesis following resistance exercise. *Medicine and Science in Sports and Exercise* 38: 667-674.

Ellsworth, N.M., B.F. Hewitt, and W.L. Haskell. 1985. Nutrient intake of elite male and female nordic skiers. *The Physician and Sportsmedicine* 13: 78-92.

Engelhardt, M., G. Neumann, A. Berbalk, and I. Reuter. 1998. Creatine supplementation in endurance sports. *Medicine and Science in Sports and Exercise* 30: 1123-1129.

Engels, H.J., M.M. Fahlman, and J.C. Wirth. 2003. Effects of ginseng on secretory IgA, performance, and recovery from interval exercise. *Medicine and Science in Sports and Exercise* 35: 690-696.

Engels, H.J., I. Kolokouri, T.J. Cieslak, and J.C. Wirth. 2001. Effects of ginseng supplementation on supramaximal exercise performance and short-term recovery. *Journal of Strength and Conditioning Research* 15: 290-295.

Eriksson, A., J. Ekholm, B. Hulten, E. Karlsson, and J. Karlsson. 1976. Anatomical, histological, and physiological factors in experienced downhill skiers. *Orthopedic Clinics of North America* 7: 159-165.

Ersoy, G. 1995. Nutrient intakes and iron status of Turkish female handball players. In *Sports Nutrition: Minerals and Electrolytes* (edited by C.V. Kies and J.A. Driskell), pp. 59-64. Boca Raton, FL: CRC Press.

Esmarck, B., J.L. Anderson, S. Olsen, E.A. Richter, M. Mizuno, and M. Kjaer. 2001. Timing of postexercise protein intake is important for muscle hypertrophy with resistance training in elderly humans. *Journal of Physiology* 535: 301-311.

Evans, G.W. 1989. The effect of chromium picolinate on insulin controlled parameters in humans. *International Journal of Biosocial and Medical Research* 11: 163-180.

Faber, M., A.J.S. Benade, and M. Van Eck. 1986. Dietary intake, anthropometric measurements and blood lipid values in weight training athletes (body builders). *International Journal of Sports Medicine* 7: 342-346.

Faber, M., and A.J. Spinnler-Benade. 1991. Mineral and vitamin intake in field athletes (discus-, hammer-, javelin-throwers and shotputters). *International Journal of Sports Medicine* 12: 324-327.

Faber, M., A.J. Spinnler-Benade, and A. Daubitzer. 1990. Dietary intake, anthropometric measurements and plasma lipid levels in throwing field athletes. *International Journal of Sports Medicine* 10: 140-145.

Falk, D.J., K.A. Heelan, J.P. Thyfault, and A.J. Koch. 2003. Effects of effervescent creatine, ribose, and glutamine supplementation on muscular strength, muscular endurance, and body composition. *Journal of Strength and Conditioning Research* 17: 810-816.

Fallon, K. 2006. Athletes with gastrointestinal disorders. In *Clinical Sports Nutrition, 3rd ed.* (edited by L. Burke and V. Deakin), pp. 721-738. Sydney, Australia: McGraw-Hill.

Fallowfield, J.L., and C. Williams. 1993. Carbohydrate intake and recovery from prolonged exercise. *International Journal of Sport Nutrition* 3: 150-164.

Faria, I.E., E.W. Faria, and D.L. Parker. 2002. Effect of cytochrome C supplementation on aerobic running performance. *Journal of Exercise Physiology* [Online] 5: 35-40. http://faculty.css.edu/tboone2/asep/fldr/fldr.htm [accessed September 7, 2006].

Febbraio, M.A., A. Chiu, D.J. Angus, M.J. Arkinstall, and J.A. Hawley. 2000. Effects of carbohydrate ingestion before and during exercise on glucose kinetics and performance. *Journal of Applied Physiology* 89: 2220-2226.

Febbraio, M.A., A. Steensberg, R. Walsh, I. Koukoulas, G. van Hall, B. Saltin, and B.K. Pedersen 2003. Reduced glycogen availability is associated with an elevation in HSP72 in contracting human skeletal muscle. *Journal of Physiology* 538: 911-917.

Federation International de Football Association. 2003. *Laws of the Game*. Zurich, Switzerland: FIFA.

Ferrauti, A., B.M. Pluim, T. Busch, and K. Weber. 2003. Blood glucose responses and incidence of hypoglycemia in elite tennis under practice and tournament conditions. *Journal of Science and Medicine in Sport* 6: 28-39.

Ferrauti, A., K. Weber, and H.K. Struder. 1997. Metabolic and ergogenic effects of carbohydrate and caffeine beverages in tennis. *Journal of Sports Medicine and Physical Fitness* 37: 258-266.

Filaire, E., F. Maso, F. Degoutte, P. Jouanel, and G. Lac. 2000. Food restriction, performance, psychological statue and lipid values in judo athletes. *International Journal of Sports Medicine* 22: 454-459.

Finn, J.P., T.R. Ebert, R.T. Withers, M.F. Carey, M. Mackay, J.W. Phillips, and M.A. Febbraio. 2001. Effect of creatine supplementation on metabolism and performance in humans during intermittent sprint cycling. *European Journal of Applied Physiology* 84: 238-243.

FIS. 2003. International Ski Federation Web site. Available www.fis-ski.com [accessed September 7, 2006].

Flynn, M.G., D.L. Costill, J.P. Kirwan, J.B. Mitchell, J.A. Houmard, W.J. Fink, J.D. Beltz, and L.J. D'Acquisto. 1990. Fat storage in athletes: Metabolic and hormonal responses to swimming and running. *International Journal of Sports Medicine* 11: 433-440.

Fogelholm, M. 1995. Indicators of vitamin and mineral status in athletes' blood: A review. *International Journal of Sport Nutrition* 5: 267-284.

Fogelholm, M. 2000. Vitamin, mineral and antioxidant needs of athletes. In *Clinical Sports Nutrition, 2nd ed.* (edited by L. Burke and V. Deakin), pp. 312-340. Sydney, Australia: McGraw-Hill.

Fogelholm, G.M., R. Koskinen, J. Laakso, T. Rankinen, and I. Ruokonen. 1993. Gradual and rapid weight loss: Effects on nutrition and performance in male athletes. *Medicine and Science in Sports and Exercise* 25: 371-377.

Fogelholm, G.M., T.K. Kukkonen-Harjula, S.A. Taipale, H.T. Sievanen, P. Oja, and I.M. Vuori. 1995. Resting metabolic rate and energy intake in female gymnasts, figure-skaters and soccer players. *International Journal of Sports Medicine* 16: 551-556.

Fogelholm, G.M., H.K. Naveri, K.T.K. Kiilavuori, and M.H.A. Harkonen. 1993. Low-dose amino acid supplementation: No effect on serum human growth hormone and insulin in male weightlifters. *International Journal of Sport Nutrition* 3: 290-297.

Fogelholm, M., S. Rehunen, C.-G. Gref, J.T. Laakso, J. Lehto, I. Ruokonen, and J.-J. Himberg. 1992. Dietary intake and thiamine, iron and zinc status in elite Nordic skiers during different training periods. *International Journal of Sports Nutrition* 2: 351-365.

Forbes, G.B., M.R. Brown, S.L. Welle, and L.E. Underwood. 1989. Hormonal responses to overfeeding. *American Journal of Clinical Nutrition* 49: 608-611.

Foster, C., D.L. Costill, and W.J. Fink. 1979. Effects of preexercise feedings on endurance performance. *Medicine and Science in Sports and Exercise* 11: 1-5.

Foster, C., and J.J. de Koning. 1999. Physiological perspectives in speed skating. In *Handbook of Competitive Speed Skating* (edited by H. Gemser, J.J. de Koning, and G.J. van Ingen Schenau), pp. 117-132. Lausanne, Switzerland: International Skating Union.

Foster, C., J.J. de Koning, K.W. Rundell, and A.C. Snyder. 2000. Physiology of speed skating. In *Textbook of Sports Medicine, Vol. 1* (edited by D.T. Kirkendall and W.E. Garrett), pp. 885-893. Philadelphia: Lippincott Williams & Wilkins.

Fotheringham, W. 1997. Tour de form. *Cycle Sport* September: 70-71.

French, C., L. McNaughton, P. Davies, and S. Tristam. 1991. Caffeine ingestion during exercise to exhaustion in elite distance runners. *Journal of Sports Medicine and Physical Fitness* 31: 425-432.

Frentsos, J.A., and J.T. Baer. 1997. Increased energy and nutrient intake during training and competition improves elite triathletes' endurance performance. *International Journal of Sport Nutrition* 7: 61-71.

Fricker, P.A., S.K. Beasley, and I.W. Copeland. 1988. Physiological growth hormone responses of throwers to amino acids, eating and exercise. *Australian Journal of Science and Medicine in Sport* 20: 21-22.

Fricker, P., S. Beasley, and I. Copeland. 1991. A preliminary study on the effects of amino acids, fasting and exercise on nocturnal growth hormone release in weightlifters. *Excel* 7: 2-5.

Friedl, K.E., R.J. Moore, R.W. Hoyt, L.J. Marchitelli, L.E. Martinez-Lopez, and E.W. Askew. 2000. Endocrine markers of semistarvation in healthy lean men in a multistressor environment. *Journal of Applied Physiology* 88: 1820-1830.

Fudge, B.W., K.R. Westerterp, F.K. Kiplamai, V.O. Onywera, M.K. Boit, B. Kayser, and Y.P. Pitsiladis. 2006. Evidence of negative energy balance using doubly labelled water in elite Kenyan endurance runners prior to competition. *British Journal of Nutrition* 95: 59-66.

Fulcher, K.Y., and C. Williams. 1992. The effect of diet on high-intensity intermittent exercise performance. *Journal of Sports Sciences* 10: 550-551A.

Gaffney, B.T., H.M. Hugel, and P.A. Rich. 2001. The effects of Eleutherococcus senticosus and Panax ginseng on steroidal hormone indices of stress and lymphocyte subset numbers in endurance athletes. *Life Sciences* 70: 431-442.

Gaitanos, G.C., C. Williams, L.H. Boobis, and S. Brooks. 1993. Human muscle metabolism during intermittent maximal exercise. *Journal of Applied Physiology* 75: 712-719.

Gallagher, P.M., J.A. Carrithers, M.P. Godard, K.E. Schulze, and S.W. Trappe. 2000. Beta-hydroxy-beta-methylbutyrate ingestion, Part I: Effects on strength and fat free mass. *Medicine and Science in Sports and Exercise* 32: 2109-2115.

Gao, J., D.L. Costill, C.A. Horswill, and S.H. Park. 1988. Sodium bicarbonate ingestion improves performance in interval swimming. *European Journal of Applied Physiology* 58: 171-174.

Garcia-Roves, P.M., N. Terrados, S.F. Fernandez, and A.M. Patterson. 1998. Macronutrients intake of top level cyclists during continuous competition—Change in feeding pattern. *International Journal of Sports Medicine* 19: 61-67.

Garcia-Roves, P.M., N. Terrados, S. Fernandez, and A.M. Patterson. 2000. Comparison of dietary intake and eating behaviour of professional road cyclists during training and competition. *International Journal of Sport Nutrition and Exercise Metabolism* 10: 82-98.

Garner, D.M., and P.E. Garfinkel. 1979. The eating attitudes test: An index of the symptoms of anorexia nervosa. *Psychological Medicine* 9: 273-279.

Garner, D.M., M.P. Olmsted, and J. Polivy. 1984. *Manual of Eating Disorder Inventory (EDI)*. Odessa, FL: Psychological Assessment Resources.

Gater, D.R., D.A. Gater, J.M. Uribe, and J.C. Bunt. 1992a. Effects of arginine/lysine supplementation and resistance training on glucose tolerance. *Journal of Applied Physiology* 72: 1279-1284.

Gater, D.R., D.A. Gater, J.M. Uribe, and J.C. Bunt. 1992b. Impact of nutritional supplements and resistance training on body

composition, strength and insulin-like growth factor-1. *Journal of Applied Sport Science Research* 6: 66-76.

Geyer, H., M. Bredehoft, U. Mareck, M.K. Parr, and W. Schanzer. 2003. High doses of the anabolic steroid metandienone found in dietary supplements. *European Journal of Sport Science* 3: 1-5.

Geyer, H., M.K. Henze, U. Mareck-Engelke, G. Sigmund, and W. Schanzer. 2000. Positive doping cases with norandosterone after application of contaminated nutritional supplements. *Deutsche Zeitschrift fur Sportmedezin* 51: 378-382.

Geyer, H., M.K. Parr, U. Reinhart, Y. Schrader, U. Mareck, and W. Schanzer. 2004. Analysis of non-hormonal nutritional supplements for anabolic-androgenic steroids - results of an international study. *International Journal of Sports Medicine* 25: 124-129.

Glazier, L.M., T. Stellingwerff, and L.L. Spriet. 2004. Effects of Microhydrin® supplementation on endurance performance and metabolism in well-trained cyclists. *International Journal of Sport Nutrition and Exercise Metabolism* 14: 560-573.

Gleeson, M., and N.C. Bishop. 2000. Elite athlete immunology: Importance of nutrition. *International Journal of Sports Medicine* 21: S44-S50.

Gleeson, M., A.K. Blannin, N.P. Walsh, N.C. Bishop, and A.M. Clark. 1998. Effect of low- and high-carbohydrate diets on the plasma glutamine and circulating leukocyte responses to exercise. *International Journal of Sport Nutrition* 8: 49-59.

Gleeson, M., G.I. Lancaster, and N.C. Bishop. 2001. Nutritional strategies to minimise exercise-induced immunosuppression in athletes. *Canadian Journal of Applied Physiology* 26: S23-S35.

Gleeson, M., D.C. Nieman, and B.K. Pedersen. 2004. Exercise, nutrition and immune function. *Journal of Sports Sciences* 22: 115-122.

Godek, S.F., A.R. Bartolozzi, and J.J. Godek. 2005. Sweat rate and fluid turnover in American football players compared with runners in a hot and humid environment. *British Journal of Sports Medicine* 39: 205-211.

Godek, S.F., J.J. Godek, and A.R. Bartolozzi. 2005. Hydration status in college football players during consecutive days of twice-a-day preseason practices. *American Journal of Sports Medicine* 33: 843-851.

Goedecke, J.H., C. Christie, G. Wilson, S.C. Dennis, T.D. Noakes, W.G. Hopkins, and E.V. Lambert. 1999. Metabolic adaptations to a high-fat diet in endurance cyclists. *Metabolism* 48: 1509-1517.

Goedecke, J.H., V.R. Clark, T.D. Noakes, and E.V. Lambert. 2005. The effects of medium-chain triacylglycerol and carbohydrate ingestion on ultra-endurance exercise performance. *International Journal of Sport Nutrition and Exercise Metabolism* 15: 15-28.

Goedecke, J.H., R. Elmer-English, S.C. Dennis, I. Schloss, T.D. Noakes, and E.V. Lambert. 1999. Effects of medium-chain triacylglycerol ingested with carbohydrate on metabolism and exercise performance. *International Journal of Sport Nutrition* 9: 35-47.

Goforth, H.W., D.A. Arnall, B.L. Bennett, and P.G. Law. 1997. Persistence of supercompensated muscle glycogen in trained subjects after carbohydrate loading. *Journal of Applied Physiology* 82: 342-347.

Goldfinch, J., L. McNaughton, and P. Davies. 1988. Induced metabolic alkalosis and its effects on 400-m racing time. *European Journal of Applied Physiology* 57: 45-48.

Gonzalez-Alonso, J., C.L. Heaps, and E.F. Coyle. 1992. Rehydration after exercise with common beverages and water. *International Journal of Sports Medicine* 13: 399-406.

Goodman, C., I. Cohen, and J. Walton. 1985. The effect of water intake on body temperature during rugby matches. *South African Medical Journal* 67: 542-544.

Gopinathan, P.M., G. Pichan, and V.M. Sharma. 1988. Role of dehydration in heat stess-induced variations in mental performance. *Archives of Environmental Health* 43: 15-17.

Gordon, B., L.A. Kohn, S.A. Levine, M. Matton, W.D. Scriver, and W.B. Whiting. 1925. Sugar content of the blood in runners following a marathon race, with especial reference to the prevention of hypoglycemia: Further observations. *Journal of the American Medical Association* 85: 508-509.

Gore, C.J., P.C. Bourdon, S.M. Woolford, and D.G. Pederson. 1993. Involuntary dehydration during cricket. *International Journal of Sports Medicine* 14: 387-395.

Goris, A.H.C., and K.R. Westerterp. 1999. Underreporting of habitual food intake is explained by undereating in highly motivated lean women. *Journal of Nutrition* 129: 878-882.

Goulet, E.D.B. 2005. Assessment of the effects of eleutherococcus senticosus on endurance performance. *International Journal of Sport Nutrition and Exercise Metabolism* 15: 75-83.

Grace Eggleton, M. 1936. *Muscular Exercise*. London: Kegan Trench Trubner and Company Limited.

Graham, L.A., and K.A. Jackson. 1998. The dietary micronutrient intake of elite Australian rules footballers: Is there a need for supplementation? Unpublished manuscript prepared for Flinders University, Adelaide, Australia.

Graham, T.E. 2001a. Caffeine and exercise: Metabolism, endurance and performance. *Sports Medicine* 31: 765-807.

Graham, T.E. 2001b. Caffeine, coffee and ephedrine: Impact on exercise performance and metabolism. *Canadian Journal of Applied Physiology* 26: S103-S109.

Graham, T.E., E. Hibbert, and P. Sathasivam. 1998. Metabolic and exercise endurance effects of coffee and caffeine ingestion. *Journal of Applied Physiology* 85: 883-889.

Graham, T.E., and L.L. Spriet. 1991. Performance and metabolic responses to a high caffeine dose during prolonged exercise. *Journal of Applied Physiology* 71: 2292-2298.

Graham, T.E., and L.L. Spriet. 1995. Metabolic, catecholamine, and exercise performance responses to various doses of caffeine. *Journal of Applied Physiology* 78: 867-874.

Grandjean, A.C. 1989. Macronutrient intake of U.S. athletes compared with the general population and recommendations made for athletes. *American Journal of Clinical Nutrition* 49: 1070-1076.

Grandjean, A. 1999. Nutritional requirements to increase lean mass. *Clinics in Sports Medicine* 18: 623-632.

Grandjean, A.C., L.J. Lolkus, R. Lind, and A.E. Schaefer. 1992. Dietary intake of female cyclists during repeated days of racing. *Cycling Science* 4: 21-25.

Grandjean, A.C., and J.S. Ruud. 1994a. Energy intake of athletes. In *Oxford Textbook of Sports Medicine* (edited by M. Harries, C. Williams, W.D. Stanish, and L.J. Micheli), pp. 53-65. New York: Oxford University Press.

Grandjean, A.C., and J.S. Ruud. 1994b. Olympic athletes. In *Nutrition in Exercise and Sport* (edited by I. Wolinsky and J.F. Hickson), pp. 447-454. Boca Raton, FL: CRC Press.

Graydon, J., S.L. Taylor, and M. Smith 1998. The effect of carbohydrate ingestion on shot accuracy during a conditioned squash match. In *Science and Racquet Sports II* (edited by A. Lees, I. Maynard, M. Hughes, and T. Reilly), pp. 68-74. London, UK: E & FN Spon.

Green, A.L., I.A. MacDonald, and P.L. Greenhaff. 1997. The effects of creatine and carbohydrate on whole body creatine retention in vegetarians. *Proceedings of the Nutrition Society* 56: 81A.

Green, A.L., E.J. Simpson, J.J. Littlewood, I.A. MacDonald, and P.L. Greenhaff. 1996. Carbohydrate ingestion augments creatine retention during creatine feeding in humans. *Acta Physiologica Scandinavica* 158: 195-202.

Green, G.A., D.H. Catlin, and B. Starcevic. 2001. Analysis of over-the-counter dietary supplements. *Clinical Journal of Sports Medicine* 11: 254-259.

Green, H.J. 1978. Glycogen depletion patterns during continuous and intermittent ice skating. *Medicine and Science in Sports* 10: 183-187.

Green, H.J., B.D. Daub, D.C. Painter, and J.A. Thomson. 1978. Glycogen depletion patterns during ice hockey performance. *Medicine and Science in Sports* 10: 289-293.

Green, H.J., J. Sutton, P. Young, A. Cymerman, and C.S. Houston. 1989. Operation Everest II: Muscle energetics during maximal exhaustive exercise. *Journal of Applied Physiology* 66: 142-150.

Greenhaff, P.L. 2000. Creatine. In *Nutrition in Sport* (edited by R.J. Maughan), pp. 367-378. Oxford, UK: Blackwell Science.

Greenhaff, P.L., M.E. Nevill, K. Soderlund, L. Boobis, C. Williams, and E. Hultman. 1994. The metabolic responses of human type I and II muscle fibres during maximal treadmill sprinting. *Journal of Physiology* 478: 149-155.

Greenleaf, J.E. 1992. Problem: thirst, drinking behaviour, and involuntary dehydration. *Medicine and Science in Sports and Exercise* 24: 645-656.

Greenwood, M., J. Farris, R. Kreider, L. Greenwood, and A. Byars. 2000. Creatine supplementation patterns and perceived effects in select Division I collegiate athletes. *Clinical Journal of Sports Medicine* 10: 191-194.

Greenwood, M., R.B. Kreider, L. Greenwood, and A. Byars. 2004. Cramping and injury incidence in collegiate football players are reduced by creatine supplementation. *Journal of Athletic Training* 38: 216-219.

Greenwood, M., R.B. Kreider, C. Melton, C. Rasmussen, S. Lancaster, E. Cantler, P. Milnor, and A. Almada. 2003. Creatine supplementation during college football training does not increase the incidence of cramping or injury. *Molecular and Cell Biochemistry* 244: 83-88.

Greer, F., C. McLean, and T.E. Graham. 1998. Caffeine, performance, and metabolism during repeated Wingate exercise tests. *Journal of Applied Physiology* 85: 1502-1508.

Greiwe, J.S., K.S. Staffey, D.R. Melrose, M.D. Narve, and R.G. Knowlton. 1998. Effects of dehydration on isometric muscular strength and endurance. *Medicine and Science in Sports and Exercise* 30: 284-288.

Grindstaff, P.D., R. Kreider, R. Bishop, M. Wilson, L. Wood, C. Alexander, and A. Almada. 1997. Effects of creatine supplementation on repetitive sprint performance and body composition in competitive swimmers. *International Journal of Sport Nutrition* 7: 330-346.

Grinspoon, S., H. Baum, V. Kim, C. Coggins, and A. Klibanski. 1995. Decreased bone formation and increased mineral dissolution during acute fasting in young women. *Journal of Clinical Endocrinology and Metabolism* 80: 3628-3633.

Gropper, S.S., L.M. Sorrels, and D. Blessing. 2003. Copper status of collegiate female athletes involved in different sports. *International Journal of Sport Nutrition and Exercise Metabolism* 13: 343-357.

Grunewald, K.K., and R.S. Bailey. 1993. Commercially marketed supplements for bodybuilding athletes. *Sports Medicine* 15: 90-103.

Gurley, B.J., P. Wang, and S.F. Gardner. 1998. Ephedrine-type alkaloid content of nutritional supplements containing Ephedra sinica (Ma Huang) as determined by high performance liquid chromatography. *Journal of Pharmaceutical Science* 87: 1547-1553.

Gutierrez, A., J.L. Mesa, J.R. Ruiz, L.J. Chirosa, and M.J. Castillo. 2003. Sauna-induced rapid weight loss decreases explosive power in women but not in men. *International Journal of Sports Medicine* 24: 518-522.

Haas, R. 1983. *Eat to Win*. New York: Rawson Associates.

Hackney, A.C. 1990. Effects of the menstrual cycle on resting muscle glycogen content. *Hormone and Metabolism Research* 22: 647.

Haff, G.G., A.J. Koch, J.A. Potteiger, K.E. Kuphal, L.M. Magee, S.B. Green, and J.J. Jakicic. 2000. Carbohydrate supplementation attenuates muscle glycogen loss during acute bouts of resistance exercise. *International Journal of Sport Nutrition and Exercise Metabolism* 10: 326-339.

Haff, G.G., M.J. Lehmkuhl, L.B. McCoy, and M.H. Stone. 2003. Carbohydrate supplementation and resistance training. *Journal of Strength and Conditioning Research* 17: 187-196.

Haff, G.G., C.A. Schroeder, A.J. Koch, K.E. Kuphal, M.J. Comeau, and J.A. Potteiger. 2001. The effects of supplemental carbohydrate ingestion on intermittent isokinetic leg exercise. *Journal of Sports Medicine and Physical Fitness* 41: 216-222.

Haff, G.G., M.H. Stone, B.J. Warren, R. Keith, R.L. Johnson, D.C. Nieman, F. Williams, and K.B. Kirksey. 1999. The effect of carbohydrate supplementation on multiple sessions and bouts of resistance exercise. *Journal of Strength and Conditioning Research* 13: 111-117.

Hagerman, F.C. 1994. Physiology and nutrition for rowing. In *Perspectives in Exercise Science and Sports Medicine* (edited by D.R. Lamb, H.G. Knuttgen, and R. Murray), pp. 221-302. Carmel, IN: Cooper.

Hahm, H., J. Kujawa, and L. Ausberger. 1999. Comparison of melatonin products against USP's nutritional supplements standards and other criteria. *Journal of the American Pharmaceutical Association* 39: 27-31.

Hall, C.J., and A.M. Lane. 2001. Effects of rapid weight loss on mood and performance among amateur boxers. *British Journal of Sports Medicine* 35: 390-395.

Hallberg, L. 1981. Bioavailability of dietary iron in man. *Annual Review of Nutrition* 1: 123-147.

Hallmark, M.A., T.H. Reynolds, C.A. deSouza, C.O. Dotson, R.A. Anderson, and M.A. Rogers. 1996. Effects of chromium and resistive training on muscle strength and body composition. *Medicine and Science in Sports and Exercise* 28: 139-144.

Hansen, A.K., C.P. Fischer, P. Plomgaard, J.L. Andersen, B. Saltin, and B.K. Pedersen. 2005. Skeletal muscle adaptation: Training twice every second day vs. training once daily. *Journal of Applied Physiology* 98: 93-99.

Hansen, R.D. 1995. Seasonal variability in physiological strain: matching performance to demand. In *Science and Racquet Sports* (edited by T. Reilly, M. Hughes, and A. Lees), pp. 15-20. London, UK: E & FN Spon.

Hansen, R.D., and J.R. Brotherhood. 1988. Prevention of heat-induced illness in squash players. *Medical Journal of Australia* 148: 100.

Hargreaves, M. 1995. Skeletal muscle carbohydrate metabolism during exercise. In *Exercise Metabolism* (edited by M. Hargreaves), pp. 41-72. Champaign, IL: Human Kinetics.

Hargreaves, M. 1999. Metabolic responses to carbohydrate ingestion: Effects on exercise performance. In *Perspectives in Exercise Science and Sports Medicine* (edited by D.R. Lamb and R. Murray), pp. 93-124. Carmel, IN: Cooper.

Hargreaves, M., D.L. Costill, A. Coggan, W.J. Fink, and I. Nishibata. 1984. Effect of carbohydrate feedings on muscle glycogen utilization and exercise performance. *Medicine and Science in Sports and Exercise* 16: 219-222.

Hargreaves, M., P. Dillo, D. Angus, and M. Febbraio. 1996. Effect of fluid ingestion on muscle metabolism during prolonged exercise. *Journal of Applied Physiology* 80: 363-366.

Hargreaves, M., J.P. Finn, R.T. Withers, J.A. Halbert, G.C. Scroop, M. Mackay, R.J. Snow, and M.F. Carey. 1997. Effect of muscle glycogen availability on maximal exercise performance. *European Journal of Applied Physiology* 75: 188-192.

Hargreaves, M., M.J. McKenna, D.G. Jenkins, S.A. Warmington, J.L. Li, R.J. Snow, and M.A. Febbraio. 1998. Muscle metabolites and performance during high-intensity, intermittent exercise. *Journal of Applied Physiology* 84: 1687-1691.

Harris, J.A., and F.A. Benedict. 1919. *A Biometric Study of Basal Metabolism in Man* (Carnegie Institute of Washington Publication No. 279). Philadelphia: Lippincott.

Harris, M.B. 2000. Weight concerns, body image, and abnormal eating in college women tennis players and their coaches. *International Journal of Sport Nutrition and Exercise Metabolism* 10: 1-15.

Harris, R.C., K. Soderlund, and E. Hultman. 1992. Elevation of creatine in resting and exercised muscle of normal subjects by creatine supplementation. *Clinical Science* 83: 367-374.

Harris, R.C., M. Viru, P.L. Greenhaff, and E. Hultman. 1993. The effect of oral creatine supplementation on running performance during maximal short term exercise in man [abstract]. *Journal of Physiology* 467: 74P.

Hassmen, P., E. Blomstrand, B. Ekblom, and E.A. Newsholme. 1994. Branched-chain amino acid supplementation during 30-km competitive run: mood and cognitive performance. *Nutrition* 10: 405-410.

Hasten, D.L., E.P. Rome, B.D. Franks, and M. Hegsted. 1992. Effects of chromium picolinate on beginning weight training students. *International Journal of Sport Nutrition* 2: 343-350.

Haussinger, D., E. Roth, F. Lang, and W. Gerok. 1993. Cellular hydration state: An important determinant of protein catabolism in health and disease. *Lancet* 342: 1330-1332.

Havemann, L., S. West, J.H. Goedecke, I.A. McDonald, A. St-Clair Gibson, T.D. Noakes, and E.V. Lambert. 2006. Fat adaptation followed by carbohydrate-loading compromises high-intensity sprint performance. *Journal of Applied Physiology* 100: 194-202.

Havenitidis, K., O. Matsouka, C.B. Cooke, and A. Theodorou. 2003. The use of varying creatine regimens on sprint cycling. *Journal of Sports Science and Medicine* 2: 88-97.

Hawley, J.A. 2000. Training techniques for successful running performance. In *Running* (edited by J.A. Hawley), pp 44-57. Oxford, UK: Blackwell Science Ltd.

Hawley, J.A., and L.M. Burke. 1997. Effect of meal frequency and timing on physical performance. *British Journal of Nutrition* 77: S91-S103.

Hawley, J.A., S.C. Dennis, and T.D. Noakes. 1992. Oxidation of carbohydrate ingested during prolonged endurance exercise. *Sports Medicine* 14: 27-42.

Hawley, J.A., G.S. Palmer, and T.D. Noakes. 1997. Effects of 3 days of carbohydrate supplementation on muscle glycogen content and utilisation during a 1-h cycling performance. *European Journal of Applied Physiology* 75: 407-412.

Hawley, J.A., E.J. Schabort, T.D. Noakes, and S.C. Dennis. 1997. Carbohydrate-loading and exercise performance: An update. *Sports Medicine* 24: 73-81.

Haymes, E.M. 1998. Trace minerals and exercise. In *Nutrition in Exercise and Sport* (edited by I. Wolinsky), pp. 197-218. Boca Raton, FL: CRC Press.

Haymes, E.M., J.L. Puhl, and T.E. Temples. 1986. Training for cross-country skiing and iron status. *Medicine and Science in Sports and Exercise* 18: 162-167.

Haymes, E.M., and D.M. Spillman. 1989. Iron status of women distance runners, sprinters, and control women. *International Journal of Sports Medicine* 10: 430-433.

Hebbelinck, M. 1963. The effects of a small dose of ethyl alcohol on certain basic components of human physical performance. *Archives in Pharmacodynamics* 143: 247-257.

Heinemann, L., and H. Zerbes. 1989. Physical activity, fitness, and diet: Behavior in the population compared with elite athletes in the GDR. *American Journal of Clinical Nutrition* 49: 1007-1016.

Heinonen, O.J. 1996. Carnitine and physical exercise. *Sports Medicine* 22: 109-132.

Heitmann, B.L., and L. Lissner. 1995. Dietary underreporting by obese individuals—Is it specific or non-specific? *British Medical Journal* 311: 986-989.

Helge, J.W. 2000. Adaptation to a fat-rich diet. *Sports Medicine* 30: 347-367.

Helge, J.W., E.A. Richter, and B. Kiens. 1996. Interaction of training and diet on metabolism and endurance during exercise in man. *Journal of Physiology* 492: 293-306.

Helge, J.W., B. Wulff, and B. Kiens. 1998. Impact of a fat-rich diet on endurance in man: role of the dietary period. *Medicine and Science in Sports and Exercise* 30: 456-461.

Hellsten, Y., B. Norman, P.D. Balsom, and B. Sjodin. 1993. Decreased resting levels of adenine nucleotides in human skeletal muscle after high-intensity training. *Journal of Applied Physiology* 75: 2523-2528.

Hellsten, Y., L. Skadhauge, and J. Bangsbo. 2004. Effect of ribose supplementation on resynthesis of adenine nucleotides after intense training in humans. *American Journal of Physiology Regulatory* 286: R182-R188.

Henson, D.A., D.C. Nieman, A.D. Blodgett, D.E. Butterworth, A. Utter, J.M. Davis, G. Sonnenfeld, D.S. Morton, O.R. Fagoaga, and S.L. Nehlsen-Cannarella. 1999. Influence of exercise mode and carbohydrate intake on the immune response to prolonged exercise. *International Journal of Sport Nutrition* 9: 213-228.

Henson, D.A., D.C. Nieman, S.L. Nehlsen-Cannarella, O.R. Fagoaga, M. Shannon, M.R. Bolton, J.M. Davis, C.T. Gaffney, W.J. Kelln, M.D. Austin, J.M.E. Hjertman, and B.K. Schilling. 2000. Influence of carbohydrate on cytokine and phagocytic responses to 2 h of rowing. *Medicine and Science in Sports and Exercise* 32: 1384-1389.

Hepburn, D., and R.J. Maughan. 1982. Glycogen availability as a limiting factor in performance of isometric exercise. *Journal of Physiology* 342: 52P-53P.

Hermansen, L., E. Hultman, and B. Saltin. 1967. Muscle glycogen during prolonged severe exercise. *Acta Physiologica Scandinavica* 71: 129-139.

Hermansen, L., and O. Vaage. 1977. Lactate disappearance and glycogen synthesis in human muscle after maximal exercise. *American Journal of Physiology - Endocrinology and Metabolism* 233: E422-E429.

Hespel, P., B. Op 't Eijnde, W. Derave, and E.A. Richter. 2001. Creatine supplementation: Exploring the role of the creatine kinase/phosphocreatine system in the human muscle. *Canadian Journal of Applied Physiology* 26: S79-S102.

Hew-Butler, T., C. Almond, J.C. Ayus, J. Dugas, W. Meeuwisse, T. Noakes, S. Reid, A. Siegel, D. Speedy, K. Stuempfle, J. Verbalis, L. Weschler, and Exercise-Associated Hyponatremia (EAH) Consensus Panel. 2005. Consensus statement of the 1st International Exercise-Associated Hyponatremia Consensus Development Conference, Cape Town, South Africa, 2005. *Clinical Journal of Sports Medicine* 15: 208-213.

Hew-Butler, T.D., K. Sharwood, M. Collins, D. Speedy, and T. Noakes. 2006. Sodium supplementation is not required to maintain serum sodium concentrations during an Ironman triathlon. *British Journal of Sports Medicine* 40: 255-259.

Heyward, V.H., W.M. Sandoval, and B.C. Colville. 1989. Anthropometric, body composition and nutritional profiles of bodybuilders during training. *Journal of Applied Sport Science Research* 3: 22-29.

Hickner, R.C., C.A. Horswill, J.M. Welker, J. Scott, J.N. Roemmich, and D.L. Costill. 1991. Test development for the study of physical performance in wrestlers following weight loss. *International Journal of Sports Medicine* 12: 557-562.

Hickson, J.F., M.A. Duke, C.W. Johnson, R. Palmer, and J.E. Stockton. 1987. Nutritional intake from food sources of high school football athletes. *Journal of the American Dietetic Association* 87: 1656-1664.

Hickson, J.F., T.E. Johnson, W. Lee, and R.J. Sidor. 1990. Nutrition and the precontest preparations of a male bodybuilder. *Journal of the American Dietetic Association* 90: 264-267.

Hickson, J.F., C.W. Johnson, J.W. Schrader, and J.E. Stockton. 1987. Promotion of athletes' nutritional intake by a university foodservice facility. *Journal of the American Dietetic Association* 87: 926-927.

Hickson, J.F., J. Schrader, and L.C. Trischler. 1986. Dietary intakes of female basketball and gymnastics athletes. *Journal of the American Dietetic Association* 86: 251-253.

Hickson, J.F., I. Wolinsky, J.M. Pivarnik, E.A. Neuman, J.F. Itak, and J.E. Stockton. 1987. Nutritional profile of football athletes eating from a training table. *Nutrition Research* 7: 27-34.

Hill, R.J., and P.S.W. Davies. 2001. Energy expenditure during 2 wk of an ultra-endurance run around Australia. *Medicine and Science in Sports and Exercise* 33: 148-151.

Hill, R.J., and P.S. Davies. 2002. Energy intake and energy expenditure in elite lightweight female rowers. *Medicine and Science in Sports and Exercise,* 34: 1823-1829.

Hilton, L.K., and A.B. Loucks. 2000. Low energy availability, not exercise stress, suppresses the diurnal rhythm of leptin in healthy young women. *American Journal of Physiology* 278: E42-E49.

Hintermeister, R.A., and G.R. Hagerman. 2000. Physiology of alpine skiing. In *Textbook of Sports Medicine, Vol. 1* (edited by D.T. Kirkendall and W.E. Garrett), pp. 695-706. Philadelphia: Lippincott Williams & Wilkins.

Hirvonen, J., A. Nummela, S. Rehunen, and M. Harkonen. 1992. Fatigue and changes in ATP, creatine phosphate and lactate during the 400 m sprint. *Canadian Journal of Sport Science* 17: 141-144.

Hirvonen, J., S. Rehunen, H. Rusko, and M. Harkonen. 1987. Breakdown of high-energy phosphate compounds and lactate accumulation during short supramaximal exercise. *European Journal of Applied Physiology* 56: 253-259.

Hitchins, S., D.T. Martin, L. Burke, K. Yates, K. Fallon, A. Hahn, and G.P. Dobson. 1999. Glycerol hyperhydration improves cycle time trial performance in hot humid conditions. *European Journal of Applied Physiology* 80: 494-501.

Hoff, J., G.O. Berdahl, and S. Braten. 2000. Jumping height development and body weight considerations in ski jumping. In *2nd International Congress on Science and Skiing* (edited by E. Muller, H. Schwameder, C. Raschner, S. Lindinger, and E. Kornexl), pp. 403-412. St. Christoph, Austria: Verlag Dr. Kovac.

Hoffman, J.R., J. Cooper, M. Wendell, J. Im, and J. Kang. 2004. Effects of beta-hydroxy-beta-methylbutyrate on power performance and indices of muscle damage and stress during high-intensity training. *Journal of Strength and Conditioning Research* 18: 747-752.

Hoffman, J.R., C.M. Maresh, R.U. Newton, M.R. Rubin, D.N. French, J.S. Volek, J. Sutherland, M. Robertson, A.L. Gomez, N.A. Ratamess, J. Kang, and W.J. Kraemer. 2002. Performance, biochemical and endocrine changes during a competitive football game. *Medicine and Science in Sports and Exercise* 34: 1845-1853.

Hoffman, J.R., H. Stavsky, and B. Falk. 1995. The effect of water restriction on anaerobic power and vertical jumping height in basketball players. *International Journal of Sports Medicine* 16: 214-216.

Hofman, Z., R. Smeets, G. Verlaan, R. van der Lugt, and P.A. Verstappen. 2002. The effect of bovine colostrum supplementation on exercise performance in elite field hockey players. *International Journal of Sport Nutrition and Exercise Metabolism* 12: 461-469.

Hood, D.A., R. Kelton, and M.L. Nishio. 1992. Mitochondrial adaptations to chronic muscle use: Effect of iron deficiency. *Comparative Biochemistry and Physiology* 101A: 597-605.

Hopkins, W.G., J.A. Hawley, and L.M. Burke. 1999. Design and analysis of research on sport performance enhancement. *Medicine and Science in Sports and Exercise* 31: 472-485.

Horswill, C.A., R.C. Hickner, J.R. Scott, D.L. Costill, and D. Gould. 1990. Weight loss, dietary carbohydrate modifications, and high intensity physical performance. *Medicine and Science in Sports and Exercise* 22: 470-477.

Horswill, C.A., S.H. Park, and J.N. Roemmich. 1990. Changes in the protein nutritional status of adolescent wrestlers. *Medicine and Science in Sports and Exercise* 22: 599-604.

Horton, T.J., H.A. Drougas, T.A. Sharp, L.R. Martinez, G.W. Reed, and J.O. Hill. 1994. Energy balance in endurance-trained female cyclists and untrained controls. *Journal of Applied Physiology* 76: 1937-1945.

Houmard, J.A., M.E. Langenfeld, R.L. Wiley, and J. Siefert. 1987. Effects of the acute ingestion of small amounts of alcohol upon 5-mile run times. *Journal of Sports Medicine* 27: 253-257.

Housh, T.J., G.O. Johnson, J. Stout, and D.J. Housh. 1993. Anthropometric growth patterns of high school wrestlers. *Medicine and Science in Sports and Exercise* 25: 1141-1150.

Houtkooper, L.B., V.A. Mullins, S.B. Going, C.H. Brown, and T.G. Lohman. 2001. Body composition profiles of elite American heptathletes. *International Journal of Sport Nutrition and Exercise Metabolism* 11: 162-173.

Howley, P., and S. Moneghetti. 1997. *In the Long Run.* Melbourne, Australia; Penguin Books Australia Ltd.

Hsu, C.C., M.C. Ho, L.C. Lin, B. Su, and M.C. Hsu. 2005. American ginseng supplementation attenuates creatine kinase level

induced by submaximal exercise in human beings. *World Journal of Gastroenterology* 11: 5327-5331.

Hubbard, R.W., P.C. Szlyk, and L.E. Armstrong. 1990. Influence of thirst and fluid palatability on fluid ingestion during exercise. In *Perspectives in Exercise Science and Sports Medicine* (edited by C.V. Gisolfi and D.R. Lamb), pp. 39-95. Carmel, IN: Benchmark Press.

Hultman, E., and P.L. Greenhaff. 2000. Carbohydrate metabolism in exercise. In *Nutrition in sport* (edited by R.J. Maughan), pp. 85-96. Oxford, UK: Blackwell Science.

Hultman, E., K. Soderlund, J.A. Timmons, G. Cederblad, and P.L. Greenhaff. 1996. Muscle creatine loading in men. *Journal of Applied Physiology* 81: 232-237.

Hultman, E., L.L. Spriet, and K. Soderlund. 1987. Energy metabolism and fatigue in working muscles. In *Exercise, Limitations and Adaptations* (edited by D. Macleod, R. Maughan, M. Nimmo, T. Reilly, and C. Williams), pp. 63-80. London, UK: E & FN Spon.

Hunter, A.M., A. St. Clair Gibson, M. Collins, M. Lambert, and T.D. Noakes. 2002. Caffeine ingestion does not alter performance during a 100-km cycling time-trial performance. *International Journal of Sport Nutrition and Exercise Metabolism* 12: 438-452.

Ihle, R., and A.B. Loucks. 2004. Dose-response relationships between energy availability and bone turnover in young exercising women. *Journal of Bone and Mineral Research* 19: 1231-1240.

Inder, W.J., M.P. Swanney, R.A. Donald, T.C.R. Prickett, and J. Hellemans. 1998. The effect of glycerol and desmopressin on exercise performance and hydration in triathletes. *Medicine and Science in Sports and Exercise* 30: 1263-1269.

International Cricket Council. 2004. ICC official playing regulations 2003/2004. Available www.cricket.org [accessed September 7, 2006].

International Olympic Committee. 2004. IOC consensus statement on sports nutrition 2003. *Journal of Sports Sciences* 22: x.

ISU. 2003. International Skating Union Web site. Available www.isu.org [accessed September 7, 2006].

Ivy, J.L., D.L. Costill, W.J. Fink, and R.W. Lower. 1979. Influence of caffeine and carbohydrate feedings on endurance performance. *Medicine and Science in Sports and Exercise* 11: 6-11.

Ivy, J.L., H.W. Goforth, B.D. Damon, T.R. McCauley, E.C. Parsons, and T.B. Price. 2002. Early post-exercise muscle glycogen recovery is enhanced with a carbohydrate-protein supplement. *Journal of Applied Physiology* 93: 1337-1344.

Ivy, J.L., A.L. Katz, C.L. Cutler, W.M. Sherman, and E.F. Coyle. 1988. Muscle glycogen synthesis after exercise: Effect of time of carbohydrate ingestion. *Journal of Applied Physiology* 64: 1480-1485.

Ivy, J.L., and C.H. Kuo. 1998. Regulation of GLUT4 protein and glycogen synthase during muscle glycogen synthesis after exercise. *Acta Physiologica Scandinavica* 162: 295-304.

Ivy, J.L., P.T. Res, R.C. Sprague, and M.O. Widzer. 2003. Effect of a carbohydrate-protein supplement on endurance performance during exercise of varying intensity. *International Journal of Sport Nutrition and Exercise Metabolism* 13: 382-395.

Izquierdo, M., J. Ibanez, J.J. Gonzalez-Badillo, and E. Gorostiaga. 2002. Effects of creatine supplementation on muscle power, endurance, and sprint performance. *Medicine and Science in Sports and Exercise* 34: 332-343.

Jacobs, I., P. Kaiser, and P. Tesch. 1981. Muscle strength and fatigue after selective glycogen depletion in human skeletal muscle fibres. *European Journal of Applied Physiology* 46: 47-53.

Jacobs, I., P. Kaiser, and P. Tesch. 1982. The effects of glycogen exhaustion on maximal short-term performance. In *Exercise and Sports Performance* (edited by P. V. Komi), pp. 103-108. Champaign, IL: Human Kinetics.

Jacobs, I., N. Westlin, J. Karlsson, M. Rasmusson, and B. Houghton. 1982. Muscle glycogen and diet in elite soccer players. *European Journal of Applied Physiology* 48: 297-302.

Jacobsen, T.L., M.A. Febbraio, M.J. Arkinstall, and J.A. Hawley. 2001. Effect of caffeine co-ingested with carbohydrate or fat on metabolism and performance in endurance-trained men. *Experimental Physiology* 86: 137-144.

Jacques, T.D., and G.R. Pavia. 1974. An analysis of the movement patterns of players in an Australian rules league football match. *Australian Journal of Sports Medicine* 5: 23-24.

James, A.P., M. Lorraine, D. Cullen, C. Goodman, B. Dawson, T.N. Palmer, and P.A. Fournier. 2001. Muscle glycogen supercompensation: Absence of a gender-related difference. *European Journal of Applied Physiology and Occupational Physiology* 85: 533-538.

Jang, K.T., M.G. Flynn, D.L. Costill, J.P. Kirwan, J.A. Houmard, J.B. Mitchell, and L.J. D'Acquisto. 1987. Energy balance in competitive swimmers and runners. *Journal of Swimming Research* 3: 19-23.

Jarvis, M., L. McNaughton, A. Seddon, and D. Thompson. 2002. The acute 1-week effects of the Zone diet on body composition, blood lipid levels, and performance in recreational endurance athletes. *Journal of Strength and Conditioning Research* 16: 50-57.

Javierre, C., J.R. Barbany, V.M. Bonjorn, M.A. Lizarraga, J.L. Ventura, and R. Segura. 2004. Creatine supplementation and performance in 6 consecutive 60 meter sprints. *Journal of Physiology and Biochemistry* 60: 265-272.

Jenkins, D.G., J. Palmer, and D. Spillman. 1993. The influence of dietary carbohydrate on performance of supramaximal intermittent exercise. *European Journal of Applied Physiology* 67: 309-314.

Jennings, S., S. Roberston, D. Jennings, J. White, and C. Gisane. 1998. Body weight loss as an indicator of dehydration in summer rugby league. *Coaching and Sport Science Journal* 3(3): 31-33.

Jensen, C.D., E.S. Zaltas, and J.H. Whittam. 1992. Dietary intakes of male endurance cyclists during training and racing. *Journal of the American Dietetic Association* 92: 986-988.

Jentjens, R.L., J. Achten, and A.E. Jeukendrup. 2004. High oxidation rates from combined carbohydrates ingested during exercise. *Medicine and Science in Sports and Exercise* 36: 1551-1558.

Jentjens, R.L.P.G., C. Cale, C. Gutch, and A.E. Jeukendrup. 2003. Effects of pre-exercise ingestion of differing amounts of carbohydrate on subsequent metabolism and cycling performance. *European Journal of Applied Physiology* 88: 444-452.

Jentjens, R.L.P.G., and A.E. Jeukendrup. 2002. Prevalence of hypoglycemia following pre-exercise carbohydrate ingestion is not accompanied by higher insulin sensitivity. *International Journal of Sport Nutrition and Exercise Metabolism* 12: 398-413.

Jentjens, R., and A.E. Jeukendrup. 2003a. Determinants of postexercise glycogen synthesis during short-term recovery. *Sports Medicine* 33: 117-144.

Jentjens, R.L.P.G., and A.E. Jeukendrup. 2003b. Effects of pre-exercise ingestion of trehalose, galactose and glucose on subsequent metabolism and cycling performance. *European Journal of Applied Physiology* 88: 449-465.

Jentjens, R.L., and A.E. Jeukendrup. 2005. High rates of exogenous carbohydrate oxidation from a mixture of glucose and fructose ingested during prolonged cycling exercise. *British Journal of Nutrition* 93: 485-492.

Jentjens, R.L.P.G., L. Moseley, R.H. Waring, L.K. Harding, and A.E. Jeukendrup. 2004. Oxidation of combined ingestion of glucose and fructose during exercise. *Journal of Applied Physiology* 96: 1277-1284.

Jentjens, R.L., L.J.C. van Loon, C.H. Mann, A.J.M. Wagenmakers, and A.E. Jeukendrup. 2001. Addition of protein and amino acids to carbohydrates does not enhance postexercise muscle glycogen synthesis. *Journal of Applied Physiology* 91: 839-846.

Jentjens, R.L.P.G., M.C. Venables, and A.E. Jeukendrup. 2004. Oxidation of exogenous glucose, sucrose, and maltose during prolonged cycling exercise. *Journal of Applied Physiology* 96: 1285-1291.

Jeukendrup, A., F. Brouns, A.J.M. Wagenmakers, and W.H.M. Saris. 1997. Carbohydrate-electrolyte feedings improve 1 h time trial cycling performance. *International Journal of Sports Medicine* 18: 125-129.

Jeukendrup, A.E., N.P. Craig, and J.A. Hawley. 2000. The bioenergetics of world class cycling. *Journal of Science and Medicine in Sport* 3: 414-433.

Jeukendrup, A.E., and R. Jentjens. 2000. Oxidation of carbohydrate feedings during prolonged exercise: Current thoughts, guidelines and directions for future research. *Sports Medicine* 29: 407-424.

Jeukendrup, A.E., W.H.M. Saris, P. Schrauwen, F. Brouns, and A.J.M. Wagenmakers. 1995. Metabolic availability of medium-chain triglycerides coingested with carbohydrates during prolonged exercise. *Journal of Applied Physiology* 79: 756-762.

Jeukendrup, A.E., J.J.H.C. Thielen, A.J.M. Wagenmakers, F. Brouns, and W.H.M. Saris. 1998. Effect of medium-chain triacylglycerol and carbohydrate ingestion during exercise on substrate utilization and subsequent cycling performance. *American Journal of Clinical Nutrition* 67: 397-404.

Johansson, L., K. Solvoll, G.A. Bjorneboe, and C.A. Drevon. 1998. Under- and overreporting of energy intake related to weight status and lifestyle in a nationwide sample. *American Journal of Clinical Nutrition* 68: 266-274.

Johnson, A., P. Collins, I. Higgins, D. Harrington, J. Connolly, C. Dolphin, M. McCreery, L. Brady, and M. O'Brien. 1985. Psychological, nutritional and physical status of Olympic road cyclists. *British Journal of Sports Medicine* 19: 11-14.

Johnson, B. 2002. Training the Kenyan way. Unpublished report. Deakin University, Melbourne, Australia.

Jones, A.M., T. Atter, and K.P. Georg. 1999. Oral creatine supplementation improves multiple sprint performance in elite ice-hockey players. *Journal of Sports Medicine and Physical Fitness* 39: 189-196.

Jones, P.J., and C.A. Leitch. 1993. Validation of doubly labeled water for measurement of caloric expenditure in collegiate swimmers. *Journal of Applied Physiology* 74: 2909-2914.

Jonnalagadda, S.S., D. Benardot, and M.N. Dill. 2000. Assessment of under-reporting of energy intake by elite female gymnasts. *International Journal of Sport Nutrition and Exercise Metabolism* 10: 315-325.

Jonnalagadda, S.S., D. Benardot, and M. Nelson. 1998. Energy and nutrient intakes of the United States national women's artistic gymnastics team. *International Journal of Sport Nutrition* 8: 331-344.

Jonnalagadda, S.S., C.A. Rosenbloom, and R. Skinner. 2001. Dietary practices, attitudes and physiological status of collegiate freshman football players. *Journal of Strength and Conditioning Research* 15: 507-513.

Jordan, A.N., R. Jurca, E.H. Abraham, A. Salikhova, J.K. Mann, G.M. Morss, T.S. Church, A. Lucia, and C.P. Earnest. 2004.

Effects of oral ATP supplementation on anaerobic power and muscular strength. *Medicine and Science in Sports and Exercise* 36: 983-990.

Jowko, E., P. Ostaszewski, M. Jank, J. Sacharuk, A. Zieniewicz, J. Wilczak, and S. Nissen. 2001. Creatine and beta-hydroxy-beta-methylbutyrate (HMB) additively increase lean body mass and muscle strength during a weight-training program. *Nutrition* 17: 558-566.

Juhn, M.S., J.W. O'Kane, and D.M. Vinci. 1999. Oral creatine supplementation in male collegiate athletes: A survey of dosing habits and side effects. *Journal of the American Dietetic Association* 99: 593-595.

Juhn, M.S., and M. Tarnopolsky. 1998a. Oral creatine supplementation and athletic performance: A critical review. *Clinical Journal of Sports Medicine* 8: 286-297.

Juhn, M.S., and M. Tarnopolsky. 1998b. Potential side-effects of oral creatine supplementation: A critical review. *Clinical Journal of Sports Medicine* 8: 298-304.

Jurimae, J., T. Jurimae, and E. Pihl. 2000. Changes in body fluids during endurance rowing training. *Annals of the New York Academy of Sciences* 904: 353-358.

Kaikkonen, J., L. Kosonen, K. Nyyssonen, E. Porkkala-Sarataho, R. Salonen, H. Korpela, and J.T. Salonen. 1998. Effect of combined coenzyme Q10 and d-a-tocopheryl acetate supplementation on exercise-induced lipid peroxidation and muscular damage: A placebo-controlled double-blind study in marathon runners. *Free Radical Research* 29: 85-92.

Kaiserauer, S., A.C. Snyder, M. Sleeper, and J. Zierath. 1989. Nutritional, physiological, and menstrual status of distance runners. *Medicine and Science in Sports and Exercise* 21: 120-125.

Karlson, K.A., C.B. Becker, and A. Merkur. 2001. Prevalence of eating disordered behaviour in collegiate lightweight women rowers and distance runners. *Clinical Journal of Sports Medicine* 11: 32-37.

Karlsson, J., A. Eriksson, A. Forsberg, L. Kallberg, and P. Tesch. 1978. *The Physiology of Alpine Skiing.* Park City, UT: United States Ski Coaches Association.

Karlsson, J., and B. Saltin. 1971. Diet, muscle glycogen, and endurance performance. *Journal of Applied Physiology* 31: 203-206.

Karvinen, E., M. Miettinen, and K. Ahlman. 1962. Physical performance during hangover. *Quarterly Journal of Studies on Alcohol* 23: 208-215.

Kavouras, S.A., L.E. Armstrong, C.M. Maresh, D.J. Casa, J.A. Herrera Soto, T.P. Scheett, J. Stoppani, G.W. Mack, and W.J. Kraemer. 2006. Rehydration with glycerol: endocrine, cardiovascular and thermoregulatory responses during exercise in the heat. *Journal of Applied Physiology* 100: 442-450.

Keen, P. 1998. The one hour track cycling record. In *Peak Performance: Training and Nutritional Strategies for Sport* (edited by J. Hawley and L. Burke), pp. 402-406. Sydney, Australia: Allen & Unwin.

Keith, R.E., M.H. Stone, R.E. Carson, R.G. Lefavi, and S.J. Fleck. 1996. Nutritional status and lipid profiles of trained steroid-using bodybuilders. *International Journal of Sport Nutrition* 6: 247-254.

Keizer, H.A., H. Kuipers, G. Van Kranenburg, and P. Guerten. 1986. Influence of liquid and solid meals on muscle glycogen resynthesis, plasma fuel hormone response, and maximal physical working capacity. *International Journal of Sports Medicine* 8: 99-104.

Kelly, V.G., and D.G. Jenkins. 1998. Effect of oral creatine supplementation on near-maximal strength and repeated sets of high-intensity bench press exercise. *Journal of Strength and Conditioning Research* 12: 109-115.

Kerksick, C., C. Rasmussen, R. Bowden, B. Leutholtz, T. Harvey, C. Earnest, M. Greenwood, A. Almada, and R. Kreider. 2005. Effects of ribose supplementation prior to and during intense exercise on anaerobic capacity and metabolic markers. *International Journal of Sport Nutrition and Exercise Metabolism* 15: 663-674.

Kern, M., L.J. Podewils, M. Vukovich, and M.J. Buono. 2001. Physiological response to exercise in the heat following creatine supplementation. *Journal of Exercise Physiology* [Online] 4: 18-27. Available: http://faculty.css.edu/tboone2/asep/fldr/fldr.htm [accessed September 7, 2006].

Kerr, D. 2006. Kinanthropometry: Physique assessment of the athlete. In *Clinical Sports Nutrition, 3rd ed.* (edited by L. Burke and V. Deakin), pp. 237-312. Sydney, Australia: McGraw-Hill.

Kerr, D., K. Khan, and K. Bennell. 2000. Bone, exercise, nutrition and menstrual disturbances. In *Clinical Sports Nutrition* (edited by L. Burke and V. Deakin), pp. 241-272. Sydney, Australia: McGraw-Hill.

Kerr, D.A., K. Khan, and K. Bennell. 2006. Bone, exercise, nutrition and menstrual disturbances. In *Clinical Sports Nutrition, 3rd ed.* (edited by L. Burke and V. Deakin), pp. 237-261. Sydney, Australia: McGraw-Hill.

Kerr, D.A., W.D. Ross, K. Norton, P. Hume, M. Kagawa, and T.R. Ackland. 2007. Olympic lightweight and open-class rowers possess distinctive physical and proportionality characteristics. *Journal of Sports Science* 25:43-53.

Khan, K.M., T. Liu-Ambrose, M.M. Sran, M.C. Ashe, M.J. Donaldson, and J.D. Wark. 2002. New criteria for female athlete triad syndrome? *British Journal of Sports Medicine* 36: 10-13.

Khoo, C.S., N.E. Rawson, M.L. Robinson, and R.J. Stevenson. 1987. Nutrient intake and eating habits of triathletes. *Annals of Sports Medicine* 3: 144-150.

Kiens, B., and E.A. Richter. 1998. Utilization of skeletal muscle triacylglycerol during postexercise recovery in humans. *American Journal of Physiology - Endocrinology and Metabolism* 275: E332-E337.

Kilduff, L.P., E. Georgiades, N. James, R.H. Minnion, M. Mitchell, D. Kingsmore, M. Hadjicharlambous, and Y.P. Pitsiladis. 2004. The effects of creatine supplementation on cardiovascular, metabolic, and thermoregulatory responses during exercise in the heat in endurance-trained humans. *International Journal of Sport Nutrition and Exercise Metabolism* 14: 443-460.

Kilduff, L.P., P. Vidakovic, G. Cooney, R. Twycross-Lewis, P. Amuna, M. Parker, L. Paul, and Y.P. Pitsiladis. 2002. Effects of creatine on isometric bench-press performance in resistance-trained humans. *Medicine and Science in Sports and Exercise* 34: 1176-1183.

Kimber, N.E., J.J. Ross, S.L. Mason, and D.B. Speedy. 2002. Energy balance during an Ironman triathlon in male and female triathletes. *International Journal of Sport Nutrition and Exercise Metabolism* 12: 47-62.

King, M.B., and G. Mezey. 1987. Eating behaviour of male racing jockeys. *Psychological Medicine* 17: 249-253.

Kipp, R., J. Seifert, and E. Burke. 2003. The influence of a carbohydrate/protein sports drink on soccer sprint performance. Abstract presented at European Congress of Sports Sciences, Salzberg, Austria.

Kirchner, E.M., R.D. Lewis, and P.J. O'Connor. 1995. Bone mineral density and dietary intake of female college gymnasts. *Medicine and Science in Sports and Exercise* 27: 543-549.

Kirchner, E.M., R.D. Lewis, and P.J. O'Connor. 1996. Effect of past gymnastics participation on adult bone mass. *Journal of Applied Physiology* 80: 226-232.

Kirkendall, D.T. 1993. Effects of nutrition on performance in soccer. *Medicine and Science in Sports and Exercise* 25: 1370-1374.

Kirkendall, D.T., C. Foster, J.A. Dean, J. Grogan, and N.N. Thompson. 1988. Effect of glucose polymer supplementation on peformance of soccer players. In *Science and Football: Proceedings of the 1st World Congress of Science and Football, Liverpool, April 13-17th 1987* (edited by T. Reilly, A. Lees, K. Davids, and W. J. Murphy), pp. 33-41. London, UK: E & FN Spon.

Kirksey, K.B., M.H. Stone, B.J. Warren, R.L. Johnson, M. Stone, G.G. Haff, F.E. Williams, and C. Proulx. 1999. The effects of six weeks of creatine monohydrate supplementation on performance measures and body composition in collegiate track and field athletes. *Journal of Strength and Conditioning Research* 13: 148-156.

Kirsch, K.A., and H. Von Ameln. 1981. Feeding patterns of endurance athletes. *European Journal of Applied Physiology* 47: 197-208.

Kirwan, J.P., D.L. Costill, J.B. Mitchell, J.A. Houmard, M.G. Flynn, W.J. Fink, and J.D. Beltz. 1988. Carbohydrate balance in competitive runners during successive days of intense training. *Journal of Applied Physiology* 65: 2601-2606.

Kleiner, S.M., T.L. Bazzarre, and B.E. Ainsworth. 1994. Nutritional status of nationally ranked elite bodybuilders. *International Journal of Sport Nutrition* 4: 54-69.

Kleiner, S.M., T.L. Bazzarre, and M.D. Litchford. 1990. Metabolic profiles, diet, and health practices of championship male and female bodybuilders. *Journal of the American Dietetic Association* 90: 962-967.

Kleiner, S.M., L.H. Calabrese, K.M. Fielder, H.K. Naito, and C.I. Skibinski. 1989. Dietary influences on cardiovascular disease risk in anabolic steroid-using and nonusing bodybuilders. *Journal of the American College of Nutrition* 8: 109-119.

Klepping, J., V. Boggio, and I. Marcer. 1984. Resultats d'enquetes alimentaires realisees chez des sportifs francais. *Schweizerische Zeitschrift fur Sportmedezin und Sporttraumatologie* 31: 15-19.

Klingshirn, L.A., R.R. Pate, S.P. Bourque, J.M. Davis, and R.G. Sargent. 1992. Effect of iron supplementation on endurance capacity in iron-depleted female runners. *Medicine and Science in Sports and Exercise* 24: 819-824.

Knitter, A.E., L. Panton, J.A. Rathmacher, A. Petersen, and R. Sharp. 2000. Effects of beta-hydroxy-beta-methylbutyrate on muscle damage after a prolonged run. *Journal of Applied Physiology* 89: 1340-1344.

Knochel, J.P. 1975. Dog days and siriasis: How to kill a football player. *Journal of the American Medical Association* 233: 513-515.

Kobayashi, Y., T. Takeuchi, T. Hosoi, and S. Takaba. 2004. Dehydration during table tennis in a hot, humid environment. In *Science and racket sports III: the proceedings of the Eighth International Table Tennis Federation Sports Science Congress and the Third World Congress of Science and Racket Sports* (edited by A. Lees, J.F. Kahn, and I.W. Maynard), pp. 15-20. London, UK: Routledge.

Koutedakis, Y., P.J. Pacy, R.M. Quevedo, D.J. Millward, R. Hesp, C. Boreham, and N.C.C. Sharp. 1994. The effects of two different periods of weight reduction on selected performance parameters in elite lightweight oarswomen. *International Journal of Sports Medicine* 15: 472-477.

Kovacs, E.M.R., R.M. Schmahl, J.M.G. Senden, and F. Brouns. 2002. Effect of high and low rates of fluid intake on post-exercise rehydration. *International Journal of Sport Nutrition and Exercise Metabolism* 12: 14-23.

Kovacs, E.M.R., J.M.G. Senden, and F. Brouns. 1999. Urine color, osmolality and specific electrical conductance are not accurate measures of hydration status during postexercise rehydration. *Journal of Sports Medicine and Physical Fitness* 39: 47-53.

Kovacs, E.M.R., J.H.C.H. Stegen, and F. Brouns. 1998. Effect of caffeinated drinks on substrate metabolism, caffeine excretion, and performance. *Journal of Applied Physiology* 85: 709-715.

Kozyrskyj, A. 1997. Herbal products in Canada. How safe are they? *Canadian Family Physician* 43: 697-702.

Kraemer, W.J., J.S. Volek, J.A. Bush, M. Putukian, and W.J. Sebastianelli. 1998. Hormonal responses to consecutive days of heavy-resistance exercise with or without nutritional supplementation. *Journal of Applied Physiology* 85: 1544-1555.

Kreider, R.B. 1998. Creatine supplementation: Analysis of ergogenic value, medical safety, and concerns. *Journal of Exercise Physiology* [Online] 1. Available http://faculty.css.edu/tboone2/asep/fldr/fldr.htm [accessed September 7, 2006].

Kreider, R.B. 1999. Dietary supplements and the promotion of muscle growth with resistance exercise. *Sports Medicine* 27: 97-110.

Kreider, R.B., M. Ferreira, M. Wilson, and A.L. Almada. 1999. Effects of calcium ß-hydroxy-ß-methylbutyrate (HMB) supplementation during resistance-training on markers of catabolism, body composition and strength. *International Journal of Sports Medicine* 20: 503-509.

Kreider, R.B., M. Ferreira, M. Wilson, P. Grindstaff, S. Plisk, J. Reinardy, E. Cantler, and A.L. Almada. 1998. Effects of creatine supplementation on body composition, strength, and sprint performance. *Medicine and Science in Sports and Exercise* 30: 73-82.

Kreider, R.B., C. Melton, M. Greenwood, C.J. Rasmussen, J. Lundberg, C. Earnest, and A.L. Almada. 2003. Effects of oral D-ribose supplementation on anaerobic capacity and selected metabolic markers in healthy males. *International Journal of Sport Nutrition and Exercise Metabolism* 13: 76-86.

Kreider, R.B., C. Melton, C.J. Rasmussen, M. Greenwood, S. Lancaster, E.C. Cantler, P. Milnor, and A.L. Almada. 2003. Long-term creatine supplementation does not significantly affect clinical markers of health in athletes. *Molecular and Cell Biochemistry* 244: 95-104.

Kristal-Boneh, E., J.G. Glusman, R. Shitrit, C. Chaemovitz, and Y. Cassuto. 1995. Physical performance and heat tolerance after chronic water loading and heat acclimation. *Aviation, Space, and Environmental Medicine* 66: 733-738.

Kuipers, H., E.J. Fransen, and H.A. Keizer. 1999. Pre-exercise ingestion of carbohydrate and transient hypoglycemia during exercise. *International Journal of Sports Medicine* 20: 227-231.

Kuipers, H., H.A. Keizer, F. Brouns, and W.H.M. Saris. 1987. Carbohydrate feeding and glycogen synthesis during exercise in man. *Pflugers Archives* 410: 652-656.

Kuipers, H., E. Van Breda, G. Verlaan, and R. Smeets. 2002. Effects of oral bovine colostrum supplementation on serum insulin-like growth factor 1 levels. *Nutrition* 18: 566-567.

Laaksonen, R., M. Fogelholm, J.J. Himberg, J. Laakso, and Y. Salorinne. 1995. Ubiquinone supplementation and exercise capacity in trained young and older men. *European Journal of Applied Physiology* 72: 95-100.

Labadarosius, D., J. Kotze, and D. Momberg. 1993. Jockeys and their practices in South Africa. In *Nutrition and Fitness for Athletes. 2nd International Conference* on Nutrition and Fitness (edited by A.P. Simopoulos and K.N. Pavlou). *World Review of Nutrition and Dietetics* 71: 97-114.

LaBotz, M., and B.W. Smith. 1999. Creatine supplement use in an NCAA Division 1 athletic program. *Clinical Journal of Sports Medicine* 9: 167-169.

Lacour, J.R., E. Bouvat, and J.C. Barthelemy. 1990. Post competition blood lactate concentrations as indicators of anaerobic energy expenditure during 400-m and 800-m races. *European Journal of Applied Physiology* 61: 172-176.

Lamanca, J.J., and E.M. Haymes. 1993. Effects of iron repletion on VO_2max, endurance, and blood lactate in women. *Medicine and Science in Sports and Exercise* 25: 1386-1392.

Lamar-Hildebrand, N., L. Saldanha, and J. Endres. 1989. Dietary and exercise practices of college-aged female body builders. *Journal of the American Dietetic Association* 89: 1308-1310.

Lamb, D.R., K.F. Rinehardt, R.L. Bartels, W.M. Sherman, and J.T. Snook. 1990. Dietary carbohydrate and intensity of interval swim training. *American Journal of Clinical Nutrition* 52: 1058-1063.

Lambert, C.P., and M.G. Flynn. 2002. Fatigue during high-intensity intermittent exercise: Application to bodybuilding. *Sports Medicine* 32: 511-522.

Lambert, C.P., M.G. Flynn, J.B. Boone, T.J. Michaud, and J. Rodriguez-Zayas. 1991. Effects of carbohydrate feeding on multiple-bout resistance exercise. *Journal of Applied Sport Science Research* 5: 192-197.

Lambert, C.P., M.G. Flynn, W.A. Braun, and D.J. Boardley. 1999. The effects of swimming and running on energy intake during 2 hours of recovery. *Journal of Sports Medicine and Physical Fitness* 39: 348-354.

Lambert, E.V., J.H. Goedecke, C.G. Van Zyl, K. Murphy, J.A. Hawley, S.C. Dennis, and T.D. Noakes. 2001. High-fat versus habitual diet prior to carbohydrate loading: Effects on exercise metabolism and cycling performance. *International Journal of Sport Nutrition and Exercise Metabolism* 11: 209-225.

Lambert, E.V., D.P. Speechly, S.C. Dennis, and T.D. Noakes. 1994. Enhanced endurance in trained cyclists during moderate intensity exercise following 2 weeks adaptation to a high fat diet. *European Journal of Applied Physiology* 69: 287-293.

Lambert, M.I., J.A. Hefer, R.P. Millar, and P.W. Macfarlane. 1993. Failure of commerical oral amino acid supplements to increase serum growth hormone concentrations in male body-builders. *International Journal of Sport Nutrition* 3: 298-305.

Landers, G.J., B.A. Blanksby, T.R. Ackland, and D. Smith. 2000. Morphology and performance of world championship triathletes. *Annals of Human Biology* 27: 387-400.

Langfort, J., R. Zarzeczny, W. Pilis, K. Nazar, and H. Kaciuba-Uscilko. 1997. The effects of a low-carbohydrate diet on performance, hormonal and metabolic response to a 30-s bout of supra-maximal exercise. *European Journal of Applied Physiology and Occupational Physiology* 76: 128-133.

Larsen-Meyer, D.E., G.R. Hunter, C.A. Trowbridge, J.C. Turk, J.M. Ernest, S.L. Torman, and P.A. Harbin. 2000. The effect of creatine supplementation on muscle strength and body composition during off-season training in female soccer players. *Journal of Strength and Conditioning Research* 14: 424-442.

Latzka, W.A., M.N. Sawka, S.J. Montain, G.S. Skrinar, R.A. Fielding, R.P. Matott, and K.B. Pandolf. 1998. Hyperhydration: Tolerance and cardiovascular effects during uncompensable exercise-heat stress. *Journal of Applied Physiology* 84: 1858-1864.

Laughlin, G.A., and S.C.S. Yen. 1997. Hypoleptinemia in women athletes: Absence of a diurnal rhythm with amenorrhea. *Journal of Clinical Endocrinology and Metabolism* 82: 318-321.

Lawrence, J.D., R.C. Bower, W.P. Riehl, and J.L. Smith. 1975. Effects of alpha-tocopherol acetate on the swimming endurance of trained swimmers. *American Journal of Clinical Nutrition* 28: 205-208.

Lawrence, J.D., J.L. Smith, R.C. Bower, and W.P. Riehl. 1975. The effect of alpha-tocopherol (vitamin E) and pyridoxone HCL (vitamin B6) on the swimming endurance of trained swimmers. *Journal of the American College Health Association* 23: 219-222.

Lawrence, S.R., D.B. Preen, B.T. Dawson, J. Beilby, C. Goodman, and N.T. Cable. 1997. The effect of oral creatine supplementation on maximal exercise performance in competitive rowers. *Sports Medicine, Training, and Rehabilitation* 7: 243-253.

Leatt, P. 1986. The effect of glucose polymer ingestion on skeletal muscle glycogen depletion during a soccer match play and its re-synthesis following a match. Unpublished thesis, University of Toronto.

Leatt, P.B., and I. Jacobs. 1989. Effect of glucose polymer ingestion on glycogen depletion during a soccer match. *Canadian Journal of Sports Science* 14: 112-116.

Lebenstedt, M., P. Platte, and K.M. Pirke. 1999. Reduced resting metabolic rate in athletes with menstrual disorders. *Medicine and Science in Sports and Exercise* 31: 1250-1260.

Leenders, N., W.M. Sherman, D.R. Lamb, and T.E. Nelson. 1999. Creatine supplementation and swimming performance. *International Journal of Sport Nutrition* 9: 251-262.

Lees, A. 2003. Science and the major racket sports: A review. *Journal of Sports Sciences* 21: 707-732.

Legaz, A., and R. Eston. 2005. Changes in performance, skinfold thicknesses, and fat patterning after three years of intense athletic conditioning in high level runners. *British Journal of Sports Medicine* 39: 851-855.

Lehmkuhl, M.J., M. Malone, B. Justice, G. Trone, E.E. Pistilli, D. Vinci, E.E. Haff, J.L. Kilgore, and G.G. Haff. 2003. The effects of 8 weeks of creatine monohydrate and glutamine supplementation on body composition and performance measures. *Journal of Strength and Conditioning Research* 17: 425-438.

Leiper, J.B., N.P. Broad, and R.J. Maughan. 2001. Effect of intermittent high-intensity exercise on gastric emptying in man. *Medicine and Science in Sports and Exercise* 33: 1270-1278.

Leiper, J.B., and R.J. Maughan. 2004. Comparison of water turnover rates in young swimmers in training and age-matched non-training individuals. *International Journal of Sport Nutrition and Exercise Metabolism* 14: 347-357.

Leiper, J.B., A.S. Prentice, C. Wrightson, and R.J. Maughan. 2001. Gastric emptying of a carbohydrate-electrolyte drink during a soccer match. *Medicine and Science in Sports and Exercise* 33: 1932-1938.

Lemon, P.W.R. 1991a. Effect of exercise on protein requirements. *Journal of Sports Sciences* 9: 53-70.

Lemon, P.W.R. 1991b. Protein and amino acid needs of the strength athlete. *International Journal of Sport Nutrition* 1: 127-145.

Lemon, P.W.R. 2000. Effects of exercise on protein metabolism. In *Nutrition in Sport* (edited by R. J. Maughan), pp. 133-152. Oxford, UK: Blackwell Science.

Lemon, P.W.R., D.T. Deutsch, and W.R. Payne. 1989. Urea production during prolonged swimming. *Journal of Sports Sciences* 7: 241-246.

Levafi, R.G. 1993. Response to GW Evans. *International Journal of Sport Nutrition* 3: 120-121.

Levafi, R.G., R.A. Anderson, R.E. Keith, G.D. Wilson, J.L. McMillan, and M.H. Stone. 1992. Efficacy of chromium supplementation in athletes: Emphasis on anabolism. *International Journal of Sport Nutrition* 2: 111-122.

Levenhagen, D.K., J.D. Gresham, M.G. Carlson, D.J. Maron, M.J. Borel, and P.J. Flakoll. 2001. Postexercise nutrient intake timing in humans is critical to recovery of leg glucose and protein homeostasis. *American Journal of Physiology* 280: E982-E993.

Levine, B.D., and J. Stray-Gundersen. 2001. The effects of altitude training are mediated primarily by acclimatization, rather than by hypoxic exercise. In *Hypoxia: From Genes to the Bedside* (edited by R.C. Roach), pp. 75-88. New York: Kluwer Academic/Plenum.

Levine, S.A., B. Gordon, and C.L. Derick. 1924. Some changes in the chemical constituents of the blood following a marathon race, with special reference to the development of hypoglycemia. *Journal of the American Medical Association* 82: 1778-1779.

Lewis, C., and J. Marx. 1996. *One More Victory Lap.* Flushing, NY: Athletics International.

Leydon, M.A., and C. Wall. 2002. New Zealand jockeys' dietary habits and their potential impact on health. *International Journal of Sport Nutrition and Exercise Metabolism* 12: 220-237.

Liang, M.T., T.D. Podolka, and W.J. Chuang. 2005. Panax notoginseng supplementation enhances physical performance during endurance exercise. *Journal of Strength and Conditioning Research* 19: 108-114.

Lindholm, C., K. Hagenfeldt, and U. Hagman. 1994. Pubertal development in elite juvenile gymnasts: Effects of physical training. *Acta Physiologica Scandinavica* 73: 269-273.

Locatelli, E., and L. Arsac. 1995. The mechanics and energetics of the 100-m sprint. *New Studies in Athletics* 10: 81-87.

Loosli, A.R., D.M. Benson, D.M. Gillien, and K. Bourdet. 1986. Nutrition habits and knowledge in competitive adolescent female gymnasts. *The Physician and Sportsmedicine* 14: 118-130.

Loucks, A.B. 2001. Physical health of the female athlete: Observations, effects, and causes of reproductive disorders. *Canadian Journal of Applied Physiology* 26: S176-S185.

Loucks, A.B. 2004. Energy balance and body composition in sports and exercise. *Journal of Sports Sciences* 22: 1-14.

Loucks, A.B. 2006. The response of luteinizing hormone pulsatility to five days of low energy availability disappears by 14 years of gynecological age. *Journal of Clinical Endocrinology and Metabolism* 91: 3158-3164.

Loucks, A.B., and A. Nattiv. 2005. The female athlete triad. *Lancet* 366: S49-S50.

Loucks, A.B., and J.R. Thuma. 2003. Luteinizing hormone pulsatility is disrupted at a threshold of energy availability in regularly menstruating women. *Journal of Clinical Endocrinology and Metabolism* 88: 297-311.

Loucks, A.B., M. Verdun, and E.M. Heath. 1998. Low energy availability, not stress of exercise, alters LH pulsatility in exercising women. *Journal of Applied Physiology* 84: 37-46.

Ludbrook, C., and D. Clark. 1992. Energy expenditure and nutrient intake in long-distance runners. *Nutrition Research* 12: 689-699.

Lugo, M., W.M. Sherman, G.S. Wimer, and K. Garleb. 1993. Metabolic responses when different forms of carbohydrate energy are consumed during cycling. *International Journal of Sport Nutrition* 3: 398-407.

Lukaski, H.C. 2001. Magnesium, zinc and chromium nutrition and athletic performance. *Canadian Journal of Applied Physiology* 26: S13-S22.

Lukaski, H.C., W.W. Bolonchuk, W.A. Siders, and D.B. Milne. 1996. Chromium supplementation and resistance training: Effects on body composition, strength, and trace element status of men. *American Journal of Clinical Nutrition* 63: 954-963.

Lukaski, H.C., B.S. Hoverson, S.K. Gallagher, and W.W. Bolonchuk.

1990. Physical training and copper, iron, and zinc status of swimmers. *American Journal of Clinical Nutrition* 51: 1093-1099.

Lundy, B., H. O'Connor, F. Pelly, and I. Caterson. 2006. Anthropometric characteristics and competition dietary intakes of professional rugby league players. *International Journal of Sport Nutrition and Exercise Metabolism* 16: 199-213.

Lutter, J.M., and S. Cushman. 1982. Menstrual patterns in female runners. *The Physician and Sportsmedicine* 10: 60-64, 69-72.

MacIntosh, B.R., and B.M. Wright. 1995. Caffeine ingestion and performance of a 1,500-metre swim. *Canadian Journal of Applied Physiology* 20: 168-177.

MacLaren, D. 1990. Court games: volleyball and basketball. In *Physiology of Sports* (edited by T. Reilly, N. Secher, P. Snell, and C. Williams), pp. 427-464. London, UK: E & FN Spon.

Madsen, K., D.A. MacLean, B. Kiens, and D. Christensen. 1996. Effects of glucose, glucose plus branched-chain amino acids, or placebo on bike performance over 100 km. *Journal of Applied Physiology* 81: 2644-2650.

Maehlum, S., and L. Hermansen. 1978. Muscle glycogen concentration during recovery after prolonged severe exercise in fasting subjects. *Scandinavian Journal of Laboratory and Clinical Investigation* 38: 557-560.

Maffulli, N. 1992. Making weight: A case study of two elite wrestlers. *British Journal of Sports Medicine* 26: 107-110.

Magal, M., M.J. Webster, L.E. Sistrunk, M.T. Whitehead, R.K. Evans, and J.C. Boyd. 2003. Comparison of glycerol and water hydration regimens on tennis-related performance. *Medicine and Science in Sports and Exercise* 35: 150-156.

Magnusson, B., L. Hallberg, L. Rossander, and B. Swolin. 1984. Iron metabolism and "sports anemia." 2. A hematological comparison of elite runners and control subjects. *Acta Medica Scandinavica* 216: 157-164.

Maisey, R., I. Perols, and M. Leydon. 2003. Does the consumption of a carbohydrate-protein beverage compared with an isoenergetic carbohydrate beverage improve time to exhaustion after recovery from glycogen-depleting exercise? *Journal of the New Zealand Dietetic Association* 57: 37-42.

Malm, C., M. Svensson, B. Ekblom, and B. Sjodin. 1997. Effects of ubiquinone-10 supplementation and high intensity training on physical performance in humans. *Acta Physiologica Scandinavica* 161: 379-384.

Malm, C., M. Svensson, B. Sjoberg, B. Ekblom, and B. Sjodin. 1996. Supplementation with ubiquinone-10 causes cellular damage during intense exercise. *Acta Physiologica Scandinavica* 157: 511-512.

Manore, M.M. 2002. Dietary recommendations and athletic menstrual dysfunction. *Sports Medicine* 32: 887-901.

Manore, M., and J. Thompson. 2006. Energy requirements of the athlete: assessment and evidence of energy efficiency. In *Clinical Sports Nutrition, 3rd ed.* (edited by L. Burke and V. Deakin), pp. 113-134. Sydney, Australia: McGraw-Hill.

Marconi, C., G. Sassi, A. Carpinelli, and P. Cerretelli. 1985. Effects of L-carnitine loading on the aerobic and anaerobic performance of endurance athletes. *European Journal of Applied Physiology* 54: 131-135.

Marcus, R., C. Cann, P. Madvig, J. Minkoff, M. Goddard, M. Bayer, M. Martin, L. Gaudini, W. Haskell, and H. Genant. 1985. Menstrual function and bone mass in elite women distance runners. *Annals of Internal Medicine* 102: 158-163.

Maresh, C.M., M.E. Bergeron, R.W. Kenefick, J.W. Castellani, J.R. Hoffman, and L.E. Armstrong. 2001. Effect of overhydration on time-trial swim performance. *Journal of Strength and Conditioning Research* 15: 514-518.

Marino, F.E., Z. Mbambo, E. Kortekaas, G. Wilson, M.I. Lambert, T.D. Noakes, and S.C. Dennis. 2000. Advantages of smaller body mass during distance running in warm, humid environments. *Pflugers Archives European Journal of Physiology* 441: 359-367.

Marr, J.W., and J.A. Heady. 1986. Within- and between-person variation in dietary surveys: Number of days needed to classify individuals. *Human Nutrition: Applied Nutrition* 40A: 347-364.

Martin, D.T., B. McLean, C. Trewin, H. Lee, J. Victor, and A.G. Hahn. 2001. Physiological characteristics of nationally competitive female road cyclists and demands of competition. *Sports Medicine* 31: 469-477.

Martin, L., A. Lambeth, and D. Scott. 2006. Nutritional practices of national female soccer players: analysis and recommendations. *Journal of Sports Science and Medicine* 5: 130-137.

Martin, M.K., D.T. Martin, G.R. Collier, and L.M. Burke. 2002. Voluntary food intake by elite female cyclists during training and racing: Effect of daily energy expenditure and body composition. *International Journal of Sport Nutrition and Exercise Metabolism* 12: 249-267.

Marylebone Cricket Club. 1992. *The Laws of Cricket, 2nd ed.* Marylebone, Australia: Marylebone Cricket Club.

Matheny, F. 1997. Scary thin: How some pros are shaving pounds. *Bicycling* October: 58.

Matson, L.G., and Z.T. Tran. 1993. Effects of sodium bicarbonate ingestion on anaerobic performance: A meta-analytic review. *International Journal of Sport Nutrition* 3: 2-28.

Maughan, R.J. 1997. Energy and macronutrient intake of professional football (soccer) players. *British Journal of Sports Medicine* 31: 45-47.

Maughan, R.J. 2000. Physiology and biochemistry of middle distance and long distance running. In *Running* (edited by J.A. Hawley), pp. 14-27. Oxford, UK: Blackwell Science Ltd.

Maughan, R.J., and S.P. Evans. 1982. Effects of pollen extract upon adolescent swimmers. *British Journal of Sports Medicine* 16: 142-145.

Maughan, R.J., and P.L. Greenhaff. 1991. High intensity exercise performance and acid-base balance: The influence of diet and induced metabolic alkalosis. In *Advances in Nutrition and Top Sport* (edited by F. Brouns), pp. 147-165. Basel, Switzerland: Karger.

Maughan, R.J., P.L. Greenhaff, J.B. Leiper, D. Ball, C.P. Lambert, and M. Gleeson. 1997. Diet composition and the performance of high-intensity exercise. *Journal of Sports Sciences* 15: 265-275.

Maughan, R.J., and E.S. Horton. 1995. Final consensus statement: Current issues in nutrition in athletics. *Journal of Sports Sciences* 13: S1.

Maughan, R.J., and J.B. Leiper. 1995. Sodium intake and post-exercise rehydration in man. *European Journal of Applied Physiology and Occupational Physiology* 71: 311-319.

Maughan, R.J., J.B. Leiper, and S.M. Shirreffs. 1996. Restoration of fluid balance after exercise-induced dehydration: Effects of food and fluid intake. *European Journal of Applied Physiology and Occupational Physiology* 73: 317-325.

Maughan, R.J., S.J. Merson, N.P. Broad, and S.M. Shirreffs. 2004. Fluid and electrolyte intake and loss in elite soccer players during training. *International Journal of Sport Nutrition and Exercise Metabolism* 14: 333-346.

Maughan, R.J., S.M. Shirreffs, S.J. Merson, and C.A. Horswill. 2005. Fluid and electrolyte balance in elite male football (soccer) players training in a cool environment. *Journal of Sports Sciences* 23: 73-79.

Maxwell, N., T. Aitchison, and M. Nimmo. 1996. The effect of climatic heat stress on intermittent supramaximal running performance in humans. *Experimental Physiology* 81: 833-845.

Mayhew, D.L., J.L. Mayhew, and J.S. Ware. 2002. Effects of long-term creatine supplementation on liver and kidney functions in American college football players. *International Journal of Sport Nutrition and Exercise Metabolism* 12: 453-460.

McCargar, L.J., and S.M. Crawford. 1992. Metabolic and anthropometric changes with weight cycling in wrestlers. *Medicine and Science in Sports and Exercise* 24: 1270-1275.

McCargar, L.J., D. Simmons, N. Craton, J.E. Taunton, and C.L. Birmingham. 1993. Physiological effects of weight cycling in female lightweight rowers. *Canadian Journal of Applied Physiology* 18: 291-303.

McCarthy, P.R., R.D. Thorpe, and C. Williams. 1988. Body fluid loss during competitive tennis match-play. In *Science and Racquet Sports II* (edited by A. Lees, I. Maynard, M. Hughes, and T. Reilly), pp. 52-55. London: E & FN Spon.

McConell, G.K., C.M. Burge, S.L. Skinner, and M. Hargreaves. 1997. Influence of ingested fluid volume on physiological responses during prolonged exercise. *Acta Physiologica Scandinavica* 160: 149-156.

McConell, G., K. Kloot, and M. Hargreaves. 1996. Effect of timing of carbohydrate ingestion on endurance exercise performance. *Medicine and Science in Sports and Exercise* 28: 1300-1304.

McGregor, S.J., C.W. Nicholas, H.K.A. Lakomy, and C. Williams. 1999. The influence of intermittent high-intensity shuttle running and fluid ingestion on the performance of a soccer skill. *Journal of Sports Sciences* 17: 895-903.

McGuine, T.A., J.C. Sullivan, and D.T. Bernhardt. 2001. Creatine supplementation in high school football players. *Clinical Journal of Sports Medicine* 11: 247-253.

McInerney, P., S.J. Lessard, L.M. Burke, V.G. Coffey, S.L. Lo Giudice, R.J. Southgate, and J.A. Hawley. 2005. Failure to repeatedly supercompensate muscle glycogen stores in highly trained men. *Medicine and Science in Sports and Exercise* 37: 404-411.

McInnes, S.E., J.S. Carlson, C.J. Jones, and M.J. McKenna. 1995. The physiological load imposed on basketball players during competition. *Journal of Sports Sciences* 13: 387-397.

McLellan, T.M., and D.G. Bell. 2004. The impact of prior coffee consumption on the subsequent ergogenic effect of anhydrous caffeine. *International Journal of Sport Nutrition and Exercise Metabolism* 14: 698-708.

McNaughton, L.R. 2000. Bicarbonate and citrate. In *Nutrition in Sport* (edited by R.J. Maughan), pp. 393-404. Oxford, UK: Blackwell Science.

McNaughton, L., K. Backx, G. Palmer, and N. Strange. 1999. Effects of chronic bicarbonate ingestion on the performance of high-intensity work. *European Journal of Applied Physiology* 80: 333-336.

McNaughton, L.R., and R. Cedaro. 1991. The effect of sodium bicarbonate on rowing ergometer performance in elite rowers. *Australian Journal of Science and Medicine in Sport* 23: 66-69.

McNaughton, L., B. Dalton, and G. Palmer. 1999. Sodium bicarbonate can be used as an ergogenic aid in high-intensity, competitive cycle ergometry of 1 h duration. *European Journal of Applied Physiology* 80: 64-69.

McNaughton, L.R., B. Dalton, and J. Tarr. 1998. The effects of creatine supplementation on high-intensity exercise performance in elite performers. *European Journal of Applied Physiology* 78: 236-240.

McNaughton, L., B. Dalton, and J. Tarr. 1999. Inosine supplementation has no effect on aerobic or anaerobic cycling performance. *International Journal of Sport Nutrition* 9: 333-344.

McNaughton, L., G. Egan, and G. Caelli. 1989. A comparison of Chinese and Russian ginseng as ergogenic aids to improve various facets of physical fitness. *International Clinical Nutrition Review* 9: 32-35.

McNaughton, L., and D. Preece. 1986. Alcohol and its effects on sprint and middle distance running. *British Journal of Sports Medicine* 20: 56-59.

McNaughton, L., N. Strange, and K. Backx. 2000. The effects of chronic sodium bicarbonate ingestion on multiple bouts of anaerobic work and power output. *Journal of Human Movement Studies* 38: 307-322.

McNaughton, L., and D. Thompson. 2001. Acute versus chronic sodium bicarbonate ingestion and anaerobic work and power output. *Journal of Sports Medicine and Physical Fitness* 41: 456-462.

Meir, R., L. Brooks, and T. Shield. 2003. Body weight and tympanic temperature change in professional rugby league players during night and day games: A study in the field. *Journal of Strength and Conditioning Research* 17: 566-572.

Meir, R.A., A.J. Davie, and P. Ohmsen. 1990. Thermoregulatory response of rugby league footballers playing in warm, humid conditions. *Sport Health* 8(4): 22-25.

Meir, R., and A. Murphy. 1998. Fluid loss and rehydration during training and competition in professional rugby league. *Coaching and Sport Science Journal* 3: 9-13.

Melby, C.L., W.D. Schmidt, and D. Corrigan. 1990. Resting metabolic rate in weight-cycling collegiate wrestlers compared with physically active, noncycling control subject. *American Journal of Clinical Nutrition* 52: 409-414.

Mendel, R.W., M. Blegen, C. Cheatham, J. Antonio, and T. Ziegenfuss. 2005. Effects of creatine on thermoregulatory responses while exercising in the heat. *Nutrition* 21: 301-307.

Mero, A., J. Kahkonen, T. Nykanen, T. Parviainen, I. Jokinen, T. Takala, T. Nikula, S. Rasi, and J. Leppaluoto. 2002. IGF-I, IgA, and IgG responses to bovine colostrum supplementation during training. *Journal of Applied Physiology* 93: 732-739.

Mero, A.A., K.L. Keskinen, M.T. Malvela, and J.M. Sallinen. 2004. Combined creatine and sodium bicarbonate supplementation enhances interval swimming. *Journal of Strength and Conditioning Research* 18: 306-310.

Mero, A., H. Mikkulainen, J. Riski, R. Pakkanen, J. Aalto, and T. Takala. 1997. Effects of bovine colostrum supplement on serum IGF-1, IgG, hormone and saliva IgA during training. *Journal of Applied Physiology* 83: 1144-1151.

Mero, A., T. Nykanen, O. Keinanen, J. Knuutinen, K. Lahti, M. Alen, S. Rasi, and J. Leppaluoto. 2005. Protein metabolism and strength performance after bovine colostrum supplementation. *Amino Acids* 28: 327-335.

Mertz, W., J.C. Tsui, J.T. Judd, S. Reiser, J. Hallfrisch, E.R. Morris, P.D. Steele, and E. Lashley. 1991. What are people really eating? The relation between energy intake derived from estimated diet records and intake determined to maintain body weight. *American Journal of Clinical Nutrition* 54: 291-295.

Meyer, N.L. 2003. Female winter sport athletes: Nutrition issues during the preparation for the 2002 Olympic winter games in Salt Lake City. Unpublished thesis, University of Utah, Salt Lake City.

Meyer, N.L., S.C. Johnson, E.W. Askew, M.L. Lutkemeier, C. Bainbridge, B.B. Shultz, and M.M. Manore. 1999. Energy and nutrient intake of elite female alpine ski racers during the preparatory phase. *Medicine and Science in Sports and Exercise* 31: S100.

Meyer, N.L., J.M. Shaw, M.M. Manore, A.W. Subudhi, E.W. Askew, B.B. Shultz, and J.A. Walker. 2003. Bone mineral density in female Olympic winter sport athletes. *Medicine and Science in Sports and Exercise* 35: S364.

Millard-Stafford, M., L.B. Rosskopf, T.K. Snow, and B.T. Hinson. 1997. Water versus carbohydrate-electrolyte ingestion before and during a 15-km run in the heat. *International Journal of Sport Nutrition* 7: 26-38.

Millard-Stafford, M., L.B. Rosskopf, and P.B. Sparling. 1989. Coronary heart disease: Risk profiles of college football players. *The Physician and Sportsmedicine* 17: 151-163.

Millard-Stafford, M.L., P.B. Sparling, L.B. Rosskopf, and L.J. Dicarlo. 1992. Carbohydrate-electrolyte replacement improves distance running performance in the heat. *Medicine and Science in Sports and Exercise* 24: 934-940.

Millard-Stafford, M., P.B. Sparling, L.B. Rosskopf, B.T. Hinson, and L.J. Dicarlo. 1990. Carbohydrate-electrolyte replacement during a simulated triathlon in the heat. *Medicine and Science in Sports and Exercise* 22: 621-628.

Miller, S.L., K.D. Tipton, D.L. Chinkes, S.E. Wolf, and R.R. Wolfe. 2003. Independent and combined effects of amino acids and glucose after resistance exercise. *Medicine and Science in Sports and Exercise* 35: 449-455.

Millward, D.J., J.L. Bowtell, P. Pacy, and M.J. Rennie. 1994. Physical activity, protein metabolism and protein requirements. *Proceedings of the Nutrition Society* 53: 223-240.

Minehan, M.R., M.D. Riley, and L.M. Burke. 2002. Effect of flavor and awareness of kilojoule content of drinks on preference and fluid balance in team sports. *International Journal of Sport Nutrition and Exercise Metabolism* 12: 81-92.

Misell, L.M., N.D. Lagomarcino, V. Schuster, and M. Kern. 2001. Chronic medium-chain triacylglycerol consumption and endurance performance in trained runners. *Journal of Sports Medicine and Physical Fitness* 41: 210-215.

Mitchell, J.B., K.J. Cole, P.W. Grandjean, and R.J. Sobczak. 1992. The effect of a carbohydrate beverage on tennis performance and fluid balance during prolonged tennis play. *Journal of Applied Sport Science Research* 6: 174-180.

Moffatt, R.J. 1984. Dietary status of elite female high school gymnasts: Inadequacy of vitamin and mineral intake. *Journal of the American Dietetic Association* 84: 1361-1363.

Mohr, M., P. Krustrup, and J. Bangsbo. 2003. Match performance of high-standard soccer players with special reference to development of fatigue. *Journal of Sports Sciences* 21: 519-528.

Monsen, E.R. 1988. Iron nutrition and absorption: Dietary factors which impact iron bioavailability. *Journal of the American Dietetic Association* 88: 786-790.

Montain, S.J., S.N. Cheuvront, and M.N. Sawka. 2006. Exercise associated hyponatremia: Quantitative analysis to understand the aetiology. *British Journal of Sports Medicine* 40: 98-106.

Montain, S.J., and E.F. Coyle. 1992. Influence of graded dehydration on hyperthermia and cardiovascular drift during exercise. *Journal of Applied Physiology* 73: 1340-1350.

Montfoort, M.C.E., L. Van Dieren, W.G. Hopkins, and J.P. Shearman. 2004. Effects of ingestion of bicarbonate, citrate, lactate, and chloride on sprint running. *Medicine and Science in Sports and Exercise* 36: 1239-1243.

Moore, J.M., A.F. Timperio, D.A. Crawford, C.M. Burns, and D. Cameron-Smith. 2002. Weight management and weight loss strategies of professional jockeys. *International Journal of Sport Nutrition and Exercise Metabolism* 12: 1-13.

Moroff, S.V., and D.E. Bass. 1980. Effects of over hydration on man's physiological responses to work in the heat. *Journal of Applied Physiology* 49: 715-721.

Morris, A.C., I. Jacobs, T.M. McLellan, A. Klugerman, L.C.H. Wang, and J. Zamecnik. 1996. No ergogenic effects of ginseng ingestion. *International Journal of Sport Nutrition* 6: 263-271.

Morris, F.L., and W.R. Payne. 1996. Seasonal variations in the body composition of lightweight rowers. *British Journal of Sports Medicine* 30: 301-304.

Morris, F.L., W.R. Payne, and J.D. Wark. 1999. Prospective decrease in progesterone concentrations in female lightweight rowers during the competition season compared with the off season: A controlled study examining weight loss and intensive exercise. *British Journal of Sports Medicine* 33: 417-422.

Morris, J., and N.S. Maxwell. 1998. Effect of a hot environment on performance of prolonged intermittent high intensity shuttle running. *Journal of Sports Sciences* 16: 677-686.

Morris, J.G., M.E. Nevill, D. Thompson, J. Collie, and C. Williams. 2003. The influence of a 6.5% carbohydrate-electrolyte solution on performance of prolonged intermittent high-intensity running at 30° C. *Journal of Sports Sciences* 21: 371-381.

Morrison, M.A., L.L. Spriet, and D.J. Dyck. 2000. Pyruvate ingestion for 7 days does not improve aerobic performance in well-trained individuals. *Journal of Applied Physiology* 89: 549-556.

Moseley, L., G.I. Lancaster, and A.E. Jeukendrup. 2003. Effects of timing of pre-exercise ingestion of carbohydrate on subsequent metabolism and cycling performance. *European Journal of Applied Physiology* 88: 453-458.

Moses, K., and M.M. Manore. 1991. Development and testing of a carbohydrate monitoring tool for athletes. *Journal of the American Dietetic Association* 91: 962-965.

Muckle, D.S. 1973. Glucose syrup ingestion and performance in soccer. *British Journal of Sports Medicine* 7: 340-343.

Muhlheim, L.S., D.B. Allison, S. Heshka, and S.B. Heymsfield. 1998. Do unsuccessful dieters intentionally underreport food intake? *International Journal of Eating Disorders* 24: 259-266.

Mujika, I., J.C. Chatard, L. Lacoste, F. Barale, and A. Geyssant. 1996. Creatine supplementation does not improve sprint performance in competitive swimmers. *Medicine and Science in Sports and Exercise* 28: 1435-1431.

Mujika, I., and S. Padilla. 2000a. Detraining: Loss of training-induced physiological and performance adaptations. Part I: Short term insufficient training stimulus. *Sports Medicine* 30: 79-87.

Mujika, I., and S. Padilla. 2000b. Detraining: Loss of training-induced physiological and performance adaptations. Part II: Long term insufficient training stimulus. *Sports Medicine* 30: 145-154.

Mujika, I., and S. Padilla. 2001. Physiological and performance characteristics of male professional road cyclists. *Sports Medicine* 31: 479-487.

Mujika, I., S. Padilla, J. Ibanez, M. Izquierdo, and E. Gorostiaga. 2000. Creatine supplementation and sprint performance in soccer players. *Medicine and Science in Sports and Exercise* 32: 518-525.

Müller, W. 2002. Unpublished report. *The Problem of Underweight Athletes: A Case Study of Ski Jumping.* Graz, Austria: University of Graz.

Mulligan, K., and G.E. Butterfield. 1990. Discrepancies between energy intake and expenditure in physically active women. *British Journal of Nutrition* 64: 23-36.

Mullins, V.A., L.B. Houtkooper, W.H. Howell, S.B. Going, and C.H. Brown. 2001. Nutritional status of US elite female heptathletes during training. *International Journal of Sport Nutrition and Exercise Metabolism* 11: 299-314.

Mustafa, K.Y., and N.E.A. Mahmoud. 1979. Evaporative water loss in African soccer players. *Journal of Sports Medicine* 19: 181-183.

Myerson, M., B. Gutin, M.P. Warren, M.T. May, I. Contento, M. Lee, F.X. Pi-Sunyer, R.N. Pierson, and J. Brooks-Gunn. 1991. Resting metabolic rate and energy balance in amenorrheic and eumenorrheic runners. *Medicine and Science in Sports and Exercise* 23: 15-22.

Nadel, E.R., G.W. Mack, and H. Nose. 1990. Influence of fluid replacement beverages on body fluid homeostasis during exercise and recovery. In *Perspectives in Exercise Science and Sports Medicine* (edited by C.V. Gisolfi and D.R. Lamb), pp. 181-205. Carmel, IN: Benchmark Press.

Nash, H.L. 1988. Sharing a water bottle: A dangerous practice? *The Physician and Sportsmedicine* 16: 29-30.

Nassis, G.P., C. Williams, and P. Chisnall. 1998. Effect of a carbohydrate-electrolyte drink on endurance capacity during prolonged intermittent high intensity running. *British Journal of Sports Medicine* 32: 248-252.

National Collegiate Athletic Association. 2003. *Wrestling Rules and Interpretations.* Indianapolis: NCAA.

Nattiv, A. 2002. New diagnostic criteria for female athlete triad syndrome? *British Journal of Sports Medicine* 36: 13.

Nattiv, A., and B.R. Mendelbaum. 1993. Injuries and special concerns in female gymnasts: Detecting, treating, and preventing common problems. *The Physician and Sportsmedicine* 21: 66-81.

Nehlsen-Cannarella, S.L., O.R. Fagoaga, D.C. Nieman, D.A. Henson, D.E. Butterworth, R.L. Schmitt, E.M. Bailey, B.J. Warren, A. Utter, and J.M. Davis. 1997. Carbohydrate and the cytokine response to 2.5 h of running. *Journal of Applied Physiology* 82: 1662-1667.

Neufer, P.D., D.L. Costill, M.G. Flynn, J.P. Kirwan, J.B. Mitchell, and J. Houmard. 1987. Improvements in exercise performance: Effects of carbohydrate feedings and diet. *Journal of Applied Physiology* 62: 983-988.

Nevill, M.E., L.H. Boobis, S. Brooks, and C. Williams. 1989. Effect of training on muscle metabolism during treadmill training. *Journal of Applied Physiology* 67: 2376-2382.

Nevill, M.E., C. Williams, D. Roper, C. Slater, and A.M. Nevill. 1993. Effect of diet on performance during recovery from intermittent sprint exercise. *Journal of Sports Sciences* 11: 119-126.

Newhouse, I.J., D.B. Clement, J.E. Taunton, and D.C. McKenzie. 1989. The effects of prelatent/latent iron deficiency on physical work capacity. *Medicine and Science in Sports and Exercise* 21: 263-268.

Nicholas, C.W. 2000. Sprinting. In *Nutrition in Sport* (edited by R.J. Maughan), pp. 535-549. Oxford, UK: Blackwell Science.

Nicholas, C.W., K. Tsintzas, L. Boobis, and C. Williams. 1999. Carbohydrate-electrolyte ingestion during intermittent high-intensity running. *Medicine and Science in Sports and Exercise* 31: 1280-1286.

Nicholas, C.W., C. Williams, H.K.A. Lakomy, G. Phillips, and A. Nowitz. 1995. Influence of ingesting a carbohydrate-electrolyte solution on endurance capacity during intermittent, high-intensity shuttle running. *Journal of Sports Sciences* 13: 283-290.

Nicklas, B.J., A.C. Hackney, and R.L. Sharp. 1989. The menstrual cycle and exercise: Performance, muscle glycogen, and substrate responses. *International Journal of Sports Medicine* 10: 264-269.

Niekamp, R.A., and J.T. Baer. 1995. In-season dietary adequacy of trained male cross-country runners. *International Journal of Sport Nutrition* 5: 45-55.

Nielsen, A.N., M. Mizuno, A. Ratkevicius, T. Mohr, M. Rohde, S.A. Mortensen, and B. Quistorff. 1999. No effect of antioxidant supplementation in triathletes on maximal oxygen uptake, 31P-NMRS detected muscle energy metabolism and muscle fatigue. *International Journal of Sports Medicine* 20: 154-158.

Nielsen, P., and D. Nachtigall. 1998. Iron supplementation in athletes: Current recommendations. *Sports Medicine* 26: 207-216.

Nieman, D.C., D.A. Henson, L.L. Smith, A.C. Utter, D.M. Vinci, J.M. Davis, D.E. Kaminsky, and M. Shute. 2001. Cytokine changes after a marathon race. *Journal of Applied Physiology* 91: 109-114.

Nikolopoulos, V., M.J. Arkinstall, and J.A. Hawley. 2004. Reduced neuromuscular activity with carbohydrate ingestion during constant load cycling. *International Journal of Sport Nutrition and Exercise Metabolism* 14: 161-170.

Niles, E.S., T. Lachowetz, J. Garfi, W. Sullivan, J.C. Smith, B.P. Leyh, and S.A. Headley. 2001. Carbohydrate-protein drink improves time to exhaustion after recovery from endurance exercise. *Journal of Exercise Physiology* [Online] 4: 45-52. Available http://faculty.css.edu/tboone2/asep/fldr/fldr.htm [accessed September 7, 2006].

Nissen, S.L., and R.L. Sharp. 2003. Effect of dietary supplements on lean mass and strength gains with resistance exercise: A meta-analysis. *Journal of Applied Physiology* 94: 651-659.

Nissen, S., R. Sharp, M. Ray, J.A. Rathmacher, D. Rice, J.C. Fuller, A.S. Connelly, and N. Abumrad. 1996. Effect of leucine metabolite ß-hydroxy-ß-methylbutyrate on muscle metabolism during resistance-exercise training. *Journal of Applied Physiology* 81: 2095-2104.

Noakes, T.D. 1997. Challenging beliefs: Ex Africa semper aliquid novi. *Medicine and Science in Sports and Exercise* 29: 571-590.

Noakes, T.D. 2002. IMMDA advisory statement of guidelines for fluid replacement during marathon running. *New Studies in Athletics: The IAAF Technical Quarterly* 17: 15-24.

Noakes, T.D. 2003a. *Lore of Running*. Champaign, IL: Human Kinetics.

Noakes, T.D. 2003b. Overconsumption of fluid by athletes. *British Medical Journal* 327: 113-114.

Noakes, T.D., B.A. Adams, K.H. Myburgh, C. Greeff, T. Lotz, and M. Nathan. 1988. The danger of an inadequate water intake during prolonged exercise. *European Journal of Applied Physiology* 57: 210-219.

Noakes, T.D., J.R. Cowling, W. Gevers, and J.P. Van Nierkark. 1982. The metabolic responses to squash including the influence of pre-exercise carbohydrate ingestion. *South African Medical Journal* 62: 721-723.

Noakes, T.D., N.J. Rehrer, and R.J. Maughan. 1991. The importance of volume in regulating gastric emptying. *Medicine and Science in Sports and Exercise* 23: 307-313.

Noakes, T.D., K. Sharwood, D. Speedy, T. Hew, S. Reid, J. Dugas, C. Almond, P. Wharam, and L. Weschler. 2005. Three independent biological mechanisms cause exercise-associated hyponatremia: Evidence from 2,135 weight competitive athletic performance. *Proceedings of the National Academy of Science* 102: 18550-18555.

Noakes, T.D., and D.B. Speedy. 2006. Case proven: exercise associated hyponatraemia is due to overdrinking. So why did it take 20 years before the original evidence was accepted? *British Journal of Sports Medicine* 40: 567-572.

Nobes, K.J., D.L. Montgomery, D.J. Pearsall, R.A. Turcotte, R. Lefebvre, and F. Whittom. 2003. A comparison of skating economy on-ice and on the skating treadmill. *Canadian Journal of Applied Physiology* 28: 1-11.

Noonan, D., K. Berg, R.W. Latin, J.C. Wagner, and K. Reimers. 1998. Effect of varying dosages of oral creatine relative to fat free body mass on strength and body composition. *Journal of Strength and Conditioning Research* 12: 104-108.

Nose, H., G.W. Mack, X.R. Shi, and E.R. Nadel. 1988. Role of osmolality and plasma volume during rehydration in humans. *Journal of Applied Physiology* 61: 325-331.

Nowak, R.K., K.S. Knudsen, and L.O. Schulz. 1988. Body composition and nutrient intakes of college men and women basketball players. *Journal of the American Dietetic Association* 88: 575-578.

Nutter, J. 1991. Seasonal changes in female athletes' diets. *International Journal of Sport Nutrition* 1: 395-407.

Nybo, L., and B. Nielsen. 2001. Hyperthermia and central fatigue during prolonged exercise in humans. *Journal of Applied Physiology* 91: 1055-1060.

Nygaard, E., P. Andersen, P. Nilsson, E. Eriksson, T. Kjessel, and B. Saltin. 1978. Glycogen depletion pattern and lactate accumulation in leg muscles during recreactional downhill skiing. *European Journal of Applied Physiology and Occupational Physiology* 38: 261-269.

O'Brien, C.P. 1993. Alcohol and sport: Impact of social drinking on recreational and competitive sports performance. *Sports Medicine* 15: 71-77.

O'Connor, D.M., and M.J. Crowe. 2003. Effects of beta-hydroxy-beta-methylbutyrate and creatine monohydrate on aerobic and anaerobic capacity of highly trained athletes. *Journal of Sports Medicine and Physical Fitness* 41: 64-68.

O'Connor, P.J., R.D. Lewis, and E.M. Kirchner. 1995. Eating disorder symptoms in female college gymnasts. *Medicine and Science in Sports and Exercise* 27: 550-555.

O'Keeffe, K.A., R.E. Keith, G.D. Wilson, and D.L. Blessing. 1989. Dietary carbohydrate intake and endurance exercise performance of trained female cyclists. *Nutrition Research* 9: 819-830.

Oliver, S.K., and M.S. Tremblay. 2002. Effects of a sports nutrition bar on endurance running performance. *Journal of Strength and Conditioning Research* 16: 152-156.

Onywera, V.O., F.K. Kiplamai, P.J. Tuitoek, M.K. Boit, and Y.P. Pitsiladis. 2004. Food and macronutrient intake of elite Kenyan distance runners. *International Journal of Sport Nutrition and Exercise Metabolism* 14: 709-719.

Oopik, V., M. Paasuke, T. Sikku, S. Timpmann, L. Medijainen, J. Ereline, T. Smirnova, and E. Gapejeva. 1996. Effect of rapid weight loss on metabolism and isokinetic performance capacity. A case study of two well trained wrestlers. *Journal of Sports Medicine and Physical Fitness* 36: 127-131.

Oopik, V., M. Paasuke, S. Timpmann, L. Medijainen, J. Ereline, and J. Gapejeva. 2002. Effect of creatine supplementation during recovery from rapid body mass reduction on metabolism and muscle performance capacity in well-trained wrestlers. *Journal of Sports Medicine and Physical Fitness* 42: 330-339.

Oopik, V., M. Paasuke, S. Timpmann, L. Medijainen, J. Ereline, and T. Smirnova. 1998. Effect of creatine supplementation during rapid body mass reduction on metabolism and isokinetic muscle performance capacity. *European Journal of Applied Physiology* 78: 83-92.

Oopik, V., I. Saaremets, L. Medijainen, K. Karelson, T. Janson, and S. Timpmann. 2003. Effects of sodium citrate ingestion before exercise on endurance performance in well-trained runners. *British Journal of Sports Medicine* 37: 485-489.

Oopik, V., I. Saaremets, S. Timpmann, L. Medijainen, and K. Karelson. 2004. Effects of acute ingestion of sodium citrate on metabolism and 5 km running performance: A field study. *Canadian Journal of Applied Physiology* 29: 691-703.

Op 't Eijnde, B., M. van Leemputte, F. Brouns, G.J. Van Der Vusse, V. Larbarque, M. Ramaekers, R. van Schuylenberg, P. Verbessem, H. Wijnen, and P. Hespel. 2001. No effects of oral ribose supplementation on repeated maximal exercise and ATP resynthesis. *Journal of Applied Physiology* 91: 2274-2281.

Op 't Eijnde, B., L. Vergauwen, and P. Hespel. 2001. Creatine loading does not impact on stroke performance in tennis. *International Journal of Sports Medicine* 22: 76-80.

Oppliger, R.A., R.D. Harms, D.E. Herrmann, C.M. Streich, and R.R. Clark. 1995. The Wisconsin wrestling minimum weight project: A model for weight control among high school wrestlers. *Medicine and Science in Sports and Exercise* 27(8): 1220-1224.

Oppliger, R.A., G.L. Landry, S.W. Foster, and A.C. Lambrecht. 1998. Wisconsin minimum weight program reduces weight-cutting practices of high school wrestlers. *Clinical Journal of Sports Medicine* 8: 26-31.

Oppliger, R.A., S.N. Steen, and J.R. Scott. 2003. Weight loss practices of college wrestlers. *International Journal of Sport Nutrition and Exercise Metabolism* 13: 29-46.

Orvanova, E. 1987. Physical structure of winter sports athletes. *Journal of Sports Science* 5: 197-248.

Ostojic, S.M. 2004. Creatine supplementation in young soccer players. *International Journal of Sport Nutrition and Exercise Metabolism* 14: 95-103.

Ostojic, S.M., and S. Mazic. 2002. Effects of a carbohydrate-electrolyte drink on specific soccer tests and performance. *Journal of Sports Science and Medicine* 1: 47-53.

O'Sullivan, S., R.L. Sharp, and D.S. King. 1994. Carbohydrate ingestion during competitive swimming training. *Journal of Swimming Research* 10: 35-40.

Otis, C.L., B. Drinkwater, M. Johnson, A. Loucks, and J. Wilmore. 1997. American College of Sports Medicine position stand. The female athlete triad. *Medicine and Science in Sports and Exercise* 29: i-ix.

Ousley-Pahnke, L., D.R. Black, and R.J. Gretebeck. 2001. Dietary intake and energy expenditure of female collegiate swimmers during decreased training prior to competition. *Journal of the American Dietetic Association* 101: 351-354.

Paddon-Jones, D., A. Keech, and D. Jenkins. 2001. Short-term β-hydroxy-β-methylbutyrate supplementation does not reduce symptoms of eccentric muscle damage. *International Journal of Sport Nutrition and Exercise Metabolism* 11: 442-450.

Palmer, G.S., M.C. Clancy, J.A. Hawley, I.M. Rodger, and L.M. Burke. 1998. Carbohydrate ingestion immediately before exercise does not improve 20 km time trial performance in well trained cyclists. *International Journal of Sports Medicine* 19: 415-418.

Palmer, T.N., E.B. Cook, and P.G. Drake. 1991. Alcohol abuse and fuel homeostasis. In *Alcoholism: A Molecular Perspective* (edited by T.N. Palmer), pp. 223-235. New York: Plenum Press.

Panton, L.B., J.A. Rathmacher, S. Baier, and S. Nissen. 2000. Nutritional supplementation of the leucine metabolite beta-hydroxy-beta-methylbutyrate (hmb) during resistance training. *Nutrition* 16: 734-739.

Papadopoulou, S.K., S.D. Papadopoulou, and G.K. Gallos. 2002. Macro- and micro-nutrient intake of adolescent Greek female volleyball players. *International Journal of Sport Nutrition and Exercise Metabolism* 12: 73-80.

Parasrampuria, J., K. Schwartz, and R. Petesch. 1998. Quality control of dehydroepiandrosterone dietary supplement products. *Journal of the American Medical Association* 280: 1565.

Parcell, A.C., J.M. Smith, S.S. Schulthies, J.W. Myrer, and G. Fellingham. 2004. Cordyceps Sinensis (CordyMax Cs-4) supplementation does not improve endurance exercise performance. *International Journal of Sport Nutrition and Exercise Metabolism* 14: 236-242.

Parkin, J.A.M., M.F. Carey, I.K. Martin, L. Stojanovska, and M.A. Febbraio. 1997. Muscle glycogen storage following prolonged exercise: effect of timing of ingestion of high glycemic index food. *Medicine and Science in Sports and Exercise* 29: 220-224.

Parr, M.K., H. Geyer, G. Sigmund, K. Kohler, and W. Schanzer. 2003. Screening of nutritional supplements for stimulants and other drugs. In *Recent Advances in Doping Analysis, Vol. 11* (edited by W. Schanzer, H. Geyer, A. Gotzmann, and U. Mareck-Engelke), pp. 67-75. Koln, Germany: Sport und Buch Stauss.

Paschoal, V.C.P., and O.M.S. Amancio. 2004. Nutritional status of Brazilian elite swimmers. *International Journal of Sport Nutrition and Exercise Metabolism* 14: 81-94.

Pasman, W.J., M.A. van Baak, A.E. Jeukendrup, and A. de Haan. 1995. The effect of different dosages of caffeine on endurance performance time. *International Journal of Sports Medicine* 16: 225-230.

Passe, D.H., M. Horn, and R. Murray. 2000. Impact of beverage acceptability on fluid intake during exercise. *Appetite* 35: 219-229.

Paton, C.D., W.G. Hopkins, and L. Vollebregt. 2001. Little effect of caffeine ingestion on repeated sprints in team-sport athletes. *Medicine and Science in Sports and Exercise* 33: 822-825.

Paul, D.R., S.M. Mulroy, J.A. Horner, K.A. Jacobs, and D.R. Lamb. 2001. Carbohydrate-loading during the follicular phase of the menstrual cycle: Effects on muscle glucogen and exercise performance. *International Journal of Sport Nutrition and Exercise Metabolism* 11: 430-441.

Pearson, D.R., D.G. Hamby, W. Russel, and T. Harris. 1999. Long-term effects of creatine monohydrate on strength and power. *Journal of Strength and Conditioning Research* 13: 187-192.

Pedersen, B.K., H. Bruunsgaard, M. Jensen, A.D. Toft, H. Hansen, and K. Ostrowski. 1999. Exercise and the immune system—Influence of nutrition and ageing. *Journal of Science and Medicine in Sport* 2: 234-252.

Peeters, B.M., C.D. Lantz, and J.L. Mayhew. 1999. Effect of oral creatine monohydrate and creatine phosphate supplementation on maximal strength indices, body composition, and blood pressure. *Journal of Strength and Conditioning Research* 13: 3-9.

Perharic, L., D. Shaw, M. Collbridge, I. House, C. Leon, and V. Murray. 1994. Toxicological problems resulting from exposure to traditional remedies and food supplements. *Drug Safety* 11: 284-294.

Perrottet, T. 2004. *The Naked Olympics*. New York: Random House.

Peters, H.P.F., L.M.A. Akkermans, and W.R. De Vries. 2001. Gastrointestinal symptoms during prolonged exercise: Incidence, etiology, and recommendations. *American Journal of Medicine and Sports* 3: 94-101, 106.

Petersen, H.L., C.T. Peterson, M.B. Reddy, K.B. Hanson, J.H. Swain, R.L. Sharp, and D.L. Alekel. 2006. Body composition, dietary intake, and iron status of female collegiate swimmers and divers. *International Journal of Sport Nutrition and Exercise Metabolism* 16: 281-295.

Peyrebrune, M.C., M.E. Nevill, F.J. Donaldson, and D.J. Cosford. 1998. The effects of oral creatine supplementation on performance in single and repeated sprint swimming. *Journal of Sports Sciences* 16: 271-279.

Peyrebrune, M.C., K. Stokes, G.M. Hall, and M.E. Nevill. 2005. Effect of creatine supplementation on training for competition in elite swimmers. *Medicine and Science in Sports and Exercise* 37: 2140-2147.

Phillips, S.M., J.W. Hartman, and S.B. Wilkinson. 2005. Dietary protein to support anabolism with resistance exercise in young men. *Journal of the American College of Nutrition* 24: 134S-139S.

Phillips, S.M., G. Parise, B.D. Roy, K.D. Tipton, R.R. Wolfe, and M.A. Tarnopolsky. 2002. Resistance-training-induced adaptations in skeletal muscle protein turnover in the fed state. *Canadian Journal of Physiology and Pharmacology* 80: 1045-1053.

Phillips, S.M., K.D. Tipton, A. Aarsland, S.E. Wolf, and R.R. Wolfe. 1997. Mixed muscle protein synthesis and breakdown after resistance exercise in humans. *American Journal of Physiology Endocrinology and Metabolism* 273: E99-E107.

Phillips, S.M., K.D. Tipton, A.A. Ferrando, and R.R. Wolfe. 1999. Resistance training reduces the acute exercise-induced increase in muscle protein turnover. *American Journal of Physiology. Endocrinology and Metabolism* 276: E118-E124.

Phinney, S.D., B.R. Bistrian, W.J. Evans, E. Gervino, and G.L. Blackburn. 1983. The human metabolic response to chronic ketosis without caloric restriction: Preservation of submaximal exercise capacity with reduced carbohydrate oxidation. *Metabolism* 32: 769-776.

Piehl, K. 1974. Time course for refilling of glycogen stores in human muscle fibres following exercise-induced glycogen depletion. *Acta Physiologica Scandinavica* 90: 297-302.

Pieralisi, G., P. Ripari, and L. Vecchiet. 1991. Effects of a standardized ginseng extract combined with dimethylaminoethanol bitartrate, vitamins, minerals, and trace elements on physical performance during exercise. *Clinical Therapeutics* 13: 373-382.

Pierce, E.F., N.W. Eastman, W.H. Hammer, and T.D. Lynn. 1992. Effect of induced alkalosis on swimming time trials. *Journal of Sports Sciences* 10: 255-259.

Pilegaard, H., T. Osada, L.T. Andersen, J.W. Helge, B. Saltin, and P.D. Neufer. 2005. Substrate availability and transcriptional regulation of metabolic genes in human skeletal muscle during recovery from exercise. *Metabolism* 54: 1048-1055.

Pitsiladis, Y.P., C. Duignan, and R.J. Maughan. 1996. Effects of alterations in dietary carbohydrate intake on running performance during a 10 km treadmill time trial. *British Journal of Sports Medicine* 30: 226-231.

Pluim, B.M., A. Ferrauti, F. Broekhof, M. Deutekom, A. Gotzmann, H. Kuipers, and K. Weber. 2006. The effects of creatine supplementation on selected factors of tennis specific training. *British Journal of Sports Medicine* 40: 507-512.

Pohl, A.P., M.W. O'Halloran, and P.R. Pannall. 1981. Biochemical and physiological changes in football players. *Medical Journal of Australia* 1: 467-470.

Potteiger, J.A., M.J. Webster, G.K. Nickel, M.D. Haub, and R.J. Palmer. 1996. The effects of buffer ingestion on metabolic factors related to distance running performance. *European Journal of Applied Physiology* 72: 365-371.

Powell, P.D., and A. Tucker. 1991. Iron supplementation and running performance in female cross-country runners. *International Journal of Sports Medicine* 12: 462-467.

Preen, D., B. Dawson, C. Goodman, J. Beilby, and S. Ching. 2003. Creatine supplementation: A comparison of loading and maintenance protocols on creatine uptake by human skeletal muscle. *International Journal of Sport Nutrition and Exercise Metabolism* 13: 97-111.

Preen, D., B. Dawson, C. Goodman, S. Lawrence, J. Beilby, and S. Ching. 2001. Effect of creatine loading on long-term sprint exercise performance and metabolism. *Medicine and Science in Sports and Exercise* 33: 814-821.

Price, M., P. Moss, and S. Rance. 2003. Effects of sodium bicarbonate ingestion on prolonged intermittent exercise. *Medicine and Science in Sports and Exercise* 38: 1303-1308.

Proctor, K.L., W.C. Adams, J.D. Shaffrath, and M.D. Van Loan. 2002. Upper-limb bone mineral density of female collegiate gymnasts versus controls. *Medicine and Science in Sports and Exercise* 34: 1830-1835.

Prouteau, S., A. Pelle, K. Collomp, L. Benhamou, and D. Courteix. 2006. Bone density in elite judoists and effects of weight cycling on bone metabolic balance. *Medicine and Science in Sports and Exercise* 38: 694-700.

Pyke, F.S., and A.G. Hahn. 1980. Body temperature regulation in summer football. *Sports Coach* 4: 41-43.

Pyne, D.B., M.E. Anderson, and W.G. Hopkins. 2006. Monitoring changes in lean mass of elite male and female swimmers. *International Journal of Sports Physiology and Performance* 1: 14-26.

Rankinen, T., S. Lyytikainen, E. Vanninen, I. Penttila, R. Rauramaa, and M. Uusitupa. 1998. Nutritional status of the Finnish elite ski jumpers. *Medicine and Science in Sports and Exercise* 30: 1592-1597.

Ransone, J., K. Neighbours, R. Lefavi, and J. Chromiak. 2003. The effect of β-hydroxy β-methylbutyrate on muscular strength and body composiiton in collegiate football players. *Journal of Strength and Conditioning Research* 17: 34-39.

Rasmussen, B.B., K.D. Tipton, S.L. Miller, S.E. Wolf, and R.R. Wolfe. 2000. An oral essential amino acid-carbohydrate supplement enhances muscle protein anabolism after resistance exercise. *Journal of Applied Physiology* 88: 386-392.

Rauch, H.G.L., J.A. Hawley, M. Woodey, T.D. Noakes, and S.C. Dennis. 1999. Effects of ingesting a sports bar versus glucose polymer on substrate utilisation and ultra-endurance performance. *International Journal of Sports Medicine* 20: 252-257.

Rawson, E.S., and J.S. Volek. 2003. Effects of creatine supplementation and resistance training on muscle strength and weightlifting performance. *Journal of Strength and Conditioning Research* 17: 822-831.

Ray, M.L., M.W. Bryan, T.M. Ruden, S.M. Baier, R.L. Sharp, and D.S. King. 1998. Effect of sodium in a rehydration beverage when consumed as a fluid or meal. *Journal of Applied Physiology* 85: 1329-1336.

Redondo, D.R., E.A. Dowling, B.L. Graham, A.L. Almada, and M.H. Williams. 1996. The effect of oral creatine monohydrate supplementation running velocity. *International Journal of Sport Nutrition* 6: 213-221.

Reed, M.J., J.T. Brozinick, M.C. Lee, and J.L. Ivy. 1989. Muscle glycogen storage postexercise: Effect of mode of carbohydrate administration. *Journal of Applied Physiology* 66: 720-726.

Reeves, S., and K. Collins. 2003. The nutritional and anthropometric status of Gaelic football players. *International Journal of Sport Nutrition and Exercise Metabolism* 13: 539-548.

Reggiani, E., G.B. Arras, S. Trabacca, D. Senarega, and G. Chiodini. 1989. Nutritional status and body composition of adolescent female gymnasts. *Journal of Sports Medicine and Physical Fitness* 29: 285-258.

Rehrer, N.J., E.J. Beckers, F. Brouns, F. Ten Hoor, and W.H.M. Saris. 1990. Effects of dehydration on gastric emptying and gastrointestinal distress while running. *Medicine and Science in Sports and Exercise* 22: 790-795.

Rehrer, N.J., M. Van Kemenade, W. Meester, F. Brouns, and W.H.M. Saris. 1992. Gastrointestinal complaints in relation to dietary intake in triathletes. *International Journal of Sport Nutrition* 2: 48-59.

Reilly, T. 1990a. Football. In *Physiology of Sports* (edited by T. Reilly, N. Secher, P. Snell, and C. Williams), pp. 371-426. London: E & FN Spon.

Reilly, T. 1990b. The racquet sports. In *Physiology of Sports* (edited by T. Reilly, N. Secher, P. Snell, and C. Williams), pp. 337-369. London: E & FN Spon.

Reilly, T., and V. Thomas. 1976. A motion analysis of work rate in different positional roles in professional football match-play. *Journal of Human Movement Studies* 2: 87-97.

Reilly, T., and V. Woodbridge. 1999. Effects of moderate dietary manipulations on swim performance and on blood lactate-swimming velocity curves. *International Journal of Sports Medicine* 20: 93-97.

Richardson, R.S., A.T. White, J.D. Seifert, J.M. Porretta, and S.C. Johnson. 1993. Blood lactate concentrations in elite skiers during a series of on-snow downhill ski runs. *Journal of Strength and Conditioning Research* 7: 168-171.

Richter, E.A., K.J. Mikines, H. Galbo, and B. Kiens. 1989. Effects of exercise on insulin action in human skeletal muscle. *Journal of Applied Physiology* 66: 876-885.

Rico-Sanz, J. 1998. Body composition and nutritional assessments in soccer. *International Journal of Sport Nutrition* 8: 113-123.

Rico-Sanz, J., W.R. Frontera, P.A. Mole, M.A. Rivera, A. Rivera-Brown, and C.N. Meredith. 1998. Dietary and performance assessment of elite soccer players during a period of intense training. *International Journal of Sport Nutrition* 8: 230-240.

Rico-Sanz, J., W.R. Frontera, M.A. Rivera, A. Rivera-Brown, P.A. Mole, and C.N. Meredith. 1996. Effects of hyperhydration on total body water, temperature regulation and performance of elite young soccer players in a warm climate. *International Journal of Sports Medicine* 17: 85-91.

Rico-Sanz, J., M. Zehnder, R. Buchli, M. Dambach, and U. Boutellier. 1999. Muscle glycogen degradation during simulation of a fatiguing soccer match in elite soccer players examined noninvasively by 13C-MRS. *Medicine and Science in Sports and Exercise* 31: 1587-1593.

Rintamäki, H., T. Makinen, J. Oksa, and J. Latvala. 1995. Water balance and physical performance in cold. *Arctic Medical Research* 54 (suppl 2): 32-36.

Risser, W.L., E.J. Lee, A. Leblanc, H.B.W. Poindexter, J.M.H. Risser, and V. Schneider. 1990. Bone density in eumenorrheic female college athletes. *Medicine and Science in Sports and Exercise* 22: 570-574.

Robergs, R.A., and S.E. Griffin. 1998. Glycerol: biochemistry, pharmacokinetics and clinical and practical applications. *Sports Medicine* 26: 145-167.

Robergs, R.A., S.B. McMinn, C. Mermier, G. Leadbetter, B. Ruby, and C. Quinn. 1998. Blood glucose and glucoregulatory hormone responses to solid and liquid carbohydrate ingestion during exercise. *International Journal of Sport Nutrition* 8: 70-83.

Robergs, R.A., D.R. Pearson, D.L. Costill, W.J. Fink, D.D. Pascoe, M.A. Benedict, C.P. Lambert, and J.J. Zachwieja. 1991. Muscle glycogenolysis during differing intensities of weight-resistance exercise. *Journal of Applied Physiology* 70: 1700-1706.

Roberts, D., and D. Smith. 1990. Serum ferritin values in elite speed and synchronized swimmers and speed skaters. *Journal of Laboratory and Clinical Medicine* 116: 661-665.

Roberts, D., and D.J. Smith. 1992. Training at moderate altitude: Iron status of elite male swimmers. *Journal of Laboratory and Cinical Medicine* 120: 387-391.

Robertson, J.D., R.J. Maughan, A.C. Milne, and R.L.J. Davidson. 1992. Hematological status of male runners in relation to the extent of physical training. *International Journal of Sport Nutrition* 2: 366-375.

Robinson, T.A., J.A. Hawley, G.S. Palmer, G.R. Wilson, D.A. Gray, T.D. Noakes, and S.C. Dennis. 1995. Water ingestion does not improve 1-h cycling performance in moderate ambient temperatures. *European Journal of Applied Physiology* 14: 153-160.

Robinson, T.M., D.A. Sewell, E. Hultman, and P.L. Greenhaff. 1999. Role of submaximal exercise in promoting creatine and glycogen accumulation in human skeletal muscle. *Journal of Applied Physiology* 87: 598-604.

Rockwell, J.A., J. Walberg-Rankin, and B. Toderico. 2001. Creatine supplementation affects muscle creatine during energy restriction. *Medicine and Science in Sports and Exercise* 33: 61-68.

Rockwell, M.S., J. Walberg-Rankin, and H. Dixon. 2003. Effects of muscle glycogen on performance on repeated sprints and mechanisms of fatigue. *International Journal of Sport Nutrition and Exercise Metabolism* 13: 1-14.

Roemmich, J.N., R.J. Richmond, and A.D. Rogol. 2001. Consequences of sport training during puberty. *Journal of Endocrinological Investigation* 24: 708-715.

Roemmich, J.N., and W.E. Sinning. 1996. Sport-seasonal changes in body composition, growth, power and strength of adolescent wrestlers. *International Journal of Sports Medicine* 17: 92-99.

Roemmich, J.N., and W.E. Sinning. 1997a. Weight loss and wrestling training: Effects on growth-related hormones. *Journal of Applied Physiology* 82: 1760-1764.

Roemmich, J.N., and W.E. Sinning. 1997b. Weight loss and wrestling training: effects on nutrition, growth, maturation, body composition, and strength. *Journal of Applied Physiology* 82: 1751-1759.

Romer, L.M., J.P. Barrington, and A.E. Jeukendrup. 2001. Effects of oral creatine supplementation on high intensity, intermittent exercise performance in competitive squash players. *International Journal of Sports Medicine* 22: 546-552.

Ronsen, O., J. Sundgot-Borgen, and S. Maehlum. 1999. Supplement use and nutritional habits in Norwegian elite athletes. *Scandinavian Journal of Medicine and Science in Sports* 9: 28-35.

Ros, J.J., M.G. Pelders, and P.A. de Smet. 1999. A case of positive doping associated with a botanical food supplement. *Pharmaceutical World Science* 21: 44-46.

Rosen, L.W., D.B. McKeag, D.O. Hough, and V. Curley. 1986. Pathogenic weight-control behaviour in female athletes. *The Physician and Sportsmedicine* 14: 79-86.

Rossiter, H.B., E.R. Cannell, and P.M. Jakeman. 1996. The effect of oral creatine supplementation on the 1000-m performance of competitive rowers. *Journal of Sports Sciences* 14: 175-179.

Roufs, J.B. 1992. Review of L-tryptophan and eosinophilia-myalgia syndrome. *Journal of the American Dietetic Association* 92: 844-850.

Rowlands, D.S., and W.G. Hopkins. 2002. Effects of high-fat and high-carbohydrate diets on metabolism and performance in cycling. *Metabolism* 51: 678-690.

Roy, B.D., and M.A. Tarnopolsky. 1998. Influence of differing macronutrient intakes on muscle glycogen resynthesis after resistance exercise. *Journal of Applied Physiology* 84: 890-896.

Roy, B.D., M.A. Tarnopolsky, J.D. MacDougall, J. Fowles, and K.E. Yarasheski. 1997. Effect of glucose supplement timing on protein metabolism after resistance training. *Journal of Applied Physiology* 82: 1882-1888.

Ruddel, H., C. Werner, and H. Ising. 1990. Impact of magnesium supplementation on performance data in young swimmers. *Magnesium Research* 3: 103-107.

Rusko, H. 2003a. Training for cross-country skiing. In *Handbook of Sports Medicine and Science—Cross-Country Skiing* (edited by H. Rusko), pp. 62-100. Oxford, UK: Blackwell Science.

Rusko, H. 2003b. Physiology of cross country skiing. In *Handbook of Sports Medicine and Science—Cross-country skiing* (edited by H. Rusko), pp. 1-31. Oxford, UK: Blackwell Science Ltd.

Ryan, A.J. 1981. Anabolic steroids are fool's gold. *Federation Proceedings* 40: 2682-2688.

Sahlin, K. 1992. Metabolic factors in fatigue. *Sports Medicine* 13: 99-107.

Saltin, B. 1973. Metabolic fundamentals in exercise. *Medicine and Science in Sports and Exercise* 5: 137-146.

Saltin, B. 1978. Fluid, electrolyte and energy losses and their replenishment in prolonged exercise. In *Nutrition, Physical Fitness and Health* (edited by J. Parizkova and V.A. Rogozkin), pp. 76-97. Baltimore: University Park Press.

Saltin, B. 1997. The physiology of competitive cross-country skiing across a four decade perspective: With a note on training induced adaptations and role of training at medium altitude. In *1st International Congress on Skiing and Science* (edited by E. Müller, H. Schwameder, E. Kornexl, and C. Raschner), pp. 435-469. St. Christoph, Austria: Chapman & Hall, UK.

Sandoval, W.M., V.H. Heyward, and T.M. Lyons. 1989. Comparison of body composition, exercise and nutritional profiles of female and male body builders at competition. *Journal of Sports Medicine and Physical Fitness* 29: 63-70.

Saris, W.H.M., M.A. Van Erp-Baart, F. Brouns, K.R. Westerterp, and F. Ten Hoor. 1989. Study on food intake and energy expenditure during extreme sustained exercise: The Tour de France. *International Journal of Sports Medicine* 10: S26-S31.

Sasaki, H., J. Maeda, S. Usui, and T. Ishiko. 1987. Effect of sucrose and caffeine ingestion on performance of prolonged strenuous running. *International Journal of Sports Medicine* 8: 261-265.

Saunders, A.G., J.P. Dugas, R. Tucker, M.I. Lambert, and T.D. Noakes. 2005. The effects of different air velocities on heat storage and body temperature in humans cycling in a hot, humid environment. *Acta Physiologica Scandinavica* 183: 241-255.

Saunders, M.J., M.D. Kane, and M.K. Todd. 2004. Effects of a carbohydrate-protein beverage on cycling endurance and muscle damage. *Medicine and Science in Sports and Exercise* 36: 1233-1238.

Sawka, M.N., and K.B. Pandolf. 1990. Effects of body water loss on physiological function and exercise performance. In *Perspectives in Exercise Science and Sports Medicine* (edited by C.V. Gisolfi and D.R. Lamb), pp. 1-38. Carmel, IN: Benchmark Press.

Schabort, E.J., G. Wilson, and T.D. Noakes. 2000. Dose-related elevations in venous pH with citrate ingestion do not alter 40-km cycling time-trial performance. *European Journal of Applied Physiology* 83: 320-327.

Schedel, J.M., P. Terrier, and Y. Schutz. 2000. The biomechanic origin of sprint performance enhancement after one-week creatine supplementation. *Japanese Journal of Physiology* 50: 273-276.

Schena, F., A. Pattini, and S. Mantovanelli. 1995. Iron status in athletes involved in endurance and prevalently anaerobic sports. In *Sports Nutrition: Minerals and Electrolytes* (edited by C.V. Kies and J.A. Driskell), pp. 65-79. Boca Raton, FL: CRC Press.

Schmidt, W.D., D. Corrigan, and C.L. Melby. 1993. Two seasons of weight cycling does not lower resting metabolic rate in college wrestlers. *Medicine and Science in Sports and Exercise* 25: 613-619.

Schneiker, K.T., D. Bishop, B. Dawson, and L.P. Hackett. 2006. Effects of caffeine on prolonged intermittent-sprint ability in team-sport athletes. *Medicine and Science in Sports and Exercise* 38: 578-585.

Schoeller, D.A. 1995. Limitations in the assessment of dietary energy intake by self-report. *Metabolism* 44: 18-22.

Schoeller, D.A., E. Ravussin, Y. Schutz, K.J. Acheson, P. Baertschi, and E. Jequier. 1986. Energy expenditure by doubly labeled water: Validation in humans and proposed calculation. *American Journal of Physiology Regulatory, Integrative and Comparative Physiology* 250: R823-R830.

Schoene, R.B., P. Escourrou, H.T. Robertson, K.L. Nilson, J.R. Parsons, and N.J. Smith. 1983. Iron repletion decreases maximal exercise lactate concentrations in female athletes with minimal iron-deficiency anemia. *Journal of Laboratory and Clinical Medicine* 102: 306-312.

Schofield, W.N., C. Schofield, and W.P.T. James. 1985. Basal metabolic rate—Review and prediction, together with an annotated bibliography of source material. *Human Nutrition Applied Nutrition* 39C: 1-96.

Schroder, H., E. Navarro, J. Mora, D. Galiano, and A. Tramullas. 2001. Effects of alpha-tocopherol, beta-carotene and ascorbic acid on oxidative, hormonal and enzymatic exercise stress markers in habitual training activity of professional basketball players. *European Journal of Nutrition* 40: 178-184.

Schroder, H., E. Navarro, A. Tramullas, J. Mora, and D. Galiano. 2000. Nutrition antioxidant status and oxidative stress in professional basketball players: Effects of a three compound antioxidative supplement. *International Journal of Sports Medicine* 21: 146-150.

Schulz, L.O., S. Alger, I. Harper, J.H. Wilmore, and E. Ravussin. 1992. Energy expenditure of elite female runners measured by respiratory chamber and doubly labeled water. *Journal of Applied Physiology* 72: 23-28.

Schwameder, H., E. Müller, C. Raschner, and F. Brunner. 1997. Aspects of technique—Specific strength training in ski jumping. In *1st International Congress on Skiing and Science* (edited by E. Müller, H. Schwameder, E. Kornexl, and C. Raschner), pp. 309-319. St. Christoph, Austria: Chapman & Hall, UK.

Schwellnus, M.P., E.W. Derman, and T.D. Noakes. 1997. Aetiology of skeletal muscle 'cramps' during exercise: a novel hypothesis. *Journal of Sport Sciences* 15: 277-285.

Schwellnus, M.P., J. Nicol, R. Laubscher, and T.D. Noakes. 2004. Serum electrolyte concentrations and hydration status are not associated with exercise associated muscle cramping (EAMC) in distance runners. *British Journal of Sports Medicine* 38: 488-492.

Scott, J.R., R.A. Oppliger, A.C. Utter, and C.G. Kerr. 2000. Body weight changes at the national tournaments—The impact of rules governing wrestling weight management [abstract]. *Medicine and Science in Sports and Exercise* 32 (5 suppl): S131.

Sears, B. 1995. *The Zone: A Dietary Road Map to Lose Weight Permanently, Reset Your Genetic Code, Prevent Disease, Achieve Maximum Physical Performance*. New York: HarperCollins Publishers.

Sears, B. 1997. *Mastering the Zone. The Next Step in Achieving SuperHealth and Permanent Fat Loss.* New York: HarperCollins Publishers.

Sears, B. 2000. The Zone diet and athletic performance [letter to editor]. *Sports Medicine* 29: 289-294.

Seifert, J.G., M.J. Luetkemeier, A.T. White, and L.M. Mino. 1998. The physiological effects of beverage ingestion during cross country ski training in elite collegiate skiers. *Canadian Journal of Applied Physiology* 23: 66-73.

Seifert, J.G., M.J. Lutkemeier, A.T. White, L.M. Mino, and D. Miller. 2000. Fluid balance during slalom training in elite collegiate alpine racers. In *2nd International Congress on Skiing and Science* (edited by E. Müller, H. Schwameder, C. Raschner, S. Lindinger, and E. Kornexl), pp. 634-640. St. Christoph, Austria: Verlag Dr. Kovac.

Selby, G.B., and E.R. Eichner. 1986. Endurance swimming, intravascular hemolysis, anemia, and iron depletion: New perspective on athlete's anemia. *American Journal of Medicine* 81: 791-794.

Selsby, J.T., K.D. Beckett, M. Kern, and S.T. Devor. 2003. Swim performance following creatine supplementation in Division III athletes. *Journal of Strength and Conditioning Research* 17: 421-424.

Shangold, M.M., and H.S. Levine. 1982. The effect of marathon training upon menstrual function. *American Journal of Obstetrics and Gynecology* 143: 862-869.

Sharman, I.M., M.G. Down, and N.G. Norgan. 1976. The effects of vitamin E on physiological function and athletic performance of trained swimmers. *Journal of Sports Medicine* 16: 215-225.

Sharman, I.M., M.G. Down, and R.N. Sen. 1971. The effects of vitamin E and training on physiological function and athletic performance in adolescent swimmers. *British Journal of Nutrition* 26: 265-276.

Sharp, N.C.C. 1979. Fitness for squash: how to build your aerobic power. *Squash Player International* 8: 15-17.

Sharwood, K., M. Collins, J. Goedecke, G. Wilson, and T. Noakes. 2002. Weight changes, sodium levels and performance in the South African Ironman™. *Clinical Journal of Sports Medicine* 12: 391-399.

Shave, R., G. Whyte, A. Siemann, and L. Doggart. 2001. The effects of sodium citrate ingestion on 3,000-meter time-trial performance. *Journal of Strength and Conditioning Research* 15: 230-234.

Shaw, D., C. Leon, S. Kolev, and V. Murray. 1997. Traditional remedies and food supplements. A 5-year toxicological study (1991-1995). *Drug Safety* 17: 342-356.

Sherman, W.M., G. Brodowicz, D.A. Wright, W.K. Allen, J. Simonsen, and A. Dernbach. 1989. Effects of 4 h preexercise carbohydrate feedings on cycling performance. *Medicine and Science in Sports and Exercise* 21: 598-604.

Sherman, W.M., D.L. Costill, W.J. Fink, F.C. Hagerman, L.E. Armstrong, and T.F. Murray. 1983. Effect of a 42.2 km footrace and subsequent rest or exercise on muscle glycogen and enzymes. *Journal of Applied Physiology* 55: 1219-1224.

Sherman, W.M., D.L. Costill, W.J. Fink, and J.M. Miller. 1981. Effect of exercise-diet manipulation on muscle glycogen and its subsequent utilisation during performance. *International Journal of Sports Medicine* 2: 114-118.

Sherman, W.M., J.A. Doyle, D.R. Lamb, and R.H. Strauss. 1993. Dietary carbohydrate, muscle glycogen, and exercise performance during 7 d of training. *American Journal of Clinical Nutrition* 57: 27-31.

Shing, C.M., D.G. Jenkins, L. Stevenson, and J.S. Coombes. 2006. The influence of bovine colostrum supplementation on exercise performance in highly trained cyclists. *British Journal of Sports Medicine* 40: 797-801.

Shirreffs, S.M., L.F. Aragon-Vargas, M. Chamorro, R.J. Maughan, L. Serratosa, and J.J. Zachwieja. 2005. The sweating response of elite professional soccer players to training in the heat. *International Journal of Sports Medicine* 26: 90-95.

Shirreffs, S.M., L.E. Armstrong, and S.N. Cheuvront. 2004. Fluid and electrolyte needs for preparation and recovery from training and competition. *Journal of Sports Sciences* 22: 57-63.

Shirreffs, S.M., and R.J. Maughan. 1997. Restoration of fluid balance after exercise-induced dehydration: Effects of alcohol consumption. *Journal of Applied Physiology* 83: 1152-1158.

Shirreffs, S.M., and R.J. Maughan. 1998. Urine osmolality and conductivity as indices of hydration status in athletes in the heat. *Medicine and Science in Sports and Exercise* 30: 1598-1602.

Shirreffs, S.M., A.J. Taylor, J.B. Leiper, and R.J. Maughan. 1996. Post-exercise rehydration in man: Effects of volume consumed and drink sodium content. *Medicine and Science in Sports and Exercise* 28: 1260-1271.

Shokman, C.P., I.H.E. Rutishauser, and R.J. Wallace. 1999. Pre- and postgame macronutrient intake of a group of elite Australian Rules football players. *International Journal of Sport Nutrition* 9: 60-69.

Short, S.H., and W.R. Short. 1983. Four-year study of university athletes' dietary intake. *Journal of the American Dietetic Association* 82: 632-645.

Simard, C., A. Tremblay, and M. Jobin. 1988. Effects of carbohydrate intake before and during an ice hockey game on blood and muscle energy substrates. *Research Quarterly for Exercise and Sport* 59: 144-147.

Simonsen, J.C., W.M. Sherman, D.R. Lamb, A.R. Dernbach, J.A. Doyle, and R. Strauss. 1991. Dietary carbohydrate, muscle glycogen, and power output during rowing training. *Journal of Applied Physiology* 70: 1500-1505.

Sims, G. 2003. *Why die? The extraordinary Percy Cerruty "maker of champions."* South Melbourne, Australia: Lothian.

Sjödin, A.M., A.B. Andersson, J.M. Hogberg, and K.R. Westerterp. 1994. Energy balance in cross-country skiers: A study using doubly labeled water. *Medicine and Science in Sports and Exercise* 26: 720-724.

Skare, O.C., O. Skadberg, and A.R. Wisnes. 2001. Creatine supplementation improves sprint performance in male sprinters. *Scandinavian Journal of Medicine and Science in Sports* 11: 96-102.

Slater, G.J., and D. Jenkins. 2000. β-hydroxy β-methylbutyrate (HMB) supplementation and the promotion of muscle growth and strength. *Sports Medicine* 30: 105-116.

Slater, G., D. Jenkins, P. Logan, H. Lee, M. Vukovich, J.A. Rathmacher, and A.G. Hahn. 2001. β-hydroxy-β-methylbutyrate (HMB) supplementation does not affect changes in strength or body composition during resistance training in trained men. *International Journal of Sport Nutrition and Exercise Metabolism* 11: 384-396.

Slater, G.J., A.J. Rice, I. Mujika, A.G. Hahn, K. Sharpe, and D.G. Jenkins. 2005. Physique traits of lightweight rowers and their relationship to competitive success. *British Journal of Sports Medicine* 39: 736-741.

Slater, G.J., A.J. Rice, K. Sharpe, I. Mujika, D. Jenkins, and A.G. Hahn. 2005. Body-mass management of Australian lightweight rowers prior to and during competition. *Medicine and Science in Sports and Exercise* 37: 860-866.

Slater, G.J., A.J. Rice, K. Sharpe, R. Tanner, D. Jenkins, C.J. Gore, and A.G. Hahn. 2005. Impact of acute weight loss and/or thermal stress on rowing ergometer performance. *Medicine and Science in Sports and Exercise* 37: 1387-1394.

Slater, G.J., A.J. Rice, R. Tanner, K. Sharpe, D. Jenkins, and A.G. Hahn. 2006a. Impact of two different body management strategies on repeat rowing performance. *Medicine and Science in Sports and Exercise* 38: 138-146.

Slater, G.J., A.J. Rice, R. Tanner, K. Sharpe, D. Jenkins, and A.G. Hahn. 2006b. Acute weight loss followed by an aggressive nutritional recovery strategy has little impact on on-water rowing performance. *British Journal of Sports Medicine* 40: 55-59.

Smith, G.J., E.C. Rhodes, and R.H. Langill. 2002. The effect of pre-exercise glucose ingestion on performance during prolonged swimming. *International Journal of Sport Nutrition and Exercise Metabolism* 12: 136-144.

Smith, J.A., and D.L. Dahm. 2000. Creatine use among a select population of high school athletes. *Mayo Clinic Proceedings* 75: 1257-1263.

Smith, M., R. Dyson, T. Hale, M. Hamilton, J. Kelly, and P. Wellington. 2001. The effects of restricted energy and fluid intake on simulated amateur boxing performance. *International Journal of Sport Nutrition and Exercise Metabolism* 11: 238-247.

Smith, M.P., J. Mendez, M. Druckenmiller, and P.M. Kris-Etherton. 1982. Exercise intensity, dietary intake, and high-density lipoprotein cholesterol in young female competitive swimmers. *American Journal of Clinical Nutrition* 36: 251-255.

Smith, M.S., R. Dyson, T. Hale, J.H. Harrison, and P. McManus. 2000. The effects in humans of rapid loss of body mass on a boxing-related task. *European Journal of Applied Physiology* 83: 34-39.

Smith, S. 2002. Marathon runner's death linked to excessive fluid intake. *New York Times* August 13, pp. 1-2.

Snider, I.P., T.L. Bazzarre, S.D. Murdoch, and A. Goldfarb. 1992. Effects of coenzyme athletic performance system as an ergogenic aid on endurance performance to exhaustion. *International Journal of Sport Nutrition* 2: 272-286.

Snow, C.M., D.P. Williams, J. LaRiviere, R.K. Fuchs, and T.L. Robinson. 2001. Bone gains and losses follow seasonal training and detraining in gymnasts. *Calcified Tissue International* 69: 7-12.

Snow, R.J., and R.M. Murphy. 2003. Factors influencing creatine loading into human skeletal muscle. *Exercise and Sport Sciences Reviews* 31: 154-158.

Snyder, A.C., L.L. Dvorak, and J.B. Roepke. 1989. Influence of dietary iron source on measures of iron status among female runners. *Medicine and Science in Sports and Exercise* 21: 7-10.

Snyder, A.C., and C. Foster. 1994. Physiology and nutrition for skating. In *Physiology and nutrition for competitive sport* (edited by D.R. Lamb, H.G. Knuttgen, and R. Murray), pp. 181-216. Carmel, IN: Cooper.

Soler, R., M. Echegaray, and M.A. Rivera. 2003. Thermal responses and body fluid balance of competitive male swimmers during a training session. *Journal of Strength and Conditioning Research* 17: 362-367.

Sovak, D., and M.R. Hawes. 1987. Anthropological status of international calibre speed skaters. *Journal of Sports Science* 5: 287-304.

Speedy, D.B., J.G. Faris, M. Hamlin, P.G. Gallagher, and R.G. Campbell. 1997. Hyponatremia and weight changes in an ultradistance triathlon. *Clinical Journal of Sports Medicine* 7: 180-184.

Speedy, D.B., T.D. Noakes, T. Boswell, J.M. Thompson, N. Rehrer, and D.R. Boswell. 2001. Response to a fluid load in athletes with a history of exercise induced hyponatremia. *Medicine and Science in Sports and Exercise* 33: 1434-1442.

Speedy, D.B., T.D. Noakes, N.E. Kimber, I.R. Rodgers, J.M.D. Thompson, D.R. Boswell, J.J. Ross, R.G.D. Campbell, P.G. Gallagher, and J.A. Kuttner. 2001. Fluid balance during and after an ironman triathlon. *Clinical Journal of Sports Medicine* 11: 44-50.

Speedy, D.B., T.D. Noakes, I.R. Rodgers, J.M.D. Thompson, R.G.D. Campbell, J.A. Kuttner, D.R. Boswell, S. Wright, and M. Hamlin. 1999. Hyponatremia in ultradistance triathletes. *Medicine and Science in Sports and Exercise* 31: 809-815.

Speedy, D.B., I.R. Rodgers, T.D. Noakes, J.M. Thompson, J. Guirey, S. Safih, and D.R. Boswell. 2000. Diagnosis and prevention of hyponatremia at an ultradistance triathlon. *Clinical Journal of Sports Medicine* 10: 52-58.

Speedy, D.B., I.R. Rodgers, T.D. Noakes, S. Wright, J.M.D. Thompson, R. Campbell, I. Hellemans, N.E. Kimber, D.R. Boswell, J.A. Kuttner, and S. Safih. 2000. Exercise-induced hyponatremia in ultradistance triathletes is caused by inappropriate fluid retention. *Clinical Journal of Sports Medicine* 10: 272-278.

Speedy, D.B., J.M.D. Thompson, I. Rodgers, M. Collins, and K. Sharwood. 2002. Oral salt supplementation during ultradistance exercise. *Clinical Journal of Sports Medicine* 12: 279-284.

Spodaryk, K. 1993. Haematological and iron-related parameters of male endurance and strength trained athletes. *European Journal of Applied Physiology and Occupational Physiology* 67: 66-70.

Spriet, L.L., D.A. MacLean, D.J. Dyck, E. Hultman, G. Cederblad, and T.E. Graham. 1992. Caffeine ingestion and muscle metabolism during prolonged exercise in humans. *American Journal of Physiology Endocrinology and Metabolism* 262: E891-E898.

Stager, J.M., L. Cordain, and T. J. Becker. 1984. Relationship of body composition to swimming performance in female swimmers. *Journal of Swimming Research* 1: 21-26.

Stanko, R.T., R.J. Robertson, R.W. Galbreath, J.J. Reilly, K.D. Greenawalt, and F.L. Goss. 1990. Enhanced leg exercise endurance with a high-carbohydrate diet and dihydroxyacetone and pyruvate. *Journal of Applied Physiology* 69: 1651-1656.

Stanko, R.T., R.J. Robertson, R.J. Spina, J.J. Reilly, K.D. Greenawalt, and F.L. Goss. 1990. Enhancement of arm exercise endurance capacity with dihydroxyacetone and pyruvate. *Journal of Applied Physiology* 68: 119-124.

Starling, R.D., T.A. Trappe, A.C. Parcell, C.G. Kerr, W.J. Fink, and D.L. Costill. 1997. Effects of diet on muscle triglyceride and endurance performance. *Journal of Applied Physiology* 82: 1185-1189.

Starling, R.D., T.A. Trappe, K.R. Short, M. Sheffield-Moore, A.C. Joszi, W.J. Fink, and D.L. Costill. 1996. Effect of inosine supplementation on aerobic and anaerobic cycling performance. *Medicine and Science in Sports and Exercise* 28: 1193-1198.

Stathis, C.G., M.A. Febbraio, M.F. Carey, and R.J. Snow. 1994. Influence of sprint training on human skeletal muscle purine nucleotide metabolism. *Journal of Applied Physiology* 76: 1802-1809.

Steen, S.N. 1991. Precontest strategies of a male body builder. *International Journal of Sport Nutrition* 1: 69-78.

Steen, S.N., and K.D. Brownell. 1990. Patterns of weight loss and regain in wrestlers: Has the tradition changed? *Medicine and Science in Sports and Exercise* 22: 762-768.

Steen, S.N., and S. McKinney. 1986. Nutrition assessment of college wrestlers. *The Physician and Sportsmedicine* 14: 100-116.

Steen, S.N., R.A. Oppliger, and K.D. Brownell. 1988. Metabolic effects of repeated weight loss and regain in adolescent wrestlers. *Journal of the American Medical Association* 260: 47-50.

Steen, S.N., K. Mayer, K.D. Brownell, and T.A. Wadden. 1995. Dietary intake of female collegiate heavyweight rowers. *International Journal of Sport Nutrition* 5: 225-231.

Stellingwerff, T., L.L. Spriet, M.J. Watt, N.E. Kimber, M. Hargreaves, J.A. Hawley, and L.M. Burke. 2006. Decreased PDH activation and glycogenolysis during exercise following fat adaptation with carbohydrate restoration. *American Journal of Physiology Endocrinology and Metabolism* 290: E380-388.

Stensrund, T., F. Ingjer, H. Holm, and S.B. Stromme. 1992. L-tryptophan supplementation does not improve running performance. *International Journal of Sports Medicine* 13: 481-485.

Stephens, F.B., D. Constantin-Teodosiu, D. Laithwaite, E.F. Simpson, and P.L. Greenhaff. 2006. Insulin stimulates L-carnitine accumulation in humans. *FASEB Journal* 20: 377-379.

Stephens, T.J., M.J. McKenna, B.J. Canny, R.J. Snow, and G.K. McConell. 2002. Effect of sodium bicarbonate on muscle metabolism during intense endurance cycling. *Medicine and Science in Sports and Exercise* 34: 614-621.

Stevenson, S.W., and G.A. Dudley. 2001. Creatine loading, resistance exercise performance, and muscle mechanics. *Journal of Strength and Conditioning Research* 15: 413-419.

Stofan, J.R., J.J. Jachwieja, C.A. Horswill, and R. Murray. 2003. Sweat and sodium losses during practice in professional football players [abstract]. *Medicine and Science in Sports and Exercise* 34: S113.

Stofan, J.R., J.J. Jachwieja, C.A. Horswill, R. Murray, E.R. Eichner, and S. Anderson. 2005. Sweat and sodium losses in NCAA football players: A precursor to heat cramps. *International Journal of Sport Nutrition and Exercise Metabolism* 15: 641-652.

Stone, M.H., K. Sanborn, L.L. Smith, H.S. O'Bryant, T. Hoke, A.C. Utter, R.L. Johnson, R. Boros, J. Hruby, K.C. Pierce, M.E. Stone, and B. Garner. 1999. Effects of in-season (5 weeks) creatine and pyruvate supplementation on anaerobic performance and body composition in American football players. *International Journal of Sport Nutrition* 9: 146-165.

Stout, J., J. Eckerson, D. Noonan, and G. Moore. 1999. Effects of 8-weeks of creatine supplementation on exercise performance and fat-free weight in football players during training. *Nutrition Research* 19: 217-225.

Stray-Gundersen, J., A. Hochstein, D. deLemos, and B.D. Levine. 1992. Failure of red cell volume to increase to altitude exposure in iron deficient runners. *Medicine and Science in Sports and Exercise* 24: S90.

Stroescu, V., J. Dragan, L. Simionescu, and O.V. Stroescu. 2001. Hormonal and metabolic response in elite female gymnasts undergoing strenuous training and supplementation with SUPRO Brand Isolated Soy Protein. *Journal of Sports Medicine and Physical Fitness* 41: 89-94.

Stuart, G.R., W.G. Hopkins, C. Cook, and S.P. Cairns. 2006. Multiple effects of caffeine on simulated high-intensity team sport performance. *Medicine and Science in Sports and Exercise* 37: 1998-2005.

Stuessi, C., P. Hofer, C. Meier, and U. Boutellier. 2005. L-carnitine and the recovery from exhaustive endurance exercise: A randomised, double-blind, placebo-controlled trial. *European Journal of Applied Physiology* 95: 431-435.

Subudhi, A.W., S.L. Davis, R.W. Kipp, and E.W. Askew. 2001. Antioxidant status and oxidative stress in elite alpine ski racers. *International Journal of Sport Nutrition and Exercise Metabolism* 11: 32-41.

Sugiura, K., I. Suzuki, and K. Kobayashi. 1999. Nutritional intake of elite Japanese track-and-field athletes. *International Journal of Sport Nutrition* 9: 202-212.

Sukala, W.R. 1998. Pyruvate: beyond the marketing hype. *International Journal of Sport Nutrition* 8: 241-249.

Sullivan, J.E. 1909. *Marathon running.* New York: American Sports Publishing Company.

Sullo, A., A. Monda, G. Brizzi, V. Meninno, A. Papa, P. Lombardo, and B. Fabbri. 1998. The effect of a carbohydrate loading on running performance during a 25-km treadmill time trial by level of aerobic capacity. *European Review for Medical and Pharmacological Sciences* 2: 195-202.

Sundgot-Borgen, J. 1993. Prevalence of eating disorders in elite female athletes. *International Journal of Sport Nutrition* 3: 29-40.

Sundgot-Borgen, J. 1994. Eating disorders in female athletes. *Sports Medicine* 17: 176-188.

Sundgot-Borgen, J. 1996. Eating disorders, energy intake, training volume, and menstrual function in high-level modern rhythmic gymnasts. *International Journal of Sport Nutrition* 6: 100-109.

Sundgot-Borgen, J. 2000. Eating disorders in athletes. In *Nutrition in Sport* (edited by R.J. Maughan), pp. 510-522. Oxford, UK: Blackwell Science.

Svensson, M., C. Malm, M. Tonkonogi, B. Ekblom, B. Sjodin, and K. Sahlin. 1999. Effect of Q10 supplementation on tissue Q10 levels and adenine nucleotide catabolism during high-intensity exercise. *International Journal of Sport Nutrition* 9: 166-180.

Sykora, C., C.M. Grilo, D.E. Wilfley, and K.D. Brownell. 1993. Eating, weight, and dieting disturbances in male and female lightweight and heavyweight rowers. *International Journal of Eating Disorders* 14: 203-211.

Syrotuik, D.G., G.J. Bell, R. Burnham, L.L. Sim, R.A. Calvert, and I.M. MacLean. 2000. Absolute and relative strength performance following creatine monohydrate supplementation combined with periodized training. *Journal of Strength and Conditioning Research* 14: 182-190.

Syrotuik, D.G., A.B. Game, E.M. Gillies, and G.J. Bell. 2001. Effects of creatine monohydrate supplementation during combined strength and high intensity rowing training on performance. *Canadian Journal of Applied Physiology* 26: 527-542.

Syrotuik, D.G., K.L. MacFadyen, V.J. Harber, and G.J. Bell. 2005. Effect of elk velvet antler supplementation on the hormonal response to acute and chronic exercise in male and female rowers. *International Journal of Sport Nutrition and Exercise Metabolism* 15: 366-385.

Szlyk, P.C., I.V. Sils, R.P. Francseconi, R.W. Hubbard, and L.E. Armstrong. 1989. Effects of water temperature and flavouring on voluntary dehydration in men. *Physiology and Behavior* 45: 639-645.

Taaffe, D.R., T.L. Robinson, C.M. Snow, and R. Marcus. 1997. High-impact exercise promotes bone gain in well-trained female athletes. *Journal of Bone and Mineral Research* 12: 255-260.

Talbot, D., and J. Jamieson. 1977. An examination of the effect of vitamin E on the performance of highly trained swimmers. *Canadian Journal of Applied Sports Science* 2: 67-69.

Talbott, S.M., and S.A. Shapses. 1998. Fasting and energy intake influence bone turnover in lightweight male rowers. *International Journal of Sport Nutrition* 8: 377-387.

Tanaka, J.A., H. Tanaka, and W. Landis. 1995. An assessment of carbohydrate intake in collegiate distance runners. *International Journal of Sport Nutrition* 5: 206-214.

Tanser, T. 1997. The Kenyan diet. In *Train hard, win easy : the Kenyan way* (edited by T. Tanser), pp. 66-73. Mountainview, CA: Tafnews.

Tarnopolsky, M.A. 1999. Introduction. In *Gender Differences in Metabolism: Practical and Nutritional Implications* (edited by M.A. Tarnopolsky), pp. 1-13. Baton Rouge, LA: CRC Press.

Tarnopolsky, M. 2006. Protein and amino acid needs for training and bulking up. In *Clinical Sports Nutrition, 3rd ed.* (edited by L. Burke and V. Deakin), pp. 90-123. Sydney, Australia: McGraw-Hill.

Tarnopolsky, M.A., S.A. Atkinson, J.D. MacDougall, A. Chesley, S. Phillips, and H.P. Schwarcz. 1992. Evaluation of protein requirements for trained strength athletes. *Journal of Applied Physiology* 73: 1986-1995.

Tarnopolsky, M.A., S.A. Atkinson, S.M. Phillips, and J.D. MacDougall. 1995. Carbohydrate loading and metabolism during exercise in men and women. *Journal of Applied Physiology* 78: 1360-1368.

Tarnopolsky, M.A., M. Bosman, J.R. MacDonald, D. Vandeputte, J. Martin, and B.D. Roy. 1997. Postexercise protein-carbohydrate and carbohydrate supplements increase muscle glycogen in men and women. *Journal of Applied Physiology* 83: 1877-1883.

Tarnopolsky, M.A., N. Cipriano, C. Woodcroft, W.J. Pulkkinen, D.C. Robinson, J.M. Henderson, and J.D. MacDougall. 1996. Effects of rapid weight loss and wrestling on muscle glycogen concentration. *Clinical Journal of Sports Medicine* 6: 78-84.

Tarnopolsky, M.A., J.D. MacDougall, and S.A. Atkinson. 1988. Influence of protein intake and training status on nitrogen balance and lean body mass. *Journal of Applied Physiology* 64: 187-193.

Tarnopolsky, M.A., and D.P. MacLennan. 2000. Creatine monohydrate supplementation enhances high-intensity exercise performance in males and females. *International Journal of Sport Nutrition and Exercise Metabolism* 10: 452-463.

Tarnopolsky, M.A., C. Zawada, L.B. Richmond, S. Carter, J. Shearer, T. Graham, and S.M. Phillips. 2001. Gender differences in carbohydrate loading are related to energy intake. *Journal of Applied Physiology* 91: 225-230.

Taub, D.E., and R.A. Benson. 1992. Weight concerns, weight control techniques, and eating disorders among adolescent competitive swimmers: The effect of gender. *Sociology of Sport Journal* 9: 76-86.

Terblanche, S., T.D. Noakes, S.C. Dennis, D.W. Marais, and M. Eckert. 1992. Failure of magnesium supplementation to influence marathon running performance or recovery in magnesium-replete subjects. *International Journal of Sport Nutrition* 2: 154-164.

Terrillion, K.A., F.W. Kolkhorst, F.A. Dolgener, and S.J. Joslyn. 1997. The effect of creatine supplementation on two 700-m maximal running bouts. *International Journal of Sport Nutrition* 7: 138-143.

Tesch, P.A., E.B. Colliander, and P. Kaiser. 1986. Muscle metabolism during intense heavy exercise. *European Journal of Applied Physiology* 55: 362-366.

Tesch, P., L. Larsson, A. Eriksson, and J. Karlsson. 1978. Muscle glycogen depletion and lactate concentration during downhill skiing. *Medicine and Science in Sports* 10: 85-90.

Tesch, P.A., L.L. Ploutz-Snyder, L. Ystrom, M. Castro, and G. Dudley. 1998. Skeletal muscle glycogen loss evoked by resistance exercise. *Journal of Strength and Conditioning Research* 12: 67-73.

Theodorou, A.S., C.B. Cooke, R.F.G.J. King, C. Hood, T. Denison, B.G. Wainwright, and K. Havenetidis. 1999. The effect of longer-term creatine supplementation on elite swimming performance after an acute creatine loading. *Journal of Sports Sciences* 17: 853-859.

Theodorou, A.S., K. Havenetidis, C.L. Zanker, J.P. O'Hara, R.F. King, C. Hood, G. Paradisis, and C.B. Cooke. 2005. Effects of acute creatine loading with or without carbohydrate on repeated bouts of maximal swimming in high-performance swimmers. *Journal of Strength and Conditioning Research* 19: 265-269.

Thiel, A., H. Gottfried, and F.W. Hesse. 1993. Subclinical eating disorders in male athletes: a study of the low weight category in rowers and wrestlers. *Acta Psychiatrica Scandinavica* 88: 259-265.

Thomas, D.E., J.R. Brotherhood, and J.C. Brand. 1991. Carbohydrate feeding before exercise: Effect of glycemic index. *International Journal of Sports Medicine* 12: 180-186.

Thompson, C.H., G.J. Kemp, A.L. Sanderson, R.M. Dixon, P. Styles, D.J. Taylor, and G.K. Radda. 1996. Effect of creatine on aerobic and anaerobic metabolism in skeletal muscle in swimmers. *British Journal of Sports Medicine* 30: 222-225.

Thompson, J., and M.M. Manore. 1996. Predicted and measured resting metabolic rate of male and female endurance athletes. *Journal of the American Dietetic Association* 96: 30-34.

Thompson, J., M.M. Manore, and J.S. Skinner. 1993. Resting metabolic rate and thermic effect of a meal in low- and adequate-energy intake male endurance athletes. *International Journal of Sport Nutrition* 3: 194-206.

Thompson, J.L., M.M. Manore, J.S. Skinner, E. Ravussin, and M. Spraul. 1995. Daily energy expenditure in male endurance athletes with differing energy intakes. *Medicine and Science in Sports and Exercise* 27: 347-354.

Thong, F.S.L., and T.E. Graham. 1999. Leptin and reproduction: Is it a critical link between adipose tissue, nutrition, and reproduction? *Canadian Journal of Applied Physiology,* 24: 317-336.

Thong, F.S.L., C. McLean, and T.E. Graham. 2000. Plasma leptin in female athletes: Relationship with body fat, reproductive, nutritional, and endocrine factors. *Journal of Applied Physiology* 88: 2037-2044.

Tilgner, S.A., and M.R. Schiller. 1989. Dietary intakes of female college athletes: The need for nutrition education. *Journal of the American Dietetic Association* 89: 967-969.

Tipton, C.M., and T.K. Tcheng. 1970. Iowa wrestling study: Weight loss in high school students. *Journal of the American Medical Association* 214: 1269-1274.

Tipton, K.D., E. Borsheim, S.E. Wolf, A.P. Sanford, and R.R. Wolfe. 2003. Acute response of net muscle protein balance reflects 24-h balance after exercise and amino acid ingestion. *American Journal of Physiology Endocrinology and Metabolism* 284: E76-E89.

Tipton, K.D., T.A. Elliott, M.G. Cree, A.A. Aarsland, A.P. Sanford, and R.R. Wolfe. 2006. Stimulation of net muscle protein synthesis by whey protein ingestion before and after exercise. *American Journal of Physiology Endocrinology and Metabolism,* Aug 8 epub ahead of print.

Tipton, K.D., T.A. Elliott, M.G. Cree, S.E. Wolf, A.P. Sanford, and R.R. Wolfe. 2004. Ingestion of casein and whey proteins results in muscle anabolism after resistance exercise. *Medicine and Science in Sports and Exercise* 36: 2073-2081.

Tipton, K.D., A.A. Ferrando, S.M. Phillips, D. Doyle, and R.R. Wolfe. 1999. Postexercise net protein synthesis in human muscle from orally administered amino acids. *American Journal of Physiology Endocrinology and Metabolism* 276: E628-E634.

Tipton, K.D., A.A. Ferrando, B.D. Williams, and R.R. Wolfe. 1996. Muscle protein metabolism in female swimmers after a combination of resistance and endurance exercise. *Journal of Applied Physiology* 81: 2034-2038.

Tipton, K.D., B.B. Rasmussen, S.L. Miller, S.E. Wolf, S.K. Owens-Stovall, B.E. Petrini, and R.R. Wolfe. 2001. Timing of amino acid-carbohydrate ingestion alters anabolic response of muscle to resistance exercise. *American Journal of Physiology Endocrinology and Metabolism* 281: E197-E206.

Tipton, K.D., and R.R. Wolfe. 2001. Exercise, protein metabolism, and muscle growth. *International Journal of Sport Nutrition and Exercise Metabolism* 11: 109-132.

Tipton, K.D., and R.R. Wolfe. 2004. Protein and amino acids for athletes. *Journal of Sports Sciences* 22: 65-79.

Tiryaki, G.R., and H.A. Atterbom. 1995. The effects of sodium bicarbonate and sodium citrate on 600 m running time of trained females. *Journal of Sports Medicine and Physical Fitness* 35: 194-198.

Toro, J., B. Galilea, E. Martinez-Mallen, M. Salamero, L. Capdevila, J. Mari, J. Mayolas, and E. Toro. 2005. Eating disorders in Spanish female athletes. *International Journal of Sports Medicine* 26: 693-700.

Trappe, S.W., D.L. Costill, B. Goodpaster, M.D. Vukovich, and W.J. Fink. 1994. The effects of L-carnitine supplementation on performance during interval swimming. *International Journal of Sports Medicine* 15: 181-185.

Trappe, T.A., A. Gastaldelli, A.C. Jozsi, J.P. Troup, and R.R. Wolfe. 1997. Energy expenditure of swimmers during high volume training. *Medicine and Science in Sports and Exercise* 29: 950-954.

Troup, J.P., D. Strass, and T.A. Trappe. 1994. Physiology and nutrition for competitive swimming. In *Perspectives in Exercise Science and Sports Medicine* (edited by D.R. Lamb, H.G. Knuttgen, and R. Murray), pp. 99-129. Carmel, IN: Cooper.

Tsintzas, K., R. Liu, C. Williams, I. Campbell, and G. Gaitanos. 1993. The effect of carbohydrate ingestion on performance during a 30 km race. *International Journal of Sport Nutrition* 3: 127-139.

Tsintzas, O.K., C. Williams, L. Boobis, and P. Greenhaff. 1996. Carbohydrate ingestion and single muscle fiber glycogen metabolism during prolonged running in men. *Journal of Applied Physiology* 81: 801-809.

Tsintzas, O.K., C. Williams, R. Singh, and W. Wilson. 1995. Influence of carbohydrate-electrolyte drinks on marathon running performance. *European Journal of Applied Physiology* 70: 154-160.

Tsintzas, O.K., C. Williams, and W. Wilson. 1993. Influence of carbohydrate ingestion on muscle glycogen utilization during prolonged running in man. *Journal of Physiology* 467: 72P.

Tsintzas, O.K., C. Williams, W. Wilson, and J. Burrin. 1996. Influence of carbohydrate supplementation early in exercise on endurance running capacity. *Medicine and Science in Sports and Exercise* 28: 1373-1379.

Vallerand, A.L., J. Zamecnik, and I. Jacobs. 1995. Plasma glucose turnover during cold stress in humans. *Journal of Applied Physiology* 78: 1296-1302.

Vallieres, F., A. Tremblay, and L. St-Jean. 1989. Study of the energy balance and the nutritional status of highly trained female swimmers. *Nutrition Research* 9: 699-708.

Van Erp-Baart, A.M.J., W.H.M. Saris, R.A. Binkhorst, J.A. Vos, and J.W.H. Elvers. 1989a. Nationwide survey on nutritional habits in elite athletes. Part I: Energy, carbohydrate, protein, and fat intake. *International Journal of Sports Medicine* 10: S3-S10.

Van Erp-Baart, A.M.J., W.H.M. Saris, R.A. Binkhorst, J.A. Vos, and J.W.H. Elvers. 1989b. Nationwide survey on nutritional habits in elite athletes. Part II: Mineral and vitamin intake. *International Journal of Sports Medicine* 10: S11-S16.

Van Essen, M., and M.J. Gibala. 2006. Failure of protein to improve time trial performance when added to a sports drink. *Medicine and Science in Sports and Exercise* 38: 1476-1483.

Van Gammeren, D., D. Falk, and J. Antonio. 2002. The effects of four weeks of ribose supplementation on body composition and exercise performance in healthy, young, male recreational

body builders: A double-blind, placebo-controlled trial. *Current Therapeutic Research* 63: 486-495.

Van Hall, G., W.H.M. Saris, P.A.I. van de Schoor, and A.J.M. Wagenmakers. 2000. The effect of free glutamine and peptide ingestion on the rate of muscle glycogen resynthesis in man. *International Journal of Sports Medicine* 21: 25-30.

Van Hall, G., S.M. Shirreffs, and J.A.L. Calbert. 2000. Muscle glycogen resynthesis during recovery from cycle exercise: No effect of additional protein ingestion. *Journal of Applied Physiology* 88: 1631-1636.

Van Handel, P.J., K.A. Cells, P.W. Bradley, and J.P. Troup. 1984. Nutritional status of elite swimmers. *Journal of Swimming Research* 1: 27-31.

van Ingen Schenau, G.J., and J.J. de Koning. 1999. Biomechanics of speed skating. In *Handbook of Competitive Speed Skating* (edited by H. Gemser, J.J. de Koning, and G.J. van Ingen Schenau), pp. 41-74. Lausanne, Switzerland: International Skating Union.

Van Loon, L.J., R. Murphy, A.M. Oosterlaar, D. Cameron-Smith, M. Hargreaves, A.J. Wagenmakers, and R. Snow. 2004. Creatine supplementation increases glycogen storage but not GLUT-4 expression in human skeletal muscle. *Clinical Science* 106: 99-106.

Van Loon, L.J.C., W.H.M. Saris, M. Kruijshoop, and A.J.M. Wagenmakers. 2000. Maximizing postexercise muscle glycogen synthesis: Carbohydrate supplementation and the application of amino acid or protein hydrolysate mixtures. *American Journal of Clinical Nutrition* 72: 106-111.

Van Nieuwenhoven, M.A., F. Brouns, and E.M.R. Kovacs. 2005. The effect of two sports drinks and water on GI complaints and performance during an 18-km run. *International Journal of Sports Medicine* 26: 281-285.

van Rensburg, A., A. van der Linde, P.C. Ackermann, A.J. Kileblock, and N.B. Strydom. 1982. Physiological profile of squash players. *South African Journal for Research in Sport, Physical Education and Recreation* 5: 25-56.

van Schuylenbergh, R., M. van Leemputte, and P. Hespel. 2003. Effects of oral creatine-pyruvate supplementation in cycling performance. *International Journal of Sports Medicine* 24: 144-150.

Van Soeren, M.H., and T.E. Graham. 1998. Effect of caffeine on metabolism, exercise endurance, and catecholamine responses after withdrawal. *Journal of Applied Physiology* 85: 1493-1501.

Van Zyl, C.G., E.V. Lambert, J.A. Hawley, T.D. Noakes, and S.C. Dennis. 1996. The effect of medium-chain triglyceride ingestion on fuel metabolism and cycling performance. *Journal of Applied Physiology* 80: 2217-2225.

Vanakoski, J., V. Kosunen, E. Merirrine, and T. Seppala. 1998. Creatine and caffeine in anaerobic and aerobic exercise: Effects of physical performance and pharmacokinetic considerations. *International Journal of Clinical Pharmacology and Therapeutics* 36: 258-263.

Vandebuerie, F., B. Vanden Eynde, K. Vandenberghe, and P. Hespel. 1998. Effect of creatine loading on endurance capacity and sprint power in cyclists. *International Journal of Sports Medicine* 19: 490-495.

Vandenberghe, K., P. Hespel, B. Vanden Eynde, R. Lysens, and E.A. Richter. 1995. No effect of glycogen level on glycogen metabolism during high intensity exercise. *Medicine and Science in Sports and Exercise* 27: 1278-1283.

Veitl, V., K. Irsigler, and E. Ogris. 1977. Body composition, glucose tolerance, serum insulin, serum lipids and eating behavior in top Austrian sportsmen. *Nutrition and Metabolism* 21 (suppl 1): 88-94.

Vergauwen, L., F. Brouns, and P. Hespel. 1998. Carbohydrate supplementation improves stroke performance in tennis. *Medicine and Science in Sports and Exercise* 30: 1289-1295.

Videman, T., I. Lereim, P. Hemmingsson, M.S. Turner, M.P. Rousseau-Bianchi, P. Jenoure, E. Raas, H. Schonhuber, H. Rusko, and J. Stray-Gundersen. 2000. Changes in hemoglobin values in elite cross-country skiers from 1987-1999. *Scandinavian Journal of Medicine and Science in Sports* 10: 98-102.

Viitasalo, J.T., H. Kyrolainen, C. Bosco, and M. Alen. 1987. Effects of rapid weight reduction on force production and vertical jumping height. *International Journal of Sports Medicine* 8: 281-285.

Viitasalo, J.T., H. Rusko, O. Pakala, P. Rahkila, M. Ahila, and H. Montonen. 1982. Endurance requirements in volleyball. *Canadian Journal of Applied Sports Science* 12: 194-201.

Villani, R.G., J. Gannon, M. Self, and P.A. Rich. 2000. L-carnitine supplementation combined with aerobic training does not promote weight loss in moderately obese women. *International Journal of Sport Nutrition and Exercise Metabolism* 10: 199-207.

Vincent, J.B. 2003. The potential value and toxicity of chromium picolinate as a nutritional supplement, weight loss agent and muscle development agent. *Sports Medicine* 33: 213-230.

Vinci, D.M. 1998. Effective nutrition support programs for college athletes. *International Journal of Sport Nutrition* 8: 308-320.

Viru, M., V. Oopik, A. Nurmekivi, L. Medijainen, S. Timpmann, and A. Viru. 1994. Effect of creatine intake on the performance capacity in middle-distance runners. *Coaching and Sport Science Journal* 1: 31-36.

Vistisen, B., L. Nybo, X. Xuebing, C.E. Hoy, and B. Kiens. 2003. Minor amounts of plasma medium-chain fatty acids and no improved time trial performance after consuming lipids. *Journal of Applied Physiology* 95: 2434-2443.

Vogt, S., L. Heinrich, Y.O. Schumacher, M. Grosshauser, A. Blum, D. Konig, A. Berg, and A. Schmid. 2005. Energy intake and energy expenditure of elite cyclists during preseason training. *International Journal of Sports Medicine* 26: 701-706.

Volek, J.S., N.D. Duncan, S.A. Mazzetti, R.S. Staron, M. Putukian, A.L. Gomez, D.R. Pearson, W.J. Fink, and W.J. Kraemer. 1999. Performance and muscle fiber adaptations to creatine supplementation and heavy resistance training. *Medicine and Science in Sports and Exercise* 31: 1147-1156.

Volek, J.S., W.J. Kraemer, J.A. Bush, M. Boetes, T. Incledon, K.L. Clark, and J.M. Lynch. 1997. Creatine supplementation enhances muscular performance during high-intensity resistance exercise. *Journal of the American Dietetic Association* 97: 765-770.

Volek, J.S., N.A. Ratamess, M.R. Rubin, A.L. Gomez, D.N. French, M.M. McGuigan, T.P. Scheett, M.J. Sharman, K. Hakkinen, and W.J. Kraemer. 2004. The effects of creatine supplementation on muscular performance and body composition responses to short-term resistance training overreaching. *European Journal of Applied Physiology and Occupational Physiology* 91: 628-637.

Vrijens, D.M.J., and N.J. Rehrer. 1999. Sodium-free fluid ingestion decreases plasma sodium during exercise in the heat. *Journal of Applied Physiology* 86: 1847-1851.

Vukovich, M.D., and G.D. Dreifort. 2001. Effect of β-hydroxy β-methylbutyrate on the onset of blood lactate accumulation and VO$_2$peak in endurance-trained cyclists. *Journal of Strength and Conditioning Research* 15: 491-497.

WADA. 2003. World Anti-Doping Association. Available www.wada.ama-org [accessed September 7, 2006].

Welsh, R.S., J.M. Davis, J.R. Burke, and H.G. Williams. 2002. Carbohydrates and physical/mental performance during intermittent exercise to fatigue. *Medicine and Science in Sports and Exercise* 34: 723-731.

Wagenmakers, A.J.M. 1991. L-carnitine supplementation and performance in man. In *Advances in Nutrition and Top Sport* (edited by F. Brouns), pp. 110-127. Basel, Switzerland: Karger.

Walberg, J.L., M.K. Leidy, D.J. Sturgill, D.E. Hinkle, S.J. Ritchey, and D.R. Sebolt. 1988. Macronutrient content of a hypoenergy diet affects nitrogen retention and muscle function in weight lifters. *International Journal of Sports Medicine* 9: 261-266.

Walberg-Rankin, J., C.E. Edmonds, and F.C. Gwazdauskas. 1993. Diet and weight changes of female bodybuilders before and after competition. *International Journal of Sport Nutrition* 3: 87-102.

Walberg-Rankin, J., C.E. Hawkins, D.S. Fild, and D.R. Sebolt. 1994. The effect of oral arginine during energy restriction in male weight trainers. *Journal of Strength and Conditioning Research* 8: 170-177.

Walberg-Rankin, J., J.V. Ocel, and L.L. Craft. 1996. Effect of weight loss and refeeding diet composition on anaerobic performance in wrestlers. *Medicine and Science in Sports and Exercise* 28: 1292-1299.

Walker, J. L., G.J.F. Heigenhauser, E. Hultman, and L.L. Spriet. 2000. Dietary carbohydrate, muscle glycogen content and endurance performance in well trained women. *Journal of Applied Physiology* 88: 2151-2158.

Walker, L.S., M.G. Bemben, D.A. Bemben, and A.W. Knehans. 1998. Chromium picolinate effects on body composition and muscular performance in wrestlers. *Medicine and Science in Sports and Exercise* 30: 1730-1737.

Wallis, J.C., and S.D.R. Galloway. 2003. The effects of carbohydrate/electrolyte drink ingestion on maintenance of skills in squash players. Abstract presented at European Congress of Sports Sciences, Salzberg, Austria.

Walsh, R., and L. McNaughton. 1989. Serum iron levels in young female swimmers during pre-season phase of competition and the effects of iron supplementation upon them. *Journal of Human Movement Studies* 17: 229-238.

Walsh, R.M., T.D. Noakes, J.A. Hawley, and S.C. Dennis. 1994. Impaired high-intensity cycling performance time at low levels of dehydration. *International Journal of Sports Medicine* 15: 392-398.

Walsh, S.J, C.B. Cooke, P.D. Davies, and R.F.G.J. King. 1995. Fluid loss and replacement in English Division One Professional Rugby League players. Conference presentation from Dehydration, Rehydration and Exercise in the Heat conference Nottingham, UK, cited in R. Meir and A. Murphy. 1998. Fluid loss and rehydration during training and competition in professional rugby league. *Coaching and Sport Science Journal* 3: 9-13.

Ward, P., T. Tellez, and R. Ward. 1976. USA discus camp: Preliminary report. *Track and Field Quarterly Review* 76: 29-39.

Watsford, M.L., A.J. Murphy, W.L. Spinks, and A.D. Walshe. 2003. Creatine supplementation and its effect on musculotendinous stiffness and performance. *Journal of Strength and Conditioning Research* 17: 26-33.

Watten, R.G. 1995. Sports, physical exercise and use of alcohol. *Scandinavian Journal of Medicine and Science in Sports* 5: 364-368.

Webster, B.L., and S.I. Barr. 1995. Calcium intakes of adolescent female gymnasts and speed skaters: Lack of association with dieting behaviour. *International Journal of Sport Nutrition* 5: 2-12.

Weight, L.M., and T.D. Noakes. 1987. Is running an analogue of anorexia? A survey of the incidence of eating disorders in female distance runners. *Medicine and Science in Sports and Exercise* 19: 213-217.

Weimann, E., W.F. Blum, C. Witzel, S. Schwidergall, and H.J. Bohles. 1999. Hypoleptinemia in female and male elite gymnasts. *European Journal of Clinical Investigation* 29: 853-860.

Weimann, E., C. Witzel, S. Schwidergall, and H.J. Bohles. 2000. Peripubertal pertubations in elite gymnasts caused by sports specific training regimes and inadequate nutritional intake. *International Journal of Sports Medicine* 21: 210-215.

Welsh, R.S., J.M. Davis, J.R. Burke, and H.G. Williams. 2002. Carbohydrates and physical/mental performance during intermittent exercise to fatigue. *Medicine and Science in Sports and Exercise* 34: 723-731.

Westerterp, K.R., W.H.M. Saris, M. Van Es, and F. Ten Hoor. 1986. Use of the doubly labeled water technique in humans during heavy sustained exercise. *Journal of Applied Physiology* 61: 2162-2167.

Weston, S.B., S. Zhou, R.P. Weatherby, and S.J. Robson. 1997. Does exogenous coenzyme Q10 affect aerobic capacity in endurance athletes? *International Journal of Sport Nutrition* 7: 197-206.

White, A.T., and S.C. Johnson. 1991. Physiological comparison of international, national and regional alpine skiers. *International Journal of Sports Medicine* 12: 374-378.

White, A.T., and S.C. Johnson. 1993. Physiological aspects and injury in elite Alpine skiers. *Sports Medicine* 15: 170-178.

Whitten, P. 1993a. Stanford's secret weapon: New nutrition program lifts Cardinal swimmers to record-breaking year. *Swimming World and Junior Swimmer* 34: 28-33.

Whitten, P. 1993b. To carbo-load or not to carbo-load? That is the question . . . *Swim* 9: 25-29.

Whitten, P. 2002. Dr. Barry Sears says, "Take lots of fish oil": The full interview. http://www.swimmingworldmagazine.com/lane9/news/3897.asp [accessed: September 7, 2006].

Wiita, B.G., and I.A. Stombaugh. 1996. Nutrition knowledge, eating practices, and health of adolescent female runners: A 3-year longitudinal study. *International Journal of Sport Nutrition* 6: 414-425.

Wilber, R. 2004. *Altitude Training and Athletic Performance.* Champaign, IL: Human Kinetics.

Wilborn, C.D., C.M. Kerksick, B.I. Campbell, L.W. Taylor, B.M. Marcello, C.J. Rasmussen, M.C. Greenwood, A. Almada, and R.B. Kreider. 2004. Effects of zinc magnesium asparate (ZMA) supplementation on training adaptations and markers of anabolism and catabolism. *Journal of the International Society of Sports Nutrition* 1: 12-20.

Wilder, N., R. Gilders, F. Hagerman, and R.G. Deivert. 2002. The effects of a 10-week, periodized, off-season resistance-training program and creatine supplementation among collegiate football players. *Journal of Strength and Conditioning Research* 16: 343-352.

Wiles, J.D., S.R. Bird, J. Hopkins, and M. Riley. 1992. Effect of caffeinated coffee on running speed, respiratory factors, blood lactate and perceived exertion during 1500-m treadmill running. *British Journal of Sports Medicine* 26: 116-120.

Wiles, J.D., D. Coleman, M. Tegerdine, and I.L. Swaine. 2006. The effects of caffeine ingestion on performance time, speed and power during a laboratory-based 1 km cycling time trial. *Journal of Sports Science* 24: 1165-1171.

Wilk, B., and O. Bar-Or. 1996. Effect of drink flavor and NaCl on voluntary drinking and hydration of boys exercising in the heat. *Journal of Applied Physiology* 80: 1112-1117.

Wiles, J.D., D. Coleman, M. Tegerdine, and I.L. Swaine. 2006. The effects of caffeine ingestion on performance time, speed and power during a laboratory-based 1 km cycling time trail. *Journal of Sports Science* 24: 1165-1171.

Wilkes, D., N. Geldhill, and R. Smyth. 1983. Effect of acute induced metabolic alkalosis on 800-m racing time. *Medicine and Science in Sports and Exercise* 15: 277-280.

Williams, A.G., M. van den Oord, A. Sharma, and D.A. Jones. 2001. Is glucose/amino acid supplementation after exercise an aid to strength training? *British Journal of Sports Medicine* 35: 109-113.

Williams, C., J. Brewer, and M. Walker. 1992. The effect of a high carbohydrate diet on running performance during a 30-km treadmill time trial. *European Journal of Applied Physiology* 65: 18-24.

Williams, C., and G. Gandy. 1994. Physiology and nutrition for sprinting. In *Perspectives in Exercise Science and Sports Medicine* (edited by D.R. Lamb, H.G. Knuttgen, and R. Murray), pp. 55-98. Carmel, IN: Cooper.

Williams, J.H., J.F. Signorile, W.S. Barnes, and T.W. Henrich. 1988. Caffeine, maximal power output and fatigue. *British Journal of Sports Medicine* 22: 132-134.

Williams, M.H. 1985. Drug foods—Alcohol and caffeine. *Nutritional Aspects of Human Physical and Athletic Performance,* 2nd ed, pp. 272-295. Springfield, IL: Charles Thomas

Williams, M.H. 1991. Alcohol, marijuana and beta blockers. In *Perspectives in Exercise Science and Sports Medicine* (edited by D.R. Lamb and M.H. Williams), pp. 331-372. Dubuque, IA: Brown & Benchmark.

Williams, M., R. Kreider, and J.D. Branch. 1998. *Creatine.* Champaign, IL: Human Kinetics.

Williams, M.H., R.B. Kreider, D.W. Hunter, C.T. Somma, L.M. Shall, M.L. Woodhouse, and L. Rokitzki. 1990. Effect of inosine supplementation on 3-mile treadmill run performance and VO_2 peak. *Medicine and Science in Sports and Exercise* 22: 517-522.

Willoughby, D.S. 2004. Effects of an alleged myostatin-binding supplement and heavy resistance training on serum myostatin, muscle strength and mass, and body composition. *International Journal of Sport Nutrition and Exercise Metabolism* 14: 461-472.

Wilmore, J.H. 1991. Eating and weight disorders in the female athlete. *International Journal of Sport Nutrition* 1: 104-117.

Wing-Gaia, S.L., A.W. Subudhi, and E.W. Askew. 2005. Effect of purified oxygenated water on exercise performance during acute hypoxic exposure. *International Journal of Sport Nutrition and Exercise Metabolism* 15: 680-688.

Wingo, J.E., D.J. Casa, E.M. Berger, W.O. Dellis, J.C. Knight, and J.M. McClung. 2004. Influence of a pre-exercise glycerol hydration beverage on performance and physiologic function during mountain-bike races in the heat. *Journal of Athletic Training* 39: 169-175.

Winnick, J.J., J.M. Davis, R.S. Welsh, M.D. Carmichael, E.A. Murphy, and J.A. Blackmon. 2005. Carbohydrate feedings during team sport exercise preserve physical and CNS function. *Medicine and Science in Sports and Exercise* 37: 306-315.

Wojtaszewski, J.P.F., P. Nielson, B. Kiens, and E.A. Richter. 2001. Regulation of glycogen synthase kinase-3 in human skeletal muscle: effects of food intake and bicycle exercise. *Diabetes* 50: 265-269.

Wolfe, R.R., and S.L. Miller. 1999. Amino acid availability controls muscle protein metabolism. *Diabetes Nutrition and Metabolism* 12: 322-328.

Wootton, S., and C. Williams. 1984. Influence of carbohydrate-status on performance during maximal exercise. *International Journal of Sports Medicine* 5: 126-127.

World Health Organization. 1985. *Energy and Protein Requirements. Report of a Joint FAO/WHO/UNU Expert Committee* (Technical Report Series 724). Geneva: World Health Organization.

Wray, N., K.A. Jackson, and L. Cobiac. 1994. Comparison of nutritional attitudes and practices between elite and less professional Australian Rules footballers. Unpublished manuscript prepared for Flinders University, Adelaide, Australia.

Wright, D.A., W.M. Sherman, and A.R. Dernbach. 1991. Carbohydrate feedings before, during, or in combination improve cycling endurance performance. *Journal of Applied Physiology* 71: 1082-1088.

Wroble, R.R., and D.P. Moxley. 1998. Weight loss patterns and success rates in high school wrestlers. *Medicine and Science in Sports and Exercise* 30: 625-628.

Wu, J., S. Ishizaki, Y. Kato, Y. Kuroda, and S. Fukashiro. 1998. The side-to-side differences of bone mass at proximal femur in female rhythmic sports gymnasts. *Journal of Bone and Mineral Research* 13: 900-906.

Yaspelkis, B.B., and J.L. Ivy. 1999. The effect of a carbohydrate-arginine supplement on postexercise carbohydrate metabolism. *International Journal of Sport Nutrition* 9: 241-250.

Yaspelkis, B.B., J.G. Patterson, P.A. Anderla, Z. Ding, and J.L. Ivy. 1993. Carbohydrate supplementation spares muscle glycogen during variable-intensity exercise. *Journal of Applied Physiology* 75: 1477-1485.

Yeager, K.K., R. Agostini, A. Nattiv, and B. Drinkwater. 1993. The female athlete triad: Disordered eating, amenorrhea, osteoporosis. *Medicine and Science in Sports and Exercise* 25: 775-777.

Ylikoski, T., J. Piirainen, O. Hanninen, and J. Penttinen. 1997. The effect of coenzyme Q10 on the exercise performance of cross-country skiers. *Molecular Aspects of Medicine* 18 (suppl): s283-s290.

Yoshimura, H. 1970. Anemia during physical training (sports anemia). *Nutrition Reviews* 28: 251-253.

Zachwieja, J.J., D.L. Costill, D.D. Pascoe, R.A. Robergs, and W.J. Fink. 1991. Influence of muscle glycogen depletion on the rate of resynthesis. *Medicine and Science in Sports and Exercise* 23: 44-48.

Zachwieja, J.J., D.M. Ezell, A.D. Cline, J.C. Ricketts, P.C. Vicknair, S.M. Schorle, and D.H. Ryan. 2001. Short-term dietary energy restriction reduces lean body mass but not performance in physically active men and women. *International Journal of Sports Medicine* 22: 310-316.

Zawadzki, K.M., B.B. Yaspelkis, and J.L. Ivy. 1992. Carbohydrate-protein complex increases the rate of muscle glycogen storage after exercise. *Journal of Applied Physiology* 72: 1854-1859.

Zeederberg, C., L. Leach, E.V. Lambert, T.D. Noakes, S.C. Dennis, and J.A. Hawley. 1996. The effect of carbohydrate ingestion on the motor skill of soccer players. *International Journal of Sport Nutrition* 6: 348-355.

Zehnder, M., J. Rico-Sanz, G. Kuhne, and U. Boutellier. 2001. Resynthesis of muscle glycogen after soccer specific performance examined by 13C-magnetic resonance spectroscopy in elite players. *European Journal of Applied Physiology and Occupational Physiology* 84: 443-447.

Ziegenfuss, T.N., M. Rogers, L. Lowery, N. Mullins, R. Mendel, J. Antonio, and P. Lemon. 2002. Effect of creatine loading on anaerobic performance and skeletal muscle volume in NCAA Division I athletes. *Nutrition* 18: 397-402.

Ziemba, A.W., J. Chmura, H. Kaciuba-Uscilko, K. Nazar, P. Wisnik, and W. Gawronski. 1999. Ginseng treatment improves psychomotor performance at rest and during graded exercise in young athletes. *International Journal of Sport Nutrition* 9: 371-377.

Zissomou, T. 2004. *The Olympic Games in Antiquity, 1st ed.* Glyfada, Greece: Tina Zissimou.

Zuliani, G., G. Baldo-Enzi, E. Palmieri, S. Volpato, E. Vitale, P. Magnanini, A. Colozzi, L. Vecchiet, and R. Fellin. 1996. Lipoprotein profile, diet and body composition in athletes practicing mixed and anaerobic activities. *Journal of Sports Medicine and Physical Fitness* 36: 211-216.

Recently added references:

Bergeron, M.F., J.L. Waller, and E.L. Marinik. 2006. Voluntary fluid intake and core temperature responses in adolescent tennis players: sports beverages versus water. *British Journal of Sports Medicine* 40: 406-441.

Burke, L.M. 2006b. Voluntary fluid intakes and sweat losses of elite basketball players during training. Unpublished report.

Burke, L.M. 2006c. Voluntary fluid intakes and sweat losses of elite cricket players during training. Unpublished report.

Collier, S.R., E. Collins, and J.A. Kanaley. 2006. Oral arginine attenuates the growth hormone response to resistance exercise. *Journal of Applied Physiology* 101: 848-852.

Eichner, E.R. 1985. Runner's macrocytosis: a clue to footstrike hemolysis. Runner's anemia as a benefit versus runner's hemolysis as a detriment. *American Journal of Medicine* 78: 321-325.

Koopman, R., A.J.M. Wagenmakers, R.J.F. Manders, A.H.G. Zorenc, J.M.G. Senden, M. Gorselink, H.A. Keizer, and L.J.C. Van Loon. 2005. Combined ingestion of protein and free leucine with carbohydrate increases postexercise muscle protein synthesis in vivo in male subjects. *American Journal of Physiology – Endocrinology and Metabolism* 288: E645-E653.

Kovacs, M.S. 2006. Applied physiology of tennis performance. *British Journal of Sports Medicine* 40: 381-385.

Paddon-Jones, D., M. Sheffield-Moore, R.J. Urban, A.P. Sanford, A. Aarsland, R.R. Wolfe, and A.A. Ferrando. 2004. Essential amino acid and carbohydrate supplementation ameliorates muscle protein loss in humans during 28 days bedrest. *Journal of Clinical Endocrinology and Metabolism* 89(9): 4351-4358.

Sharp, N. 1998. Physiological demands and fitness for squash. In *Science and racket sports II* (edited by A. Lees, I. Maynard, M. Hughes, and T. Reilly), pp. 3-13. London, UK: E & FN Spon.

index

Note: Page numbers followed by an italicized *f* or *t* indicate a figure or table will be found on that page. Italicized *ff* or *tt* indicates multiple figures or tables, respectively.

A

absolute aerobic capacity 144-145
acetyl-CoA production 68
adenine nucleotide 64
adenosine triphosphate 64, 265
adolescent eating habits 148-149
aerials 348
aerobic capacity 144-145, 170, 244
aid stations 103
Akt pathway 272
alcohol
    abuse by athletes 205
    acute effects on exercise 209-210
    affect on performance 210
    daily intake by Australian Rules football players 206
    drinking practices of athletes 205-206
    and effective fluid replacement 211
    effect on judgment and behavior 211
    and hydration status 10
    intake guidelines 212-213
Allen, Mark 103
Allison, Annette 297
Alpine skiing 342*t*, 343-347
alpine skiing 326*t*
amenorrhea 16, 117, 329
American College of Sports Medicine (ACSM) 98, 135-137, 210
American Psychiatric Association 332
amino acid delivery 282
amino acids
    following resistance exercise 14
    postexercise intake of 272-273
anaerobic energy 265
anaerobic glycolysis 123, 170
androstenedione 48-49
anemia 119
anorexia athletica 117, 332
anorexia nervosa 332
antioxidants 56
appetite management 166*t*
Armstrong, Lance 81, 82
Around Oahu Bike race 102-103
athletes. *See also* specific sports
    alcohol intake by 205-207
    alcohol intake guidelines 212-213
    binge drinking patterns of 205-206
    disordered eating among 150
    energy requirements of 1-3
    fat storage in 162

female
    body image issues 5, 149-150, 226
    carbohydrate-energy ratio, correlation to total carbohydrate intake 99-100
    dietary causes of menstrual disturbances 329-331
    dietary intakes, court and indoor games 448*t*
    dietary intakes, cyclists 363*t*
    dietary intakes, gymnasts 481*t*
    dietary intakes, racket sports 463*t*
    dietary intakes, strength and power 470*t*
    energy availability calculations 36*f*
    energy balance 146
    energy intake 133-134, 195
    energy requirements of 1-2
    energy-restriction strategies 81-82
    female athlete triad 16, 118
    increased calcium intake 57
    menstrual disturbances 7, 16, 117-118
    menstrual status affect on glycogen storage 126
    metabolic rates 134
    overhydration in 23
    protein intake guidelines 5-6, 5*t*
    reported dietary intakes 432*t*-433*t*
    restricted energy intake by 16
    training diets 77, 78-79, 78*f*
    weight concerns 245-247
food preparation skills 213*t*-214*t*
hypoglycemic 21
immune status 15-16
iron status in 6-7
issues and strategies for traveling 259*t*-262*t*
male
    carbohydrate intake 77
    daily energy intakes 1-2
    dietary intakes, court and indoor games 447*t*
    dietary intakes, cyclists 362*t*
    dietary intakes, gymnasts 480*t*
    dietary intakes, strength and power 467*t*-469*t*
    energy availability calculations 36*f*

energy intake and expenditure 132*t*
    muscle hypertrophy 4
    protein intake guidelines 5-6, 5*t*
    reported dietary intakes 430*t*-431*t*
    sever energy restriction 16
physical characteristics 3-5
athlete villages 237-238
Australian football 187*t*, 190. *See also* field and court sports
    players daily alcohol intake 206
Australian Institute of Sport (AIS) 200
    high-fat, high carbohydrate studies 102
    list of identified problems with supplements 43
    supplement program 50-51, 51*t*-52*t*
Australian Institute of Sport Guidelines 417*t*-420*t*
Australian National Swimming Team 152
Australian Rowing Championships 309
Australian rules football
    opportunities for fluid intake 234*t*
Australian Rules Football League 206
Australian Therapeutic Goods Act (1989) 42
Australian women's road cycling team 77

B

badminton 234*t*, 241-242
balance studies 360*t*-361*t*
Ballantine, D. 205
bananas 94*t*
banned substances 44, 48
Baptiste, Andre 290
Barcelona Olympic games 256
basal metabolic rate (BMR) 33
basketball. *See also* court and indoor sports
    fuel utilization patterns 222
    opportunities for fluid intake 234*t*
    playing courts 223-224
    typical activity patterns 221-222
Bekele, Kenenisa 110*t*
Bergeron, M. 255
Bergeron, Michael 262-264
β-hydroxy β-methylbutyrate (HMB) 63

about the author

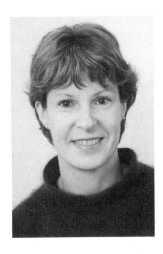

Louise Burke, PhD, APD, FACSM, is a sports dietitian who has worked with elite athletes for more than 25 years. She is founder of the department of sports nutrition at the Australian Institute of Sport and has served as head for the last 17 years. She was appointed dietitian to the Australian Olympic team for the 1996, 2000, and 2004 Summer Olympic Games. She is a member of the International Olympic Committee Working Group on Nutrition and the Medical and Anti-Doping Commission of the International Association of Athletics Foundations.

Dr. Burke is a fellow of the American College of Sports Medicine, Sports Medicine Australia, and Sports Dietitians Australia. An accredited practicing dietitian, she is an editor of the *International Journal of Sport Nutrition and Exercise Metabolism* and is on the editorial board of *Medicine and Science in Sports and Exercise.* She earned her PhD in 1990 from Deakin University, Melbourne, Australia. Also, a former tri-athlete, Dr. Burke represented Australia in the Ironman Team Cup at the 1985 and 1986 Hawaii Ironman World Championships.

Nanna L. Meyer is originally from Switzerland and currently employed as a Research Associate and Sports Dietitian at The Orthopedic Specialty Hospital (TOSH Sport Science) in Salt Lake City, Utah, She has been the sports dietitian of U.S. Speed Skating since 1999. In 2001 she received funding through the IOC Medical Commission to study the diets of winter sports athletes in preparation for the Salt Lake City Olympic Winter Games. Prior to her position at TOSH, she worked with the Swiss Ski Team. Nanna is also an adjunct faculty in the Division of Nutrition at the University of Utah in Salt Lake City and a visiting professor at the University of Salzburg in Austria, teaching both undergraduate and graduate courses in nutrition for exeircse and sport.

Susie Parker-Simmons is a Sports Dietitian and Physiologist for the United States Ski and Snowboard Association (USSA). Prior to working at the USSA, she resided in Australia lecturing in Sports Science and Nutrition at RMIT University and worked in private practice at Olympic Park Sports Medicine Center where she consulted with a variety of athletes. Susie has worked at three Olympic Games and five World Champoiships.

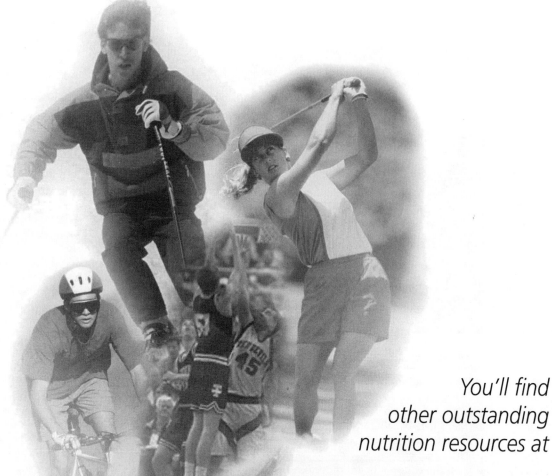